Dedicated to those seeking the truth,

and fighting to make this world a better place

Edition 5.0 - March 2023 - © Prof. Marcello Allegretti
Cover Design: Marco Allegretti

Legal Notice & Disclaimer

This book is to be considered as a notional aid for the knowledge of techniques and application methods of electronic devices, which use electromagnetic fields for various purposes. The information contained herein is not intended as, and should not be used for, therapeutic, diagnostic or prescriptive purposes, nor to prevent, treat or cure disease, but for education and responsible experimentation only.

The information this book contains can in no way replace the work of a medically trained professional. Please consult a licensed health practitioner for medical advice.

The author cannot guarantee the reliability of the information contained herein nor errors and/or omissions. The information and concepts within this guide must not be considered or construed in any way to be medical advice or treatment.

The author of this book cannot be held liable for any consequences, harmful or otherwise, that may occur by using the information contained in this book.

Thanks

This manual is a useful tool for all those who like to experience the effects of electromagnetic fields to achieve a condition of "physical and mental balance" and "well-being."

The frequency programs proposed are the result of international scientific studies, research with sophisticated bioresonance systems and empirical experiments. Therefore, they are suitable for applications with any electromagnetic frequency generator, especially with Rife Machines, as they are known for their flexibility of use.

*I owe special thanks to **John White**, creator of **Spooky2**, a great scientist who is revolutionizing the world of Rifing and made it possible for me to create this book, since the first edition.*

*A warm thank you to the Managers of **ETDFL** and **Biomedis**, to all scientific researchers, to friends from all over the world who have given their contributions and to thousands of readers, who in recent years have stimulated me to new studies and research and who, with their suggestions and indications, helped me make this manual even better.*

CONTENTS

Introduction

Rifing is a technology that takes its name from Dr. Royal Raymond Rife, a great scientist, researcher and inventor who, in the early decades of the last century, managed to discover an unfailing method to devitalize pathogens (viruses, bacteria and fungi). Rife was one of the first in the world to use electromagnetic frequencies for therapeutic use and certainly the first to use this technology for the treatment of infectious diseases caused by pathogens.

More than 80 years after his first successes, the technology invented by Dr. Rife has evolved in an extraordinary way. Today, we can find many modern electronic devices being sold that are programmed with software and provide for an excellent user experience. The modern Rife equipment cannot only apply the frequencies for disabling individual microorganisms (**killing** frequencies), but also an immense number of frequencies able to provide health benefits and/or well-being (**healing**) and detoxification (**detox**).

Therefore, Rifing means the exposure to electromagnetic fields, characterized by precise frequencies and harmonics, by means of various transmission devices, which are connected to a Rife Machine: i.e., to a frequency generator. This technology offers the most extensive and complete application of electromagnetic waves for therapeutic purposes.

In Germany and South Africa, as well as some other countries, frequency devices (such as *Rife Machines*) are legally authorized as medical instruments. In all other countries, according to the legislation in force, such frequency systems can be legally used only for testing, energy balancing, life extension, relaxation and experiments on bacterial cultures or laboratory animals.

In addition to providing support to Researchers from all over the world, the main purpose of this manual is to is to facilitate the identification of a *Subject* and the corresponding program of frequencies, according to logic and origin criteria, to be then used with a frequency device. Essentially, it aims to remove confusion from the process of choosing the right frequencies to use.

More than 10000 frequency programs are listed. They cover the human body organs, pathogens, diseases, homeopathic products, minerals, vitamins, chakras and more. They are sorted and catalogued in a way that makes it much easier to locate the information that will allow the best program choices.

Thanks to the *Notes* and the fact that all of the programs related to a topic are listed together and when necessary, repeated in additional paragraphs, it is possible to deal with a *complex* situation, following different logical paths and then experimenting with various programs of frequencies, until reaching satisfactory or conclusive results. Basically, this means that there are many situations you can try. If this does not work, an alternative approach can be followed, using factors that may be considered marginal at the beginning or those that are radical and profound. For this reason, the condition to be treated should always be studied well, with close attention paid to the written Notes.

Even when it comes to a simple case or a case with limited choices, comparing two programs of nearly identical frequencies or locating an Author that is considered more reliable, the reader will be able to perform choices that will be more and more targeted and effective as time goes by.

Among the features of this manual there is the reference (in the Notes) of the most known pathogens that could cause any kind of health problem. It is in fact now established that fungi, bacteria and viruses are almost always involved in all diseases. Sometimes they are the cause of the disease, in other cases they others may arise or proliferate where a disease is located. Therefore, whatever the cause, the devitalization of the possible pathogens involved, can represent the temporary or permanent solution of the health problem. When you understand and can test the effectiveness of this methodology, with a frequency device, it is then possible to achieve increasingly satisfactory results. There are thousands of pathogens that can cause very serious damage to an organism. In the Notes section, you will find listed only the best known or those involved in the most common or serious health problems, so the list is not complete and for many diseases it may be missing a precise reference. For this reason, especially when a frequency program does not achieve results, it is always advisable to perform all possible research and techniques (e.g., Biofeedback, Bioresonance, etc.), in order to identify which pathogens may be present in any condition of discomfort. You may be amazed to discover that even a problem that we cannot even imagine can be caused by pathogens (e.g., mental problems or back pain), which may actually be caused by them.

New in this edition

Among the many new features of this 5th edition, we highlight:
- Updates of about 1,300 frequencies with the **EDTFL** abbreviation
- Introduction of about 2,000 frequencies resulting from Russian researchers (**Biomedis**), which greatly enriched the extensive amount of information in this manual
- Elimination of entries with identical frequencies;
- References to the various Sections of the manual and graphical expedients that make it increasingly easier and faster to locate the items you intend to consult (subdivision of the topics covered in 30 numbered Sections, colored columns with precise references, etc.)
- New subdivision and sequence of Sections and topics so as to facilitate more and more, the search for an entry.

In addition, several entries that had been placed in incorrect Sections or positions have been corrected. So, this latest edition has achieved a much higher degree of accuracy and its usability than previous versions, so that those doing research can experience all the best available frequencies.

If read or simply leafed through carefully and patiently, this manual can very quickly increase the skills needed to use any frequency generator and contribute to the research being done around the world.

The evolution of the Rife Machine

Dr. Royal Rife, thanks to his discoveries, opened a path whose evolution had been surprising and unimaginable, especially considering the sad conditions in which this great scientist had left the medical-scientific community. The current use of electromagnetic waves in the therapeutic field has evolved to the point of including: *Therapies with light radiation, Electrostatic Therapies, Electrotherapy or Electrostimulation, Thermotherapies, Ultrasound, Shockwaves, Neuroacoustics, Magnetotherapy, Rifing*, as well as a series of new applications that use increasingly advanced technologies with results that were unthinkable until a few years ago.

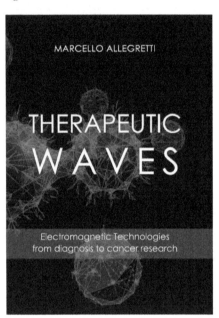

The book, "**Therapeutic Wave**s," describes all these technologies in the most accurate and understandable possible way, offering clarity on the techniques used, therapeutic applications and the extraordinary effects that are obtained on organic tissues, cells and organelles and on the DNA. In addition, there are many pages dedicated to diagnostic equipment, water energy properties, electromagnetic pollution harmful effects and finally cancer, with a dedicated chapter about the relevant studies carried out all over the world. These technologies, in many cases, have evolved into recognized and approved applications for the treatment or ablation of cancer.

This book is useful for informing everyone, both professionals and those interested in learning more about these concepts, methodologies and discoveries, whose existence is almost always unknown.

Reading this book, one finally clearly understands how it is possible that the thousands of frequencies mentioned and collected in this manual, applied in an appropriately, can act in such a way, as to induce a long series of biological reactions ranging from the restoration of the potential cellular membrane, up to gene stimulation.

Rife Machines, almost always excluded from medical-scientific environments, due to the vastness of the field of application that characterize them, have evolved in an extraordinary way. Thanks to the possibility of choosing a considerable number of electrical parameters, modern Rife Machines have proven to be an ideal tool for those who do research.

In the following paragraphs I will describe the products of some Companies that have particularly caught my attention in recent years.

Spooky2

The Spooky2 journey started in March 2011 when an experienced Rife user and experimenter Johann Stegmann experienced something that changed the course of his life.

After buying a new Rife machine, Johann's friend made the astonishing claim that the DNA contained in fingernails or hair could transmit energy frequencies directly to the owner of that DNA, simply by placing the samples between the machine's electrodes - without applying the usual contacts to the person's skin. Johann was skeptical, but together with his friend decided to test this theory on his daughter, Tania, who is particularly sensitive to energy. To his astonishment, he discovered that it worked perfectly.

How do you explain this phenomenon? Albert Einstein called it "*spooky action at a distance.*" Modern physics calls it "*quantum entanglement.*" In simple words, this means that if any part of a single system is removed from that system and placed in a different location, any action performed on the part will instantly affect the system as well and vice versa.

In this case, the system is the human body from which the DNA sample is taken. With the exception of mature red blood cells, all human cells contain DNA, which is absolutely unique to every single person. So, when the energy of the frequencies is transmitted to a small sample containing DNA (like a piece of fingernail), the effects will be instantly transmitted to the entire living organism from which the sample was taken.

Over the following 18 months, Johann continued to experiment and discovered a way to monitor and verify the effects of the frequencies remotely. In every case, his experiments worked perfectly. Thus, it was necessary to identify a suitable frequency generator for this purpose and to create a powerful and flexible software, capable of having all the means useful for experimentation.

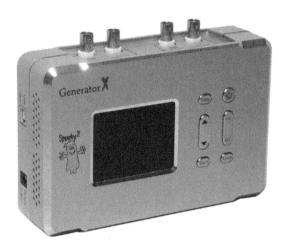

John White, an engineer and software developer, had been following these developments with growing interest and excitement. Thanks to him, the Spooky2 software was born. Primarily designed as a remote Rife system, it could also be used with a simple contact device or plasma tube when coupled with an amplifier.

In the years to follow, an international team of electronic engineers, design technicians, software developers and Rife professionals was formed, whose goal is the worldwide diffusion of a system based on Royal Rife's technology, with affordable prices for all.

Nowadays, thanks to modern technologies, making the hardware, ie a frequency generator up to 40MHz, is not a problem (even in economic terms). But the real power of a Rife Machine lies in the software, which creates the waveforms, durations, amplitudes, and other essential parameters.

In May 2013, the Spooky team presented their first system, simply called Spooky. The software for this was completely free, while the hardware cost less than a nice evening out.

After gaining useful experience with Spooky, the team developed a new system that includes a state-of-the-art frequency generator, the Spooky2-XM and then the new **GX Pro**, with software designed to allow the best use of all hardware capabilities, equipped with a very rich database with more than 60,000 Frequency Programs.

In addition to the Spooky Remote described above, a series of accessories of fundamental importance have now been added to the system, to name a few:

- A plasma tube (very similar to the first used by Rife to devitalize pathogens),
- The electrodes designed for the contact mode,
- A scalar wave device,
- Cold laser devices.

For further information: https://www.spooky2.com/

Rife Digital Professional V3 - EDTFL

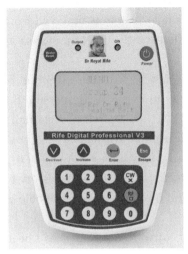

The Electro Therapy Device Frequency List (**EDTFL**) is an ongoing project by 12 Clinics across the planet who use the *Quantum SCIO* Bioresonance machine to record Disease frequencies of actual clients, and then produce the 10 most accurate frequencies which are deemed suitable for treatment with the *Royal Rife Machine.* The accuracy of the frequencies is seen in the positive results of the clients who use this Frequencies in clinics and homes in every country.

This project began in 2006 when the original CAFL frequency list was discontinued. ETDFL is a list of Frequency Programs used by the thousands of **Rife Digital Professional V3** users around the planet. The compact size, easy-to-read menu, and large display in 3 built-in languages, as well as the instruction booklet in 12 languages, make this Rife machine suitable for people in all places and countries. The Frequency Programs of this Rife Machine are designed according to the highest standards in Germany and are applicable in various modes, including contact mode, magnetic mat and infrared led mat.

For further information: https://www.etdfl.com/

Biomedis

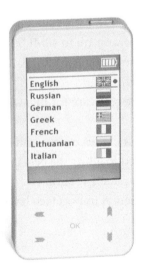

Biomedis is a Research and Production Company established in Russia in 2008, which uses advanced technologies to build devices and appliances that can correct and support a high level of health and energy of the body for health and well-being. Specifically, the **BIOMEDIS TRINITY** is a device that emits electromagnetic waves in multifrequency and synchronization, which can enhance body functions and systems, improve organ working capacity, prevent premature aging, and maintain natural balance. The device comes with about 3000 Frequency Programs and can be connected to a PC for complex sequence programming (software can be downloaded free of charge from the website).

For further information: https://www.biomedis.life/

Power-Waves

It is a new company located in Italy, that produces electronic devices, the result of years of research in the field of electromagnetic waves for scientific and therapeutic use. Two of the innovative devices made by this company are described below.

Tesla Coil Imprinter

The **Tesla Coil Imprinter** uses a very special Tesla coil, which is the result of years of study and experimentation in the field of electromagnetic and scalar waves.

Thanks to these theories and studies, the first **Tesla Coil Imprinter** was born. This is the first Tesla coil that, exploits the electrical characteristics of the construction parameters and is able to modulate the frequency, which is intended to be imprinted in a solution of water and alcohol, on a carrier of about 1.5 MHz.

The combination of a precise high frequency with an equally high voltage, allows to obtain an imprinting with characteristics and results never achieved before.

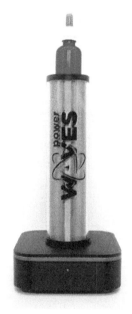

In fact, an electric field is able to hook water molecules and structure them in the direction of the field, in an orderly way. But, the energy of an electric field is proportional to the voltage! So this is how the high voltage that is established on the top of a Tesla coil can be decisive for the purpose. Similarly, the energy of an electromagnetic wave is directly proportional to its frequency, so as the frequency increases, the energy transported increases.

Combining a high electric field with a high frequency through a resonant Tesla coil was the winning idea for this unique device.

The main function for which this coil was designed and built is to be able to store in Clusters and Water Coherence Domains, electromagnetic frequencies for any scientific purpose.

Spooky2 signal generators, thanks to the sophisticated software included, are the best means of driving a Tesla Coil Imprinter. In fact, just setting the carrier value and the value of the frequencies to be imprinted correctly is enough to achieve outstanding results.

Scalar Wave Generator

Power Waves is one of the very few companies in the world to produce and market a pair of scalar antennas executed according to the original patent of Tesla, who for a long time studied a system capable of transporting electrical energy and signals, through the ether without the use of any electrical conductor.

By electrically resonating the Tx antenna (at a specific frequency), the energy is picked up by the Rx antenna, which, being identical, also resonates, creating an equal and opposite electromagnetic wave (180° out of phase) that cancels the transmission wave. From the suppression of the electromagnetic

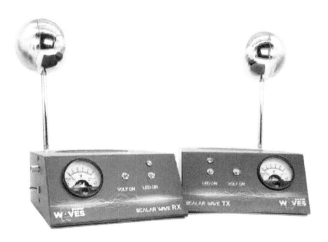

field, a scalar field is created that follows totally different laws from those enunciated by physics about electromagnetic waves. This is how Tesla was able to send both energy and frequency signals (thanks to amplitude modulation) from the Tx to the Rx.

So, the **Scalar Wave Generator** lends itself very well to experimentation in the areas of Physics, **Radionics**, Imprinting and Rifing, in fact with this kit it is possible to:

- Demonstrate the existence of scalar waves

- Create a scalar field capable of carrying energy and frequency signals

- Perform an imprinting of a substance by placing an active ingredient on the receiver plane and a flask or glass of water on the transmitter plane

- Use the power of scalar waves for an infinite number of applications in the world of **Radionics**.

The careful selection of the construction materials for these devices were carried out so that the possible use includes a target, ranging from those who intend to carry out experiments on electromagnetism, up to the companies that produce these devices for scientific and therapeutic use.

In fact, they are the result of a continuous investigation, aimed at identifying the safest, most effective and quickest ways to regain a condition of physical, mental and spiritual well-being.

Power-Waves' electromagnetic devices are compatible with any arbitrary wave function generator that works according to the principle of Direct Digital Synthesis (DDS), such as the **Spooky2**. Compatibility tests with other equipment and Rife Machines will be performed soon.

Power-Waves is a company full of ideas and projects that promises to develop high-tech products with unique characteristics. In addition, it is increasingly expanding the distribution of its products outside national borders.

*For further information: https://**www.power-waves.com***

Guide to Using this Manual

This manual has been designed so that it can be easily used for the identification and choice of frequency programs that can be utilized on frequency generators and electronic equipment of any kind.

Frequency Programs have been grouped into **30** separate **Sections** by topic to simplify the search.. The pages have been set up according to the description below.

First column, *Subject / Argument*

Indicates the Argument or Subject of the frequency Program. Except for a few special applications such as homeopathic remedies, minerals, vitamins, etc., it is almost always the name of a disease or pathogen.

In some cases, to facilitate the identification of items of particular importance or belonging to the same topic, colors other than black and colored boxes are used.

The items that have Subjects in common are repeated several times in different Sections.

Second column, *Author*

Refers to the origin of the programs:

- Rife are the original frequencies of **Dr. Royal Raymond Rife**.
- CAFL is the list of "Consolidated Annotated Frequency" based on years of experience of many Rife investigators. Many of these frequencies, can be found in hundreds of scientific publications that report studies and experiments carried out all over the world. These frequencies have been widely tested and very often have been used in therapeutic systems of all types (machines for magnetotherapy, electrotherapies, bioresonance, etc.).
- The Electro Therapy Device Frequency List (**ETDFL**) is a large list with frequencies obtained through a well-known bioresonance machine called *Quantum SCIO*. The most important aspect of EDTFLs is that they include Frequency Programs to try to give an answer even to little known and widespread health problems.
- KHZ is a collection of Frequency Programs that, like the ETDFL, start from a few tens of Hz to finish at a few hundred kHz. In this edition, the KHZ frequencies have almost all been replaced by ETDFLs.
- **BIOM** is the acronym for the Frequency Programs used by Biomedis equipment (described in a paragraph above). These are normally low frequencies, which could be considered as an evolution of CAFLs.
- RL: is a collection of frequencies identified by **Dr. Richard Loyd**, thanks to a series of tests performed on people suffering from infectious diseases.
- **PROV** has produced consistent results in almost all the subjects with which it was used.
- BIO and VEGA are research-based Russian frequencies, both very valid.
- XTRA are programs of varied origin, chosen for their reputation and effectiveness.
- **ALT** consists of programs based on the knowledge and practice of Ayurvedic, Solfeggio and planetary frequencies.
- HC is the database of **Dr. Hulda Clark**. When using these frequency sets, the frequency generator should be set with Positive Offset of 100%, Square Wave, and Amplitude of 9.5 volts.
- CUST they are new frequencies of various nature and origin.

Third column, *Frequencies*

This is the proposed Frequency Program.

Please note that the symbol "=" followed by a number indicates the proposed execution time in seconds (e.g.: = 900 means to execute for 900 seconds). Furthermore, two frequencies separated by the sign "-" indicate a scan that starts from the first frequency and ends with the second.

Fourth column, *Notes*

This contains the description, details or explanations of what is written in the first column. Highlighted in *red* or in *blue* sometimes are notes of particular importance, while the **Blue** bold highlighting notes the pathogens that could be involved in the health problem in question. It is reiterated that if no pathogen is reported in the Notes, it does not mean that these microorganisms cannot be present, therefore it is always advisable to try to carry out research on this, especially if the desired results are not achieved with the proposed program.

Some notes indicate the settings that must be given to the software for effective application of the frequencies program or contain information on how to apply accessories to specific Rife Machines.

Fifth and Sixth Column, *Origin / Target*

They contain information that allows quick identification of the topic to be consulted.

How to Search

To quickly perform a search, always consult the index of this manual. If you do not know the origin of the item to search for, it is advisable to search the web. For example, if you know the name of a pathogen but not the type (virus, bacterium, fungus, etc.), find the exact entries in this manual, as it is essential to know what it is.

Most electronic devices capable of generating electromagnetic frequencies have the ability to enter frequencies not included in their database. In this case, this manual becomes an indispensable tool for experimentation or comparison of effectiveness.

This should also be considered:

- The running time of each frequency is almost always determined by the equipment used. Normally the minimum time is 180 seconds (3 minutes) for each frequency.

- When there are several frequency Programs concerning the same Topic, to decide which one to use, attention must be paid to the content of the Notes, and the frequencies used.

In this case:

- It could be the case to first try a Program written by an Author considered more reliable (e.g., **CAFL**, **ETDFL** or **Biomedis** than others).

- If a Program differs from another for one or two more frequencies (the rest are identical), you could decide to choose the one that offers more possibilities.

- Try one Program at a time and put a mark next to the item that was most effective.

For further information on this topic, it may be useful to read the book "**Therapeutic Waves**" (by the same author), in which an entire chapter has been dedicated on Royal Rife, on Rifing and on how to apply frequencies.

Facebook and Messenger can be used (for contact with) to contact the Author.

Subject / Argument	Author	Frequencies	Notes	Origin	Target
	**1 - Various Conditions**

Subject / Argument	Author	Frequencies	Notes	Origin	Target
Spine Problems A=432 Hz	XTRA	128.43,144.16,161.82,171.44,192.43,216,242.45 ,136.07,152.74,181.63,203.88,228.84,	See "The Spine Frequencies". Based on A=432Hz tuning. Waveform=square. Repeat Program=0.		Various c.
Spine Problems A=440 Hz	XTRA	130.81,146.83,164.81,174.61,196,220.2,246.94, 138.57,155.56,185,207.65,233.08,	See "The Spine Frequencies". Based on A=440Hz tuning. Waveform=square. Repeat Program=0.	Nerve	Various c.
General Program Blaster 5	CAFL	80,400,500,600,622,666,690,727,740,776,784,7 87,800,880,1500,1550,1560,1570,1600,1800,18 40,1998,2000,2008,2128,2489,	Medley of useful frequencies taken from Rife machine.		Various c.
General Comprehensive	CAFL	10000,5000,4412,3176,3040,2145,2128,2112,20 08,1998,1862,1550,1500,1488,880,832,802,786, 776,766,760,740,732,728,712,688,683,676,666, 660,644,464,450,444,428,422,128,120,95,66.5,2 0,			Various c.
General Demo	CAFL	10000,4412,3040,2128,2112,1862,1550,880,800 ,786,732,728,712,688,676,644,464,422,128,120, 20,	Greatest hits! Medley of useful frequencies from CAFL database.		Various c.
Greatest Hits	XTRA	20,120,128,422,464,644,676,688,712,728,732,7 86,800,880,1550,1862,2112,2128,3040,4412,10 000,	Medley of useful frequencies taken from Rife machine.		Various c.
Self-assembly of Body	XTRA	9,187,948,181			Various c.
40KHz General	XTRA	40000	Helps with lesions, pathogens, cell oxygenation, circulation, immune system, thyroid.		Various c.
General Balancing	CAFL	1130,1131,33			Various c.
Overall Balance	XTRA	6.88			Various c.
General Cleanser	XTRA	337,464,467,576,688,728,786,803,856,882,912, 1554,1862,2128,3337,5762,6667,			Various c.
General Health 1	XTRA	263.1			Various c.
General Health 2	XTRA	59.29			Various c.
Health improvement	BIOM	20; 26; 38; 39; 45.7; 83; 6.8			Various c.
General Malady	CAFL	40000,10000,5000,			Various c.
General Prophylaxis	CAFL	20,64,95,125,225,427,440,664,728,784,880,802, 832,680,760,1550,464,10000,676,1488,			Various c.
Regeneration and Healing	CAFL	47,2720		Healing	Various c.
Healing and Regeneration 1	CAFL	2720,266,47		Healing	Various c.
Regeneration and Healing 1	CAFL	2720,2,20.5,3.9,4,50.5,6.3,148,7,		Healing	Various c.
Regeneration and Healing	XTRA	20.5		Healing	Various c.
Healing and Regeneration 2	XTRA	47,2720=1800		Healing	Various c.
Healing and Regeneration	BIOM	2; 3.9; 4; 6.3; 7; 47; 148; 266		Healing	Various c.
Healing	XTRA	10.5,360		Healing	Various c.
Healing 1	XTRA	1026,1537,2029		Healing	Various c.
Healing 2	XTRA	1549,3642,7055		Healing	Various c.
Healing 3	XTRA	8		Healing	Various c.
Healing center	BIOM	4; 10; 11; 12.5; 15; 18; 23; 28		Healing	Various c.
Healing Centre-4	BIOM	12.5; 18.0; 23.0; 28.0		Healing	Various c.
Accelerate Healing	XTRA	7.83	Healing of wounds, scars, bruises, trauma, fractures, surgery.	Healing	Various c.
Healing Acceleration	XTRA	20,26,33,39,45,78.29,140,200,300,330,450,783, 900,		Healing	Various c.
Speeding-up of healing	BIOM	7.83; 26.4; 33.39; 7; 34; 10; 324; 528; 97; 135; 150; 200; 140; 330; 450; 160; 500; 783; 10000; 5000; 1600; 70		Healing	Various c.
Poor healing process	BIOM	11; 19; 26; 84.5; 97.5		Healing	Various c.
Accelerate Injury Healing	XTRA	47	As mentioned above	Healing	Various c.
Accelerate Scar Healing	XTRA	5.9	See also Section 11a - Skin	Healing	Various c.
Regeneration and heal-over	BIOM	47; 2720		Healing	Various c.
Repair - Regeneration	BIOM	2720; 266; 47		Healing	Various c.
Regeneration	BIOM	47; 2720; 2; 20.5; 3.9; 4; 50.5; 6.3; 148; 7		Healing	Various c.
Tissue Healing and Regeneration	XTRA	47,266,1360,2128,2720,5000,		Healing	Various c.
Self-healing 1	XTRA	10		Healing	Various c.
Healing Special	XTRA	5.8,8.01,9.6,59.3,148,216,266,2720,3000,20000,		Healing	Various c.
Healing Enhanced	XTRA	7.83	Schumann frequency.	Healing	Various c.
Healing Frequency Russian	XTRA	59.3		Healing	Various c.
Healing General	XTRA	9,8		Healing	Various c.

Subject / Argument	Author	Frequencies	Notes	Origin	Target
Healing Infinite	XTRA	1638,2444,3127		Healing	Various c.
Organ Healing	XTRA	7		Healing	Various c.
Recovery after illness	BIOM	664; 1488; 3000		Healing	Various c.
Recovering from Sickness	BIOM	10000; 3000; 2720; 2489; 1800; 1600; 1550; 1500; 1488; 880; 832; 802; 787; 784; 776; 760; 728; 727; 680; 676; 666; 664; 650; 600; 465; 464; 440; 427; 225; 190; 125; 95; 64; 47.5; 20		Healing	Various c.
Recovery Process	BIOM	12.5; 23.0		Healing	Various c.
Recovery Acceleration	BIOM	7.83; 26.4; 33.0; 39.0; 7.34; 10.0; 324.0; 528.0; 97.0; 135.0; 150.0; 200.0; 140.0; 330.0; 450.0; 160.0; 500.0; 783.0; 10000.0; 5000.0; 1600.0; 70.0		Healing	Various c.
Development 1	BIOM	2.2; 10.0; 12.5; 19.5; 26.0; 49.0; 55.0; 92.5			Various c.
Development 2	BIOM	2.5; 4.59; 5.5; 9.6; 10.0; 11.0; 15.0; 17.5; 19.0; 21.5; 30.0; 42.5; 47.5; 55.0			Various c.
Development 3	BIOM	57.5; 60.0; 62.5; 72.0; 77.5; 80.0; 80.5; 82.5; 92.5; 93.5; 97.5; 98.5; 99.0; 100.0			Various c.
Crinkle Lines, Culique™ Anti Aging Multiple IR MAT	EDTFL	200,22500,132800,158630,429300,533900,678210,834630,888760,942320,			Various c.
Mickie's Magic Three	XTRA	324,528,15	From Bruce Stenulso. Reputed to help arthritis, diabetes, hypertension, muscle spasms and more.		Various c.
PEMF Pulsed Electromagnetic Field MAT GP20 (Stress Relief)	EDTFL	140,680,2500,60000,122530,300000,496010,655200,750000,9123300			Various c.
Coma	EDTFL	230,450,850,7500,93500,212590,528530,625200,752330,921700		Coma	Various c.
Coma	BIOM	63.5		Coma	Various c.
Chronic Disease	EDTFL	120,230,970,15190,63770,86440,132800,302300,452500,825000			Various c.
Systemic Conditions	XTRA	3.89,4.9,20,72,95,125,422,450,660,690,727,5,664,676,784,787,802,1550,832,880,1552,2008,2127.5,	Disorders which affect a number of organs and tissues, or the body as a whole.		Various c.
Weather susceptibility	BIOM	33; 50.5; 68.2; 99; 99.5			Various c.
Heat Exchange	XTRA	5.35	.		Various c.
Heat Generation	XTRA	5.5,6			Various c.
Hypothermia [Loosing Body Heat]	EDTFL	90,120,680,800,32750,107500,321550,350000,476290,605680,	Core body temperature below 35C (95F) as a result of exposure to cold.		Various c.
Frostbite	CAFL	880,787,727			Various c.
Frostbite	BIOM	880; 787; 727; 465			Various c.
Frostbite 1	XTRA	727,787,880,5000=420,			Various c.
Frostbite 2	XTRA	660,690,727.5,787,880,			Various c.
Fever	CAFL	1552,880,800,832,422,2112,787,727,20,	Addresses some causes.	Fever	Various c.
Fever All Kinds	CAFL	20,727,787,880,5000,		Fever	Various c.
Fever (of various aetiologies)	BIOM	2112; 1552; 880; 832; 800; 787; 727; 20		Fever	Various c.
Posttraumatic fever	BIOM	234; 278; 568; 672; 677; 702		Fever	Various c.
Fever	EDTFL	110,240,650,830,2500,27480,55370,87500,125520,322060		Fever	Various c.
Hyperthermia	EDTFL	40,500,680,870,5580,7500,95540,323010,326150,426900		Fever	Various c.
Hyperpyrexia, Malignant	EDTFL	60,260,570,9000,12850,35540,324050,424370,760000,812910	Rare genetic condition where certain anesthetic drugs, and sometimes exercise or hot environments can trigger life-threatening oxidative changes.	Fever	Various c.
Hyperthermia, Malignant	EDTFL	30,400,680,870,5580,7500,95540,323010,326150,719340		Fever	Various c.
Pyrexia	EDTFL	60,260,570,9000,12850,35540,324050,424370,760000,812910,		Fever	Various c.
Fever 2	XTRA	20,727,787,880,5000,		Fever	Various c.
Fever 3	XTRA	20,422,660,690,727.5,787,800,832,880,2112,		Fever	Various c.
High Fever Acute Pyrexia	XTRA	20,727,787,880,		Fever	Various c.
Heat Stress [Disorders]	EDTFL	80,130,350,7500,85000,193930,237500,487500,706210,946500,		Fever	Various c.
Heat Cramps [Muscle Spasms]	EDTFL	90,410,15090,87500,122060,312390,532410,655200,752000,927200,		Fever	Various c.
Mediterranean Fever, Familial	EDTFL	50,900,1520,55150,375030,479930,523000,662710,789000,987230	As mentioned above	Fever	Various c.
Periodic Disease [Familial Mediterranean fever]	EDTFL	50,900,1520,55150,375030,479930,523000,662710,789000,987230,	As mentioned above	Fever	Various c.

Subject / Argument	Author	Frequencies	Notes	Origin	Target
Pain General	CAFL	3000,95,666,80	Look under name of condition causing pain.	Pain	Various c.
Pain, General	EDTFL	160,350,950,5260,27500,52500,225470,522530,682020,750000		Pain	Various c.
Suffering, Physical	EDTFL	60,260,650,5710,7000,42500,92500,478900,527000,667000		Pain	Various c.
Pain	XTRA	95,3040		Pain	Various c.
Acute Pain	CAFL	3000,95,1550,802,880,787,727,690,666,26,160,333,522,555.1,	Sudden onset of pain.	Pain	Various c.
Pain Acute	CAFL	3000,95,10000,1550,802,880,787,727,690,666	See Acute Pain set. Look under name of condition causing pain.	Pain	Various c.
Pain Control	XTRA	9		Pain	Various c.
Pain Decrease	XTRA	10		Pain	Various c.
Pain Relief	CAFL	304,6000,3000,666,80,		Pain	Various c.
Pain Relief	XTRA	2.5		Pain	Various c.
Pain Relief	EDTFL	160,350,950,5260,27500,52500,225470,522530,682020,750000		Pain	Various c.
Anti-pain	BIOM	3.8; 4.0; 4.9; 5.5; 8.0; 9.4; 9.5; 9.6		Pain	Various c.
PEMF Pulsed Electromagnetic Field MAT GP19 (Pain Relief)	EDTFL	160,350,950,5260,27500,52500,225470,522530,682020,750000		Pain	Various c.
Sedation and Pain Relief	CAFL	304,6000		Pain	Various c.
Sedation and Pain Relief	XTRA	304		Pain	Various c.
Sedative Effect	CAFL	2.5	Reported use also on bleeding, bruises, insomnia, and sinusitis.	Pain	Various c.
Sedative Effect	BIOM	2.5; 304; 6000		Pain	Various c.
Analgesia	EDTFL	40,570,10530,95050,210250,424370,563190,671290,707260,985900,	Pain relief.	Pain	Various c.
Analgesic	XTRA	10	Pain relief.	Pain	Various c.
Analgesic effect	BIOM	0.5; 0.8; 1; 1.5; 2.5; 3; 3.6; 3.9; 9.7		Pain	Various c.
Analgesic Pain Relief	XTRA	90=1800,		Pain	Various c.
Surgical Pain Post Op	CAFL	95,2720,3000		Pain	Various c.
Complex pain	BIOM	10000; 3040; 3000; 2720; 1550; 95; 802; 787; 727; 690; 666; 90; 80; 40		Pain	Various c.
Complex Regional Pain Syndrome Type I	EDTFL	140,550,850,7470,120000,315500,472500,725750,852000,975930	Severe pain, swelling, and skin changes in parts or all of the body. Also see Causalgia.	Pain	Various c.
Complex Regional Pain Syndrome Type II	EDTFL	140,550,850,7470,120000,315500,472500,725750,852000,975930		Pain	Various c.
Pain of Infection	CAFL	3000,95,880,1550,802,787,776,727,4.9,	Look under name of condition causing pain.	Pain	Various c.
Pain and inflammation basic	BIOM	1.2; 2.5; 3.6; 3.8; 3.9; 7.5; 33; 79; 2.5; 9.6; 9.69; 68.5; 69; 84.5; 96; 100		Pain	Various c.
Pain in case of inflammation	BIOM	3040; 95; 880; 1550; 802; 787; 776; 727; 4.9		Pain	Various c.
Inflammation General	CAFL	3, 3.6	See Infections sets.	Inflammation	Various c.
Inflammation General	XTRA	1.5		Inflammation	Various c.
Anti-Inflammatory Effect	BIOM	1.7		Inflammation	Various c.
Anti-inflammatory effect	BIOM	1; 1.5; 2; 3.6; 29		Inflammation	Various c.
Inflammation	BIOM	75.5		Inflammation	Various c.
Inflammation 1	XTRA	1.5,3,3.6,2720,		Inflammation	Various c.
Inflammation 2	XTRA	1.3,3.6,6.29,10.5,148,2720,		Inflammation	Various c.
Inflammation	BIOM	1664.0; 1550.0; 962.0; 880.0; 802.0; 787.0; 727.0; 120.0; 80.0; 60.0; 40.0; 30.0; 28.0; 26.0; 25.0; 20.0; 30.0; 150.0; 100.0; 96.0; 93.9; 76.9		Inflammation	Various c.
Inflammation 1-2	BIOM	53.0; 53.5; 62.0; 62.5; 75.0; 75.5; 85.0; 86.0		Inflammation	Various c.
Inflammation 2-2	BIOM	3.6; 73.5; 87.5; 90.0; 91.5; 94.5; 98.0		Inflammation	Various c.
Inflammation	EDTFL	70,120,850,9500,88000,141200,297500,425950,675310,827000		Inflammation	Various c.
Systemic Inflammatory Response Syndrome	EDTFL	120,170,300,890,6910,141200,297500,425950,513760,675310,	Serious condition related to systemic inflammation, organ dysfunction, and organ failure.	Inflammation	Various c.
Infections			See Section 19 - Pathogens	Infections	Various c.
Abscesses	CAFL	2720,2170,880,787,727,500,200,190,	Build-up of pus caused by bacterial infection. Many types may be involved. Use Staphylococcus Aureus (MRSA), and see Listeriose.	Abscess	Various c.
Abscess	BIOM	2720; 2160; 787; 727; 190; 500; 465; 428; 444; 450; 500; 760; 802; 880; 1550; 1865; 2170		Abscess	Various c.
Abscesses Secondary	CAFL	1550,802,760,660,465,450,444,428,	As mentioned above	Abscess	Various c.

Subject / Argument	Author	Frequencies	Notes	Origin	Target
Abscesses 2	XTRA	2720,2170,1865,1550,880,802,787,727,500,444, 190,	As mentioned above	Abscess	Various c.
Abscesses 3	XTRA	2720,2170,1865,1550,880,802,787,760,727,690, 660,500,465,450,444,428,190,	As mentioned above	Abscess	Various c.
Abscess Nocardia Asteroides	XTRA	228,231,237,694,710,887,2890,11092.19,11096. 87,17679.38,	Bacterium producing pulmonary infections. Also see Streptothrix.	Abscess	Various c.
Edema 1	CAFL	6.3,148,440,444,465,522,727,787,880,	See Section 5 - Lymphatic System	Edema	Various c.
Edema 2	CAFL	6.3,20,40,146,148,440,444,465,522,727,787,880 ,5000,10000,		Edema	Various c.
Edema and Swelling	CAFL	6.3,20,146,148,440,444,465,522,727,787,880,50 00,10000,		Edema	Various c.
Edema Swelling	CAFL	6.3,20,440,444,465,522,727,787,880,5000,1000 0,		Edema	Various c.
Edema	BIOM	6.3; 148; 440; 522; 146; 444; 440; 880; 787; 727		Edema	Various c.
Edema 1	XTRA	6.29,20,24.3,146,148,440,444,465,522,660,690, 727.5,787,880,1865,3000,5000,10000,		Edema	Various c.
Edema	EDTFL	130,520,900,8500,12530,145850,262500,39750 0,633910,825170		Edema	Various c.
Lymphatic edema	BIOM	38; 38.5; 69; 79; 17; 56.25; 56; 63.5; 74.5		Edema	Various c.
Cellular Edema	BIOM	22.5		Edema	Various c.
Cellular Edema	BIOM	97.5		Edema	Various c.
Dropsy	XTRA	727,787,10000	Also called Edema - see sets.	Edema	Various c.
Hydrops [Edema]	EDTFL	130,520,900,8500,12530,145850,262500,39750 0,633910,825170,	Abnormal accumulation of interstitial fluid beneath skin and in body cavities. Also see Kidney insufficiency, and appropriate Lymph sets.	Edema	Various c.
Arthrogenous effect	BIOM	9.6		Edema	Various c.
Swelling Edema 2	XTRA	522,146,6.3,148,444,440,880,787,727,	Also see Kidney Insufficiency, and Lymph Stasis sets.	Edema	Various c.
Swelling	CAFL	522,146,6.3,148,444,440,880,787,727,20,10000, 5000,3000,	Edema. See Kidney insufficiency, and Lymph Stasis sets.	Edema	Various c.
Swelling	XTRA	787,1000	As mentioned above	Edema	Various c.
Swelling Legs and Feet	XTRA	20,727,787,880,5000,10000,	As mentioned above	Edema	Various c.
Fluid in Joints and Tissues	XTRA	15,24.3	Also see Edema.	Edema	Various c.
Fluid Retention	XTRA	24.3	Reduce excess fluid in joints and tissues. Also see Edema.	Edema	Various c.
Drainage	BIOM	645.0; 632.0; 635.0; 1335.0; 662.0; 537.0; 763.0; 654.0; 751.0; 625.0; 696.0; 835.0			Various c.
Drainage-1	BIOM	645; 632; 635; 1335; 662; 537; 763; 654; 751; 625; 696; 835			Various c.
Drainage-2	BIOM	15; 17; 337; 537; 625; 635; 654; 669; 676; 696; 751; 764; 835; 1335; 1434; 1524; 2452			Various c.
Decongest	XTRA	400			Various c.
Hernia	EDTFL	180,560,950,7500,22500,42500,125220,275560, 533630,652430	Protrusion of organ through wall of its containing cavity.		Various c.
Hernia General	XTRA	9.09,110,660,690,727.5,787,2720,5000,10000,	Protrusion of organ through wall of its containing cavity.		Various c.
Colic	CAFL	1550,832,802,787,727,20,	Use Cramping and Nausea, and General antiseptic sets.	Colic	Various c.
Colic	EDTFL	40,240,650,850,2500,13060,119500,695000,722 700,932410		Colic	Various c.
Colic 1	XTRA	10,20,422,465,660,690,727.5,787,802,832,1550, 6766,		Colic	Various c.
Colic Intestinal	XTRA	8,123,457		Colic	Various c.
Colic Stomach and Colon Pain	XTRA	20,727,787,800,880,		Colic	Various c.
Cramp	EDTFL	20,200,900,20000,55000,92500,224700,475110, 527000,987230,		Cramps	Various c.
Cramps General	CAFL	36,727,787,880,10000,		Cramps	Various c.
Cramping and Nausea	CAFL	72,95,190,880,832,787,727,20,4.9,		Cramps	Various c.
Cramps General	CAFL	36,727,787,880,10000,		Cramps	Various c.
Ulcers General	CAFL	676,664,802,784,2489,2170,2127,1800,1600,88 0,832,802,787,776,727,73,		Ulcers	Various c.
Ulcer, General	EDTFL	150,240,650,830,2500,127500,255470,387500,6 96500,825910,		Ulcers	Various c.
Ulcer, basic	BIOM	2489; 2170; 2160; 2127; 1800; 1600; 880; 832; 802; 787; 784; 727; 96; 93; 73; 60.5		Ulcers	Various c.
Ulcers 1	XTRA	1.2,73,727,776,787,802,832,880,1600,1800,212 7,2170,2489,		Ulcers	Various c.
Ulcers 2	XTRA	727,776,787,832,880,1600,1800,2127,2170,248 9,		Ulcers	Various c.
Ulcers 3	XTRA	727,776,787,880		Ulcers	Various c.
Ulcers 4	XTRA	73,664,676,727,776,784,787,802,832,880,1600, 1800,2127,2170,2489,		Ulcers	Various c.

Subject / Argument	Author	Frequencies	Notes	Origin	Target
Ulcer Disease 1	BIOM	2.2; 10; 12.5; 19.5; 26; 49; 55; 92.5		Ulcers	Various c.
Ulcer Disease 2	BIOM	3.6; 3.8; 7; 8; 8.6; 9.4; 9.44; 10; 23.5; 46; 59; 61; 61.5; 63; 67; 73; 74; 79.5; 83; 95.5; 96		Ulcers	Various c.
Ulcer Disease 4	BIOM	2.8; 3.3; 8.1; 9.19; 54.0; 54.25; 54.5		Ulcers	Various c.
Ulcer Disease 5	BIOM	0.7; 0.9; 2.5; 2.65; 3.3; 9.8; 56.0; 69.0		Ulcers	Various c.
Ulcer Disease 6	BIOM	2.5; 3.6; 3.9; 5.0; 8.1; 34.0; 92.0		Ulcers	Various c.
Ulcer Repair	BIOM	2489; 2170; 2127; 1800; 1600; 880; 832; 787; 776; 727; 1.2; 73		Ulcers	Various c.
Fistula Ulcer	CAFL	880,832,787,727	Complication of fistula in GI tract, found in Crohn's Disease (see sets). Also use appropriate Staphylococcus set(s).	Fistula	Various c.
Fistula, General	ETDFL	180,240,10530,27500,35000,57500,96500,3251 10,475160,527000,	Abnormal connection between two hollow organs, intestines, or blood vessels.	Fistula	Various c.
Fistula	XTRA	660,690,727.5,787,832,880,	As mentioned above	Fistula	Various c.
Postoperative pain	BIOM	95; 3000; 3040		Surgery	Various c.
Endoscopy	EDTFL	20,120,950,13390,22500,51300,261020,491510, 619340,875350	Medical procedure that uses a small camera on a tube to look inside the body. Purpose of set unknown.	Surgery	Various c.
Catheterization	EDTFL	40,500,700,970,5760,7500,37500,96500,225910 ,425370		Surgery	Various c.
Cannulation	EDTFL	50,530,14330,31230,56720,63440,231270,4348 20,622180,653500		Surgery	Various c.
Reconstructive Surgical Procedures	EDTFL	150,1370,16750,81930,118850,131500,237500, 415700,725000,825950	Includes cosmetic surgeries.	Surgery	Various c.
Reconstructive Surgical Procedures, Cosmetic	EDTFL	70,500,970,9000,11090,131500,237500,415700, 725000,825950		Surgery	Various c.
Cosmetic Reconstruction (Post)	EDTFL	80,350,5750,12930,63470,182500,435290,5625 00,793500,995750		Surgery	Various c.
Oral Surgical Procedures	EDTFL	40,180,700,2250,5590,47500,342190,472500,55 1220,819340		Surgery	Various c.
Suture Techniques	EDTFL	140,260,900,125000,376290,404330,515160,68 7620,712810,992000		Surgery	Various c.
Graft vs Host Disease	EDTFL	80,320,730,3870,19180,150000,475000,527000, 663710,776500	Common disorder after tissue graft/transplant where white blood cells in the graft tissue attack the host body.	Surgery	Various c.
Homologous Wasting Disease	EDTFL	20,150,910,19390,28500,43220,49340,81500,20 4110,305440	As mentioned above	Surgery	Various c.
Runt Disease	EDTFL	80,350,5500,35190,72500,93500,387450,52437 0,655200,754190	As mentioned above	Surgery	Various c.
Prosthesis Implantation	EDTFL	240,730,870,7600,30000,67500,92400,95900,52 4370,650000	An artificial device used to replace a body part.	Surgery	Various c.
Acid-Base Balance Regulation	BIOM	21.5			Various c.
Sensitivity disfunction	BIOM	10000; 1550; 880; 802; 800; 787; 727; 465; 100; 20			Various c.
Electrolyte Levels	CAFL	8.1,20,10000	Improves electrical conductivity in the body.		Various c.
Lack of Conductivity	XTRA	20,727,787,880,10000,	Useful for dry skin in long Contact Mode sessions.		Various c.
Wounds and Injuries			See Section 11a - Skin		Various c.
Trauma			See Section 9c - Pain and Inflammation		Various c.

2 - Substances, Toxins and Intoxicants, Cells, Rare Diseases

2a - Vitamins

Subject / Argument	Author	Frequencies	Notes	Origin	Target
Avitaminosis	EDTFL	40,260,460,7500,37500,57500,210250,326510,436420,561930,			Vitamins
Vitamin Deficiency	EDTFL	40,260,460,7500,37500,57500,210250,326510,436420,561930,			Vitamins
Vitamin Deficiency (Avitaminosis)	XTRA	2400,4420,7360,15000,37500,28750,33333,26875,22530,38797,			Vitamins
Vitamag Complete Set	CAFL	1,2,3,4,5,6,7,7.8,9,10,13,16,19.5,22.5,24,	Magnesium, zinc and vitamin B complex supplement.		Vitamins
Hypervitaminosis A	EDTFL	70,460,830,7500,32100,85230,313630,405790,429700,535590	Toxicity from ingestion of excess pre-formed vitamin A. Eat carotenoid precursors instead.	A	Vitamins
Vitamin A Deficiency	XTRA	2100,9120,15200,23500,33297,28750,26440,22530,38183,33170,	CAFL Anecdotal.	A	Vitamins
Vitamin A Deficiency	EDTFL	120,250,930,2750,30000,155680,262100,315670,527500,725370		A	Vitamins
Vitamin B Deficiency	EDTFL	190,780,12710,55300,90000,175050,426000,571000,822000,934000		B	Vitamins
Vitamin B12 Deficiency	XTRA	50,6560,16000,22500,32500,35925,36400,38279,37240,38705,	CAFL Anecdotal. Use also for Vitamin B Deficiency.	B	Vitamins
Vitamin B12 Deficiency	EDTFL	50,410,1000,45000,97500,324370,410250,566410,709830,930120,	It can be caused by **Helicobacter Pylori**.	B	Vitamins
Beriberi	EDTFL	120,220,5810,5500,40000,67500,150000,269710,749000,987230,	Primarily due to thiamine deficiency (**vitamin B1**) with CNS, neuro, cardiac, motor, and psych problems.	B	Vitamins
Beriberi, Cerebral	EDTFL	170,17850,27500,45470,148000,230500,472500,719000,725710,903320,		B	Vitamins
Biotinidase Deficiency	EDTFL	130,230,730,850,5250,137250,545760,687500,895270,976290	Enzyme deficiency caused by failure to process biotin (**vitamin B7**) in food.	B	Vitamins
Pellagra	EDTFL	130,540,770,2520,7500,50000,187500,455300,672230,775870	Due to **B3** / niacin or tryptophan deficiency. Causes Diarrhea, Dermatitis, and Dementia (see sets). Also see Avitaminosis, and Vitamin Deficiency (Avitaminosis) sets.	B	Vitamins
Vitamin C Deficiency	XTRA	2100,11680,29500,23750,15420,34065,5009,39375,36000,39923,	CAFL Anecdotal.	C	Vitamins
Vitamin C Deficiency	EDTFL	140,650,25050,87300,125370,222530,479930,527000,667000,987230		C	Vitamins
Vitamin D Deficiency	XTRA	2890,3740,9920,33270,40000,28750,25000,37233,34000,	CAFL Anecdotal.	D	Vitamins
Vitamin D Deficiency	EDTFL	120,900,5620,93500,222700,425000,522530,689920,752600,923700		D	Vitamins

2b - Toxins

Subject / Argument	Author	Frequencies	Notes	Origin	Target
Autointoxication	BIOM	10000.0; 1550.0; 880.0; 800.0; 787.0; 727.0; 522.0; 146.0; 100.0; 20.0			Toxins
Auto Intoxication	CAFL	20,333,522,555.1,727,787,800,880,1550,10000,	Build-upof toxins in the intestines/colon.		Toxins
Autointoxication	CAFL	522,146,1550,10000,800,880,787,727,20,	Build-upof toxins in the intestines/colon.		Toxins
Detox Autointoxication	XTRA	20,146,522,727,787,800,880,1550,10000,	Also see Constipation, Auto Intoxication, and Autointoxication.		Detox
Intoxication	XTRA	10000,			Toxins
Chronic intoxication	BIOM	1370; 633; 639; 578; 866; 136; 255; 975; 2688; 771; 5419; 6007; 1365; 7755; 533; 435; 253; 392; 714; 837			Toxins
Food Poisoning	CAFL	1552,802,832	Some classes. Use **Salmonella typhimurium** set. See General Antiseptic, Abdominal Pain, and Inflammation sets.	Food	Toxins
Food Poisoning	BIOM	5553.5; 1552; 972; 802; 832; 727; 718; 717; 713; 664; 643; 787; 880; 10000		Food	Toxins
Food Poisoning [Gastro]	EDTFL	120,200,900,47500,110250,322540,332410,684810,712230,992000,		Food	Toxins
Food Poisoning 1	XTRA	59,92,165,420,643,664,707,711,717,719,752,947.62,954.32,956.79,958.15,972,1244,1522,6787,7771,11946.87,12031.25,12062.5,12079.69,19168.02,19217.81,		Food	Toxins
Food Poisoning 2	XTRA	546,693,754,762,773,947.62,954.32,956.79,958.15,1634,8656,11946.87,12031.25,12062.5,12079.69,19168.02,19217.81,		Food	Toxins
Food Poisoning 4	XTRA	10000		Food	Toxins
Food Poisoning Distilled Water	XTRA	727,787,880,10000,		Food	Toxins
Addiction	XTRA	230,290,440,1500,2300,3300,83350,184000,283000,303400,	Alcohol addiction.	Addiction	Toxins
Alcoholism	CAFL	10000	See Liver enlargement and Liver support.	Addiction	Toxins
Addiction Alcoholism	CAFL	727,787,880,10000,	See Liver enlargement and Liver support.	Addiction	Toxins

Subject / Argument	Author	Frequencies	Notes	Origin	Target
Addictions, Alcohol, General	EDTFL	230,290,440,1500,2300,3300,83350,184000,283000,303400,		Addiction	Toxins
Detox in case of alcohol intoxicatyion	BIOM	10000; 522; 146; 100		Addiction	Detox
Hangover	CAFL	10000,522,146	See Kidney support and Liver support sets.	Addiction	Toxins
Hangover	XTRA	10		Addiction	Toxins
Drug Addiction	CAFL	20,727,787,880,5000,		Addiction	Toxins
Antidrug	BIOM	3.5; 18.5; 29.5; 49.5; 61.5; 90		Addiction	Toxins
Withdrawal symptoms control	BIOM	1.2; 6.8; 9.2; 9.4; 9.6; 18.5; 29.5; 49.5		Addiction	Toxins
Removal of addictive drug (Phase 1)	BIOM	19; 24.5; 35.5; 36; 37.5; 94.5; 98.5		Addiction	Toxins
Removal of addictive drug (Phase 2)	BIOM	2; 5.5; 12; 26; 26.5; 66; 75.5; 94		Addiction	Toxins
Addiction Drugs	XTRA	5,333,353		Addiction	Toxins
Addiction Drugs	XTRA	20,727,787,880,5000,		Addiction	Toxins
Addictions, Drug, General	EDTFL	280,350,470,1880,4340,5200,43420,143040,234040,343450,		Addiction	Toxins
Adverse Drug Reaction	EDTFL	140,200,330,420,440,520,550,730,760,1860,			Toxins
Detox Depression Drug Toxin	XTRA	1.1,30.5,73			Toxins
Depression Drugs Or Toxins	CAFL	1.1,73	Detox.		Toxins
Depression, toxicological (caused by medicines, narcotic drugs, etc.)	BIOM	1.1; 3.5; 7.73; 428; 444; 660; 700; 35; 787; 800; 5000			Toxins
Depression caused by Medications	BIOM	1000.0; 5000.0; 3176.0; 800.0; 787.0; 73.0; 35.0; 33.0; 26.0; 14.0; 7.83; 3.5; 1.1			Toxins
Depression of Infectious Toxic Origin	BIOM	5711.5; 5414.5; 4064.6; 3791.2; 2032.0; 2363.0; 1865.0; 2995.0; 2198.0; 1763.0; 2571.0; 2035.0; 2356.0; 1870.0; 1626.0; 2644.0; 2795.0; 2151.0			Toxins
Plant Poisoning [Gastro]	EDTFL	120,200,900,47500,110250,322540,332410,684810,712230,992000,			Toxins
Konzo	EDTFL	30,520,620,930,7500,12710,96500,225540,300000,324540	Form of epidemic paralysis that occurs almost exclusively from consumption of the "bitter" cassava plant (with a high percentage of cyanide).		Toxins

2c - Detox

Subject / Argument	Author	Frequencies	Notes	Origin	Target
General Cleanser	XTRA	337,464,467,576,688,728,786,803,856,882,912,1554,1862,2128,3337,5762,6667,			Detox
Deep Cleansing	BIOM	0.7; 0.9; 2.5; 2.65; 3.3; 9.8; 56.0; 69.0			Detox
Matrix Detoxification	BIOM	10000; 3176; 3040; 880; 787; 751; 727; 625; 522; 465; 444; 440; 1505; 1035.9; 3176; 676; 635; 146; 250; 304; 306; 148; 152; 63			Detox
Detox All Purpose	XTRA	6.29,9.18,9.19,15=900,20.5,146,148,333,428,444,522,523,528,555,660,690,727.5,768,786,787,802,880,1550,1865,3176,10000,			Detox
Detox	EDTFL	20,200,900,5950,8500,125690,262500,592500,758570,823440,			Detox
Elimination of Toxins	BIOM	0.5; 522.0; 146.0; 1552.0; 800.0			Detox
Detoxification	BIOM	10000.0; 3176.0; 3040.0; 880.0; 787.0; 751.0; 727.0; 625.0; 522.0; 465.0; 444.0; 440.0; 1505.0; 1035.9; 3176.0; 676.0; 635.0; 304.0; 306.0; 250.0; 148.0; 152.0; 63.0			Detox
Detoxication of organism	BIOM	0.9; 2.5; 2.65; 3.3; 6; 8; 9.8; 56			Detox
Deep cleaning of organism	BIOM	0.7; 0.9; 2.5; 2.65; 3.3; 9.8; 56.0; 69			Detox
Deep cleaning of organism (special)	BIOM	3.5; 5.0; 2.5; 12.5; 45.5; 53.5; 57.0; 90.0; 95.0			Detox
Detox Assist	CAFL	10000,3176	Also see Blood Purify sets.		Detox
Detox Antiseptic Effect	XTRA	14,333,428,444,450,465,523,555,590,660,690,727.5,760,768,786,787,802,804,880,1360,1550,1770,1865,2000,2720,3176,5000,10000,			Detox
Detox Toxins Elimination 1	XTRA	0.5,146,522,800,1552,			Detox
Detox Toxins Elimination 2	XTRA	0.5,2.5,6.29,9.18,9.19,20,146,148,333,428,444,522,523,555,660,690,727.5,768,786,787,802,880,1550,1865,10000,			Detox
Toxin Elimination	CAFL	0.5,522,146,1552,800,	See Detox 4 toxins throughout the body, and Blood Purify sets.		Detox
Elimination of toxins	BIOM	0.5; 0.8; 1.1; 4.9; 6; 522; 1552; 800; 7344			Detox

Subject / Argument	Author	Frequencies	Notes	Origin	Target
Blood Purify 1	CAFL	3.92		Blood	Detox
Blood Purification	XTRA	66.5	Use for all types of cancer.	Blood	Detox
Blood Purification	BIOM	2; 727; 787; 800; 880; 5000; 2008; 2127		Blood	
Blood Cleanser	PROV	727,787,880,2008,2127,5000,	Use for all types of Cancer sets.	Blood	Detox
Blood Plasma Cleaner	CAFL	800		Blood	Detox
Purification of blood and plasma	BIOM	727; 787; 800; 880; 5000; 2008; 2127		Blood	Detox
Blood Cleanser Cancer	XTRA	727,787,880,2008,2127,5000,10000,		Blood	Detox
Detox and Lymphs	CAFL	2.5,6,3,7.83,10.10,10.36,15.05,15.2,146,148,304 ,306,440,444,465,522,625,635,676,727,751,787, 880,3040,3176,10000,	Also see Blood Purify sets.	Lymphs	Detox
Detox and Lymphs	XTRA	2.5,6.29,7.83,10,10.35,15.05,15.19,146,148,304, 306,440,444,465,522,625,635,676,727,751,787, 880,3040,3176,10000,	Also see Blood Purify sets.	Lymphs	Detox
Detox Lymphs	XTRA	2.5,6.29,7.83,10,10.35,15.05,15.19,146,148,304, 440,444,465,522,625,635,676,727,751,787,880, 3175,3176,3177,10000,		Lymphs	Detox
Lymph and Detoxification	BIOM	10000; 3177; 3176; 3175; 3040; 880; 787; 751; 727; 676; 635; 625; 522; 465; 444; 440; 304; 152; 150.5; 148; 146; 150.5; 103.6; 100; 63; 25; 15.2; 15.05; 10.36; 10; 7.83; 6.3; 2.5		Lymphs	Detox
Detox - lymph and intercellular space	BIOM	10000; 3177; 3040; 880; 787; 727; 676; 635; 625; 522; 465; 444; 440; 304; 306; 148; 146; 15.2; 15.5; 10.36; 10; 7.84; 6.3; 2.5		Lymphs	Detox
Detox Adrenal Gland	XTRA	20,10000,12000		Lymphs	Detox
Detox 1	XTRA	24,89,164,522,3176,10000,	Also see Blood Purify sets.		Detox
Detox 1 Toxins in the Intestines	CAFL	2.4,2.68,5.8,6.3,10,20,40,60,72,95,125,165,200, 333,428,444,465,522,555,600,625,650,666,690, 727,787,802,832,880,1250,1500,1865,	Also see Blood Purify sets.		Detox
Detox 2 Parasites in the Intestines	CAFL	9.6,15,26,35,48,60,95,125,160,200,230,410,440, 465,588,760,776,1000,2000,2127,	Also see Blood Purify sets.		Detox
Detox 3 Toxins in the Kidneys and Liver	PROV	2.4,6.3,7.8,9.2,14,20,35,60,72,95,126,160,200,2 40,440,444,465,522,600,625,666,690,727,787,8 02,832,880,1500,1550,1865,2000,	Also see Blood Purify sets.		Detox
Detox 4 Toxins Throughout the Body	CAFL	2.4,5.8,6.3,7.8,20,26,35,60,72,125,165,200,444, 465,522,588,600,625,650,666,685,690,727,760, 776,787,802,832,880,1250,1500,1550,1850,212 7,	Also see Blood Purify sets.		Detox
Detox [Toxin extraction]	EDTFL	190,200,7250,45750,96500,325000,519340,655 200,750000,922530,			Detox
Detox (Liver, Kidneys, Lymph, Intestine, Lung)	EDTFL	50,180,1520,5350,8520,125690,324520,637500, 721620,852090,			Detox
Detoxication of liver	BIOM	0.9; 2.5; 3.3; 9.2; 69; 79; 95.5			Detox
Detox in case of acute infection	BIOM	20; 232; 622; 822; 2112; 4211			Detox
Detox in case of mycotic infection	BIOM	336; 337; 146; 148			Detox
Fungus Detoxification	BIOM	336; 337; 146; 148; 152; 10000; 3176; 3040; 880; 787; 751; 727; 625; 522; 1505; 1035.9; 3176; 676; 635; 465; 444; 440; 304; 306; 250; 63			Detox
Parasite Detoxification	BIOM	20; 64; 72; 96; 112; 120; 125; 128; 152; 240; 334; 422; 442; 465; 524; 651; 688; 728; 732; 751; 784; 800; 854; 880; 1864			Detox
Detox Anesthesia 1	XTRA	146,522			Detox
Detox Anesthesia 2	XTRA	0.5,2.5,6.29,146,148,333,522,523,555,768,786			Detox
Surgery Anaesthesia Detox	CAFL	522,146	Use Liver support set.		Detox
Vaccine Toxins	XTRA	1048551.1993	From Newport. Neutralizes vaccine toxins. Based on Dr. Hulda Clark's frequency.		Detox
Detox Tetanus	XTRA	363,458	Infectious disease of central nervous system caused by Clostridium Tetani - see program.		Detox
Detox Methotrexate	XTRA	584	Chemotherapy drug that inhibits folic acid production and induces abortion.		Detox
Detox Headache Toxicity 1	XTRA	1.19,4.9,20,146,160,250,522,660,690,727.5,787, 880,3000,			Detox
Detox Headache Toxicity 2	XTRA	4.9,20,146,522,727,787,880,3000,			Detox

Subject / Argument	Author	Frequencies	Notes	Origin	Target
Detox Mental Disorders	XTRA	4.9,20,72,95,125,146,428,522,550,802,10000,			Detox
Detox SSRI Benzo	XTRA	7676767.6666,7676767.66,7676767.67,7676767 .2-7676768.2=1000, 7776765.6666,7776765.66,7776765.67,7776765 .2-7776766.2=1000,	Psychoanalgesic detox: benzodiazepines and selective serotonin reuptake inhibitors.		Detox
Detox Toxic Proteins	XTRA	9887			Detox
Detox Uremic Poison	XTRA	911	Also called Uremia. Excessive nitrogenous waste in the blood, as in kidney failure. Use Kidney Insufficiency, and Lymph Stasis - Secondary sets. See Blood Purify sets.		Detox
Detox Urticaria	XTRA	4.9,6.29,95,125,146,148,444,522,660,690,727.5, 787,880,1800,1865,	Also called Hives - see sets.		Detox
Heavy Metals	CAFL	30000		Heavy Met.	Toxins
Mercury Toxicity V	CAFL	47,48,49,75	Toxic metal element.	Heavy Met.	Toxins
Heavy Metal Toxicity	XTRA	317,1902,4202.3,5333.69,9887,14164.1,15952.7 9,19007.15,19007.2,19169.38,19516.29,21822.1 5,		Heavy Met.	Toxins
Arsenic Poisoning	EDTFL KHZ	100,830,5500,52500,342060,458500,515090,68 7620,712230,995380,		Heavy Met.	Toxins
Metals	CAFL	30000	Detox of metals from cells.	Heavy Met.	Detox
Intoxication Heavy Metals Salts	BIOM	4202.2; 5333.5; 9886.5; 1902.0; 317.0		Heavy Met.	Detox
Detox Heavy Metals 1	XTRA	528,945,1121,1183,1211,1343,1354,1425,2154,		Heavy Met.	Detox
Detox Heavy Metals 2	XTRA	63,146,148,152,250,304,306,440,444,465,522,6 25,635,676,727.5,751,787,880,1036,1505,3040, 3176,10000,		Heavy Met.	Detox
Detox Heavy Metals 3	XTRA	317,1902,4202.3,5333.69,9887,14164.1,15952.7 9,19007.15,19007.2,19169.38,19516.29,21822.1 5,		Heavy Met.	Detox
Detox Heavy Metals 4	XTRA	15000		Heavy Met.	Detox
Detox in case of heavy metals	BIOM	6887; 4202.3; 5333.7; 1902; 317		Heavy Met.	
Detox Aluminum	XTRA	15952.79		Heavy Met.	Detox
Detox Barium	XTRA	19516.29,21822.15	Heavy metal.	Heavy Met.	Detox
Detox Mercury 1	XTRA	14164.1,19007.15		Heavy Met.	Detox
Mercury excretion	BIOM	47,48,49,75		Heavy Met.	Detox
Detox Lead	XTRA	4202.3,19007.15		Heavy Met.	Detox
Detox Green Dye Chemical	XTRA	563,2333	Remove toxins from exposure to green dye.	Chemical s.	Detox
Detox of chemical substances	BIOM	664; 7344; 2842; 1146.9; 686.6; 684.1; 1113; 779.9; 829.3; 679.2; 865; 970; 1067; 783.6; 800.4; 1045; 1062; 673.9; 690.7		Chemical s.	Detox
Chemical Sensitivity	CAFL	727	As mentioned above	Chemical s.	Detox
Detox Chemical Sensitivity	XTRA	440,443	Also see Multiple Chemical Sensitivity, and Morgellons sets.	Chemical s.	Detox
Detox Pesticide	XTRA	1,6,26,73		Chemical s.	Detox
Pesticide Detox	CAFL	73,26,6,1	Also use Liver, and Kidney support, Circulatory, and Lymph stasis sets.	Chemical s.	Detox
Detoxication from pesticides	BIOM	73; 26; 6; 0.8		Chemical s.	Detox
Glyphosate	XTRA	23355767.753	Experimental. May destroy toxic mutagenic pesticide.	Chemical s.	Detox
Ammonia Remove	XTRA	1719,51	Removes ammonia and 'vinegar' in Lyme Disease.	Chemical s.	Detox
Detox Fluoride	XTRA	19169.38		Chemical s.	Detox
Detox Fluoride 2	XTRA	158.87,56656.4		Chemical s.	Detox
Detox Acrylamide	XTRA	21822.15	Carcinogenic constituent of polymers. Used in water treatment, food production, cosmetics, and pesticides. Also produced when food is grilled, fried, or baked too long.	Chemical s.	Detox
Perfluorooctanoic Acid Detox	XTRA	3574961.94	Experimental. Persistent toxic carcinogen found in Teflon.	Chemical s.	Detox
Plastics Detox	XTRA	7755766.6555,67553.6343,54423.7760	Dowsed by Newport, BPA frequency from Dr. Jeff Sutherland. Use for activated and dormant Morgellons.	Chemical s.	Detox
Detox Plastics 2	XTRA	67553.63,67553.64,1055.52,1055.53,54423.77,5 4423.78	Bisphenol A, and Phthalates (DEHP, DINP, and DIDP).	Chemical s.	Detox
Silicone Detox	XTRA	787998.7877	Apply=Frequencies Directly. Use after Smart Dust set. Dowsed by Newport. Use for activated and dormant Morgellons.	Chemical s.	Detox
Smart Dust	XTRA	55454.5454	Duty Cycle=67, Apply=Frequencies Directly. Dowsed by Newport. Use Silicone Detox after this. Use for activated and dormant Morgellons.	Chemical s.	Detox
Chemical Spray-Related Illness	XTRA	113,279.19,664,673.89,684.1,686.6,690.7,779.8 9,783.6,800.39,829.29,865,969.89,1045,1062,10 67,1147,2842,7344,	Also use Chemtrail sets.	Chemical s.	Detox
Detox Respiratory	XTRA	6.29,9.18,9.19,20.5		Chemtrail	Detox
Detox - lungs and antrum	BIOM	338; 783; 932; 1035; 1160; 1630; 712; 713; 715; 1244		Chemtrail	Detox

Subject / Argument	Author	Frequencies	Notes	Origin	Target
Chemtrail Detox	CAFL	664,7344,2842,1147,686.6,684.1,1113,779.9,82 9.3,679.2,865,969.9,1067,783.6,800.4,1045,106 2,673.9,690.7,	Addresses aerially-sprayed toxic metals and biological agents. Also useful for lung and sinus problems.	Chemtrail	Detox
Chemtrail Detox 2	XTRA	16542.41	Addresses aerially-sprayed toxic metals and biological agents. Also useful for lung and sinus problems.	Chemtrail	Detox
Detox Chemtrail 1	XTRA	664,7344,2842,1147,686.6,684.1,1113,779.9,82 9.3,679.2,865,969.9,1067,783.6,800.4,1045,106 2,673.9,690.7,	Addresses aerially-sprayed toxic metals and biological agents. Also useful for lung and sinus problems. See Chemtrail Detox.	Chemtrail	Detox
Detox Chemtrail 2	XTRA	16542.41,16939.43	As mentioned above	Chemtrail	Detox
Detox Chemtrail 3	XTRA	16542.41	As mentioned above	Chemtrail	Detox
Nicotine Cravings	XTRA	38		Nicotine	Detox
Nicotine Cravings 2	XTRA	111		Nicotine	Detox
Nicotine Withdrawal	XTRA	10		Nicotine	Detox
Detox Nicotine	XTRA	10000		Nicotine	Detox
Anti-smoking	BIOM	3.5		Nicotine	Detox
Electrical Sensitivity Reduce	XTRA	657	Symptoms may include headache, fatigue, stress, sleep disturbance, skin prickling, burning, rashes, muscle ache and other problems on exposure to EMFs.	Radiation	Detox
Detox EMF	XTRA	99.5	Experimental.	Radiation	Detox
Electro Magnetic Field Radiation (EMF) and Detox EMF Exposure (with Detox frequencies) Radiation Detox Radiation General	EDTFL	60,330,900,85750,150000,223700,225000,4545 00,515170,687620		Radiation	Detox
Detox in case of electric smog	BIOM	99.5	Symptoms may include headache, fatigue, stress, sleep disturbance, skin prickling, burning, rashes, muscle ache and other problems on exposure to EMFs.	Radiation	Detox
Radiation Remove All	XTRA	6,847,972,437		Radiation	Detox
Detox in case of radiation emissions	BIOM	144; 147; 174		Radiation	Detox

2d - Cells, Amino acids, Enzymes, etc.

Subject / Argument	Author	Frequencies	Notes	Origin	Target
Human Body Cell	XTRA	11875			Cell
Cell Regeneration	XTRA	111			Cell
Cell Regeneration	BIOM	97.5			Cell
Cell frequencies	BIOM	22.5; 17.5; 29.0; 79.5; 99.5			Cell
Biological charging	BIOM	49; 10; 12.5			Cell
Oxygenation and Mitochondria					Cell
Hypoxia	CAFL	727,787,880,10000	Low oxygen. Use Circulatory stasis.	Oxygenation	Cell
Hypoxia	BIOM	50.5; 50; 787; 10000			Cell
Hypoxia	EDTFL	30,460,600,850,2500,5250,17500,93500,224940 ,425610		Oxygenation	Cell
Anoxia Anoxia, Brain	EDTFL	150,180,800,5500,17500,32500,151270,257460, 413910,692270	Extreme form of Hypoxia.	Oxygenation	Cell
Cerebral Anoxia	EDTFL	120,230,7200,13610,96500,175000,327750,682 450,753070,927100		Oxygenation	Cell
Blood Hemoglobin Production	XTRA	2452	Improve blood oxygen transport ability.	Oxygenation	Cell
Blood Flow and Oxygen Supply	BIOM	50; 50.5; 55		Oxygenation	Cell
Methemoglobinemia	EDTFL	150,680,2100,62410,122530,305000,327740,65 5200,755000,805120	Due to methemoglobin, a form of hemoglobin with ferric rather than ferrous iron, leading to impaired oxygen delivery to tissues.	Oxygenation	Cell
Oxygenate Cells	XTRA	16,	Also allows cells to take in calcium.	Oxygenation	Cell
Oxygen Intake	BIOM	50; 55			Cell
Oxygenation	XTRA	5.35	Also allows cells to take in calcium.	Oxygenation	Cell
Oxygen	XTRA	5.772		Oxygenation	Cell
Oxidative Phosphorylation [Hypertrophic]	EDTFL	70,230,880,35230,63020,125030,235680,39650 0,575610,751770,		Oxygenation	Cell
Respiratory Failure Acute	XTRA	1,257,814	Abnormal levels of oxygen or carbon dioxide in blood. Also see Anoxia, Hypoxia, Cyanosis, Circulation, and Circulatory sets.	Oxygenation	Cell
Minerals - Iron	XTRA	416=600	Oxygen to cells, circulation, digestion, elimination, respiration, tissue oxidation, liver, hemoglobin, immunological response.	Minerals	Cell
ATP Generate	XTRA	9.6	Helps mitochondria produce ATP, essential for transport of chemical energy in cells.		Cell

Subject / Argument	Author	Frequencies	Notes	Origin	Target
Mitochondrial Diseases	EDTFL	40,250,460,520,780,900,42500,87500,132410,376290			Cell
Respiratory Chain Deficiencies, Mitochondrial	EDTFL	40,250,460,520,780,900,42500,87500,132410,376290,	Deficiencies in electron transport chain in mitochondria that converts oxygen to enable ATP generation. Also see Electron Transport Chain Def.		Cell
Electron Transport Chain Deficiency	EDTFL	80,120,850,58870,224030,410200,585830,626070,725340,826900			Cell
Inosine Production Stimulate	XTRA	2642	Nucleoside which increases the energy levels of the body producing good amount of ATP. Is essential for correct translation of genetic code. May be useful for MS, post-stroke, or spinal cord insults. May cause kidney stones.		Cell
Carnitine Disorders	EDTFL	140,260,900,125000,376290,404370,515160,687620,712810,992000	Amino acids-derived compound necessary for mitochondrial health.		Cell
Carnitine Disorders	KHZ	30,520,7500,30000,225160,475190,527000,667000,789000,988900,	Amino acids-derived compound necessary for mitochondrial health.		Cell
L Lysine	CAFL	195.5,391,782,1564.1,3128.2,6256.4,	Essential amino acid precursor of carnitine. Stimulation. Plays a major role in calcium absorption, building muscle, recovery from injuries; and production of hormones, enzymes, and antibodies.		Cell
Lysine Stimulate	XTRA	391,782,1564.09,1950.5,3128.19,6256.39,	Amino acid necessary for production of protein.		Cell
Stimulation of lysin	BIOM	195.5; 391; 782; 1564; 3128.2; 6255.5			Cell
Acidemia	EDTFL	490,730,800,2500,132600,347500,377650,597500,775950,925310	Inherited disorder with inability to process lysine, hydroxylysine, and tryptophan, leading to brain and organ damage. May cause carnitine deficiency - see Carnitine Disorders.		Cell
Glutaric Acidemia	EDTFL	490,730,800,2500,132600,347500,377650,597500,775950,925310,	As mentioned above		Cell
Glutaric Acidemia	EDTF KHZ	120,550,950,5290,95520,142500,362500,402500,590000,822530,	As mentioned above		Cell
Mitochondrial Myopathy	EDTFL	40,250,460,520,780,900,87500,93400,224940,497610	Mitochondrial Encephalomyopathy, Lactic acidosis, and Stroke-like episodes. Genetic disorder affecting brain/CNS and muscles.	Genetic disorder	Cell
MELAS Syndrome	EDTFL	140,220,620,7500,15700,41090,465700,597500,722700,875930	As mentioned above	Genetic disorder	Cell
Interleukin	PROV	3448,2929,4014,5611,2867,2855,2791,	Vital to immune system. Use to stimulate lymphocyte production.		Cell
Interleukin	BIOM	3448; 2929; 4014; 5611; 2867; 2855; 2791	As mentioned above		Cell
N-Acetylcysteine NAC	XTRA	3985210.11	Experimental. May boost glutathion, loosen thick respiratory mucus, and treat paracetamol overdose.		Cell
Amyloidosis	EDTFL	60,7500,10830,322530,452590,519679,689410,712000,833210,995380,	Caused by misfolded proteins, most commonly in kidneys and heart.		Cell
Antioxidant effect	BIOM	9.45			Cell
Endorphin Release	XTRA	38	Pain-killing morphine-like neuropeptide produced by the CNS and pituitary gland.		Cell
Serotonin	XTRA	2.5,10,80,160	Regulatory neurotransmitter found in GI tract, blood platelets, and nervous system, with many functions including mood, sleep, appetite, and blood clotting.		Cell
Serotonin	XTRA	2.5,10,22.027,80,160,	As mentioned above		Cell
Antiserotonergic	BIOM	8.1; 9.6			Cell
Serotonin Syndrome	EDTFL	120,900,5620,93500,222700,425000,522530,689930,752630,923700	Excessive levels of serotonin that may occur after drug administration, combination, overdose of particular drugs, or recreational use of certain drugs.		Cell
Dopamine Stimulate Production	XTRA	38	Important neurotransmitter that performs many essential body functions.		Cell
Trophism	BIOM	727.0; 787.0; 880.0; 5000.0	General state of nutrition of an organism or part of an organism.		Metabolism
Metabolic Syndrome		Can be caused by the bacteria Chlamydia pneumoniae and Helicobacter pylori, as well as the viruses Cytomegalovirus and Herpes simplex virus 1.			
Metabolism	BIOM	46			Metabolism
Malabsorption Syndrome	XTRA	660,690,727.5,787,800,802,880,1550,1552,3000	Abnormal absorption of nutrients in GI tract. May lead to malnutrition. Also use Parasites General.		Metabolism
Malabsorption Syndrome	BIOM	880; 1552; 3000			Metabolism
Malabsorption Syndrome 1	CAFL	727,787,880,800,1552,3000,	As mentioned above		Metabolism
Short Bowel Syndrome	EDTFL	110,750,2600,63000,87200,236410,327550,561910,714840,978090	Malabsorption disorder mainly caused by surgical removal of small intestine.		Metabolism
Metabolic Stress [Group 20]	EDTFL	140,680,2500,60000,122530,300000,496010,655200,750000,912330,	Disorder due to metabolic reaction to stress produced by events, substances, activities, worries, or the like.		Metabolism
Hepatolenticular Degeneration [Wilsons Disease]	EDTFL	30,500,900,13610,37500,117500,322520,497500,715700,842060,	Genetic disorder with accumulation of copper in tissues.	Genetic disorder	Metabolism
Wilson Disease	EDTFL	30,500,900,13610,37500,117500,322520,497500,715700,842060	As mentioned above	Genetic disorder	Metabolism
Metabolic Diseases Metabolic Syndrome X	EDTFL	60,530,49930,172500,287500,313980,455230,607500,811520,903540	Large class of genetic diseases involving congenital disorders of metabolism.	Genetic disorder	Metabolism

Subject / Argument	Author	Frequencies	Notes	Origin	Target
Reaven Syndrome X	EDTFL	170,250,20000,125160,377910,414170,515169, 683000,712000,993410,	Associated with obesity, raised BP, high fasting plasma glucose, high serum triglycerides, and low HDL, with risk of cardiovascular disease or diabetes.	Genetic disorder	Metabolism
Thesaurismosis	EDTFL	120,2500,15750,52500,96500,225160,524370,6 50000,753070,927100		Genetic disorder	Metabolism
Magnesium deficit	BIOM	62.5; 480		Magnesium	Metabolism
Potassium metabolism	BIOM	10		Potasssium	Metabolism
Sodium/potassium, balance	BIOM	5.5; 8.1			Metabolism
Calcium Metabolism Improve	XTRA	9.59,326,328,673.1,771,4760.5,10000,	Regulation of movement of calcium in the body, normally handled by the thyroid and parathyroid.	Calcium	Metabolism
Calcium Metabolism	XTRA	328	Stimulate normalization. Regulation of movement of calcium in the body, normally handled by the thyroid and parathyroid.	Calcium	Metabolism
Calcium deficit	BIOM	15; 52.5		Calcium	Metabolism
Calcium deposit	BIOM	326		Calcium	Metabolism
Calcium Uptake Reduce	XTRA	16	Opens potassium ion channels of cell membranes, reducing influx of calcium ions.	Calcium	Metabolism
Fat Cells	XTRA	295.8		Fat	Metabolism
Fat Energy Metabolism	XTRA	285,295.8,612,5219,5797,5859,6140,8875,		Fat	Metabolism
Fat metabolism, adiposity	BIOM	2; 4.9; 32; 34.5; 35; 35.5		Fat	Metabolism
Fat Burn	CAFL	2.5,4,6.3,7.83,10,10.36,15.05,15.2,146,148,304, 440,444,456,522,625,635,676,727,751,787, 880,3175,3176,3177,10000,	Also run Hypophyseal Disturbances, Lymph Stasis Secondary, and appropriate Detox sets.	Fat	Metabolism
Fat Burn 1	XTRA	124,333,523,666,768,786,950,958,959,959.6,96 0.39,962,967.6,969.29,	As mentioned above	Fat	Metabolism
Fat Burn 2	XTRA	6028.98	As mentioned above	Fat	Metabolism
Fat Burn 3	XTRA	20,26,48,60,72,95,125,160,180,300,333,444,522 ,523,555,660,690,727.5,768,787,802,880,942,95 1,952,959,960,962,968,969,1009,1034,1060,106 2,1395,1500,1550,1865,2050,2720,4868,5000,6 989,7001,7009,7702,7762,7767,10000,	Also run Hypophyseal Disturbances, Lymph Stasis Secondary, and appropriate Detox sets.	Fat	Metabolism
Fat Burn 4	XTRA	5218.75,5796.86,5859.36,6140.25,8875,	Also run Hypophyseal Disturbances, Lymph Stasis Secondary, and appropriate Detox sets.	Fat	Metabolism
Fat Cells	XTRA	295.8		Fat	Metabolism
Constitutional excessive weight	BIOM	10000; 465; 100		Fat	Metabolism
Fat Burn Hypophyseal Lymph Detox	XTRA	2.5,4=240,6.29,7.53,10,10.35,15.05,15.19,146,1 48,304,440,444,456,465=240,522,625,635,676, 727,751,787,880,3175,3176,3177,10000=240,	.	Fat	Metabolism
Fatty Acid Oxidation Disorders [Hypoglycemia]	EDTFL	160,540,850,5450,32500,125790,270000,49250 0,658570,824940,	Group of genetic disorders caused by inability to produce or use one enzyme needed for fatty acid oxid oxidation.	Fat	Metabolism
Leucine Metabolism Disorders	EDTFL	60,370,870,870,8000,62500,95560,325870,4730 00,742060	Genetic metabolic disorder affecting processing of leucine amino acid. Also see Branched-Chain Ketoaciduria, and Maple Syrup Urine Disease.	Amino Acid	Metabolism
Branched-Chain Ketoaciduria	EDTFL	40,550,970,93500,210500,453720,515190,6830 00,712230,993430	Genetic metabolic disorder affecting processing of branched-chain amino acids.	Amino Acid	Metabolism
Thiamine Responsive Maple Syrup Urine Disease	EDTFL	50,35750,60000,93300,225150,454330,517500, 687620,712000,992000	As mentioned above	Amino Acid	Metabolism
Carbohydrate metabolism regulation basic	BIOM	3.3; 4; 7; 9.19; 9.44; 9.69; 11.5; 12.5; 23; 25.5; 26.5; 46; 52; 79.5; 85.5; 92; 94.5		Carbohydrate	Metabolism
Amino Acid Metabolism Amino Acid Transport Disorder Amino Acidopathies, Congenital	EDTFL	170,2500,20000,92400,310250,450000,517500, 687620,712230,993410,	Normalisation.	Amino Acid	Metabolism
Neutral Amino Acid Transport	EDTFL	170,2500,20000,92400,310250,450000,517500, 687620,712230,993410,	Genetic metabolic disorder affecting absorption of essential amino acids.	Amino Acid	Metabolism
Hartnup Disease	EDTFL	450,620,640,4970,7500,15310,317900,325930,3 85900,504370	As mentioned above	Amino Acid	Metabolism
Phenylketonurias {Amino Specific]	EDTFL	40,500,890,2750,82850,122010,237500,422530, 635350,873530,	Inborn metabolic error with impaired metabolism of the amino acid phenylalanine. Sufferers must never ingest aspartame.	Amino Acid	Metabolism
Histidinemia	EDTFL	20,500,870,172400,207500,315230,425620,691 220,735540,962070	Originally believed to be linked to developmental disorders, but now classed as a 'benign inborn error of metabolism.'	Amino Acid	Metabolism
Phenylalanine Hydroxylase Deficiency Disease	EDTFL	160,550,950,17500,93980,137500,396300,5758 30,824370,963190		Amino Acid	Metabolism
Dihydropteridine Reductase	EDTFL	180,220,650,2480,7500,40000,157000,325550,3 75630,519350	As mentioned above	Amino Acid	Metabolism

Subject / Argument	Author	Frequencies	Notes	Origin	Target
Tetrahydrobiopterin Deficiency	EDTFL	60,7500,67500,95000,367350,376290,475050,665340,761850,987230	Rare metabolic disorder that increases blood levels of phenylalanine, causing problems ranging from low muscle tone to intellectual disability.	Amino Acid	Metabolism
Tyrosine Transaminase Deficiency	EDTFL	370,750,20500,23900,31500,141640,316500,431300,685670,739390	Disorder with metabolic error where the body cannot process the amino acid tyrosine.	Amino Acid	Metabolism
Tyrosinemias [Tyrosine disorder]	EDTFL	370,750,20500,23900,31500,139000,141640,415170,506000,637000,		Amino Acid	Metabolism
Fumarylacetoacetase Deficiency	EDTFL	130,230,900,8530,17500,72570,155290,396500,437480,828570	As mentioned above	Amino Acid	Metabolism
Multiple Carboxylase [Biotinidase Deficiency]	EDTFL	130,230,730,850,5250,137250,545760,687500,895270,976290,		Amino Acid	Metabolism
Cystinuria	EDTFL	100,230,680,830,190890,312400,452500,687500,795690,892500,	Genetic disorder causing cystine stones in kidneys, bladder, and ureters.	Amino Acid	Metabolism
Homocystinuria	EDTFL	30,120,960,13400,22500,50000,60000,93500,234110,475870,	Multisystemic, hereditary metabolic disease characterized by the deficiency of an enzyme involved in the metabolic pathway of the amino acid methionine.	Amino Acid	Metabolism
Cystathionine Deficiency Disease [Homocystinuria]	EDTFL	30,120,960,13400,22500,50000,60000,93500,234110,475870,		Amino Acid	Metabolism
Galactose-1-Phosphate U.T.D	EDTFL	120,200,900,47800,96500,275030,534250,691270,753070,927100			Metabolism
Galactosemias	EDTFL	180,550,910,5150,13980,137500,362500,697500,775000,922530	Rare genetic disorder affecting the ability to metabolize galactose, leading to serious liver, brain, kidney, ovarian, and systemic problems.	Genetic disorder	Metabolism
Galactokinase Deficiency	EDTFL	200,460,600,2250,12850,27500,42500,96500,236420,455230	As mentioned above	Genetic disorder	Metabolism
UDPglucose 4-Epimerase Deficiency Disease	EDTFL	310,750,23900,49000,96500,202590,522530,655200,750000,923700		Genetic disorder	Metabolism
UDPglucose-Hexose-1-Phosphate Uridylyltransferase Deficiency	EDTFL	310,750,23900,49000,96500,405750,523880,667500,825280,915700		Genetic disorder	Metabolism
Triosephosphate Isomerase Deficiency	EDTFL	240,750,950,95000,358570,475160,527000,667000,742000,987230	The deficiency of this enzyme causes a multisystemic disease characterized by hemolytic anemia and neurodegeneration.		Metabolism
Lesch-Nyhan Syndrome	EDTFL	100,570,950,7500,17500,37300,95540,225690,536420,689930	Congenital defect of purine metabolism. It is caused by the insufficiency of the hypoxanthine-guanine phosphoribosyltransferas enzyme.		Metabolism
Hypoxanthine-Phosphoribosyl-Transferase Deficiency Disease	EDTFL	20,240,850,39500,101320,221100,419340,562910,709830,976900	Also called juvenile gout. Hereditary disease of purine metabolism associated with an overproduction of uric acid.		Metabolism
Carbohydrate-Deficient Glycoprotein Syndrome	EDTFL	130,830,5230,17300,32120,71500,320300,434400,642910,983170	Now called Congenital Disorder of Glycosylation. Can cause serious organ system failure in infants.		Metabolism
Glycoprotein Syndrome	EDTFL	130,830,5230,17300,32119,71500,320300,434400,642910,983170,			Metabolism
Hyperphenylalaninemia, Non-Phenylketonuric	EDTFL	30,460,600,8850,72500,115780,324450,493500,723010,825790	As mentioned above		Metabolism
Trimethylaminuria	EDTFL	140,490,730,950,2500,7500,20000,136420,376290,458500	Also known as Fish Odor Syndrome. Metabolic disease that causes a defect in the normal production of the flavin monooxygenase enzyme.		Metabolism
Zellweger Syndrome	EDTFL	110,2500,32500,125000,275050,451170,515160,684810,712810,997870	Rare congenital disorder with reduction or absence of functional peroxisomes in cells. Also see Peroxisomal Disorders, Adrenoleukodystrophy, Leukodystrophy, Refsum Disease, and Lysosomal Storage Diseases.	Genetic disorder	Metabolism
Peroxisomal Disorders	EDTFL	170,290,7220,8600,132280,427300,555980,691000,874000,936440	Conditions caused by defects in peroxisome functions which may be due to defects in single enzymes.	Genetic disorder	Metabolism
Cerebrohepatorenal Syndrome	EDTFL	230,780,930,7500,10890,95900,322530,415700,563910,742060	Congenital disorder with multiple organ and system problems. Also called Zellweger Syndrome.	Genetic disorder	Metabolism
Hyperpipecolic Acidemia	EDTFL	490,730,800,2500,132600,347500,377650,597500,775950,925310,	Pain which starts and stops abruptly, usually due to contractions of tubular structure. Use Cramping and Nausea, and General Antiseptic programs.	Genetic disorder	Metabolism
Adrenoleukodystrophy [AMN]	EDTF	160,190,750,5160,30000,229320,323400,564280,714820,978050,	Fatty acid oxidation disorder.	Genetic disorder	Metabolism
Adrenomyeloneuropathy [AMN]	EDTF	160,190,750,5160,30000,229320,323400,564280,714820,978050,	As mentioned above	Genetic disorder	Metabolism
Schilder-Addison [Adrenoleukodystrophy]	EDTFL	160,190,750,5160,30000,229320,323400,564280,714820,978050,		Genetic disorder	Metabolism
X-Linked Adrenoleukodystrophy	EDTFL	160,190,750,5160,30000,229320,323400,564280,714820,978050,	As mentioned above	Genetic disorder	Metabolism
Refsum Disease	EDTFL	480,930,17000,38000,87000,96200,150000,433000,592000,850000	Genetic neurological condition caused by excessive phytanic acid in cells and tissues.	Genetic disorder	Metabolism
Heredopathia Atactica Polyneuritiformis	EDTFL	40,2860,5220,27400,45530,92220,202500,312430,353070,512300	As mentioned above	Genetic disorder	Metabolism

Subject / Argument	Author	Frequencies	Notes	Origin	Target
Phytanic Acid Storage Disease	EDTFL	170,240,1500,34850,62250,102750,232500,425540,725360,862710	As mentioned above	Genetic disorder	Metabolism

Lysosomal Storage Diseases or LSD: *are a large family of pathologies of genetic origin, having the characteristic of causing an accumulation of metabolites or substances in the lysosomes with consequent loss of cellular functionality.*

Subject / Argument	Author	Frequencies	Notes	Origin	Target
Lysosomal Storage Diseases	EDTFL	20,120,950,13390,22500,50000,93500,234110,322900,470210	Internal cell enzyme disorders disrupting metabolism. Also see Leukodystrophy Metachromatic.	Genetic disorder	Cell
Lysosomal Enzyme Disorders	EDTFL	20,120,950,13390,22500,50000,93500,234110,321800,470210		Genetic disorder	Cell
Angiokeratoma Corporis Diffusum	EDTFL	70,220,730,2700,5200,48000,475110,527000,667000,987230	Rare genetic lysosomal storage disorder with a wide range of systemic symptoms.	Genetic disorder	Cell
Anderson-Fabry Disease	EDTFL	100,500,700,2970,15870,37500,77500,157500,326500,722010,	As mentioned above	Genetic disorder	Cell
Arylsulfatase A Deficiency	EDTFL	140,550,820,7160,32500,35540,317560,376290,515700,689980	Lysosomal storage disease affecting the growth and development of myelin nerve sheath. See Lysosomal Storage Diseases.	Myelin	Cell
Leukodystrophy Metachromatic	EDTFL	70,220,620,2600,7500,41010,119340,475690,527000,665000	As mentioned above	Myelin	Cell
Mucolipidosis	EDTFL	20,240,950,2500,25780,172500,296500,475580,576290,772200	Genetic disorder affecting normal turnover of various materials within cells.	Genetic disorder	Cell
Cherry Red Spot Myoclonus Syndrome	EDTFL	130,490,600,870,2250,5260,113980,545870,735000,805070,	As mentioned above	Genetic disorder	Cell
I-Cell Disease	EDTFL	80,850,2500,43000,97230,175000,388000,791000,853000,972200	As mentioned above	Genetic disorder	Cell
Lipomucopolysaccharidosis	EDTFL	20,120,850,7500,32500,40000,60000,92500,150000,426900	As mentioned above	Genetic disorder	Cell
Sialidosis	EDTFL	180,300,45750,72500,92500,375190,477500,527000,662710,727050	As mentioned above	Genetic disorder	Cell
Pseudo-Hurler Polydystrophy	EDTFL	160,350,950,5500,27500,47500,357300,478500,527000,717000	As mentioned above	Genetic disorder	Cell
Mucopolysaccharidoses	EDTFL	50,320,730,3950,17510,125230,162520,275870,523520,671220	Metabolic disorders affecting ability to build bone, cartilage, tendons, corneas, skin, and connective tissue.	Genetic disorder	Cell
Hurler's Syndrome [Mucopolysaccharidoses]	EDTFL	50,320,730,3950,17510,125230,162520,275870,523520,671220,		Genetic disorder	Cell
Scheie Syndrome	EDTFL	240,700,5500,7500,10890,142500,372500,490000,825270,919340		Genetic disorder	Cell
Sanfilippo Syndrome	EDTFL	80,1350,17500,125300,145000,223060,307830,404630,522320,636550	Mucopolysaccharidosis 3	Genetic disorder	Cell
Cerebroside Sulphatase Deficiency Disease	EDTFL	190,260,570,7700,12690,35340,322060,425710,564280,930120	Disease which leads to an accumulation of cerebroside sulphate in the nervous system and other organs.	Genetic disorder	Cell
Diffuse Globoid Body Sclerosis	EDTFL	40,250,680,2250,10890,145220,329150,425910,657770,825220,	As mentioned above	Genetic disorder	Cell
Cystinosis [Lysosomal storage disease]	EDTFL	20,120,950,13390,22500,50000,93500,234110,322900,470210,	Genetic lysosomal storage disorder with abnormal amounts of cystine.	Genetic disorder	Cell
Neuronal Ceroid-Lipofuscinoses [lysosomal storage disease]	EDTFL	20,120,950,13390,22500,50000,93500,234110,322900,470210,	Multiple neurodegenerative disorders that result from excessive accumulation of lipopigments (lipofuscin) in tissues. Also see Lysosomal Storage Diseases.	Genetic disorder	Cell
Ceroid-Lipofuscinosis, Neuronal	EDTFL	50,240,840,950,2500,7500,32500,125370,319300,519340		Genetic disorder	Cell
Cerebroside Lipidosis [Gaucher]	EDTFL	90,520,710,930,2560,33180,215490,402530,592500,725370,	Genetic disorder with bruising, fatigue, anemia, low platelet count, and enlarged liver and spleen.	Genetic disorder	Cell
Glucocerebrosidase Deficiency	EDTFL	150,240,670,830,32500,197500,332500,555370,696500,875520	As mentioned above	Genetic disorder	Cell
Neuronopathic Gaucher Disease	EDTFL	90,520,710,930,2560,33180,215490,402530,592500,725370,		Genetic disorder	Cell
Pseudo-Gaucher Disease	EDTFL	90,520,710,930,2560,33180,215490,402530,592500,725370,	Genetic disorder in which glucocerebroside accumulates in cells and certain organs, with bruising, fatigue, anemia, low blood platelet count, and enlargement of liver and spleen.	Genetic disorder	Cell
Glucosylceramide Beta-Glucosidase Deficiency Disease	EDTFL	30,130,600,930,2250,217500,387500,475000,575520,726900		Genetic disorder	Cell
Galactosylceramidase Deficiency	EDTFL	130,250,620,2750,10890,25260,125370,245450,393500,505100	Diseases that have the characteristic of causing an accumulation of metabolites or substances in the lysosomes with consequent loss of cellular functionality.	Genetic disorder	Cell
Krabbe Disease [Lysosomal storage disease]	EDTFL	20,120,950,13390,22500,50000,93500,234110,322900,470210,	As mentioned above	Genetic disorder	Cell
Leukodystrophy, Globoid Cell	EDTFL	70,240,10570,37290,132810,313750,437500,520500,631940,771000	Also called Krabbe Disease. Rare demyelinating and nerve degenerating disorder.	Myelin	Cell

Subject / Argument	Author	Frequencies	Notes	Origin	Target
Niemann-Pick Diseases	EDTFL	100,570,800,7500,15400,52500,95110,655800,750000,923700	Group of severe genetic metabolic disorders that allow the fat sphingomyelin to accumulate in cells. Also see Lysosomal Storage Diseases.	Genetic disorder	Cell
alpha-Mannosidosis	EDTFL	750,7500,57500,122530,269710,479500,527000,667000,742000,986220,	Genetic enzymatic disease causing inability to process sugars.	Genetic disorder	Cell
Mannosidosis, alpha B, Lysosomal	EDTFL	100,410,880,5500,130000,255610,362000,492680,597500,654370	As mentioned above	Genetic disorder	Cell
Fucosidosis	EDTFL	120,580,38000,53770,202000,390610,502330,581260,638190,708920,	Rare genetic lysosomal storage disorder with accumulation of complex sugars in body parts, leading to multiple progressive dysfunctions.	Genetic disorder	Cell
Fucosidase Deficiency Disease [Fucosidosis]	EDTFL	120,580,38000,53770,202000,390610,502330,581260,638190,708920,	As mentioned above	Genetic disorder	Cell
Sandhoff Disease	EDTFL	40,2070,5520,9120,10380,22730,59330,95360,125540,233690	Rare lysosomal genetic lipid storage disorder with progressive nervous system destruction.	Genetic disorder	Cell
Hexosaminidase B Deficiency	EDTFL	550,950,291250,292000,293050,345500,434000,495250,734270,824370		Genetic disorder	Cell
Ganglioside Sialidase Deficiency [Lysosomal Disorder]	EDTFL	20,120,950,13390,22500,50000,93500,234110,322900,470210,	As mentioned above	Genetic disorder	Cell
Gangliosidosis G[M2], Type I [Lysosomal Disorder]	EDTFL	20,120,950,13390,22500,50000,93500,234110,322900,470210,	As mentioned above	Genetic disorder	Cell
Gangliosidosis G[M2], Type II [Lysosomal Disorder]	EDTFL	20,120,950,13390,22500,50000,93500,234110,322900,470210,	As mentioned above	Genetic disorder	Cell
Gangliosidosis, B Variant [Lysosomal Disorder]	EDTFL	20,120,950,13390,22500,50000,93500,234110,322900,470210,	As mentioned above	Genetic disorder	Cell
Glycogenosis	EDTFL	110,240,650,830,2500,27530,55370,87500,125520,322060	Genetic or acquired defects in processing of glycogen synthesis or breakdown in muscles, liver, and other cells.	Genetic disorder	Cell
Glycogen Storage Disease	EDTFL	50,270,950,950,2000,7500,32500,125370,319340,519340		Genetic disorder	Cell
McArdle Disease [Glycogen storage disease]	EDTFL	50,270,950,950,2000,7500,32500,125370,319340,519340,		Genetic disorder	Cell
Pompe's Disease	EDTFL	40,250,500,2700,13550,41000,175880,709840,842500,985900		Genetic disorder	Cell
Tay-Sachs Disease	EDTFL	70,500,1000,7300,17500,127500,335290,525140,705220,813670	Rare childhood genetic disorder with progressive deterioration of nerve cells and of mental and physical abilities.	Genetic disorder	Cell
Tay-Sachs Disease, B Variant	EDTFL	70,500,1000,7300,17500,127500,335290,475440,525140,527000		Genetic disorder	Cell
Wolman Disease	EDTFL	200,770,2570,3400,5590,95870,175910,343920,425870,571400,	Under-production of active lysosomal acid lipase (LAL) enzyme, with serious digestive problems, usually in infants.	Genetic disorder	Cell
Adenomatous Polyposis Coli (APC)	EDTFL	40,250,500,2400,322060,422530,561930,709830,842500,985900,	Protein encoded by APC gene, a tumor suppressor.		Protein
DNA and DNA Nucleotides + WBC RBC etc	ALT	528,731,732,537.8=300,543.4=300,545.6=300,550=300,637=600,999=300,1434=600,1524=600,2452=600,1056,2008,9999,	Repairs DNA and stimulates creation of red and white blood cells. DNA frequencies Solfeggio-based, so use with caution.		DNA
DNA Heal	XTRA	5333.69			DNA
DNA Integrity Stimulate	XTRA	528	Solfeggio Frequency.		DNA
DNA Repair	CAFL	528,731,732	Experimental. Contains Solfeggio frequency.		DNA
RNA Integrity Stimulate	XTRA	637			RNA
DNA Create New	XTRA	7	Used by Dr. Luc Montagnier for DNA replication in water		DNA
Chromosome 5p- Syndrome	EDTFL	180,190,620,42500,97500,175000,475190,527000,661710,742000	Rare genetic disorder with many problems and organ/system defects.	Genetic disorder	DNA
Cri-du-Chat Syndrome	EDTFL	70,380,850,900,5690,7250,30000,55540,93500,322060		Genetic disorder	DNA
Chromosome 16 Abnormalities	EDTFL	70,220,620,2400,7500,41010,119340,475630,527000,667000	Include Trisomy 16, FMF, Crohn's Disease, Thalassemia, PKD-1, Autism, Schizophrenia, ADHD, and Synesthesia.	Genetic disorder	DNA
Chromosome 17 Abnormalities	EDTFL	180,240,700,830,2500,17500,432500,555910,625290,775530		Genetic disorder	DNA
Chromosome 18 Abnormalities	EDTFL	130,570,870,10890,95190,300000,436420,563190,707260,978850		Genetic disorder	DNA
Chromosome 20 Abnormalities	EDTFL	200,460,17500,47500,95190,357300,452590,515270,683000,995380		Genetic disorder	DNA
Chromosome 22 Abnormalities	KHZ	120,230,970,15190,63770,86440,132800,302300,452500,825000,		Genetic disorder	DNA
Autosomal Chromosome	EDTFL	190,230,370,15190,63770,258230,326900,452500,833000,975750,		Genetic disorder	DNA
Chromosome Abnormality	EDTFL	130,250,730,42500,97500,377910,475270,527000,667000,749000		Genetic disorder	DNA

Subject / Argument	Author	Frequencies	Notes	Origin	Target
Chromosome Disorders	EDTFL	130,350,950,5500,27500,47500,352930,426900, 571000,846000		Genetic disorder	DNA
Genetic Chromosome Disorders Symptoms	EDTFL	130,350,950,5500,27500,47500,352930,426900, 571000,846000		Genetic disorder	DNA
Klinefelter Syndrome	EDTFL	150,420,18210,89100,115180,220050,375000,5 32510,615200,713870	Symptoms arising from presence of two or more X chromosomes in males, primarily sterility.	Genetic disorder	DNA
XXY Males XYY Karyotype [Jacobsen Syndrome]	EDTFL	60,490,9650,57500,219510,357590,370400,625 310,725870,871000,	Genetic condition where a male has one extra male chromosome, associated with increased early growth, slightly lower IQ, and learning difficulties.	Genetic disorder	DNA
Fragile X Syndrome	EDTF KHZ	900,920,32750,293700,329050,415830,423470, 472120,512140,629900	Genetic syndrome with intellectual disability and physical characteristics, mostly in males.	Genetic disorder	DNA
FRAXA Syndrome	EDTFL	80,550,570,7500,18000,121090,242090,360000, 596500,975430	As mentioned above	Genetic disorder	DNA
Martin-Bell Syndrome	EDTFL	20,240,900,9850,201750,364000,423010,69730 0,873930,979530	As mentioned above	Genetic disorder	DNA
Turner Syndrome	EDTFL	60,320,2250,32500,67500,96500,97500,150000, 682020,752630	Disorder where a female is partly or completely missing an X chromosome, leading to many physical, developmental, and reproductive problems.	Genetic disorder	DNA
Bonnevie-Ullrich Syndrome [Turner F]	EDTFL	60,320,2250,32500,67500,96500,97500,150000, 682020,752630,	As mentioned above	Genetic disorder	DNA
Gonadal Disorders Gonadal Dysgenesis, 45, X	EDTFL	30,370,950,2500,7500,72500,96500,269740,375 370,377910	As mentioned above	Genetic disorder	DNA
Gonadal Dysgenesis, XO [congenital reproductive disorder] O	EDTFL	30,370,950,2500,7500,72500,96500,269740,375 370,377910,	As mentioned above	Genetic disorder	DNA
Turner Syndrome [Male][Noonan Syndrome]	EDTFL	50,370,850,2500,7500,122530,328550,611210,7 15220,852930,	Congenital disorder with heart defects, short stature, learning and blood clotting problems.	Genetic disorder	DNA
Noonan Syndrome	EDTFL	50,370,850,2500,7500,122530,328550,611210,7 15220,852930	As mentioned above	Genetic disorder	DNA
Monosomy	EDTFL	200,460,750,8890,12780,57500,301600,617500, 747500,891350	Chromosomal abnormality with presence of just one chromosome from a pair.	Genetic disorder	DNA

2e - Rare, genetic and multisystem diseases

Subject / Argument	Author	Frequencies	Notes	Origin	Target
Aicardi Syndrome	EDTFL	780,8000,92500,125000,355080,452590,515160 ,687620,712810,997870	Genetic syndrome with partial or complete absence of corpus callosum and eye abnormalities.	Genetic disorder	Rare diseases
Arteriohepatic Dysplasia	EDTFL	170,520,620,850,20700,97500,155270,562500,7 53200,850000,	As mentioned above	Genetic disorder	Rare diseases
Aldrich Syndrome	EDTFL	200,770,2530,3400,5590,95870,175910,343920, 425870,571400,	Also called Wiskott-Aldrich Syndrome. Genetic disorder - skin, blood, and immune problems.	Genetic disorder	Rare diseases
Wiskott-Aldrich Syndrome	EDTFL	140,410,8000,30000,57540,125000,357770,689 980,750000,934250	As mentioned above	Genetic disorder	Rare diseases
Alexander Disease	EDTFL KHZ	140,780,2500,97500,357770,475050,527000,65 7110,749000,987230,	Genetic neurodegenerative disease.		Rare diseases
Alpha 1-Antitrypsin Deficiency	EDTFL KHZ	40,120,7500,40000,132410,342060,419340,560 000,642910,930120,	Genetic disorder of respiratory system.	Genetic disorder	Rare diseases
Alpers Syndrome	EDTFL	250,780,930,7500,10890,95900,321530,415700, 562910,742060	Mitochondrial DNA depletion syndrome		Rare diseases
Alport's Syndrome	EDTFL	30,370,700,780,5140,12690,32700,73500,39250 0,575560,	Genetic condition characterized by progressive loss of renal and auditory function. It can also affect the eyes.	Genetic disorder	Rare diseases
Alstrom Syndrome	EDTFL	70,370,950,7500,82000,193930,237500,487500, 706210,946500,	Rare multisystemic disease		Rare diseases
Anhidrotic Ectodermal Dysplasia	EDTFL	150,520,900,8500,12530,145880,262500,39750 0,633910,825170,	Group of genetic disorders manifesting in skin, sweat glands, teeth, hair, eyes and other craniofacial features.	Genetic disorder	Rare diseases
Ectodermal Defect, Congenital	EDTFL	70,520,700,930,337050,372500,375000,382850, 519340,791280	As mentioned above	Genetic disorder	Rare diseases
Ectodermal Dysplasia	EDTFL	110,550,800,23500,117500,252500,462500,596 500,797500,975340	As mentioned above	Genetic disorder	Rare diseases
Hidrotic Ectodermal Dysplasia [Clouston Syndrome]	EDTFL	130,400,620,900,5580,117290,442520,657510,7 22590,865870,		Genetic disorder	Rare diseases
Clouston's Syndrome	EDTFL	130,400,620,900,5580,117290,442520,657510,7 22590,865870	Also known as hydrotic ectodermal dysplasia, it is a rare genetic disease resulting in nail dystrophy, alopecia and palmar-plantar hyperkeratosis.	Genetic disorder	Rare diseases
Ankyloglossia	EDTFL KHZ	80,780,5810,67500,350000,475000,527000,665 340,742000,985670,	Also called Tongue-Tie. Congenital, due to a short frenulum.		Rare diseases
Antiphospholipid Syndrome	EDTFL	50,730,1550,13390,22500,247000,361150,5710 00,827000,937410,	Promotes thrombosis and pregnancy-related complications.		Rare diseases
Hughe's Syndrome [Antiphospholipid]	EDTFL	50,730,1550,13390,22500,247000,361150,5710 00,827000,937410,	As mentioned above		Rare diseases
Arnold-Chiari Malformation	EDTFL KHZ	60,830,2500,20000,65000,207460,479930,5270 00,749000,986220,	Brain condition with many symptoms, including tinnitus and numbness/tingling of extremities.		Rare diseases

Subject / Argument	Author	Frequencies	Notes	Origin	Target
Bannayan-Zonana Syndrome [Riley BZS]	EDTFL	60,260,900,9000,10890,45910,125290,526160,652480,750000,	Genetic disease with overgrowth of lipomas, hemangiomas, and head enlargement.	Genetic disorder	Rare diseases
Barth Syndrome	EDTFL KHZ	50,180,17500,45000,70000,125750,377910,475160,527000,753230,	Genetic disorder affecting multiple body systems, found only in males.	Genetic disorder	Rare diseases
Beckwith-Wiedemann Syndrome	EDTFL	550,900,290050,292000,293200,375500,414000,495220,730250,824300	Overgrowth disorder with increased risk of childhood cancer.		Rare diseases
Birt-Hogg-Dube Syndrome	EDTFL	80,350,500,600,2750,5500,50000,62500,90000,95670	Genetic disorder causing predisposition to kidney cancer, cysts, and fibrofolliculomas.	Genetic disorder	Rare diseases
Bloom Syndrome	EDTFL	70,520,30000,47500,150000,225160,357850,527000,663710,742000	Genetic condition with short stature and predisposition to cancer and genomic instability.	Genetic disorder	Rare diseases
BOR [Branchio-Oto-Renal]	EDTFL	170,410,620,850,2500,25000,109320,362570,621680,775670,	Genetic disorder with absent or insufficient renal function and ear malformations.	Genetic disorder	Rare diseases
Branchio-Oto-Renal Syndrome	EDTFL	170,410,620,850,2500,25000,109320,362570,621680,775670	As mentioned above	Genetic disorder	Rare diseases
Branchio-Otorenal Dysplasia	EDTFL	20,40,650,85710,90000,375110,496000,682000,750000,911400	As mentioned above	Genetic disorder	Rare diseases
Branchio-Oculo-Facial Syndrome	EDTFL	170,180,800,5500,17600,32500,151270,257440,413910,692270	As mentioned above	Genetic disorder	Rare diseases
Cat Eye Syndrome	EDTFL	70,120,900,20000,40000,134250,357770,510210,752630,923700	Genetic disorder causing lower GI, cardiac, kidney, skeletal, intellectual and other problems.	Genetic disorder	Rare diseases
CHARGE Syndrome	EDTFL	390,400,430,650,6870,7930,8330,8480,8630,8820	Genetic disorder with eye, ear, nose, heart, genito-urinary, and growth problems.	Genetic disorder	Rare diseases
Chediak-Higashi Syndrome	EDTFL	240,700,7500,72500,119340,324370,515700,682020,754190,941000	Genetic disorder with increased infection susceptibility, partial albinism, and peripheral neuropathy.	Genetic disorder	Rare diseases
Chondroectodermal Dysplasia	EDTFL	130,350,950,159220,243050,451170,515190,688290,712230,993410	Also called Ellis-van Creveld Syndrome. Genetic skeletal and cardiac disorder.	Genetic disorder	Rare diseases
Ellis-Van Creveld Syndrome	EDTFL	2080,4620,6870,8880,235000,323070,549330,627330,741120,803910	As mentioned above	Genetic disorder	Rare diseases
Congenital Abnormalities Congenital Defects Congenital Disorders	EDTFL	150,230,620,950,7500,212850,455950,557500,796500,891500	Structural or functional anomalies		Rare diseases
Deformities	EDTFL	70,210,700,7100,13520,45530,137500,572500,715400,903500,	Structural or functional anomalies		Rare diseases
Costello Syndrome	EDTFL	190,250,710,1150,2750,14530,32500,92300,356750,425580	Also called FCS Syndrome. Rare genetic disorder that affects many part of the body.	Genetic disorder	Rare diseases
Cushing Disease [Syndrome]	EDTFL	110,200,1710,12810,82500,112500,235950,657500,802500,925290,	Caused by prolonged exposure to cortisol, either from medications or due to a tumor.		Rare diseases
Cystic Fibrosis	CAFL	523,557,478,776,660,727,778,787,802,880,	Use Pseudomonas Aeruginosa, Breathing Deep, and General Antiseptic sets. See Parasites General, and Roundworm sets if no progress.	Genetic disorder	Rare diseases
Cystic Fibrosis	EDTFL	50,230,950,13390,121590,285430,325510,472500,612500,930000,	As mentioned above	Genetic disorder	Rare diseases
Cystic Fibrosis 2	XTRA	333,478,523,557,660,690,727.5,768,775,776,778,786,787,802,880,1550,	As mentioned above	Genetic disorder	Rare diseases
Cystic Fibrosis 3	XTRA	660,727,778,787,802,880,	As mentioned above	Genetic disorder	Rare diseases
Cystic Fibrosis Pseudomonas Aeruginosa	XTRA	174,178,191,405,482,633,731,785,1132,3965,5311,6646,16579.09,20703.13=1800,20812.5,	As mentioned above	Genetic disorder	Rare diseases
Mucoviscidosis [Pancreatic Fibrosis]	EDTFL	50,230,950,13390,121590,285430,325510,472500,612500,930000,	As mentioned above	Genetic disorder	Rare diseases
Mucoviscidosis	BIO	523	As mentioned above	Genetic disorder	Rare diseases
Mucoviscidosis	CAFL	478,523,557,660,727,776,778,787,802,880,	As mentioned above	Genetic disorder	Rare diseases
Brachmann-De Lange Syndrome	EDTFL	70,200,850,9500,98000,141200,297500,425950,675310,827000,	Genetic disorder with multiple physical, cognitive, and medical challenges.	Genetic disorder	Rare diseases
Cornelia De Lange Syndrome	EDTFL	1420,6990,57200,112500,201190,335310,402050,513230,809820,829230	As mentioned above		Rare diseases
De Lange Syndrome	EDTFL	70,200,850,9500,98000,141200,297500,425950,675310,827000,	As mentioned above		Rare diseases
DiGeorge Syndrome	EDTFL	220,780,930,7100,10890,95900,322530,415700,562910,747060	Genetic condition with multiple birth defects and disabilities.	Genetic disorder	Rare diseases
Distal Trisomy	EDTFL	50,410,620,2750,7500,40000,275650,475680,527000,667000	Genetic condition with slow postnatal growth and serious intellectual problems.	Genetic disorder	Rare diseases
Down Syndrome Palliative	CAFL	20			Rare diseases
Down Syndrome	XTRA	20,5000	Palliative.		Rare diseases
Mongolism (Symptoms only)	EDTFL	150,890,1700,6970,12890,62300,421000,468000,895000,951300			Rare diseases
Downs Syndrome (Symptoms only)	EDTFL	70,500,970,9000,12850,132800,337500,524370,758570,955720	Also see Down Syndrome sets.		Rare diseases

Subject / Argument	Author	Frequencies	Notes	Origin	Target
Albright's Syndrome	EDTFL	200,460,600,2250,12850,144900,323720,602530,726820,918280,	Genetic disorder of bones, skin pigmentation, and hormone problems with premature puberty.	Genetic disorder	Rare diseases
McCune-Albright Syndrome	EDTFL	70,240,780,12500,57500,112050,361280,367750,596500,888200	As mentioned above	Genetic disorder	Rare diseases
Fibrous Dysplasia, Polyostotic	EDTFL	850,900,980,17530,213260,321290,423690,597200,862500,915540	As mentioned above	Genetic disorder	Rare diseases
Freeman-Sheldon Syndrome	EDTFL	160,200,620,112600,230890,412500,615000,752500,802500,925520	Rare severe form of multiple congenital contracture (MCC) syndromes affecting eyes, ears, face, with slow hearing loss, walking difficulties, and Scoliosis (see set).		Rare diseases
Gulf War Syndrome 1	XTRA	136,253,255,392,435,533,578,633,639,714,771,837,866,975,1365,1370,2688,5419,6007,7755,	Chronic multisymptom disorder affecting military veterans and civilians in Gulf War.		Rare diseases
Goldenhar Syndrome	EDTFL	170,550,850,2190,20000,47300,72300,125170,379930,475190			Rare diseases
Oculoauriculovertebral Syndrome [Goldenhar]	EDTFL	170,550,850,2190,20000,47300,72300,125170,379930,475190,	Rare congenital defect with incomplete development of ear, nose, soft palate, lip, and mandible, and organ problems.		Rare diseases
Neurohepatic Degeneration	EDTFL	140,540,730,13610,125290,255560,372580,551230,673290,713720		Genetic disorder	Rare diseases
Hermanski-Pudlak Syndrome	EDTFL	150,180,870,5290,27500,45560,65290,95220,182500,233450	It is a rare autosomal recessive disease that leads to oculocutaneous albinism, bleeding problems and hemorrhages due to changes in platelet function		Rare diseases
Hirudo Med.	VEGA	128	Medical leech whose saliva contains anticoagulant.		Rare diseases
Miosis, Innervational Defect	EDTFL	110,490,14730,82500,217500,344020,671520,753280,871020,975870	Symptoms appearing when the sympathetic trunk nerve group is damaged, mostly ocular.		Rare diseases
Oculosympathetic Syndrome {Horner}	EDTFL	240,730,830,7800,30000,57500,95870,97500,424960,562910,	As mentioned above		Rare diseases
Giant Platelet Syndrome	EDTFL	150,890,12400,77000,134200,235870,312500,420350,465300,872900	As mentioned above		Rare diseases
Horner Syndrome Horner's Syndrome	EDTFL	240,730,830,7800,30000,57500,95870,97500,424960,562910	As mentioned above		Rare diseases
Bernard-Soulier Syndrome	EDTFL	60,490,680,7300,102500,231700,472500,625690,705800,857200	As mentioned above		Rare diseases
Ivemark Syndrome	EDTFL	20,40,650,85740,90000,375110,496000,682000,750000,911200	Uncommon congenital heterotaxy syndrome with defects in heart, spleen, and paired organs.		Rare diseases
Jacobsen Syndrome	EDTFL	60,490,9650,57500,219510,357590,370400,625310,725870,871000	Rare congenital disorder with intellectual disabilities, facial/skeletal and heart defects, and a variety of other problems.		Rare diseases
Hyperimmunoglobulin E-Recurrent [Skin Staph. Infections]	EDTFL	140,300,950,178720,375170,477500,527000,667000,761850,988900,	Group of genetic immune disorders with recurrent staphylococcal and severe lung infections as well as facial, dental, and skeletal abnormalities.	Genetic disorder	Rare diseases
Job's Syndrome	EDTFL	130,230,620,970,7500,12060,152500,293900,315620,496010	As mentioned above	Genetic disorder	Rare diseases
Kallmann Syndrome	EDTFL	110,240,570,38830,222720,317600,431200,572500,695670,905620	Genetic condition with failure to start or complete puberty, leading to Hypogonadism and Infertility - see sets. The sense of smell is also altered.	Genetic disorder	Rare diseases
Klippel-Trenaunay-Webe	EDTFL	130,410,650,970,7500,10470,95540,323010,328250,426900	Rare congenital condition where blood and/or lymph vessels fail to properly form.		Rare diseases
Klippel-Trenaunay Disease	EDTFL	130,410,650,970,7500,10470,398450,401000,404650,419000			Rare diseases
Trichorhinophalangeal Type II	EDTFL	130,550,850,72420,125750,375130,477400,527000,667000,752700	Rare genetic disorder caused by deletion of chromosomal material, associated with mild/moderate learning difficulties.	Genetic disorder	Rare diseases
Langer-Giedion Syndrome	EDTFL	150,220,630,7280,11030,32130,232500,355690,430000,855080	As mentioned above	Genetic disorder	Rare diseases
Giedion-Langer Syndrome	EDTFL	70,410,730,850,7500,20000,57500,151000,225370,342060	As mentioned above	Genetic disorder	Rare diseases
Larsen Syndrome	EDTFL	120,230,830,5250,97000,128210,162200,338030,511940,631410	Congenital disorder with dislocation of large joints and facial abnormalities.		Rare diseases
Laurence-Moon Syndrome Laurence-Moon-Biedl	EDTFL	30,500,870,7500,13520,27500,35000,125690,297500,437500	Rare genetic disorder with retinitis pigmentosa, extra digits, spastic paraplegia, hypogonadism, and mental retardation.	Genetic disorder	Rare diseases
Bardet-Biedel Syndrome	EDTFL	310,500,680,860,35250,164270,204190,325690,521290,662520,	As mentioned above		Rare diseases
Melorheostosis	EDTFL	160,350,930,2500,130000,355650,419340,651100,723030,868430	Developmental disorder and mesenchymal dysplasia in which the bony cortex widens and becomes very dense.		Rare diseases
Mucous Membrane General Inflammation	CAFL	380	See Leukoplakia, Mouth Eruptions white patches, EBV, BX virus, Papilloma, Cancer BX virus, and Carcinoma sets.	Mouth	Rare diseases
Osteo-Onychodysplasia	EDTFL	140,300,830,7500,128000,202430,340000,450000,575370,719370	Genetic disorder with poorly developed nails and kneecaps. Can also affect other areas of body, such as elbows, chest, and hips.	Genetic disorder	Rare diseases
Pelvic Horn Syndrome [Congestion]	EDTFL	80,400,830,5470,105000,357300,424390,561930,642910,930120,	As mentioned above	Genetic disorder	Rare diseases

Subject / Argument	Author	Frequencies	Notes	Origin	Target
Nail-Patella Syndrome	EDTFL	180,540,2620,6820,29830,58710,347700,58948 0,701200,812000	As mentioned above	Genetic disorder	Rare diseases
Osterreicher Syndrome [Patella Hypoplasia]	EDTFL	180,540,2620,6820,29830,58710,347700,58948 0,701200,812000,	As mentioned above	Genetic disorder	Rare diseases
Ochoa Syndrome	EDTFL	150,220,630,58450,215500,327850,442010,617 300,869710,975390	Congenital condition with urinary obstructive problems and inverted facial expressions - smiling looks like crying. Related to Hydronephrosis - see set.		Rare diseases
Cerebrooculorenal Syndrome	EDTFL	90,120,900,15170,96500,225000,425160,57100 0,841000,937410	Rare genetic disorder with congenital Cataracts, Hypotonia and areflexia, intellectual disability, proximal tubular Acidosis, aminoaciduria, phosphaturia, and proteinuria - see appropriate sets.	Genetic disorder	Rare diseases
Oculocerebrorenal Syndrome	EDTFL	70,320,950,5500,47500,434030,527000,667000, 752700,988900		Genetic disorder	Rare diseases
Lowe Syndrome [Oculocerebrorenal]	EDTFL	70,320,950,5500,47500,434030,527000,667000, 752700,988900,	As mentioned above	Genetic disorder	Rare diseases
Pallister-Killian Syndrome	EDTFL	80,490,680,6350,11980,17900,70100,214600,45 5900,518799,	Very rare genetic disorder with developmental disability, epilepsy, hypotonia, both hypopigmentation and hyperpigmentation, and other symptoms.	Genetic disorder	Rare diseases
Peutz-Jeghers Syndrome	EDTFL	40,320,700,840,5780,32500,181910,621690,705 540,815700	Genetic disease with benign hamartomatous polyps in GI tract and hyperpigmented macules on lips and oral mucosa (Melanosis - see set).	Genetic disorder	Rare diseases
Poland Syndrome	EDTFL	50,350,750,930,5710,7500,345830,465340,5934 00,725000	Rare birth defect with underdevelopment or absence of chest muscle on one side of body, and also usually webbed fingers.		Rare diseases
Progeria Progeria, Adult	EDTFL	60,120,710,39030,135550,253790,316500,5231 10,604220,625790	Rare genetic disorder in which symptoms resembling aging manifest at a very early age.	Genetic disorder	Rare diseases
Hutchinson-Gilford Syndrome	EDTFL	40,320,570,850,30250,173210,301800,402850,4 10700,475470	As mentioned above	Genetic disorder	Rare diseases
Werner Syndrome	EDTFL	180,240,700,1930,112750,217600,435270,6575 00,895000,925270	As mentioned above	Genetic disorder	Rare diseases
Proteus Syndrome [Wiedemann]	EDTFL	550,900,290050,292000,293200,375500,414000 ,495220,730250,824300,	Rare congenital disorder causing skin overgrowth and atypical bone development, often accompanied by tumors over half the body.		Rare diseases
Rhabdomyolysis	EDTFL	70,460,650,900,71220,110630,321000,637090,8 05800,972200	Condition where damaged skeletal striated muscle breaks down rapidly, which can lead to kidney failure. Caused by trauma, strenuous exercise, and statin or fibrate drugs.		Rare diseases
Robinow Syndrome	EDTFL	120,570,950,5580,20000,145790,262500,39350 0,734540,919340	Very rare genetic disorder with short-limbed dwarfism, abnormalities in head, face, and external genitalia, and vertebral segmentation.	Genetic disorder	Rare diseases
Royer Syndrome [hyperbilirubinemia]	EDTFL	150,180,800,5500,33200,172300,471200,55785 0,603440,921880,	Also called Prader-Willi Syndrome. Rare genetic disorder with low muscle tone, short stature, incomplete sexual development, cognitive disabilities, behavior problems, and chronic insatiable hunger.	Genetic disorder	Rare diseases
Prader Willi Syndrome (Symptoms)	EDTFL	130,350,950,5500,27500,47500,352930,426900, 571000,846000	As mentioned above	Genetic disorder	Rare diseases
Rubinstein-Taybi Syndrome	EDTFL	180,410,5670,10090,22120,98180,122310,2240 70,355900,451110	Genetic condition with short stature, learning difficulties, distinctive facial features, and broad thumbs and first toes.	Genetic disorder	Rare diseases
Russell Silver Syndrome	EDTFL	150,230,650,930,7500,11090,52500,172510,383 500,516510	Type of dwarfism.		Rare diseases
SAPHO Syndrome	EDTFL	30,250,2780,37930,115710,237500,495000,734 250,852560,915350	Autoinflammatory disease, characterized by the association between skin neutrophil involvement and chronic osteomyelitis		Rare diseases
Schnitzler Syndrome	EDTFL	570,680,880,2500,5710,32500,92500,322530,51 9340,653690	Rare disease with chronic Hives/Urticaria (see sets) and periodic fever, bone pain and joint pain/inflammation, weight loss, malaise, fatigue, swollen lymph glands, and enlarged spleen and liver.		Rare diseases
Septo-Optic Dysplasia	EDTFL	60,260,650,5150,7500,42500,92500,475950,527 000,661720	Rare congenital malformation syndrome with underdevelopment of optic nerve, pituitary gland dysfunction, and absence of septum pellucidum (part of brain). Also see Schizencephaly.		Rare diseases
Sick Building Syndrome	EDTFL	70,8000,13980,42500,97200,325170,515700,65 0000,750000,927100	Condition where occupants experience acute health and comfort effects that appear linked to time spent in a building, but no illness or cause can be identified.		Rare diseases
Situs Inversus	EDTFL	20,770,2500,3000,92500,357300,425170,57100 0,845000,937410	Congenital condition where major visceral organs are reversed or mirrored from their normal positions.		Rare diseases
Smith-Magenis Syndrome	EDTFL	40,410,620,2790,7500,40000,275650,475680,52 7000,667000	Developmental disorder affecting body and brain, including intellectual disability, broad face, difficulty sleeping, and various behavioral problems.		Rare diseases
Stickler Syndrome	EDTFL	170,420,18410,89100,115180,220050,375000,5 32510,615200,713870	Genetic disorders affecting connective tissue, specifically collagen, with distinctive facial abnormalities, eye problems, hearing loss, and joint problems.	Genetic disorder	Rare diseases
Neuroretinoangiomatosis	EDTFL	70,460,470,620,2730,132280,265000,533630,65 7770,834250	Rare congenital neurological and skin disorder, with port-wine stains of face, glaucoma, seizures, mental retardation, and cerebral malformations and tumors.		Rare diseases
Thanatophoric Dysplasia	EDTFL	30,240,840,2500,5870,85000,96500,175870,357 770,452590	Severe skeletal disorder with extremely short limbs with extra folds of skin, and small ribcage.		Rare diseases
Trichothiodystrophy [Brittle Hair]	EDTFL	20,450,650,2210,6150,10230,15940,30280,7750 0,327110,	Inherited disorders with brittle hair/nails, short stature, and intellectual impairment. Photosensitivity is also present in many cases.		Rare diseases

Subject / Argument	Author	Frequencies	Notes	Origin	Target
Usher Syndrome	EDTFL	20,460,680,970,2500,210500,500000,652430,75 9830,923700	Rare genetic disorder with gene mutation causing hearing loss and visual impairment.	Genetic disorder	Rare diseases
Uveomeningoencephalitic Syndrome	KHZ	150,930,5090,17500,35750,73300,125000,3750 90,830000,932000,	Multisystem disorder with Uveitis (see set), dysacousia, Leukodermia (see set), Alopecia (see set), canities (whitened hair), poliosis (whitened eyebrows and eyelashes), acute encephalitic signs, and meningeal symptoms.		Rare diseases
Uveomeningoencephalitic	EDTFL	40,400,680,5090,7500,35000,96500,177160,753 230,985670			Rare diseases
Uveomeningoencephalitis [Vogt]	EDTFL	40,260,460,7500,37500,57500,210250,328050,4 36420,561930,			Rare diseases
Vogt-Koyanagi-Harada	EDTFL	40,260,460,7500,37500,57500,210250,328050,4 36420,561930	As mentioned above		Rare diseases
Cerebelloretinal Angiomatosis	EDTFL	150,230,7900,13610,96500,175000,327950,682 450,753070,927100	Genetic disorder affecting vision, heart, and circulatory system, with possible brain and spine tumors.	Genetic disorder	Rare diseases
Lindau Disease [Von Hippel]	EDTFL	140,520,2500,12850,35160,97500,200000,4765 00,665340,986220,	As mentioned above	Genetic disorder	Rare diseases
Lindau Disease	EDTFL	50,490,620,950,10470,32710,317540,402800,69 2100,775090		Genetic disorder	Rare diseases
Waardenburg's Syndrome	EDTFL	140,350,820,6550,115280,347500,347500,5925 00,675910,775550	Rare genetic disorder with varying degrees of deafness, minor defects in neural crest structures, and pigmentation anomalies, sometimes with differently colored eyes.	Genetic disorder	Rare diseases
Klein-Waardenburg	EDTFL	300,1000,5500,13330,45000,234510,475160,52 7000,752300,987230,		Genetic disorder	Rare diseases
Elfin Facies Syndrome	EDTFL	20,240,680,870,2500,17500,197500,315700,328 550,419340	Rare neurodevelopmental disorder with heart defects, unusual facial features, and overt sociability.	Genetic disorder	Rare diseases
Contiguous Gene Syndrome, Williams	EDTFL	170,520,600,850,225530,327500,455950,76000 0,850000,969710	As mentioned above		Rare diseases
Williams Syndrome	EDTFL	30,520,570,800,10530,30000,72500,225330,425 160,571000	As mentioned above		Rare diseases
William-Beuren Syndrom	EDTFL	870,2500,7530,32500,97500,250000,328400,52 7000,789000,987230	As mentioned above		Rare diseases
Wolf-Hirschhorn Syndrome	EDTFL	160,550,950,7500,22500,42600,125220,275560, 533630,652430	Genetic disorder with distinct craniofacial features, heart defects, intellectual impairment, seizures, and growth restriction.	Genetic disorder	Rare diseases
Zadik–Barak–Levin syndrome	EDTFL	190,4200,22300,224200,395020,653210,715220 ,804820,837210,901240	Is a congenital disorder in humans. It is the result of an embryonic defect in the mesodermal-ectodermal midline development.	Genetic disorder	Rare diseases

3 - Respiratory System

3a - Nose

Subject / Argument	Author	Frequencies	Notes	Origin	Target
Nose	XTRA	10.3			Nose
Nose	BIOM	12; 74			Nose
Nose Diseases	EDTFL	60,180,970,5830,22000,47280,87220,97500,355 720,434000			Nose
Nasal Diseases	EDTFL	70,400,900,12850,20140,67110,135520,325000, 475540,612530			Nose
Nose Disorders	XTRA	20,440,727,787,880,			Nose
Respiratory passages, nose - Circulation and inflammation	BIOM	17.5; 20; 22.5; 99.5; 15.5; 70; 72.5; 75			Nose
Accessory sinuses of the nose	BIOM	2.5; 2.9; 57; 58			Nose
Accessory sinuses, fistula	BIOM	19; 98			Nose
Sinus trouble	BIOM	2.9; 53.5; 160; 440; 615; 618; 625; 650; 660; 741; 784; 802; 820; 942; 952; 1150; 1234; 1395; 1552; 1862			Nose
Frontal sinus	BIOM	74			Nose
Sinus Congestion	XTRA	1.8			Nose
Sinusitis	CAFL	952,741,682,320,160,	Inflammation of mucous membrane that lines paranasal sinuses. Also see Lung Sinus Bacteria, and Sinus Bacteria. Use Streptococcus Pneumoniae, and appropriate Sinusitis and Rhinitis sets.	Sinusitis	Nose
Sinusitis 1	CAFL	728,784,880,20,72,120,146,400,440,464,524,54 8,660,712,732,802,1500,1552,1600,1862,683,	As mentioned above	Sinusitis	Nose
Sinusitis 2	CAFL	125,160,367,472,600,615,625,650,820,952,1150 ,1520,1865,2000,4392,4400,4412,	As mentioned above	Sinusitis	Nose
Sinusitis 3	CAFL	60,95,128,225,414,427,432,456,610,614,618,12 34,2600,5500,304,	As mentioned above	Sinusitis	Nose
Sinusitis 4	CAFL	107,160,952,942,320,741,682,1395,	As mentioned above	Sinusitis	Nose
Sinusitis	EDTFL	130,400,57500,92500,175190,479920,527000,6 67000,742000,988900	As mentioned above	Sinusitis	Nose

Subject / Argument	Author	Frequencies	Notes	Origin	Target
Sinusitis	XTRA	72,120	As mentioned above	Sinusitis	Nose
Sinusitis	BIOM	1.7; 2; 2.5; 2.9; 3.6; 7.5; 9.19; 9.4; 10; 12; 26; 26.5; 50; 53.5; 57; 58; 68.5; 74; 79; 81; 96; 95.5		Sinusitis	Nose
Sinusitis, persistent	BIOM	10000; 7344; 5000; 2950; 2900; 2650; 2600; 1550; 1234; 880; 787; 740; 727; 330; 165; 82.6; 41.8; 30; 20.9		Sinusitis	Nose
Sinusitis (complex)	BIOM	5499.5; 4412; 4400; 4392; 2600; 2000; 1862; 1552; 1520; 1395; 1234; 1150; 952; 942; 732; 728; 712; 682; 614; 610; 600; 548; 524; 472; 456; 432; 427; 414; 400; 367; 304; 160		Sinusitis	Nose
Sinusitis Frontalis	CAFL	952,320,682	Inflammation of frontal sinuses located behind eyebrow ridges.	Sinusitis	Nose
Sinusitis Frontalis	BIO	952	Inflammation of frontal sinuses located behind eyebrow ridges.	Sinusitis	Nose
Frontal sinusitis	BIOM	952; 741; 682; 320; 160; 79; 74; 69; 58; 26; 19.5; 2.5		Sinusitis	Nose
Sinusitis Maxillaris	CAFL	160,741	Inflammation of maxillary sinuses located beneath eyes.	Sinusitis	Nose
Sinusitis Maxillariss	BIO	160	As mentioned above	Sinusitis	Nose
Sinus Bacteria	PROV	548	Use for running nose. See Lung sinus bacteria set. Use Streptococcus pneumoniae and the appropriate Sinusitis sets.	Sinusitis	Nose
Lung Sinus Bacteria	CAFL	244,1466,597,1311	Run after any Sinusitis set. See Chemtrail detox and Alternaria tenuis sets.	Sinusitis	Nose
Lung Sinus Bacteria	BIO	548	Use for running nose. See Lung sinus bacteria set. Use Streptococcus pneumoniae and the appropriate Sinusitis sets.	Sinusitis	Nose
Coryza Nose Disorder	XTRA	727,787,880,5000	Also called Rhinitis. Inflammation of nasal mucous membranes, causing runny nose.	Rhinitis	Nose
Coryza, Acute	EDTFL	370,430,620,970,7500,145830,262500,397500,6 33910,825170,		Rhinitis	Nose
Rhinitis, general	BIOM	10000; 5000; 2127; 2008; 1550; 1500; 880; 802; 787; 776; 727; 690; 666; 522; 465; 444; 440; 146; 120; 100; 20		Rhinitis	Nose
Rhinitis	CAFL	20,120,1550,802,1500,880,787,727,465,522,146	Runny nose. See Sinusitis, and Cold sets.	Rhinitis	Nose
Rhinitis	BIOM	2; 12; 26; 26.5; 66; 75.5; 94; 95.5		Rhinitis	Nose
Rhinitis	EDTFL	40,480,780,7500,118000,215430,362510,42206 0,608410,751200		Rhinitis	Nose
Vasomotor rhinitis	BIOM	2.5; 2.6; 2.9		Rhinitis	Nose
Coryza, Acute	EDTFL	370,430,620,970,7500,145830,262500,397500,6 33910,825170,		Rhinitis	Cold
Ozena	BIOM	184; 222; 439	It is a form of chronic rhinitis characterized by progressive atrophy of the nasal mucosa, which becomes thin and dysfunctional.	Rhinitis	Nose
Sinus Congestion	XTRA	1.8		Rhinitis	Nose
Nasal Catarrh	EDTFL	50,370,950,2750,7500,22500,47500,607500,834 560,911870		Rhinitis	Nose
Runny Nose (Rhinitis)	XTRA	5,189,912		Rhinitis	Nose
Allergic Rhinitis	EDTFL	40,480,780,7500,118000,215430,362510,42206 0,608410,751200,		Rhinitis	Nose
Rheum	CAFL	952,436,595,775	Watery discharge from nose or eyes.		Nose
Rheum	VEGA	952	As mentioned above		Nose
Rheum Special	XTRA	1744,952,333,376,436,595,775,	As mentioned above		Nose
Nasal defluviums	BIOM	1550; 802; 1500; 880; 787; 727; 465; 522; 146			Nose
Snoring	BIOM	28.5; 80.5; 83.5; 98.5			Nose
Rhinoscleroma	EDTFL	160,550,990,5710,13930,137500,262500,49750 0,626070,822530	Chronic granulomatous bacterial disease of nose that can sometimes infect the upper respiratory tract, usually due to subspecies of Klebsiella Pneumoniae - see sets.		Nose
Scleroma [Rhinoscleroma]	EDTFL	160,550,990,5710,13930,137500,262500,49750 0,626070,822530,	As mentioned above		Nose
Epistaxis [Nosebleeds]	EDTFL	140,570,730,7500,14500,327030,555910,66502 0,756720,875290,	Commonly called a nosebleed.		Nose
Ozaena	CAFL	184,222,439	Chronic inflammation of nose with atrophy of mucosa, glands, and nerves.		Nose
Anosmia Smell Sense Loss Of	CAFL	20,10000	Loss of sense of smell		Nose
Anosmia	EDTFL	110,490,570,5270,13390,20000,35520,60000,93 500,315700,	Derangement of sense of smell. Includes Anosmia, and Hyperosmia.		Nose
Olfaction Disorders [Hyposmia]	EDTFL	120,400,520,42700,57500,92500,177000,47517 0,527000,667000,			Nose
Smell Disorders	EDTFL	120,400,520,42700,57500,92500,177000,47517 0,527000,667000			Nose
Paraosmia [Smell Disorder]	EDTFL	120,400,520,42700,57500,92500,177000,47517 0,527000,667000,	Smell disorder in which one smell is misperceived or mistaken for another.		Nose

Subject / Argument	Author	Frequencies	Notes	Origin	Target
Hyperosmia	CAFL	20,10000,522,146	Overacute smell and taste		Nose
Hyperosmia	BIOM	522; 10000	As mentioned above		Nose
Hyperosmia	XTRA	727,787,800,880,10000,	As mentioned above		Nose
Hyperosmia	XTRA	20,146,522,812,10000,	As mentioned above		Nose
Polyp Nasal	CAFL	542,1436	Benign growth inside the nasal passage.		Nose
Nasal Polyp	VEGA	1436	As mentioned above		Nose

3b - Larynx - Trachea

Subject / Argument	Author	Frequencies	Notes	Origin	Target
Larynx	BIOM	13.5			Larynx
Larynx	CAFL	10,440,465,444,1550,880,802,787,727,28,7.69,3,1.2,250,9.6,9.39,			Larynx
Laryngeal Diseases	EDTFL	110,320,970,2600,11090,35780,137090,490210,822500,935220			Larynx
Laryngeal Perichondritis	EDTFL	110,320,970,2600,11090,7250,30000,55540,93500,322060			Larynx
Laryngitis	EDTFL	30,240,620,830,183390,315620,328530,691500,822540,923010	Can be caused by measles, mumps, varicella Zoster and candida or aspergillosis infections.	Laryngitis	Larynx
Laryngitis	XTRA	660,690,727.5,760,880,		Laryngitis	Larynx
Laryngitis, complex	BIOM	4192; 3552; 2720; 2489; 2154; 1800; 1600; 1550; 802; 885; 880; 875; 787; 776; 727; 46.5; 766; 222; 262; 73.5; 13.5			Larynx
Laryngomalacia	EDTFL	80,120,15330,85000,90000,357300,527000,657110,833700,987230	Condition where the larynx collapses during inhalation, causing airway obstruction. Most common in infancy.		Larynx
Laryngostenosis [Airway Disorder]	EDTFL	110,320,970,2600,11090,97500,434610,560000,840940,985900,	Narrowing or stricture of the larynx.		Larynx
Laryngeal Stenosis	EDTFL	110,320,970,2600,11090,97500,434610,560000,840940,985900			Larynx
Subglottic Stenosis	EDTFL	180,1070,4330,15250,58210,109420,326800,387020,434270,611050			Larynx
Larynx Infection	XTRA	1.19,3,7.69,7.7,9.39,9.4,9.59,10,28,230,250,440,444,465,660,690,727.5,787,802,880,1550,1865,2720,			Larynx
Laryngeal edema (Croup)	BIOM	728; 766; 787; 880; 1234; 5000; 7344			Larynx
Laryngeal Nerve Palsy [Vocal Cord Paralysis] Laryngeal Paralysis	EDTFL	50,730,2950,47500,222530,324530,452590,683000,712000,993410,			Larynx
Laryngeal Polyp	CAFL	202,765			Larynx
Trachea	BIOM	84			Trachea
Tracheitis	BIOM	9.5			Trachea
Tracheal Stenosis	EDTFL	180,220,55000,62500,132410,210500,475150,527000,667000,749000	Narrowing of airways, causing breathlessness, with many causes. See Breathing Difficulty (Dyspnea), and Dyspnea sets.		Trachea
Tracheoesophageal Fistula	EDTFL	180,240,10530,27500,35000,57500,96500,325110,475160,527000	Abnormal connection between trachea and esophagus.		Trachea

3c - Bronchi

Subject / Argument	Author	Frequencies	Notes	Origin	Target
Bronchopulmonary system	BIOM	0.9; 4; 8; 9.4; 9.44			Bronchi
Upper respiratory tracts	BIOM	9.4			Bronchi
Respiratory tracts - Pilot frequencies	BIOM	17.5; 20; 22.5; 99.5; 15.5; 70; 72.5; 75			Bronchi
Bronchi - Pilot frequencies	BIOM	32.5; 46; 76.5; 86; 92			Bronchi
Bronchial Diseases	EDTFL	20,460,5120,18800,85000,95710,150000,434710,682420,753090			Bronchi
Bronchitis	CAFL	7344,3672,1234,880,743,727,683,464,452,333,72,20,9.39,9.35,	Can be caused by Mycoplasma pneumoniae, Chlamydia pneumoniae and Bordetella pertussis.	Bronchitis	Bronchi
Bronchitis Bronchiolitis	EDTFL	20,460,5120,18800,85000,95710,150000,434710,682420,753090		Bronchitis	Bronchi
Bronchitis	BIOM	0.9; 2.5; 3.8; 4; 5.9; 6.5; 7.5; 7.7; 8; 9.4; 9.44; 11.5; 21.5; 32.5; 46; 65.5; 75; 76.5; 86; 89; 92; 98.5; 95.5		Bronchitis	Bronchi
Bronchitis 1	XTRA	9.34,9.39,727,880		Bronchitis	Bronchi
Bronchitis 2	XTRA	9.34,9.39,9.4,20,72,333,344,452,464,510,514,523,660,683,690,727.5,743,768,786,880,943,1234,3672,		Bronchitis	Bronchi
Bronchitis Secondary	XTRA	688,766,776		Bronchitis	Bronchi
Acute bronchitis (ARD)	BIOM	0.9; 4; 8; 9.4; 9.45; 46; 86			Bronchi
Bronchitis, chronic	BIOM	330; 340; 688; 766; 776; 1998			Bronchi

Subject / Argument	Author	Frequencies	Notes	Origin	Target
Bronchitis of virus-mycotic aetiology	BIOM	9.35; 9.39; 86; 452; 464; 684; 727; 743; 880; 1234; 3672; 7344			Bronchi
Bronchitis caused by acute respiratory viral infection	BIOM	0.9; 4; 8; 9.4; 9.45; 46; 86			Bronchi
Broncho Pulmonary Dysplasia	KHZ	40,230,950,7500,10890,55150,376290,534250,6 55200,904100,	Chronic lung disease of the newborn		Bronchi
Broncho Pneumonia Borinum	CAFL	452,550,578,727,776,787,802,880,1474,	See Pneumonia bronchial.	Broncho P.	Bronchi
Broncho Pneumonia Borinum	VEGA	452,1474		Broncho P.	Bronchi
Bronchial Pneumonia	CAFL	452,550,578,727,776,787,802,880,1474,	See Pneumonia bronchial.	Broncho P.	Bronchi
Bronchopneumonia	BIOM	452; 550; 578; 727; 776; 787; 880; 1474		Broncho P.	Bronchi
Bronchial Pneumonia 1	XTRA	452,550,578,727,776,787,802,880,1474,1550,		Broncho P.	Bronchi
Bronchial Pneumonia 2	XTRA	727,776,787,802,880,1550,		Broncho P.	Bronchi
Bronchial Pneumonia 3	XTRA	20,412,450,452,550,578,600,625,650,660,683,6 88,690,709.2,727.5,766,776,787,802,880,975,12 38,1474,1550,1862,2688,2838,		Broncho P.	Bronchi
Bronchiectasis	CAFL	342,510,778	Chronic dilatation of the bronchi.		Bronchi
Bronchiectasis	EDTFL	370,750,23900,45000,96500,202590,522530,64 5200,750000,923700	As mentioned above		Bronchi
Bronchiectasis	BIOM	342; 510; 778			Bronchi
Bronchiectasis	BIO	342	As mentioned above		Bronchi
Bronchiectasis	XTRA	342,344,510,778,943,	As mentioned above		Bronchi
Cryptogenic Pneumonia	EDTFL	20,220,920,7500,22500,85370,155470,285000,4 16500,605410,	Now called Bronchiolitis Obliterans Organizing Pneumonia. Non-infectious, with many possible causes.		Bronchi
Bronchospasm	BIOM	3.8; 5.9; 7.7; 9.4; 50; 55			Bronchi

3d - Lung and Respiratory Diseases

Subject / Argument	Author	Frequencies	Notes	Origin	Target
Lung General	CAFL	9,20,3672	See Chemtrail Detox, Nocardia Asteroides, and Alternaria Tenuis sets.		Lung
Lungs	BIOM	58.5; 59; 72			Lung
Lung	XTRA	9,3672			Lung
Lungs	XTRA	5.35,12			Lung
Lung General 1	XTRA	9,20,72,95,125,444,450,727,776,787,802,880,15 50,1865,			Lung
Lung General 2	XTRA	9,3672,			Lung
Lung General 3	XTRA	9,20,72,95,125,444,450,727,776,787,880,1550,1 865,			Lung
Lung General 4	XTRA	14160.15			Lung
Lung General 5	XTRA	220			Lung
Lung General Conditions	XTRA	20,72,95,125,444,450,590,660,690,727.5,776,78 7,802,880,1550,1800,1865,			Lung
Lung General Tonic	XTRA	307.89,318,568			Lung
Lung Breathing	XTRA	727,787,880	See Chemtrail detox sets.		Lung
Respiratory Diseases	XTRA	5,823,214		Respiratory	Lung
Croup	EDTFL	70,220,750,930,15090,24400,417500,505000,79 1500,995150,	Respiratory condition due to viral infection of upper airway.	Respiratory	Lung
Croup	XTRA	20,72,95,278,290,333,444,523,580,666,683,688, 712,728,766,776,786,870,880,960,1165,1234,15 50,3672,3702,7344,10000,	Respiratory condition due to viral infection of upper airway.	Respiratory	Lung
Respiratory Syndrome, Severe Acute	EDTFL	550,610,780,970,5870,57050,152030,524370,60 1270,781090	Also called SARS, or Sars. Also see Sars, and use Streptococcus Pneumoniae sets.	Respiratory	Lung
SARS (Preventative)	EDTFL	50,200,33400,72540,305370,443220,507000,62 1730,735000,900400		Respiratory	Lung
Respiratory Distress Syndrome, Newborn	EDTFL	40,550,780,970,5870,57050,152030,592500,602 530,953720	Syndrome in premature newborns due to structural immaturity in lungs, or to neonatal infection. Can also be genetic.	Respiratory	Lung
Respiratory Failure Acute	XTRA	1,257,814	Abnormal levels of oxygen or carbon dioxide in blood. Also see Anoxia, Hypoxia, Cyanosis, Circulation, and Circulatory sets.	Respiratory	Lung
Respiratory Hypersensitivity	EDTFL	40,550,780,970,5870,15750,232500,492500,826 070,925950		Respiratory	Lung
Asbestosis	EDTFL KHZ	40,970,7500,87500,175330,475160,527000,657 110,742000,985670,	Caused by inhalation and retention of asbestos fibres.	Asbestos	Lung
Asbestos in Lungs	PROV	5111,	See Asbestosis.	Asbestos	Lung
Berylliosis	EDTFL	230,950,12860,25050,97500,110250,322800,53 6420,650000,752630	Chronic lung disease due to beryllium exposure.	Beryllium	Lung

Subject / Argument	Author	Frequencies	Notes	Origin	Target
Beryllium Disease	EDTFL	230,950,12860,25050,97500,110250,322800,536420,650000,752630,	As mentioned above	Beryllium	Lung
Silicosis	EDTFL	200,250,650,2780,3000,7500,95500,326160,534250,652430	Lung disease caused by inhalation of crystalline silica dust, marked by inflammation and scarring with lesions in upper lobes of lungs.	Silicon	Lung
Lung Diseases	EDTFL	70,370,950,3520,28100,123980,407920,627280,736220,816610			Lung
Pulmonary Diseases	EDTFL	140,890,1920,5850,52200,135500,434500,525310,734250,878500	Disorders involving the respiratory tract.		Lung
Diffuse Parenchymal Lung	EDTFL	70,370,830,2500,3000,62500,195310,375000,575310,875690			Lung
Lung Abscess	CAFL	228,231,237,694,719,887,2890,	See Chemtrail Detox, Nocardia Asteroides, and Alternaria Tenuis sets.	Abscess	Lung
Lung Abscess	EDTFL	40,370,950,3520,28100,123980,342510,721200,823100,919340	As mentioned above	Abscess	Lung
Lung Abscess	BIOM	1.7; 86		Abscess	Lung
Lung Abscess 2	XTRA	228,231,237,694,719,747,887,2890,		Abscess	Lung
Lung Abscess 3	XTRA	880.2,17679.38,		Abscess	Lung
Atelectasis Pulmonary	EDTFL	50,730,950,5700,17500,37500,322060,563190,714820,930120,	Collapse of lung with alveoli deflation.		Lung
Atelectasis, Congestive	EDTFL	50,730,950,5000,17500,37500,322060,563190,714820,930120,	As mentioned above		Lung
Lung Collapse	EDTFL	40,370,950,3520,376290,452590,522390,687620,712420,995380	As mentioned above		Lung
Chronic obstructive pulmonary disease		*Includes both chronic bronchitis and emphysema; can be caused by Chlamydia pneumoniae and Epstein-Barr virus.*			
Pulmonary Disease, Chronic Obstructive	EDTFL	140,890,1920,5850,67100,135500,432500,525310,734250,878500		COPD	Lung
COPD (Chronic Obstructive Pulmonary Diease)	EDTFL	170,410,980,5800,28500,42500,161980,234070,396800,673980		COPD	Lung
COPD Chronic Obstructive Pulmonary Disease	XTRA	100	As mentioned above	COPD	Lung
Chronic Airflow Obstruction [Group 2]	EDTFL	40,370,570,850,2500,27500,52500,95750,375790,871000,	Also called Chronic Obstructive Pulmonary Disease (COPD) or Emphysema - see sets.	COPD	Lung
Chronic Obstructive Airway Disease - COAD	EDTFL	40,370,570,850,2500,27500,52500,95750,375790,871000,		COPD	Lung
Emphysema	CAFL	1234,3672,7344,880,787,727,120,20,80,	Also called Emphysema or COPD. Also see Chemtrails and Parasites.	Emphysema	Lung
Emphysema 2	XTRA	20,75.09,80,120,128,150.3,240,300.5,422,601,650,660,683,688,709.2,727,766,777,787,880,975,1234,2404.19,2688,2838.5,3672,7344,	As mentioned above	Emphysema	Lung
Pulmonary Emphysema	EDTFL	180,650,930,9500,17510,162810,292100,317300,433950,805190,	As mentioned above	Emphysema	Lung
Emphysema, complex	BIOM	7659.5; 7344; 3672; 2838.4; 2688; 2.2; 1234; 975; 880; 787; 777; 766; 727; 709.2; 688; 683; 660; 650; 601; 422; 300.5; 240; 150.3; 128; 120; 80; 75.1; 20		Emphysema	Lung
Lung Inflammation Pulmonary Inflammation	EDTFL	40,370,950,3520,11090,45000,62500,168300,335620,443160		Pneumonia	Lung
Experimental Lung Inflammation	EDTFL	110,550,47400,92500,375750,475160,527000,667000,752700,987230		Pneumonia	Lung
Pneumonia	CAFL	20,412,450,660,683,688,727,766,776,787,802,880,975,1238,1550,1862,2688,	See Pneumonia Klebsiella, Mycoplasma, Bronchial, Pneumocytis carnii, and Bronchial pneumonia sets. Always use Streptococcus pneumoniae set.	Pneumonia	Lung
Pneumonia	Rife	1200000,381901		Pneumonia	Lung
Pneumonia	XTRA	3414900	Hoyland MOR. Also use for Spinal Meningitis.	Pneumonia	Lung
Pneumonia	EDTFL	20,220,920,7500,22500,85370,155470,285000,416500,605410		Pneumonia	Lung
Pneumonia, Interstitial	EDTFL	20,220,920,7500,22500,85370,155470,285000,850000,919340	Lung conditions affecting the tissue and spaces around air sacs.	Pneumonia	Lung
Pneumonia General	CAFL	5000,2688,1862,1550,1238,975,880,802,787,780,778,776,774,772,770,768,766,727,688,683,660,450,412,20,	See Pneumonia Klebsiella, Mycoplasma, Bronchial, Pneumocytis carnii, and Bronchial pneumonia sets. Always use Streptococcus pneumoniae set.	Pneumonia	Lung
Pneumonia General V	CAFL	6007,5423,5421,5420,5419,2688,2581,2356,967,877,838,765,748,746,568,542,532,522,520,440,	As mentioned above	Pneumonia	Lung
Pneumonia General	BIOM	7659.5; 7344; 5000; 3702; 3672; 2688; 1862; 1550; 1238; 1234; 1200; 975; 880; 802; 787; 780; 778; 776; 774; 772; 770; 768; 766; 727; 688; 683; 660; 450; 412; 352; 20		Pneumonia	Lung

Subject / Argument	Author	Frequencies	Notes	Origin	Target
Pneumonia Bronchial	CAFL	550,802,880,787,776,727,452,1474,578,	Inflammation of the bronchii and lungs.	Pneumonia	Lung
Atypical pneumonia	BIOM	162; 499.25; 524; 47; 563; 597; 68; 648; 654.4; 689.14; 701.6; 720.36; 769.62; 778.12; 937.7; 998.5; 1001.86; 1048.94; 1143; 1556; 1559; 2286; 3735; 5235; 5513; 5763; 6157; 9563		Pneumonia	Lung
Pneumonia, Lobar	EDTFL	20,220,920,7500,22500,85370,357530,495340,533910,661200		Pneumonia	Lung
Pneumonia, postinfluenzal	BIOM	5548.6; 5449.2; 5554.7; 5554.8; 5558.8; 5560.8; 5562.5; 6654.7; 6752; 7118.2; 7255; 7284.1; 7414.3; 7631.1; 7632.7; 7667.4; 7676.4; 8045.8; 8082.6; 8911.3; 9113.5; 9141.5; 9393.1		Pneumonia	Lung
Pneumonia of mycotic aetiology	BIOM	780; 877; 986; 987; 988		Pneumonia	Lung
Pneumonia of bacterial aetiology	BIOM	20; 352; 542; 746; 768; 72; 774		Pneumonia	Lung
Pneumonia of virus aetiology	BIOM	520; 1200; 1238; 1862; 3672; 3702; 5419; 5420; 5423		Pneumonia	Lung
Pneumonia Klebsiella Pneumoniae	BIO	412,766	Bacterium causing acute bacterial pneumonia. See Tuberculosis Klebsiella set.	Pneumonia	Lung
Pneumonia Klebsiella	CAFL	412,413,746,765,766,776,779,783,818,840,	Causes an acute, bacterial pneumonia. See Tuberculosis Klebsiella.	Pneumonia	Lung
Pneumonia caused by Klebsiella	BIOM	412; 413; 746; 765; 766; 818; 840; 993.98; 1038.6		Pneumonia	Lung
Pneumonia Mycoplasma	BIO	688	Also called Walking Pneumonia - see Pneumonia Walking set, and also use Streptococcus Pneumoniae.	Pneumonia	Lung
Pneumonia caused by Mycoplasma	BIOM	660; 688; 709.2; 777; 688; 709.2; 975; 2688; 2838.5		Pneumonia	Lung
Pneumonia Walking	CAFL	660,688,777,975,2688,	Caused by Pneumonia Mycoplasma. Also use Streptococcus Pneumoniae.	Pneumonia	Lung
Pneumonitis	EDTFL	50,350,2750,30930,75810,187500,324510,715000,803510,905320	General inflammation of lung tissue, not of bacterial or viral origin.	Pneumonitis	Lung
Pneumonitis, Interstitial	EDTFL	50,350,750,930,5710,7500,345900,465340,593500,725000,		Pneumonitis	Lung
Pneumothorax [Collapsed Lung]	EDTFL	40,370,950,3520,376290,452590,522390,687620,712420,995380,	Abnormal accumulation of air or gas in pleural spaces. Also see Pleural Diseases.		Lung
Pulmonary Alveolar Proteinosis	EDTFL	80,2180,17930,71500,121800,217500,431690,615850,791520,923310	Rare lung disease in which abnormal accumulation of pulmonary surfactant occurs within the alveoli, interfering with gas exchange.		Lung
Pulmonary Atresia	EDTFL	220,750,850,10840,32500,62030,225540,410500,719340,865360,	Congenital malformation of pulmonary valve where the valve orifice fails to develop, obstructing outflow of blood from heart to lungs.		Lung
Pulmonary Valve Atresia	EDTFL	70,620,650,4970,7500,15310,322000,325930,759830,926700			Lung
Pulmonary heart disease	BIOM	318; 10; 568			Lung
Pulmonary Edema	EDTFL	130,520,900,8500,12530,145850,262500,397500,633910,825170,	Fluid accumulation in air spaces and parenchyma of lungs.	Edema	Lung
Wet Lung	EDTFL	90,330,5490,37000,203830,381430,481930,614820,763000,797230	As mentioned above	Edema	Lung
Pulmonary edema	BIOM	72.5		Edema	Lung
Pulmonary Embolism	EDTFL	20,400,900,20000,55000,92500,222700,475110,527000,987230,	Blockage of a pulmonary artery with accumulation of circulating solid material (embolus), usually a blood clot (thrombus) or, rarely, other material.	Embolism	Lung
Pulmonary Thromboembolism	EDTFL	20,400,900,20000,55000,92500,222700,475110,527000,987230,		Embolism	Lung
Pulmonary Fibrosis	CAFL	27.5,220,410	Respiratory disease in which scars are formed in the lung by connective tissues, leading to serious breathing problems. Use Parasites Roundworm sets. See Fibrosis of Lung, and General Antiseptic sets.	Fibrosis	Lung
Pulmonary Fibrosis [Lung]	EDTFL	50,230,950,13390,121590,285430,325510,472500,612500,930000,	As mentioned above	Fibrosis	Lung
Pulmonary Fibrosis	BIOM	7.5; 27.5; 220; 410			Lung
Alveolitis Fibrosing	EDTFL	410,620,630,4970,7500,15310,325930,385900,397800,504370	As mentioned above	Fibrosis	Lung
Besnier-Boeck [Lung Fibrosis]	EDTFL	50,230,950,13390,121590,285430,325510,472500,612500,930000,	As mentioned above	Sarcoidosis	Lung
Hamman-Rich Syndrome [acute interstitial pneumonia]	EDTFL	20,220,920,7500,22500,85370,155470,285000,850000,919340,	As mentioned above	Fibrosis	Lung

Subject / Argument	Author	Frequencies	Notes	Origin	Target
Pulmonary Sarcoidosis	EDTFL	120,550,940,5150,13980,137500,362500,697500,775000,922530,	Disease with abnormal inflammatory cells forming lumps (Granulomas - see set), usually starting in lungs, skin, or lymph nodes, sometimes eyes, liver, heart, or brain. Any organ can be affected. Also see Cancer Lymphogranuloma, and Lymphogranuloma.	Sarcoidosis	Lung
Eczema Vascular and Lung Disturbances	CAFL	9.39	Also called Dermatitis - see sets. Skin condition with itchy, weeping, crusting patches. Can also cause blood vessel and lung problems.	Eczema	Lung
Eczema Vascular and Lung	CAFL	9.19,727,787,1550		Eczema	Lung
Eczema Vascular and Lung	XTRA	9.18,9.39,727,787,1550,		Eczema	Lung
Ciliary Dyskinesia, Primary	EDTFL	140,250,850,5250,7260,325000,587500,745310,815900,927000,	Rare genetic disorder where respiratory cilia action is defective, causing poor mucus clearance and consequent lung infections.	Genetic disorder	Lung
Kartagener Triad	EDTFL	130,230,750,800,5250,7200,35000,95400,226320,422530	Genetic disease	Genetic disorder	Lung
Kartagener Syndrome	EDTFL	130,230,750,800,5250,175750,426300,571000,843000,937410	As mentioned above	Genetic disorder	Lung
Meconium Aspiration [Newborn Disorder]	EDTFL	40,240,950,3120,5820,178500,326500,571540,705870,827230,	Lung problems caused by inhalation during birth of fetal stool material in amniotic fluid.		Lung
Lung Infection	XTRA	10.3,10.5,11.8,11.9,12.09,12.4,		Infection	Lung
Lung Infection Gordona Sputi	XTRA	381.19,400.6,429.1,435.39,762.29,801.2,858.2,870.7,1524.7,1602.29,1716.4,3049,3204.59,3432.8,3483,17410.5	Gordonia Sputi (see set) is commonly hospital-acquired, usually from medical devices like catheters.	Infection	Lung
Lung Sinus Bacteria	CAFL	244,1466,597,1311	Run after any Sinusitis set. See Chemtrail detox and Alternaria tenuis sets.	Infection	Lung
Lung Sinus Bacteria	BIO	548	vedi sopra	Infection	Lung
Respiratory Tract Infections	EDTFL	70,550,650,870,7500,16020,42010,190000,675290,826900		Infection	Lung
Upper Respiratory Tract Infections	EDTFL	70,550,650,870,7500,16020,42010,190000,675290,826900,		Infection	Lung
Pneumovirus	CAFL	278,336,712	Causes Bronchiolitis and pneumonia in infants. See Respiratory Syncytial Virus, and Cryptogenic Organizing Pneumonia.	Virus	Lung
Respiratory Syncytial Virus			See Section 17d - Virus and Diseases	Virus	Lung
Pneumocystis	VEGA	340,742	As mentioned above	Fungus	Lung
Pneumocystis Carinii	BIOM	204; 340; 742		Fungus	Lung
Pneumocystis Carinii	HC	405750-409150=3600,	Fungally-induced pneumonia usually developing in the immunosuppressed presence of AIDS.	Fungus	Lung
Parasites: Pneumocystis carinii (lung)	EDTFL	680,900,2500,5500,13930,93500,428800,437000,441000,444150	As mentioned above	Fungus	Lung
Pleura	BIOM	31.5; 82.5; 84.5			Pleura
Empyema, Thoracic	EDTFL	50,530,1730,5940,85120,117150,443200,662230,814370,952000,	Accumulation of pus in pleural cavity, usually in Pneumonia.		Pleura
Empyema, Pleural	EDTFL	40,240,910,1000,12050,177710,234000,594000,683160,849340	Accumulation of pus in pleural cavity, usually in Pneumonia.		Pleura
Pyothorax	EDTFL	50,530,1730,5940,85120,117150,443200,662230,814370,952000			Pleura
Pleural Diseases	EDTFL	40,240,910,1000,12050,177710,234000,594000,683160,849340,	Disorders affecting the thin fluid-filled space between the two pulmonary pleurae (visceral and parietal) of each lung, including Pneumothorax (see set), Pleural Effusion (see sets), and pleural tumors.	Pleurisy	Pleura
Pleural Effusion	XTRA	787,474,612,361	Excess fluid accumulating in the pleural cavity.	Pleurisy	Pleura
Pleural Effusion [Lung Edema]	EDTFL	130,520,900,8500,12530,145850,262500,397500,633910,825170,	As mentioned above	Pleurisy	Pleura
Pleuritis, complex	BIOM	1550; 1466; 1311; 802; 880; 787; 776; 727; 244; 125; 95; 72; 444; 1865; 450; 5000		Pleurisy	Pleura
Pleurisy	CAFL	1550,802,880,787,776,727,125,95,72,20,444,1865,450,	Inflammation of the lung membrane and abdominal lining. Use Bronchitis, Streptococcus Pneumoniae, and General Antiseptic sets.	Pleurisy	Pleura
Pleurisy	EDTFL	40,240,910,1000,12050,177710,234000,594000,683160,849340	As mentioned above	Pleurisy	Pleura

3e - Breathing

Subject / Argument	Author	Frequencies	Notes	Origin	Target
Breathing	XTRA	10.3			Breathing
Center of breathing	BIOM	75			Breathing
Breathing	XTRA	727,787,880,5000			Breathing
Breathe Easier	XTRA	1234,3672,7344			Breathing
Breathing Deep	CAFL	1234,3702,3672,7344			Breathing
Breathing Difficulty (Dyspnea)	XTRA	100			Breathing
Respiratory Tract Disease	EDTFL	250,550,780,970,5870,57050,152030,651100,723030,868430		Infection	Breathing

Subject / Argument	Author	Frequencies	Notes	Origin	Target
Respiratiry Tract Inflammation 1	BIOM	52.75; 53.0; 53.5; 62.0; 62.5; 75.5; 85.0; 86.0			Breathing
Respiratiry Tract Inflammation 2	BIOM	**87.5; 90.0; 91.5**			Breathing
Congenital Central Hypoventilation Syndrome	EDTFL	130,5810,25000,87500,225000,458300,522390, 683000,712230,992000,			Breathing
Central Sleep Apnea	EDTFL	60,830,970,5160,20000,65000,476500,527000,7 42000,987230,	Suspension of external breathing during sleep.		Breathing
Sleep Disorder [Breathing]	EDTFL	40,550,780,970,5870,15750,232500,492500,826 070,925950,	Suspension of external breathing during sleep.		Breathing
Hypoventilation, Central Alveolar	EDTFL	130,5810,25000,87500,225000,458300,522390, 683000,712230,992000	As mentioned above		Breathing
Ondine Curse [Central hypoventilation syndrome]	EDTFL	130,5810,25000,87500,225000,458300,522390, 683000,712230,992000,	As mentioned above		Breathing
Dyspnea	XTRA	**100**	Shortness of breath or air hunger.		Breathing
Asphyxia	EDTFL KHZ	30,700,2500,5070,40000,72500,125000,275160, 829000,937410,	Severe deficiency of oxygen due to abnormal breathing.		Breathing
Hyperventilation	EDTFL	140,580,920,6250,25300,37500,62500,93500,15 0000,478500	Excessive and inappropriate removal of carbon dioxide from the body via the lungs.		Breathing
Bad Breath	CAFL	20,727,787,802,880,1550,	Use Halitosis set, and see Streptococcus pneumonia, aureus; Pharyngitis, dental; Parasites general, and General antiseptic sets.		Breathing
Asthma		*Can be caused by Rhinovirus, Human respiratory syncytial virus and the bacterium Chlamydia Pneumoniae.*			
Bronchial Asthma	CAFL	20,72,444,522,727,787,810,880,1233,1500,1600 ,1800,2170,2720,	Chronic inflammatory disease of airways - see Asthma sets.	Asthma	Breathing
Bronchial Asthma	EDTFL	40,370,570,850,2500,95750,150000,377300,534 200,871000,	As mentioned above	Asthma	Breathing
Asthma Bronchial	XTRA	**8,943,548**	As mentioned above	Asthma	Breathing
Bronchial asthma, basic	BIOM	3.8; 4; 5.9; 7.7; 8; 9.4; 9.44; 30.9	As mentioned above	Asthma	Breathing
Asthma Bronchial	BIOM	0.5; 0.9; 4; 8; 9.45; 4.7; 47; 82; 82.5; 128; 172; 322	As mentioned above	Asthma	Breathing
Bronchial Asthma 1	XTRA	0.5,20,72,95,125,146,444,522,727,787,880,1233 ,1234,1283,1500,1600,1800,2170,2720,3672,37 02,7344,	As mentioned above	Asthma	Breathing
Bronchial Asthma 3	XTRA	0.5,20,72,95,125,146,444,522,660,690,727.5,78 7,810,880,1233,1234,1283,1500,1600,1800,186 5,2170,2720,	As mentioned above	Asthma	Breathing
Bronchial Asthma 4	XTRA	0.5,20,72,95,125,146,444,522,	As mentioned above	Asthma	Breathing
Bronchial Asthma 5	XTRA	47,120,727,787,880,1234,3672,7346,10000,	As mentioned above	Asthma	Breathing
Bronchial Asthma 6	XTRA	128,172,263,322,411,434,487,515,521,633,665, 712,756,782,822,871,886,890,3124,3125,	As mentioned above	Asthma	Breathing
Asthma	CAFL	7344,3702,3672,2720,2170,1800,1600,1500,128 3,1234,1233,880,787,727,522,444,146,125,95,7 2,20,0.5,	See Liver Support, and Parasites Roundworm and Ascaris sets.	Asthma	Breathing
Asthma 1	CAFL	**1283,1233,4.7**	As mentioned above	Asthma	Breathing
Asthma 2	CAFL	1234,3672,7346,727,787,880,10000,47,120,	As mentioned above	Asthma	Breathing
Asthma V	CAFL	3125,3124,890,886,871,822,782,756,712,665,63 3,521,515,487,434,411,322,263,172,128,	As mentioned above	Asthma	Breathing
Asthma Specific	EDTFL	40,370,570,850,2500,95750,150000,377300,534 200,871000	As mentioned above	Asthma	Breathing
Asthma Bronchial	EDTFL	40,370,570,850,2500,27500,150000,387400,534 200,871000	As mentioned above	Asthma	Breathing
Asthma	BIO	**1233,1283**	As mentioned above	Asthma	Breathing
Asthma 1	XTRA	0.5,20,72,95,125,146,444,522,727,787,880,1233 ,1283,1500,1600,1800,2170,2720,	As mentioned above	Asthma	Breathing
Asthma 3	XTRA	0.5,20,72,95,125,146,444,522,660,690,727.5,78 7,810,880,1233,1234,1283,1500,1600,1800,186 5,2170,2720,	As mentioned above	Asthma	Breathing
Asthma 4	XTRA	4.7,1233,1234,1283,3672,7344,	As mentioned above	Asthma	Breathing
Asthma 5	XTRA	727,787,880,1500,1600,1800,2170,2720,	As mentioned above	Asthma	Breathing
Allergic asthma	BIOM	0.9; 1.75; 2.5; 2.9; 4.0; 8.0; 9.45; 82; 82.5		Asthma	Breathing
Bacterial-mycotic asthma	BIOM	2720; 2170; 1800; 1600; 1500; 1283; 1234; 880; 787; 727; 465		Asthma	Breathing
Neurogenic asthma	BIOM	**3.5; 3.6; 6.3**		Asthma	Breathing
Mixed ethiology asthma	BIOM	47; 120; 128; 172; 263; 322; 411; 434; 487; 515; 521; 633; 665; 712; 727; 756; 782; 787; 822; 871; 880; 886; 890; 1234; 3124; 3125; 3672; 7346; 10000		Asthma	Breathing

Subject / Argument	Author	Frequencies	Notes	Origin	Target
Asthmatic attack	BIOM	128; 172; 263; 322; 411; 444; 434; 487; 515; 521; 633; 665; 712; 756; 782; 822; 871; 886; 890; 3124; 3672		Asthma	Breathing
Allergies, Asthma RDPV3 Group 2 Asthma & Allergies Comprehensive	EDTFL	40,370,570,850,2500,27500,52500,95750,37579 0,871000,	Allergic asthma or allergy-induced asthma.	Asthma	Breathing
Samter's Syndrome	EDTFL	70,360,920,5120,13920,139300,303500,473320, 526770,600380	Condition where asthma is induced by aspirin or other NSAIDs. Also see Asthma and related sets.	Asthma	Breathing
Stridor	EDTFL	150,700,2500,5250,47500,70000,369750,38540 0,842000,932000	High-pitched breath sound resulting from turbulent air flow in the larynx or lower.		Breathing

3f - Colds Diseases

Subject / Argument	Author	Frequencies	Notes	Origin	Target
Rhinitis			See Section 3a - Nose	Nose	Cold
Sinusitis			See Section 3a - Nose	Nose	Cold
Catarrh	CAFL	1550,802,800,880,787,727,444,20,	Inflammation of mucous membranes causing thick mucus exudate.	Throat	Cold
Catarrh	Rife	1800000,1713100	As mentioned above	Throat	Cold
Catarrh 1	XTRA	20,380,444,660,690,727.5,787,800,802,880,155 0,1865,	As mentioned above	Throat	Cold
Catarrh 4	XTRA	175,13383.59,14062.5	As mentioned above	Throat	Cold
Rheum	CAFL	952,436,595,775	Watery discharge from nose or eyes.	Throat	Cold
Rheum Special	XTRA	1744,952,333,376,436,595,775,	As mentioned above	Throat	Cold
Cough	EDTFL	60,170,230,730,12030,13200,85520,150300,221 360,572820		Cough	Cold
Cough	XTRA	1234,514		Cough	Cold
Cough, dry	BIOM	1666.4; 2543.4; 3444.6; 3665.7; 4672		Cough	Cold
Coughing	CAFL	522,524,525,146,1500,1550,0.5,514,530,432,44 0,444,720,1234,3702,20,125,72,95,7.7,		Cough	Cold
Cough Lingering	XTRA	1666.34,2543.34,2444,55,3665.65,4664.44,		Cough	Cold
Cough, reflex	BIOM	75; 81		Cough	Cold
Cough with labored breathing	BIOM	7760; 7344; 3702; 3672; 1550; 1500; 123; 776; 766; 728; 720; 688; 683; 530; 525; 524; 522; 514; 444; 440; 432; 146; 125; 95; 72; 20; 7.7		Cough	Cold
Cold Coughing	CAFL	727,10000	See Coughing set.	Cough	Cold
Cough in case of catarrhal diseases	BIOM	7.7; 432; 440; 444; 522; 684; 688; 766; 959; 962; 1234; 1550; 1666; 3672; 3702; 7344		Cough	Cold
Cough, postvaccinal	BIOM	453; 514; 524; 525; 530; 674; 720; 728; 1089; 1109; 1234; 7760		Cough	Cold
Hemoptysis	EDTFL	50,460,3800,18890,175200,212970,321510,471 240,647060,815560	Coughing up blood.		Cold
Whooping Cough - Pertussis			See Bacteria Bordetella Pertussis		Cold
Sneezing	CAFL	880,787,727,465,146,			Cold
Hoarseness	CAFL	880,760,727			Cold
Head Cold	XTRA	72,120			Cold
Cold In Head Or Chest 1	CAFL	20,444,727,776,787,880,1550,5000,10000,			Cold
Cold In Head Or Chest 2	CAFL	20,333,444,727,766,776,787,802,880,1550,4412 ,7344,10000,			Cold
Cold Feet and Hands	CAFL	20,125,146,200,727,787,880,5000,			Cold
Perniosis	BIO	232,622,822,4211	A disorder of the blood vessels caused by prolonged exposure to cold. Also see Chilblains set.		Cold
Tonsillitis			See Section 12e - Throat		Cold
Fever			See Chapter 1 - Various conditions		Cold

3g - Cold

Subject / Argument	Author	Frequencies	Notes	Origin	Target
Cold 1	CAFL	5500,4400,802,787,727,720,552,440,400,125,72 ,800,880,			Cold
Cold 2	CAFL	652,725,746,751,768,1110,333,666,542,522,			Cold
Cold 3	CAFL	20,120,146,440,444,465,727,776,787,880,1500, 1550,5000,1000,	Fall '99.		Cold
Cold 4	CAFL	3176,2489,880=600,800=600,728,			Cold
Cold 5	CAFL	7728=600,4888=600,8238,2413,880,787,776,72 7,440,746,567,7880,787,300,310,1234,9999,			Cold
Cold 6	CAFL	352,412,450,660,683,688,727,766,768,770,772, 774,776,778,780,787,802,880,975,1200,1234,12 28,1550,1862,2400,2688,3672,3702,5000,7344, 7660,			Cold

Subject / Argument	Author	Frequencies	Notes	Origin	Target
Cold 1	BIOM	12.0; 12.5; 18.0			Cold
Common Col	EDTF	120,550,850,7500,120000,315500,472500,7257 50,850000,975980			Cold
Common Cold [GROUP 10]	EDTFL	120,550,850,7500,12500,77500,120000,307250, 320000,615000,			Cold
Cold and Flu	CAFL	250,465,8210,8700,7760,	Fall '98.		Cold
Cold and Flu	PROV	13916.02			Cold
Cold, [Cold and Flu] GROUP 10	EDTFL	120,550,860,7500,12500,77500,120000,307250, 320000,615000,			Cold
Cold and Flu Basic	XTRA	959,962,8700			Cold
Winter Vomiting [Cold/Flu]	EDTFL	150,260,5250,7000,37500,60000,119340,21050 0,458500,684810,			Cold

3h - Flu

Subject / Argument	Author	Frequencies	Notes	Origin	Target
Influenza	Rife	1674000,1946704			Flu
Influenza	CAFL	7766,7760,7344,5000,3672,2720,2050,2008,155 0,1500,1234,885,880,875,800,786,728,683,512, 464,440,304,20,	Mutates to new strains constantly but these may be helpful. Also see Flu and Grippe sets.		Flu
Grippe	BIO	343,500,512,541,862,1000,1192,3012,3423,102 23,	Influenza, flu.		Flu
Grippe	VEGA	343,512,862,3012,3423,10223,	Influenza, flu.		Flu
Grippe [Intestinal Flu]	EDTFL	120,200,900,47500,110250,322540,332410,684 810,712230,992000,			Flu
Influenza, General Parainfluenza Parainfluenza Virus Infections	EDTFL	40,320,700,850,5610,32500,60000,125230,2256 80,375610	Also see Flu and Influenza sets.		Flu
Flu	CAFL	20,727,787,880,1550,	Influenza mutates to new strains.		Flu
Flu 2	CAFL	20,304,440,464,727,728,787,800,885,1234,1500 ,1550,2008,3672,5000,7344,7760,			Flu
Flu Grippe Influenza	CAFL	727,787,800,880,			Flu
Influenza Grippe General	CAFL	343,500,512,541,862,1000,1192,3012,3423,102 23,			Flu
Human Flu Human Influenza	EDTFL	740,800,920,7630,32500,51500,90170,97500,12 4140,537620			Flu
Flu Virus	PROV	88,728,800,2050,2180,2452,7760,8000,8250,	Use with cold & flu.		Flu
Grippe Virus	CAFL	861	Influenza, flu.		Flu
Grippe Virus 3	CAFL	550,553	Influenza, flu.		Flu
Grippe Virus 4	CAFL	232,352	Influenza, flu.		Flu
Grippe Virus 5	CAFL	945	Influenza, flu.		Flu
Influenza Virus General	CAFL	728,800,880,7760,8000,8250,			Flu
Flu Triple Nosode	VEGA	421,632,1242,1422,1922,3122,			Flu
Influenza With Fever Virus	CAFL	332,341,425,461,469,482,513,523,742,753,763, 787,841,889,954,			Flu
Influenza Aches and Respiratory	CAFL	440,512,683,728,784,787,800,875,880,885,2050 ,2720,5000,7760=600,7766=600,304,			Flu
Influenza A	EDTFL	70,330,750,840,3700,8510,307590,314950,4050 70,517020			Flu
Influenza A	RL	366	From Dr. Richard Loyd.		Flu
Influenza Virus A	PROV	322,332,776			Flu
Influenza B	EDTFL	160,430,7000,13980,132410,275770,512330,65 0000,753070,926500			Flu
Influenza B	XTRA	250,10530,12500,40000,170000,313350,315000 ,323900,320000,615000,			Flu
Influenza Virus B 1	PROV	468,530,532,536,537,568,679,722,740,742,744, 746,748,750,1186,			Flu
Influenza Virus B 2	PROV	530,532,536,537			Flu
Influenza A and B_1	HC	313350-323900=3600,			Flu
Flu Virus A	VEGA	332			Flu
Flu Virus B	CAFL	530,532,536,537			Flu
Influenza V Grippe	CAFL	861			Flu
Influenza V2 Grippe	CAFL	324,652,653			Flu
Influenza V3 Grippe	CAFL	550,553			Flu
Influenza V4 Grippe	CAFL	232,352,2558			Flu
Influenza V5 Grippe	CAFL	518,945			Flu
Influenza Va2 Grippe	CAFL	334,472,496,728,833,836,922,			Flu

Subject / Argument	Author	Frequencies	Notes	Origin	Target
Grippe Va 2	CAFL	833	Influenza, flu.		Flu
Grippe Va 2 L	CAFL	447	Influenza, flu.		Flu
Influenza Grippe Vapch	CAFL	153,343			Flu
Influenza V75 Victoria	CAFL	316,343,1020			Flu
Spanish Flu	VEGA	462,787	Caused by H1N1 influenza virus - see H1N1 - Swine Flu set.		Flu
Influenza Virus British	CAFL	558,932			Flu
Flu Virus British	VEGA	932			Flu
Influenza Asian Grippe A	CAFL	516,656,434			Flu
Influenza 1957 A Asian	CAFL	768,574			Flu
Flu Virus B Hong Kong	CAFL	555			Flu
Influenza Virus A Port Chalmers	BIO	332			Flu
Influenza Virus A Port Chalmers	CAFL	622,863			Flu
Influenza Haemophilus	CAFL	542,552,885,959,734,633.1,2532.4,			Flu
Haemophilus Influenzae	HC	336410	Gram-negative bacterium causing Bacteremia, Pneumonia, Epiglottitis, Meningitis, Cellulitis, Osteomyelitis, and Arthritis - see sets.		Flu
Haemophilus Influenzae	EDTFL	30,470,17500,27500,40000,85160,95000,150000,210500,434170	As mentioned above		Flu
Haemophilus influenzae	BIOM	483; 542; 552; 633.1; 652; 731; 734; 746; 885; 942; 959; 2532.4			Flu
Haemophilus Influenzae 1	XTRA	832.86,833.87,21000,21025.63,	As mentioned above		Flu
Haemophilus Influenzae 2	XTRA	832.86,16728.45	As mentioned above		Flu
Haemophilus Influenzae 3	XTRA	542	As mentioned above		Flu
Haemophilus Influenzae B	XTRA	652,942	As mentioned above		Flu
Influenza Haemophilus Type B	CAFL	483,652,731,746,942,	Can cause a type of meningitis.		Flu
Avian Influenza	EDTFL	30,500,830,5710,79300,192500,467500,652200,802510,912560,	Bird flu.		Flu
Influenza, Avian H5N1	EDTFL	30,500,830,5710,79300,192500,467500,652200,802510,912560			Flu
H5N1- Bird Flu	EDTFL	30,500,830,5710,79300,192500,467500,652200,802510,912560,			Flu
Influenza Virus Swine	CAFL	413,432,663,839,995,			Flu
Swine infuenza	BIOM	2257; 488			Flu
Swine Flu 1	BIOM	725; 2432; 243; 6352.5; 732; 844; 646			Flu
Swine Flu 2	BIOM	725; 1229.9; 245; 314; 965			Flu
Swine Flu 3	BIOM	633; 1219.9; 6229.5; 8224.5; 111; 392; 776; 837; 1675; 2664; 3806; 714			Flu
Swine Flu 5	BIOM	83; 235; 645; 2323; 3432; 4093; 5531.5			Flu
Swine Flu 6	BIOM	702; 747; 2245; 183			Flu
Swine Flu [H1N1]	EDTFL	70,320,600,850,2250,225000,329570,527000,742000,987230,			Flu
Swine Flu	VEGA	432,839	As mentioned above		Flu
Influenza, SARS, Covid, etc.			See Section 17d - Virus and Diseases		Flu

4 - Cardiovascular System

Subject / Argument	Author	Frequencies	Notes	Origin	Target
Cardio-Vascular System Spasm	BIOM	3.8; 8.0; 9.44			

4a - Blood

Subject / Argument	Author	Frequencies	Notes	Origin	Target
Blood	XTRA	4.6,10.5			Blood
Blood Purify 1	CAFL	3.92		Detox	Blood
Blood Plasma Cleaner	CAFL	800		Detox	Blood
Blood Purification	XTRA	66.5	Use for all types of cancer.	Detox	Blood
Blood Cleanser	PROV	727,787,880,2008,2127,5000,	Use for all types of Cancer sets.	Detox	Blood
Blood Cleanser Cancer	XTRA	727,787,880,2008,2127,5000,10000,		Detox	Blood
Blood Supply Centre	BIOM	50			Blood
Red blood cells	BIOM	94.5			Blood
Blood Red Cell Production	XTRA	1524			Blood
Blood Hemoglobin Production	XTRA	2452	Improve blood oxygen transport ability.		Blood
Erythropenia	BIOM	94.5	Reduction in the number of red blood cells in the blood (anemia).		Blood
White blood cells	BIOM	84.5			Blood
Blood White Cell Production	XTRA	1434			Blood
White Blood Cell Stimulation	CAFL	432,1862,2008,2128,2180,2791,2855,2867,2929,3347,3448,4014,5611,	See Immune System Stimulation and Leukocytogenesis sets.		Blood
Lymphocytes Stimulate	XTRA	2791,2855,2867,2929,3347,3448,4014,5611,	Type of white blood cell including T cells, B cells, and natural killer cells. Use in immune stimulation.		Blood
Leukocytogenesis Stimulate	XTRA	30,727	Stimulate creation of white blood cells: basophils, eosinophils, lymphocytes, monocytes, neutrophils (vital for immune response). Also see Leukopenia, and other White Blood Cell sets.		Blood
Leukopoiesis	BIOM	0.6; 0.9; 1; 6			Blood
Leukopenia	EDTFL	180,550,850,2500,5500,27500,37500,123010,327250,533690	Low white blood cell count. Also use Leukocytogenesis Stimulate, and other White Blood Cell sets.		Blood
Leukopenia	BIOM	84.5			Blood
Leukocytopenia [Low White Blood Cells]	EDTFL	180,550,850,2500,5500,27500,37500,123010,327250,533690,			Blood
Erdheim-Chester Disease	EDTFL	190,1770,5320,7830,8970,10230,31500,76330,474720,694330	Abnormal multiplication of histiocyte white blood cells affecting bones and bone marrow.		Blood
Granulomatosis, Lipid	EDTFL	30,500,700,970,88000,370500,547500,656400,725370,825520	As mentioned above		Blood
Leucosis	BIO	612,633,653,3722,41224,	Proliferation of tissues that form white blood cells. Considered to be foundational stage of leukemia.		Blood
Leukocytosis	XTRA	612,633,644,653,3722,	White blood cell count above normal range, normally a sign of inflammation following infection, parasite infestation, or bone tumor.		Blood
Leukocytosis	BIOM	59.5			Blood
Lymphoproliferative Disorders	EDTFL	120,350,930,7500,17500,35000,87500,93500,224950,497610	Pathological condition in which lymphocytes are produced in excessive quantities.		Blood
Hypovolemic Shock	EDTFL	130,570,730,850,13930,45520,132020,255100,775610,813630	It is the shock caused by the acute decrease in circulating blood mass, caused by hemorrhage or fluid loss.		Blood
Blood Conduction	XTRA	3481	Blood conditions.		Blood
Bone Marrow	BIOM	9.0; 93.0			Blood
Bone Marrow Stimulation	BIOM	95.5; 96.5; 100.0			Blood
Blood Diseases	CAFL	880,787,727,5000			Blood
Blood Diseases	EDTFL	70,250,22500,42500,125000,324520,377910,650000,759830,926700			Blood
Blood Disorder	BIOM	5000.0; 727.0; 787.0; 880.0; 5000.0			Blood
Hematologic Diseases	EDTFL	30,370,970,2750,81500,172500,396500,475290,533630,876290	Disorders primarily affecting the blood.		Blood
Hematoma	BIOM	62.5; 65; 67.5; 96; 96.5			Blood
Hematoma-2	BIOM	9.1; 110.0; 727.0; 787.0; 880.0; 2720.0; 10000.0			Blood
Anemia	EDTFL KHZ	80,550,5970,23000,50500,80500,97530,210500,533210,909260,	Deficiency of red blood cells.	Anemia	Blood
Anemia	XTRA	5000	Deficiency of red blood cells.	Anemia	Blood
Anemia	BIOM	5000; 727; 787; 880; 5000		Anemia	Blood
Anemia Aplastic	KHZ	650,7500,2500,62500,150000,319340,425330,571000,823000,937410,	Damages bone marrow and blood stem cells. Can be caused by Hepatitis B and C, Dengue, Parvovirus B19, Epstein-Barr virus, cytomegalovirus and HIV.	Anemia	Blood

Subject / Argument	Author	Frequencies	Notes	Origin	Target
Addison's Anemia Anemia, Aplastic Anemia, Fanconi Anemia, Hemolytic Anemia, Hypoplastic Anemia, Iron-Deficiency Anemia, Microangiopathic Anemia, Pernicious Anemia, Sickle Cell	EDTFL	20,120,5160,62500,110250,332410,517500,684810,712230,992000,	Abnormal breakdown of red blood cells.	Anemia	Blood
Hemolytic Anemia	EDTFL	120,350,850,27500,141590,189590,467500,591290,619340,897090		Anemia	Blood
Hemolytic-Uremic Syndrome	EDTFL	90,350,850,27500,141590,189590,301270,453020,783800,825030,	Disease with hemolytic anemia, acute kidney failure, and low platelet count, usually in children. Also use E Coli and Shigella sets.	Anemia	Blood
Gasser's Syndrome [Hemolytic uremic]	EDTFL	90,350,850,27500,141590,189590,301270,453020,783800,825030,	As mentioned above	Anemia	Blood
Anemia Iron-Deficiency	KHZ	100,320,2500,57200,125000,175000,525710,682020,759830,932410,	Decreased red blood cells and hemoglobin due to insufficient iron.It can be caused by Helicobacter Pylori.	Anemia	Blood
Iron-Deficiency Anemia	EDTFL	40,200,650,85750,90000,322510,375110,689930,753070,983220		Anemia	Blood
Anemia Megaloblastic	EDTFL	110,5160,62500,110250,332410,475050,517500,527000,657110,753230,	Due to inhibition of DNA synthesis in red blood cell production.	Anemia	Blood
Thalassemia	EDTFL	80,320,650,7500,37500,67500,96500,527000,663710,986220	Genetic disorder with abnormal formation of hemoglobin. Also see Chromosome 16 Abnormalities.	Anemia	Blood
Cooley's Anemia	EDTFL	80,550,5970,23000,50500,80500,97530,210500,533210,909260,	As mentioned above	Anemia	Blood
Fanconi Anemia	EDTFL	120,570,1120,7400,27600,42500,96500,325430,415700,562910	Very rare genetic defect in proteins responsible for DNA repair.	Anemia	Blood
Pernicious Anemia	BIOM	232; 622; 822; 4211		Anemia	Blood
Refractory Anemia	CAFL	435,	Deficiency of red blood cells and hemoglobin which fails to respond to medical treatment.	Anemia	Blood
Hemochromatosis	EDTFL	110,580,730,2580,5780,145910,372520,428010,511190,605590	Also called Iron overload. May be hereditary, genetic, or due to repeated blood transfusions. Also see Hemosiderosis.	Iron	Blood
Hemochromatosis	XTRA	5000	As mentioned above	Iron	Blood
Diabetes, Bronze	EDTFL	150,890,1700,6970,12890,62300,421000,465000,895000,951300	Genetic disorder caused by an excess of iron in the body leading to damage to the pancreas which ultimately results in diabetes.	Iron	Blood
Hemosiderosis	EDTFL	40,550,780,162120,210500,453720,515190,683000,712230,993410	Form of Iron overload disorder resulting in accumulation of hemosiderin. Also see Hemochromatosis.	Iron	Blood
Hypercapnia	EDTFL	40,240,580,17500,86530,132750,342510,721200,823100,919340	Abnormally high blood levels of carbon dioxide. See appropriate Lung, Breathe, and Breathing sets.	Carbon dioxide	Blood
Hyperkalemia	EDTFL	460,950,11090,65230,115790,342500,431220,535580,603160,805790	Excess potasssium levels in the blood.	Potasssium	Blood
Hyperpotassemia	EDTFL	30,320,620,800,2500,7500,90000,317580,322060,524940	As mentioned above	Potasssium	Blood
Hypokalemia	EDTFL	190,300,520,2500,7500,8000,55230,150000,324600,325540	Low levels of potassium in the blood. See Minerals - Potassium, and Potassium k sets.	Potasssium	Blood
Hypopotassemia	EDTFL	130,240,730,870,2250,5780,30000,150000,175610,534250	As mentioned above	Potasssium	Blood
Hypercalcemia	KHZ	110,490,14730,82500,217500,344010,671520,753210,871020,975870,	Excess calcium in the blood. See appropriate Calcium sets, and Calcifications.	Calcium	Blood
Milk-Alkali Syndrome	EDTFL	120,650,25090,87500,125320,222530,479930,527000,667000,987230		Calcium	Blood
Hypocalcemia	EDTFL	120,510,950,5580,27330,145790,262500,393500,734510,919350	Low calcium levels in blood.	Calcium	Blood
Hypocupremia, Congenital	EDTFL	120,230,850,5500,22500,35580,73300,92500,352930,523010	Copper deficiency as a result of heredity.	Copper	Blood
Menkes Syndrome	EDTFL	40,230,2750,32050,107500,352500,393220,444950,525630,653740	As mentioned above	Copper	Blood
Hyponatremia	EDTFL	150,350,620,930,7500,115090,252500,472500,693510,825790	Low levels of sodium in blood.	Sodium	Blood
Uric acid	BIOM	95.5			Blood
Uric acid, excess	BIOM	74			Blood
Acidosis	CAFL	10000,880,802,787,776,727,146,20,	Increased acidity in blood and tissue. See Heartburn, Hernia, and Hyperacidity sets.	Acidosis	Blood
Acidosis	BIOM	10000; 880; 802; 787; 776; 727; 465; 146; 20		Acidosis	Blood
Acidosis	EDTFL	490,730,800,2500,132600,347500,377650,597500,775950,925310	As mentioned above	Acidosis	Blood
Alkalosis	EDTFL	50,750,2250,72500,110250,379930,424370,561930,642060,978050,	May be respiratory, metabolic, or combined.		Blood
Cyanosis	EDTFL	70,190,850,2500,3000,62500,95750,375290,633910,875000,	Bluish coloration of tissue due to low oxygen saturation. See Hypoxia, and Circulatory Stasis.		Blood

Subject / Argument	Author	Frequencies	Notes	Origin	Target
Cryoglobulinemia	EDTFL	60,170,730,830,2750,17500,195950,320720,491 000,769710,	Causes proteins in blood to clump and become insoluble at low temperature.		Blood
Diabetes 1		Can be caused by **Echovirus 4, Coxsackie B1** and **B4 virus** and **Human Parechovirus** infection.			
Diabetes 2		Can be caused by **Human Papiloma virus 6 and 11, Cytomegalovirus, Hepatitis C virus, Enteroviruses** and **Ljungan virus.**			
Diabetes 1	CAFL	5000=900,2127,2080,2050,2013,2008,2003,200 0,1850,880,803,800,787,727,660,484,465,440,3 5,20,6.8,	Warning: can cause large drop in blood sugar level.	Diabetes	Blood
Diabetes 2	CAFL	4200,2128,1865,1850,1550,787,465,444,125,95, 72,48,302,	Warning: can cause large drop in blood sugar level.	Diabetes	Blood
Diabetes	BIOM	19.9; 52; 92; 444; 465; 500; 800; 2003; 2008; 5000		Diabetes	Blood
Diabetes	BIOM	10000.0; 5000.0; 2720.0; 2170.0; 1800.0; 1550.0; 880.0; 802.0; 787.0; 727.0; 500.0; 465.0; 100.0; 35.0; 20.0		Diabetes	Blood
Diabetes 1-1	BIOM	5000; 2127; 2080; 2050; 2013; 2008; 2003; 2000; 1850; 880; 803; 800; 787; 727; 660; 484; 465; 440; 35; 20; 6.8		Diabetes	Blood
Diabetes 2-1	BIOM	4200; 2128; 1865; 1850; 1550; 787; 465; 444; 125; 95; 72; 48; 302		Diabetes	Blood
Diabetes 3-1	BIOM	5; 787; 10000; 20; 727; 787; 800; 880; 5000		Diabetes	Blood
Diabetes Secondary	CAFL	10000,2720,2170,1800,1550,880,802,727,465,2 0,	Warning: can cause large drop in blood sugar level.	Diabetes	Blood
Diabetes Tertiary	CAFL	1850,32000,4000,500	Warning: can cause large drop in blood sugar level.	Diabetes	Blood
Tertiary Diabetes	BIOM	1850; 4000; 500		Diabetes	Blood
Diabetes Type 1 [Alternate Set]	EDTFL	150,200,1700,6970,12890,62300,347510,47823 0,895000,951300,	Run for 1-2 hours per day.	Diabetes	Blood
Diabetes Type 2 [Alternate Set]	EDTFL	150,200,1700,6970,12890,62300,465000,65750 0,895000,951300,	Run for 1-2 hours per day.	Diabetes	Blood
Diabetes Type 3 [Alternate Set]	EDTFL	160,240,680,110970,202500,367000,420350,42 2300,792900,935310,	Run for 1-2 hours per day.	Diabetes	Blood
Diabetes Mellitus Type 1	EDTFL	150,200,1700,6970,12890,62300,429700,47823 0,895000,951300,		Diabetes	Blood
Diabetes Mellitus Type 2	EDTFL	150,200,1700,6970,12890,62300,429700,46500 0,895000,951300,		Diabetes	Blood
Diabetes Gestational	EDTFL	150,200,1700,6970,12890,62300,429700,47823 0,895000,951300,	Condition where women without diabetes exhibit high blood glucose levels during pregnancy.	Diabetes	Blood
Diabetes Hyperglycemia symptoms	EDTFL	20,150,180,200,240,440,520,540,640,750,	High blood glucose. Run for 1 hour.	Diabetes	Blood
Diabetes Insipidus	EDTFL	150,200,1700,6970,12890,62300,421000,46500 0,895000,951300,		Diabetes	Blood
Diabetes Insulin-Dependent	EDTFL	150,200,1700,6970,12890,62300,421000,46500 0,895000,951300,		Diabetes	Blood
Diabetes Juvenile-Onset	EDTFL	150,200,1700,6970,12890,62300,421000,46500 0,895000,951300,		Diabetes	Blood
Diabetes Kidney Disease	EDTFL	150,200,12700,77000,134500,235870,312500,4 20350,465300,872900,		Diabetes	Blood
Diabetes Maturity-Onset	EDTFL	150,200,1700,6970,12890,62300,429700,47823 0,895000,951300,		Diabetes	Blood
Maturity-Onset Diabetes Mellitus - MODY	EDTFL	150,890,1700,6970,12890,62300,421000,46500 0,895000,951300		Diabetes	Blood
Diabetes Mellitus, Slow-Onset	EDTFL	150,200,1700,6970,12890,62300,429700,47823 0,895000,951300,		Diabetes	Blood
Diabetes Mellitus, Stable	EDTFL	150,200,1700,6970,12890,62300,421000,46500 0,895000,951300,		Diabetes	Blood
Diabetes Mellitus, Sudden-Onset	EDTFL	150,200,1700,6970,12890,62300,421000,46500 0,895000,951300,		Diabetes	Blood
IDDM (Insulin Dependent Diabetes Mellitus)	EDTFL	340,600,7000,32500,67500,97500,325750,5193 40,691270,754190		Diabetes	Blood
Diabetes Non-Insulin-Dependent - NIDDM	EDTFL	150,200,1700,6970,12890,62300,429700,47823 0,895000,951300,		Diabetes	Blood
Insulin-independent diabetes	BIOM	3.3; 4; 7; 9.19; 9.44; 9.69; 11.5; 12.5; 23; 25.5; 26.5; 46; 52; 79.5; 85.5; 92; 94.5		Diabetes	Blood
Diabetes associated with infection	BIOM	19.9; 302; 786; 1550; 1850; 2013; 2020; 2050; 2080; 4000; 4200		Diabetes	Blood
Diabetes complicated with angiopathy	BIOM	10000; 5000; 2720; 2170; 2112; 1800; 1550; 880; 802; 787; 727; 500; 465; 100; 35; 20		Diabetes	Blood
Diabetes, Autoimmune	EDTFL	150,890,1700,6970,12890,62300,421000,46500 0,895000,951300,		Diabetes	Blood

Subject / Argument	Author	Frequencies	Notes	Origin	Target
Constitutional Diabetes	BIOM	700; 35		Diabetes	Blood
Diabetic Amyotrophy	EDTFL	150,890,1700,6970,12890,62300,421000,465000,895000,951300,		Diabetes	Blood
Diabetic Autonomic Neuropathy	EDTFL	150,890,1700,6970,12890,62300,429700,478230,895000,951300,		Diabetes	Blood
Diabetic Neuralgia	EDTFL	150,890,1700,6970,12890,62300,429700,478230,895000,951300,		Diabetes	Blood
Diabetic Neuropathies	EDTFL	150,890,1700,6970,12890,62300,421000,465000,895000,951300,		Diabetes	Blood
Diabetic Neuropathies	KHZ	160,410,770,8930,32250,43010,112520,212500,647500,802590,	Nerve-damaging disorders associated with Diabetes.	Diabetes	Blood
Diabetic Neuropathy	XTRA	73	As mentioned above	Diabetes	Blood
Diabetic Polyneuropathy	EDTFL	150,890,1700,6970,12890,62300,421000,465000,895000,951300,		Diabetes	Blood
Diabetic polyneuropathy	BIOM	1250; 932.5; 880; 833; 787; 776; 727; 650; 625; 600; 565.5; 470; 464; 393.5; 304; 222; 194; 125; 110; 90.88; 72; 57.5; 47.5; 40; 35; 33; 2		Diabetes	Blood
Diabetic [Chronic Fatigue & Obesity]	EDTFL	50,120,600,3870,72250,125430,387500,525910,712500,825440,	Associated with Type 2. Run for 1-2 hours per day.	Diabetes	Blood
Diabetic Eye Disease] [Retyne™ Light mat]	EDTFL	150,890,1700,6970,12890,62300,421000,465000,895000,951300,	Use Retyne™ Light mat	Diabetes	Blood
Diabetic Retinopathy [Eye Disease] [Retyne™ Light mat]	EDTFL	150,890,1700,6970,12890,62300,421000,465000,895000,951300,	Use Retyne™ Light mat	Diabetes	Blood
Diabetes, Bronze	EDTFL	150,890,1700,6970,12890,62300,421000,465000,895000,951300,	Genetic disorder caused by an excess of iron in the body leading to damage to the pancreas which ultimately results in diabetes.	Diabetes	Blood
Diabetic Acidosis	EDTFL	150,890,1700,6970,12890,62300,421000,465000,895000,951300,		Diabetes	Blood
Diabetic Ketoacidosis	EDTFL	150,890,1700,6970,12890,62300,429700,478230,895000,951300,		Diabetes	Blood
Diabetes Ketosis-Prone	EDTFL	150,200,1700,6970,12890,62300,421000,465000,895000,951300,		Diabetes	Blood
Diabetes Ketosis-Resistant	EDTFL	150,200,1700,6970,12890,62300,421000,465000,895000,951300,		Diabetes	Blood
Ketosis, Diabetic	EDTFL	150,200,1700,6970,12890,62300,421000,465000,895000,951300,		Diabetes	Blood
Diabetes Associated Infection	CAFL	2020,800,727,786,190,80,20,		Diabetes	Blood
Children Diabetes	XTRA	5023		Diabetes	Blood
Diabetic Loading	CAFL	35,700		Diabetes	Blood
Diabetic Foot Infection	XTRA	48,72,95,125,304,444,465,787,802,1865,2000=900,		Diabetes	Blood
Diabetic foot; ulcer	BIOM	2489; 2160; 2127; 1800; 1600; 1050; 880; 832; 802; 787; 727; 73; 1.2		Diabetes	Blood
Diabetic adiposity	BIOM	35; 700; 787; 5000; 10000; 2720; 2160; 1800; 1550; 880; 802; 727; 465; 700		Diabetes	Blood
DIDMOAD [Wolfram Syndrome]	EDTFL	60,490,570,2500,7500,30000,225750,320540,419340,561930,	Rare genetic disorder, causing Diabetes Mellitus (see sets), optic atrophy, and Deafness (see related sets) as well as various other symptoms.	Diabetes	Blood
Wolfram Syndrome	EDTFL	60,490,570,2500,7500,30000,225750,320540,419340,561930	As mentioned above	Diabetes	Blood
High Blood Sugar	XTRA	324=240,528=240,15=240,1.2,250,6.79,9.39,9.4,15,20,35,40,48,72,95,125,240,302,440,465,484,500,522,600,625,650,700,787,800,802,1550,803,880,440,444,1865,428,1000,1550,1800,1850,1865,2000,2003,2008,2013,2050,2080,2127.5,2170,2720=360,4000,4200,5000=900,10000,	See Hyperglycemia sets.	Glycemia	Blood
Hyperglycemia	XTRA	324=240,528=240,15=240,1.19,250,6.79,9.39,9.4,15,20,35,40,48,72,95,125,340,302,440,465,484,500,522,600,625,650,700,787,800,802,1550,803,880,440,444,1865,428,1000,1550,1800,1850,1865,2000,2003,2008,2013,2050,2080,2127.5,2170,2720,4000,4200,5000=900,10000,	See High Blood Sugar set.	Glycemia	Blood
Hyperglycemic Hyperosmolar Nonketotic Coma	EDTFL	230,450,850,7500,47500,72510,93500,126330,275560,528530,	Serious complication that can arise when diabetes is not being properly controlled.	Glycemia	Blood
Coma, Hyperglycemic/molar Nonketotic	EDTFL	230,450,850,7500,47500,72510,93500,126330,275560,528530,		Glycemia	Blood

Subject / Argument	Author	Frequencies	Notes	Origin	Target
Low Blood Sugar	XTRA	1.19,3,10,20,26,72,95,125,230,250,444,465,600,625,650,660,690,727.5,776,787,802,832,880,1500,1550,1600,1800,1865,2008,2127.5,2127,2489,2720,	See Hypoglycemia sets.	Glycemia	Blood
Hypoglycemia	EDTFL	160,540,850,5450,32500,125790,270000,492500,658570,824940	See Low Blood Sugar set.	Glycemia	Blood
Hypoglycemia	XTRA	1.19,3,10,20,26,72,95,125,230,250,444,465,600,625,650,660,690,727.5,776,787,802,832,880,1500,1550,1600,1800,1865,2008,2127.5,2170,2489,2720,	See Low Blood Sugar set.	Glycemia	Blood
Hypoglycaemia- cf1	BIOM	25; 26; 26.5; 27.5; 30; 47.5; 50; 52		Glycemia	Blood
Hypoglycaemia- cf2	BIOM	2; 6; 52.5; 52.75; 53; 53.5; 56; 62.5		Glycemia	Blood
Hypoglycaemia- cf3	BIOM	64.5; 65; 67.5; 74.5; 79; 85; 87; 87.5		Glycemia	Blood
Hypoglycaemia- cf4	BIOM	90; 91.5; 94; 94.5; 96; 97.5; 98; 99.5		Glycemia	Blood
Insulin, lack	BIOM	52; 92		Insulin	Blood
Adenoma Beta-Cell	XTRA	40,320,700,870,5250,32500,60000,125680,225650,275680,	Also called congenital hyperinsulinism. Causes Hypoglycemia - see sets.	Insulin	Blood
Insulin, excess	BIOM	97.5		Insulin	Blood
Hyperinsulinism [Pre Diabetes 2]	EDTFL	150,200,1700,6970,12890,62300,429700,465000,895000,951300,	Excess insulin levels in the blood.	Insulin	Blood
Hyperinsulinism	XTRA	1.19,3,10,20,26,72,95,125,230,250,444,465,600,625,650,660,690,727.5,776,787,802,832,880,1500,1550,1600,1800,1865,2008,2127.5,2127,2489,2720,	Excess insulin levels in the blood.	Insulin	Blood
Dyslipidemias	EDTFL	170,900,5250,27500,57500,222530,425130,571000,838000,937410	Abnormal amounts of lipids in the blood.	Lipids	Blood
Dyslipoproteinemias	EDTFL	230,970,5830,7250,17500,67500,234250,522530,655200,751870	As mentioned above	Lipids	Blood
Hyperlipidemia, Familial	EDTFL	60,120,850,7500,32500,40000,133630,226320,475580,527000	Genetic disorder with abnormally high levels of lipids and lipoproteins in the blood.	Lipids	Blood
Hyperlipidemia [Lipoprotein]	EDTFL	60,120,850,7500,32500,40000,133630,226320,475580,527000,	As mentioned above	Lipids	Blood
Atheroembolism [Cholesterol Embolism]	EDTFL	40,230,850,5750,20000,125190,350000,450000,775170,927000,	Usually caused by atherosclerotic plaque break-up.	Lipids	Blood
Embolism, Cholesterol	EDTFL	40,230,850,5750,20000,125190,350000,450000,775170,927000,		Cholesterol	Blood
Cholesterol-2	BIOM	2.0; 4.0; 4.9; 25.5; 26.0; 32.0; 34.5; 35.5		Cholesterol	Blood
Cholesterol-3	BIOM	1386.0; 173.0; 620.0; 635.0; 780.0		Cholesterol	Blood
Hypercholesterolemia	EDTFL	80,260,780,2500,17500,255870,362540,453020,775910,925580	High levels of cholesterol in the blood.	Cholesterol	Blood
Hypercholesterolemia	BIOM	25.5; 26		Cholesterol	Blood
Hypercholesterin-lipidemia	BIOM	4; 20; 25.5; 26; 173; 620; 635; 780; 1386		Cholesterol	Blood
Analphalipoproteinemia	EDTFL	120,410,8200,17700,87500,95750,323850,476500,527000,662710,	Rare inherited disorder with severe reduction in HDL (good cholesterol) in blood.	Cholesterol	Blood
Tangier Disease	EDTFL	120,690,2500,10530,92500,355720,479930,527000,761850,987230	As mentioned above	Cholesterol	Blood
Tangier Disease Neuropathy	EDTFL	120,650,2500,10580,92500,355720,479930,527000,761850,987230		Cholesterol	Blood
Smith-Lemli-Opitz [Development Disorder]	EDTFL	30,180,930,940,7500,13520,95000,322590,454370,517500,	Inborn error of cholesterol synthesis causing multiple physical malformations.	Cholesterol	Blood
RSH Syndrome [Smith-Lemli-Opitz]	EDTFL	30,180,930,940,7500,13520,95000,322590,454370,517500,	As mentioned above	Cholesterol	Blood
Haemophilia	BIO	845	Hereditary bleeding disorder in which the blood does not readily clot.	Haemophilia	Blood
Hemophilia 1	XTRA	603,751,778,845	Hereditary blood clotting disorder.	Haemophilia	Blood
Hemophilia 2	CAFL	603	As mentioned above	Haemophilia	Blood
Hemophilia	EDTFL	80,410,1890,145560,297250,315290,407500,562530,735680,854380	As mentioned above	Haemophilia	Blood
Hemophilia	BIOM	603; 751; 778; 845		Haemophilia	Blood
Hemophilia A	EDTFL	190,230,3050,62500,297250,315290,407500,562530,735680,854380	As mentioned above	Haemophilia	Blood
Hemophilia B	EDTFL	20,120,3050,62500,297250,315290,407500,562530,735680,854380	As mentioned above	Haemophilia	Blood
Hemophilia C	EDTFL	50,180,4820,65000,297250,315290,407500,562530,735680,854380	As mentioned above	Haemophilia	Blood
Hemophilia [Vascular]	EDTFL	80,410,1890,145560,162500,219110,328100,562530,735680,833910,	As mentioned above	Haemophilia	Blood
Haemophilia Tonic	XTRA	751,778,845	As mentioned above	Haemophilia	Blood

Subject / Argument	Author	Frequencies	Notes	Origin	Target
Factor V [Protein] Deficiency [Coagulation]	EDTFL	600,870,2260,5170,93500,475160,485000,5270 00,697500,856720,		Haemophilia	Blood
Factor VII Deficiency [Coagulation]	EDTFL	80,320,610,2270,44250,115710,245480,486000, 697500,856720,		Haemophilia	Blood
Factor IX Deficiency [Clotting, Coagulation]	EDTFL	100,830,5000,45110,93500,475160,527000,650 000,759830,926700,		Haemophilia	Blood
Christmas Disease [Hemophilia B]	EDTFL	20,120,3050,62500,297250,315290,407500,562 530,735680,854380,		Haemophilia	Blood
PTA Deficiency	EDTFL	70,240,30650,78520,197250,267000,321950,60 2210,733630,925000		Haemophilia	Blood
Rosenthal Syndrome	EDTFL	90,320,950,3110,25000,45000,95000,100500,21 5790,414000	Relatively common but mild form of Haemophilia - see sets.	Haemophilia	Blood
Platelet Storage Pool Deficiency	EDTFL	50,260,960,2200,12850,35340,57500,96500,322 060,475870	Blood coagulation disorder.	Coagulation	Blood
Storage Pool Deficiency	EDTFL	130,630,950,5750,8200,26410,307450,471990,7 39000,936220	As mentioned above	Coagulation	Blood
Parahemophilia [Owrens Disease]	EDTFL	600,870,2260,5170,93500,475160,485000,5270 00,697500,856720,	Coagulation system protein deficiency leading to predisposition for hemorrhage.	Coagulation	Blood
Owren Disease [Factor V Deficiency]	EDTFL	600,870,2260,5170,93500,475160,485000,5270 00,697500,856720,		Coagulation	Blood
Hypoproconvertinemia	EDTFL	40,220,950,5580,17500,25680,42500,60000,952 30,125680		Coagulation	Blood
Hageman Trait	EDTFL	190,230,950,2250,112500,227500,252200,3225 00,421000,826320		Coagulation	Blood
Factor VIII Deficiency [Coagulation]	EDTFL	240,730,870,7700,92500,93500,95500,475160,5 24370,650000,		Coagulation	Blood
Factor X Deficiency [Coagulation]	EDTFL	60,230,970,7500,93500,321510,471210,475160, 647070,815560,	Coagulation system deficiency of enzyme necessary for blood clotting.	Coagulation	Blood
Factor XI Deficiency [Coagulation]	EDTFL	40,320,620,940,60000,90000,93500,325370,475 160,863650,		Coagulation	Blood
Factor XII Deficiency	EDTFL	70,520,30000,47500,150000,225160,367750,52 7000,663710,742000	Coagulation system deficiency of enzyme necessary for blood clotting.	Coagulation	Blood
Afibrinogenemia	EDTFL	150,180,2500,322060,458500,515049,684810,7 12420,785530,995380,	Blood clotting disorder.	Coagulation	Blood
Fibrinogen Deficiency	EDTFL	130,350,850,5750,17500,42500,221020,425430, 771000,815910	As mentioned above	Coagulation	Blood
Angiohemophilia	EDTFL	20,250,7500,51000,67500,95000,275020,47509 0,667000,985670,	Blood coagulation disorder, usually hereditary.	Coagulation	Blood
Von Willebrand Disease	EDTFL	80,160,15500,85200,92000,321350,357300,657 110,833200,987230	As mentioned above	Coagulation	Blood
Thrombasthenia	EDTFL	120,400,800,830,5750,7250,142500,557500,792 500,893000	Congenital hereditary bleeding disorder characterized by reduced or absent platelet aggregation.	Coagulation	Blood
Glanzmann Thrombasthenia	EDTFL	160,230,12850,55750,125000,210500,479950,5 93200,761850,987230	As mentioned above	Coagulation	Blood
Thrombocytopenia	EDTFL	20,400,900,20000,53000,92500,222700,475110, 527000,987230	Blood platelet deficiency. See Platelet Storage Pool Deficiency, and Blood Platelet Disorders sets.	Coagulation	Blood
Thrombocytopenia	BIOM	778.0; 845.0; 751.0	As mentioned above	Coagulation	Blood
Thrombopenia	EDTFL	20,400,900,20000,55000,92500,222500,475110, 527000,987230	As mentioned above	Coagulation	Blood
Hemorrhage 1	CAFL	1550,802		Hemorrhage	Blood
Hemorrhage 2	XTRA	800,802,1550,10000		Hemorrhage	Blood
Bleeding	BIOM	9.5		Hemorrhage	Blood
Bleeding control	BIOM	9.5; 751; 778; 845		Hemorrhage	Blood
Hemorrhagic Shock	EDTFL	40,550,910,93500,210500,212960,325430,5157 00,682450,755480	Life-threatening condition with low blood distribution to tissues, causing cell injury and inadequate tissue function.	Hemorrhage	Blood
Hemostatič	BIOM	2.5			Blood
Hemodilution	BIOM	2720.0; 2170.0; 1550.0; 802.0; 880.0; 787.0; 776.0; 760.0; 727.0; 660.0; 190.0	Decrease in the amount of cellular elements and proteins relative to the volume of blood plasma.		Blood
Blood Clots	XTRA	685		Clots	Blood
Blood Clots	XTRA	6,28,59,685		Clots	Blood
Clotting Disorders, Coagulation General	EDTFL	100,830,5000,45110,93500,475160,527000,650 000,759830,926700,		Clots	Blood
Clotting Disorders, Coagulation [Post Immunization]	EDTFL	190,200,7250,45750,96500,325000,519340,655 200,750000,922530,		Clots	Blood
Blood Platelet Disorders	KHZ	10,520,11090,55750,60000,125000,275160,571 000,834000,932000,		Clots	Blood

Subject / Argument	Author	Frequencies	Notes	Origin	Target
Blood Platelet Disorders	EDTFL	120,230,730,830,5620,7250,32500,42500,90000,175110		Clots	Blood
Factor V Leiden	EDTFL	80,320,610,2270,44250,115710,245480,486000,697500,856720	It is a variant of the human Factor V protein that increases the risk of venous thrombosis.	Thrombosis	Blood
Consumption Coagulopathy	EDTFL	190,520,650,9080,112830,217500,335000,5475 00,725280,925000		Thrombosis	Blood
Disseminated [Intravascular] Coagulation	EDTFL	100,830,5000,45110,93500,475160,527000,650 000,759830,926700,	Formation of blood clots throughout the body, usually in critical illnesses.	Thrombosis	Blood
Thrombosis	EDTFL	100,580,780,5250,21800,322530,479500,52700 0,667000,987230,	Formation of blood clot affecting blood flow.	Thrombosis	Blood
Thrombosis	BIOM	44.5; 45.5		Thrombosis	Blood
Thrombus [blood clot]	EDTFL	100,830,5000,45110,93500,475160,527000,650 000,759830,926700,		Thrombosis	Blood
Arterial Thrombosis	BIOM	43.5; 44.0; 65.5; 89.5		Thrombosis	Blood
Deep Vein Thrombosis	EDTFL	100,580,780,5250,21800,322530,479500,52700 0,667000,987230,		Thrombosis	Blood
Vein Thrombosis	CAFL	685,776,1500,	Formation of blood clot inside vein. See Thrombophlebitis.	Thrombosis	Blood
Thrombosis, Retinal Vein	EDTFL	100,580,780,5250,21800,322530,479500,52700 0,667000,987230		Thrombosis	Blood
Thrombophlebitis	CAFL	1500,776,685	Inflammation of vein walls from clotting. Use on lab animals only! See Circulatory Stasis.	Thrombosis	Blood
Thrombophlebitis	EDTFL	100,580,780,5250,21800,322530,479500,52700 0,667000,987230,	As mentioned above	Thrombosis	Blood
Thrombophlebitis	BIOM	1500; 776; 685	As mentioned above	Thrombosis	Blood
Thrombosis of herpetic aetiology	BIOM	2720; 2489; 2170; 1800; 1550; 802; 880; 87; 727; 444; 125; 95; 72; 20; 444; 1865; 1489		Thrombosis	Blood
Phlegmasia Alba Dolens [Thrombosis]	EDTFL	100,580,780,5250,21800,322530,479500,52700 0,667000,987230,		Thrombosis	Blood
Antithrombin III Deficiency	EDTFL	50,650,1000,5620,7000,377910,400000,563190, 642060,985900,	Hereditary disorder with recurring venous thrombosis, pulmonary embolism, and fetal death.	Thrombosis	Blood
Thrombosis Infective Herpes Type	CAFL	2720,2489,2170,1800,1550,802,880,787,727,44 4,125,95,72,20,444,1865,1489,	Formation of blood clot affecting blood flow, associated with Herpesviridae infections (see sets). Not to be used with Arrhythmia.	Thrombosis	Blood
Favism	EDTFL	40,250,950,7500,12850,29030,157500,381020,5 95420,875000	Also called G6PD Deficiency. Genetic disorder with predisposition to hemolysis (red blood cell destruction) and consequent jaundice with multiple triggers.	Genetic disorder	Blood
Glucosephosphate DHG Deficiency	EDTFL	30,120,400,930,2240,217500,387500,475000,57 5520,726900	As mentioned above	Genetic disorder	Blood
Glucosephosphate Dehydrogenase Deficiency	KHZ	100,240,650,830,2500,27500,55370,87500,1255 20,322060,519340,652430,751870,926160,	Also called G6PD Deficiency, or Favism. As mentioned above.	Genetic disorder	Blood
Hemoglobinopathies	EDTFL	110,490,780,2250,77500,115710,255480,48500 0,697500,856720	Genetic defects causing abnormal hemoglobin molecule structure.	Genetic disorder	Blood
Hemoglobinuria, Paroxysmal	EDTFL	500,680,77500,87500,95030,115710,255480,48 5000,697500,997870			Blood
Paroxysmal Cold Hemoglobinuria [Anemia]	EDTFL	20,120,5160,62500,110250,332410,517500,684 810,712230,992000,			Blood
Paroxysmal Nocturnal Hemoglobinuria	EDTFL	20,120,5160,62500,110250,332410,517500,684 810,712230,992000,			Blood
Hemoglobin S Disease	EDTFL	80,320,630,2270,44250,115710,255480,485000, 697500,856720			Blood
Prolactin Hypersecretion Syndrome	EDTFL	20,250,950,9000,13390,15000,67500,92200,307 700,569710	Abnormally high levels of prolactin in blood.		Blood
Prolactin, Inappropriate Secretion	EDTFL	80,240,920,1800,2250,127500,255310,693200,8 93500,926070	As mentioned above		Blood
Hyperprolactinemia	EDTFL	70,410,730,5850,72500,138000,367500,550300, 725340,920320	As mentioned above		Blood
Jaundice	CAFL	5000,1600,1550,1500,880,802,650,625,600,444, 1865,146,250,125,95,72,20,	Excessive increase in the levels of bilirubin in the blood.	Jaundice	Blood
Jaundice	EDTFL	160,490,620,850,7500,162500,281200,492520,6 75620,825230	See Liver Support, Gallbladder, Leptospirosis, Parasites General, and Flukes sets. Also see Icterus Haemolytic.	Jaundice	Blood
Icterus [Juvenile Jaundice]	EDTFL	160,490,620,850,7500,162500,281200,492520,6 75620,825230,	As mentioned above	Jaundice	Blood
Jaundice 1	XTRA	1.19,10,20,72,95,125,146,250,444,600,625,649, 650,717,726,731,734,802,863,880,1500,1550,16 00,1865,9305,	As mentioned above	Jaundice	Blood
Jaundice, Chronic Idiopathic	EDTFL	160,490,620,850,7500,162500,281200,492520,6 91270,859830		Jaundice	Blood
Dubin-Johnson Syndrome	EDTFL	410,570,800,102350,175140,475330,560060,60 0770,797680,891220		Jaundice	Blood

Subject / Argument	Author	Frequencies	Notes	Origin	Target
Icterus Haemolytic	CAFL	243,768,	A chronic form of jaundice involving anemia. See Jaundice set.	Jaundice	Blood
Jaundice Hemolytic	EDTFL	160,490,620,850,7500,162500,281200,492520,859830,922530	As mentioned above	Jaundice	Blood
Posthepatic jaundice	BIOM	243; 768		Jaundice	Blood
Kernicterus	EDTFL	70,550,700,870,5250,7250,30000,55230,93500,325620	A pathological neonatal jaundice with deposit of free bilirubin in the brain tissue. Also see Bilirubinemia and Hyperbilirubinemia Hereditary.	Jaundice	Blood
Spinal Cord Myelodysplasia	EDTFL	180,320,950,7500,25750,52500,425160,571000,841000,932000	Inability of bone marrow cells to grow and mature, so they are unable to produce enough red blood cells, white blood cells and platelets.		Blood
Myelodysplastic Syndromes	EDTFL	130,400,600,830,5820,47250,142500,357520,702510,882110	Disorder of bone marrow stem cells, causing ineffective blood cell production.		Blood
Dysmyelopoietic Syndromes	EDTFL	190,250,5310,18500,41500,126510,387200,472000,538100,614010,			Blood
Myeloproliferative Disorders	EDTFL	80,460,3290,7500,117500,327500,367750,662020,896500,981000	Bone marrow diseases in which excess blood cells are produced.		Blood
Paraproteinemias	EDTFL	140,490,800,830,2250,17750,95470,319340,327350,533630	Excessive amounts of paraprotein or single monoclonal gammaglobulin in blood, usually due to underlying immunoproliferative disorder.		Blood
Paraimmunoglobulinemias	EDTFL	140,300,950,178720,375170,477500,527000,667000,761850,988900,			Blood
Plasma Cell Dyscrasias [neoplasms]	EDTFL	570,900,15750,62500,95000,250000,434000,524370,682020,753070,			Blood
Monoclonal Gammopathies	EDTFL	140,210,780,950,5240,7230,32369,91960,205300,514000,			Blood
Gammapathy, Monoclonal	EDTFL	140,210,780,950,5240,7230,32370,91960,205300,514000			Blood
Erythremia [Chronic Polycythemia]	EDTFL	50,750,900,9000,11090,55330,326550,425710,642910,980000,	Increase in the mass of red blood cells caused by an uncontrolled proliferation. Neoplasm in which bone marrow makes too many red blood cells, and possibly white cells and platelets, causing thickening of blood.		Blood
Polycythemia Vera	EDTFL	50,750,900,9000,11090,55330,326550,425710,642910,980000	As mentioned above		Blood
Osler-Vaquez Disease	EDTFL	510,2350,25730,42300,75330,255370,427500,675230,858590,915380	As mentioned above		Blood
Porphyria	BIO	698,	It is a set of rare diseases, due to an alteration of the activity of one of the enzymes that synthesize the heme group in the blood.		Blood
Porphyria	BIOM	698; 780			Blood
Porphyrias	EDTFL	120,490,780,12500,43000,122400,262500,555340,692500,819340	Several rare disorders of the nervous system and skin.		Blood
Porphyria, Erythropoietic [Gunther]	EDTFL	40,320,960,12500,43000,122400,262500,555340,692500,819340,	Enzyme deficiency in red blood cells.		Blood
Porphyria, Erythropoietic, Congenital	EDTFL	40,320,960,12500,43000,122400,262500,555340,692500,819340,			Blood
Gunther's Disease [erythropoietic porphyria]	EDTFL	40,320,960,12500,43000,122400,262500,555340,692500,819340,	As mentioned above		Blood
Spherocytosis Hereditary	EDTFL	500,680,87600,95030,234510,367200,452590,684810,712230,997870	Genetic disorder of erythrocytes with anemia, jaundice, splenomegaly, and fatigue. See appropriate sets.	Genetic disorder	Blood
Urea Cycle Disorders	EDTFL	180,220,730,5580,13390,150000,475850,736420,819340,915700	Genetic disorder with deficiency of enzyme to remove ammonia from blood.	Genetic disorder	Blood
Uremia	CAFL	911	Also called uremic poisoning. Excessive nitrogenous waste in the blood, as in kidney failure. Use Kidney Insufficiency, and Lymph Stasis - See Blood Purify sets.		Blood
Xanthemia	CAFL	20,72,95,125,146,250,444,600,625,650,802,880,1500,1550,1600,1865,	Also called carotenemia. High levels of carotene in blood, causing skin discoloration.		Blood
Bacteremia	KHZ	350,870,2500,11090,40000,90000,275160,425710,564280,640000,	Presence of bacteria in the blood.	Bacteria	Blood
Blood Flukes	XTRA	329,419,635,847,867,5516,7391,9889,	Also see Schistosomiasis and Bilharzia.	Parasites	Blood
Schistosomiasis	KHZ	130,230,730,850,5250,137250,545750,687500,895270,976290,	Blood fluke infection. Also see Blood Flukes, Bilharzia, Schistosoma Haematobium, Parasites Schistosoma Haematobium, Schistosoma Mansoni, and Parasites Schistosoma Mansoni.	Parasites	Blood
Schistosomiasis [Katayama Flatworm]	ETDFL	680,900,2500,5500,13930,93500,386400,429500,434000,436250,	As mentioned above	Parasites	Blood
Bilharzia	XTRA	329,9889,1035.49,1087.17,1089.25,1238.74,1257.39,1261.5,1272.83,1350.21,1431.24,1564.68,1734.89,1799.56,1910.33,11031.25,	Caused by Schistosoma parasitic flatworms, commonly called Blood Flukes. Also see Schistosomiasis.	Parasites	Blood

4b - Blood vessels

Subject / Argument	Author	Frequencies	Notes	Origin	Target
Aorta	BIOM	95			Blood Vessels
Heart Arteries	BIOM	44.0			Blood Vessels

Subject / Argument	Author	Frequencies	Notes	Origin	Target
Heart arteries (coronary vessels)	BIOM	43.5; 44; 95.5			Blood Vessels
Artery Stimulator	XTRA	727,787,800,880	Blood circulation improve.		Blood Vessels
Arterioles	BIOM	94.5; 5.7			Blood Vessels
Capillaries-1	BIOM	7.0; 94.5			Blood Vessels
Capillaries Healing	XTRA	15.19			Blood Vessels
Capillaries Stimulate Healing	XTRA	15.2			Blood Vessels
Peripheral Vessels	BIOM	3.3; 4.0; 5.55; 6.0; 9.25; 9.5; 10.0			Blood Vessels
Veins	BIOM	84.5; 92; 94; 99		Veins	Blood Vessels
Veins regeneration	BIOM	2.5; 9.4; 10; 25.5; 47.5; 50; 89; 94		Veins	Blood Vessels
Vein regeneration (acute condition)	BIOM	2.5; 9.4; 10; 33.5; 46.5; 84.5; 85; 99.5		Veins	Blood Vessels
Venous Insufficiency	EDTFL	80,90,700,820,7500,17500,185750,350000,4251 70,510500	Disorder where veins can't pump enough blood back to heart. Includes Varicose Veins - see set.	Veins	Blood Vessels
Inflammation of Vein	BIOM	28.5; 89		Veins	Blood Vessels
Phlebitis	CAFL	1500,776	Vein inflammation.	Veins	Blood Vessels
Phlebitis [Thrombosis]	EDTFL	100,580,780,5250,21800,322530,479500,52700 0,667000,987230,	As mentioned above	Veins	Blood Vessels
Phlebitis	BIOM	10		Veins	Blood Vessels
Periphlebitis	EDTFL	50,370,900,2750,3000,70000,95220,175160,275 000,357300		Veins	Blood Vessels
Varicose Veins	EDTFL	110,220,730,3750,7050,51280,137500,236420,4 72290,851170	Enlarged and twisted veins, usually on leg, due to valve defects.	Veins	Blood Vessels
Varicosis -Veins	BIOM	94		Veins	Blood Vessels
Varicose veins, circulation	BIOM	40; 9.4		Veins	Blood Vessels
Varicoses 1	CAFL	1.2,20,28	As mentioned above	Veins	Blood Vessels
Varicoses 2	CAFL	2.4,9.39,20,28,33,40,72,95,148,224,300.5,685,7 76,1250,1500,1520,	As mentioned above	Veins	Blood Vessels
Varices	EDTFL	100,420,930,5250,35000,82600,178000,519340, 689930,931000	Varicose Veins	Veins	Blood Vessels
Varix	BIOM	45.5; 60.5; 66.5; 68.0; 68.5; 84.5; 85.0; 99.0		Veins	Blood Vessels
Varicosis 1	BIOM	2.2; 10; 12.5; 15; 19.5; 26; 77.5; 92.5		Veins	Blood Vessels
Varicosis 2	BIOM	1.2; 4; 6.8; 10; 47.5; 50; 52.5; 99.5		Veins	Blood Vessels
Varicosis 3	BIOM	7; 9.44; 19.5; 19.75; 40.5; 48; 85.5		Veins	Blood Vessels
Varicosis 4	BIOM	2.8; 3.3; 8.1; 9.19; 54; 54.25; 54.5		Veins	Blood Vessels
Varicosis 5	BIOM	0.7; 0.9; 2.5; 2.65; 3.3; 9.8; 56; 69		Veins	Blood Vessels
Varicosis 6	BIOM	2.5; 4.9; 9.4; 10; 28.5; 33.5; 50; 45.5; 46.5; 47.5; 84; 84.5; 85; 89; 94; 99; 99.5		Veins	Blood Vessels
Varicose veins, acute condition	BIOM	2.5; 9.4; 10; 33.5; 46.5; 84.5; 85; 99.5		Veins	Blood Vessels
Varicose ulcer	BIOM	730; 700; 727; 784; 786			Blood Vessels
Vascular Diseases	EDTFL	70,220,730,75250,117220,237020,451900,5615 10,698100,812770,	Narrowing of arteries other than those that supply the heart or brain. Includes Raynaud's Disease and coagulation disorders - see appropriate sets.	Bloodstream	Blood Vessels
Vascular Diseases, Peripheral	EDTFL	70,220,730,75250,117220,237020,451900,5615 10,698100,812770,		Bloodstream	Blood Vessels
Peripheral Angiopathies	EDTFL	140,320,650,37500,67500,96500,325590,47650 0,527000,667000		Bloodstream	Blood Vessels
Angio-Spasm	BIOM	1.2; 6.3		Bloodstream	Blood Vessels
Vasculitis		Can be caused by Hepatitis C, HIV, Parvovirus B19, hepatitis B virus and the protozoan Sarcocystis.			
Vasculitis Vasculitis Hemorrhagic	EDTFL	80,350,5500,35170,62500,93500,225000,49609 0,682450,753070	Group of disorders that destroy veins and arteries by inflammation, occurring anywhere in the body, with resultant bleeds, pain, fever, weight loss, and other symptoms.	Vasculitis	Blood Vessels
Angiitis	EDTFL	80,220,730,2500,5810,50000,322450,532410,68 9930,750000	Inflammatory vascular disease	Vasculitis	Blood Vessels
Allergic Angiitis	EDTFL	190,520,650,1000,13930,110570,380000,44750 0,728980,825270,	Type of vasculitis which destroys blood vessels by inflammation.	Vasculitis	Blood Vessels
Churg-Strauss Syndrome	EDTFL	40,230,730,850,5870,73250,324530,342500,596 500,875270	As mentioned above	Vasculitis	Blood Vessels
Allergic Granulomatous Angiitis	EDTFL	190,520,750,1780,13930,110530,380000,44750 0,728980,825270,	Type of vasculitis which destroys blood vessels by inflammation.	Vasculitis	Blood Vessels
Giant Cell Arteritis	EDTFL	70,240,600,7290,132250,427500,555950,69000 0,875000,936420	It is a vasculitis that involves the large arteries. Inflammation damages the arteries, causing them to narrow up to obstruction.	Vasculitis	Blood Vessels
Horton Giant Cell Arteritis	EDTFL	70,240,600,7290,132250,427500,555950,69000 0,875000,936420,		Vasculitis	Blood Vessels

Subject / Argument	Author	Frequencies	Notes	Origin	Target
Horton Disease [Giant Cell Arteritis]	EDTFL	70,240,600,7290,132250,427500,555950,690000,875000,936420,		Vasculitis	Blood Vessels
Cranial Arteritis	EDTFL	70,240,600,7290,132250,427500,555950,690000,875000,936420,		Vasculitis	Blood Vessels
Necrotizing Arteritis	EDTFL	70,240,600,7290,132250,427500,555950,690000,875000,936420,		Vasculitis	Blood Vessels
Essential Polyarteritis	EDTFL	200,250,650,2500,3000,25500,96500,326160,534250,651300,		Vasculitis	Blood Vessels
Periarteritis Nodosa	EDTFL	70,240,600,7290,132250,427500,555950,690000,875000,936420,		Vasculitis	Blood Vessels
Aortic Arteritis, Giant Cell	EDTFL	70,240,600,7290,132250,427500,555950,690000,875000,936420,		Vasculitis	Blood Vessels
Aortitis Syndrome Aortitis, Giant Cell	EDTFL	130,230,750,800,5250,7250,35000,95400,226320,422530,	Large vessel granulomatous vasculitis (see set) with Fibrosis (see set) and Stenosis (see sets). Mainly affects aorta and its branches, and pulmonary arteries.	Vasculitis	Blood Vessels
Pulseless Disease	EDTFL	80,350,37500,115700,175000,322060,347750,475190,527000,834500	As mentioned above	Vasculitis	Blood Vessels
Juvenile Temporal Arteritis [Infantile]	EDTFL	70,240,600,7290,132250,427500,555950,690000,875000,936420,	As mentioned above	Vasculitis	Blood Vessels
Temporal Arteritis	EDTFL	80,350,5500,35170,62500,93500,225000,496090,682450,753070,	As mentioned above	Vasculitis	Blood Vessels
Takayasu Arteritis	EDTFL	80,350,5500,35170,62500,93500,225000,496090,682450,753070,	As mentioned above	Vasculitis	Blood Vessels
Obliterating Endarteritis	BIOM	39.5; 93.5; 99.5		Vasculitis	Blood Vessels
Thromboangiitis Obliterans	EDTFL	180,17850,27500,47500,150000,225000,452590,684000,713000,993410,	Is defined as a form of vasculitis with progressive inflammation and clot formation in small and medium blood vessels of hands and feet, usually in smokers.	Vasculitis	Blood Vessels
Buerger Disease [Thromboangiitis]	EDTFL	180,17850,27500,47500,150000,225000,452590,684000,713000,993410,	As mentioned above	Vasculitis	Blood Vessels
Polyarteritis Nodosa	EDTFL	200,250,650,2500,3000,25500,96500,326160,534250,651300,	Systemic vasculitis of small- or medium-sized muscular arteries, usually involving renal and visceral vessels but not pulmonary circulation.	Vasculitis	Blood Vessels
Behcet Syndrome	EDTFL	240,900,9000,13580,85000,92500,250000,376290,425750,845100,	Rare immune-related systemic vasculitis with mucous membrane ulcers and eye problems.	Vasculitis	Blood Vessels
Silk-Road Disease	EDTFL	240,900,9000,13580,85000,92500,250000,376290,425750,845100	As mentioned above	Vasculitis	Blood Vessels
Triple-Symptom Complex		150,32500,52300,72500,95110,175750,347600,518920,684810,964000	As mentioned above	Vasculitis	Blood Vessels
Granulomatosis Wegener's	XTRA	90,330,5490,37000,203830,381410,481930,614820,763000,797230,	Also called Granulomatosis with polyangiitis (GPA). Serious systemic vasculitis that involves granulomatosis and polyangiitis.	Vasculitis	Blood Vessels
Wegener Granulomatosis	EDTFL	30,500,700,970,88000,370500,547500,656400,725370,825520		Vasculitis	Blood Vessels
Purpura			See Section 16a - Skin		Blood Vessels
Carotid Stenosis	KHZ	20,240,2750,17500,35190,97500,269710,424370,563190,875960,	Also see Carotid Artery Narrowing.		Blood Vessels
Carotid Artery Narrowing [Stenosis] Carotid Stenosis [Heart & Arterial]	EDTFL	130,230,750,800,5250,7250,35000,95400,759830,926700,			Blood Vessels
Anti-Angiospastic	BIOM	5.55; 9.5			Blood Vessels
Carotid Ulcer	EDTFL	150,240,650,830,2500,127500,255470,387500,696500,825910,			Blood Vessels
Blue Rubber Bleb Nevus Syndrome	EDTFL	30,400,780,1000,2500,33390,185580,367150,425790,719340	Venous malformations in the GI tract and on skin.		Blood Vessels
Aneurysm	CAFL	880,787,760,727,465,125,95,72,444,1865,20,727,	Bulge in weak blood vessel wall.	Aneurysm	Blood Vessels
Aneurysm	BIOM	880; 787; 760; 727; 465; 444; 1865; 125; 95; 72; 20		Aneurysm	Blood Vessels
Saccular Aneurysm	EDTFL	80,240,570,7500,10720,36210,142500,321000,415400,775680,	The most common type and accounts for 90% of all brain aneurysms. This type of aneurysm resembles a berry with a thin stem.	Aneurysm	Blood Vessels
Brain Aneurysm	EDTFL	80,240,570,7500,10720,36210,142500,321000,415400,775680,		Aneurysm	Blood Vessels
Intracranial Aneurysm [I. Vascular Disorders]	EDTFL	160,570,780,930,2750,7500,22500,40000,125000,433770,		Aneurysm	Blood Vessels
Basilar Artery Aneurysm	EDTFL	80,240,570,7500,10720,36230,142500,321000,415700,775680		Aneurysm	Blood Vessels
Berry Aneurysm	EDTFL	80,240,570,7500,10720,36210,142500,321000,415400,775680,		Aneurysm	Blood Vessels
Giant Intracranial Aneurysm	EDTFL	80,240,570,7500,10720,36210,142500,321000,415400,775680,		Aneurysm	Blood Vessels

Subject / Argument	Author	Frequencies	Notes	Origin	Target
Atherosclerosis		*Can be caused by Cytomegalovirus, and the bacteria Helicobacter pylori and Chlamydia pneumoniae.*			
Arteriosclerosis	CAFL	10000,2720,2170,1800,1600,1500,880,787,776, 727,20,	Hardening of the small arteries. Regeneration takes time. Try CMV sets.	Atheroscler.	Blood Vessels
Atherosclerosis	EDTFL	70,730,5000,7250,92500,352930,451170,51967 9,684810,712810,	Hardening of medium and large caliber arteries.	Atheroscler.	Blood Vessels
Atherosclerosis	XTRA	134,223,333,345,411,423,425,436,446,453,470. 89,471.66,479,542,554,563,572,573,574,576,62 0,643,668,686,716,718,738,786,787,934,940,94 1.79,943.29,958,1544,1577,1880,1886,2323,243 1,3343,3760.3,3767.3,3773.3,4710.5,7160,7520. 5,7543.39,20443.5,	Artery wall thickening due to white blood cells.	Atheroscler.	Blood Vessels
AtheroSclerosis	BIOM	7542.5; 7520.5; 4710.4; 3773.2; 3760.2; 1886; 1880; 943.3; 940; 620; 479; 471.6; 470.9; 941.8; 3767.2; 7159.5; 3343; 2431; 2323; 1577; 1544; 958; 934; 787; 786; 738; 718; 716; 686; 668; 643; 576; 574; 573; 572; 563; 554; 542; 453; 446; 436; 425; 423; 411; 345; 333; 223; 134		Atheroscler.	Blood Vessels
ArterioSclerosis	BIOM	10000; 5000; 2720; 2170; 1800; 1600; 1500; 880; 787; 776; 727; 20		Atheroscler.	Blood Vessels
Atherosclerosis of infectious nature	BIOM	10000; 2720; 2160; 1800; 1600; 1500; 880; 787; 465; 20; 1865; 522; 465		Atheroscler.	Blood Vessels
Arteriovenous Malformations	EDTFL	100,830,5070,12330,12710,225000,519340,655 200,752630,923700,	Abnormal artery-vein connections, bypassing capillaries, normally in the CNS.	Bloodstream	Blood Vessels
Artery Plaque	XTRA	4632,5364,5885	Usually atheroma - swelling in arteries full of pus.	Arteries	Blood Vessels
Fibromuscular Dysplasia	EDTFL	770,830,920,12320,176080,287330,488320,510 200,620300,841090	Disease of blood vessels with abnormal growth in artery walls, most commonly renal and carotid.	Arteries	Blood Vessels
Hemangioma			See Section 16c - Tumor		Blood Vessels
Perniosis	BIO	232,622,822,4211	A disorder of the blood vessels caused by prolonged exposure to cold. Also see Chilblains set.	Bloodstream	Blood Vessels
Raynaud's Disease	CAFL	727,20	Markedly reduced blood flow due to cold or emotional stress, causing discoloration of fingers, toes, and sometimes other areas.	Bloodstream	Blood Vessels
Raynaud Disease	EDTFL	570,780,900,5250,7000,115710,255830,485430, 691500,825000	As mentioned above	Bloodstream	Blood Vessels
Sneddon-Champion Syndrome	EDTFL	80,420,5500,35190,60000,62500,92500,93500,2 25000,315700	Arterial disease with severe transient neurological symptoms or Stroke (see sets) and blue/purple skin mottling.		Blood Vessels
Livedo Reticularis, Systemic	EDTFL	120,150,830,15500,127500,302500,545530,601 820,713140,847400,			Blood Vessels
Telangiectasis	EDTFL	130,200,900,47500,96500,275030,534250,6912 70,753070,927100	Abnormal small dilated blood vessels on skin or mucous membranes, most common near nose, cheeks, and chin, and also on legs.		Blood Vessels
Spider Veins	EDTFL	180,1070,4820,15250,58210,109420,325700,38 7020,434270,611050	As mentioned above		Blood Vessels
Telangiectasia, Hereditary Hemorrhagic	EDTFL	160,5500,20000,37500,96500,312330,475150,5 27000,662710,789000	Genetic disorder with abnormal blood vessel formation in skin, mucous membranes, and often in lungs, liver, and brain.	Genetic disorder	Blood Vessels
Osler-Rendu Disease	EDTFL	70,460,650,112970,295870,347500,427500,695 300,750000,875950	As mentioned above	Genetic disorder	Blood Vessels
Intracranial Vascular Disorders	EDTFL	160,570,780,930,2750,7500,22500,40000,12500 0,433770,		Cerebral arteries	Blood Vessels
Vascular Diseases, Intracranial	EDTFL	80,350,5500,35170,62500,93500,225000,49609 0,682450,753070		Cerebral arteries	Blood Vessels
Angiospasm Intracranial	EDTFL	190,260,570,7600,12690,35380,322060,425710, 564280,930120,	Stenosis of artery in brain which may cause tissue damage. May indicate subarachnoid hemorrhage - see Cerebral Hemorrhage, and other Hemorrhage sets.	Cerebral arteries	Blood Vessels
Vasospasm, Intracranial	EDTFL	150,570,15160,52500,119340,357300,424370,5 61930,642910,930120,	As mentioned above	Cerebral arteries	Blood Vessels
Cerebral Vasospasm	EDTFL	40,550,900,93500,210600,453720,515190,6830 00,712230,993410	As mentioned above	Cerebral arteries	Blood Vessels

4c - Blood Circulation

Subject / Argument	Author	Frequencies	Notes	Origin	Target
Circulation	XTRA	586			Bloodstream
Circulatory System	XTRA	10.5			Bloodstream
Circulation regulation	BIOM	7; 9.4; 9.45; 19.5; 40.5; 46; 50			Bloodstream
Blood Circulation-1	BIOM	7; 9.4; 19.5; 40.5; 46; 50			Bloodstream
Local Blood Circulation 1	BIOM	85.5			Bloodstream
Blood Flow and Circulation	BIOM	48.0; 58.0; 93.5			Bloodstream
Blood Circulation Complex 1	BIOM	7.0; 19.5; 19.75; 25.5; 40.5; 46.0; 50.0; 85.5			Bloodstream
Blood Circulation Complex 2	BIOM	95.5			Bloodstream

Subject / Argument	Author	Frequencies	Notes	Origin	Target
Blood Circulation - Control Frequencies	BIOM	47.5; 50; 52.5; 99.5			Bloodstream
Regulation of Blood Circulation	BIOM	10000.0; 5000.0; 3176.0; 2720.0; 2489.0; 2145.0; 2127.0; 2112.0; 2008.0; 880.0; 802.0; 787.0; 727.0; 690.0; 666.0; 650.0; 625.0; 600.0; 465.0; 125.0; 95.0; 73.0; 72.0; 40.0; 20.0; 9.39; 679.2; 644.0; 20.0			Bloodstream
Circulatory System Diseases (General)	EDTFL	70,730,5000,7250,92500,352930,451170,519680,684810,712810			Bloodstream
Circulatory Collapse	EDTFL	70,730,5000,7250,92500,352930,451170,519679,684810,712810,			Bloodstream
Heart and Circulation	BIOM	10000; 2720; 2489; 2145; 2112; 880; 787; 727; 465; 162; 160; 125; 100; 95; 81; 80; 73; 20; 4; 1.2			Bloodstream
Hyperemia	EDTFL	110,490,14730,82500,217500,344030,671520,753210,871020,975870	Increase in blood flow to different tissues.		Bloodstream
Blood Circulation Stimulate Normal	XTRA	337			Bloodstream
Circulation Stimulate Increased	XTRA	17			Bloodstream
Blood Circulation Sluggish	XTRA	9.39,9.4,16,17,40,			Bloodstream
Circulatory Stasis	CAFL	40,2112,2145,2720,2489,	Stimulates blood circulation throughout the body. See Circulation disturbances sets.		Bloodstream
Circulation Diabetic	XTRA	2000			Bloodstream
Circulation Disturbances	CAFL	9.39,9.5,20,40,2112,2145,2489,2720,	See Circulatory stasis set.		Bloodstream
Circulation Disturbances	XTRA	9.39,9.5,40,95,125,160,200,2112,2145,2489,2720,			Bloodstream
Blood Circulation Disorders	BIOM	7.0; 9.4; 46; 93.5			Bloodstream
Numbness	CAFL	10000,2720,2489,2170,1800,1600,1550,802,880,787,727,650,625,600,440,660,	Also use Circulatory Stasis.		Bloodstream
Numbness	XTRA	1600	As mentioned above		Bloodstream
Numbness	BIOM	10000; 2720; 2489; 2170; 1800; 1600; 1550; 802; 880; 787; 727; 660; 650; 625; 600; 440; 98.5			Bloodstream

4d - Blood Pressure

Subject / Argument	Author	Frequencies	Notes	Origin	Target
Blood Pressure-1	BIOM	48			Pressure
Blood Pressure Balance 1	XTRA	10.5			Pressure
Blood Pressure Balance 2	XTRA	15			Pressure
Blood Pressure Reduce	XTRA	4		High	Pressure
Blood Pressure, High	CAFL	6,7.83,9.19,20,304,727,728,787,10000,	Can be caused by Coxsackie virus B5, Echovirus, Nanobacteria.	High	Pressure
Blood Pressure, High [Hypertension]	EDTFL	30,400,780,1000,2500,33390,75790,185580,425790,719340,		High	Pressure
Blood Pressure High	XTRA	6,7.83,9.18,15,20,95,304,324,528,727,787,880,2112,3176,10000,		High	Pressure
Blood Hypertension	XTRA	6,9.18,9.19,20,65,72,95,304,660,690,727.5,787,880,10000,	High blood pressure.	High	Pressure
High Blood Pressure Hypertension	XTRA	9.18,727,787,880,10000,		High	Pressure
Hypertension	EDTFL	30,400,780,1000,2500,33390,75790,185580,425790,719340		High	Pressure
Hypertension basic	BIOM	6; 8.1; 9.19; 9.44; 9.5; 19.75; 24.5; 25.5; 26; 44.5; 48; 50.5; 58; 62.5; 85.5; 85.7; 93.5; 95.5		High	Pressure
Hypertension	BIOM	10000.0; 5000.0; 3176.0; 2112.0; 880.0; 787.0; 9.19; 727.0; 528.0; 324.0; 304.0; 95.0; 150.0; 7.83; 20.0; 15.0; 6.0		High	Pressure
Hypertension	BIOM	3.3; 3.9; 5.55; 7; 9.4; 19.5; 40.5; 46		High	Pressure
Hypertension 3	BIOM	6.0; 8.1; 9.19; 9.44; 9.5; 19.75; 24.5; 25.5; 26.0; 44.5; 48.0; 50.5; 58.0; 62.5; 85.5; 85.7; 93.5; 95.5		High	Pressure
Hypertension 4	BIOM	2.8; 3.3; 8.1; 9.19; 54.0; 54.25; 54.5		High	Pressure
Hypertension 5	BIOM	0.7; 0.9; 2.5; 2.65; 3.3; 9.8; 56.0; 69.0		High	Pressure
Hypertension 6	BIOM	2.5; 3.6; 3.9; 5.0; 6.3; 8.1; 34.0; 92.0		High	Pressure
Hypertension 1	XTRA	6,9.18	See Blood Pressure High.	High	Pressure
Hypertension 2	CAFL	2112,20,95,324,528,15,9.19,7.83,6,10000,880,787,727,304,	As mentioned above	High	Pressure
Hypertension 3	XTRA	6,7.83,9.18,15,20,95,304,324,528,727,787,880,2112,3176,10000,	As mentioned above	High	Pressure

Subject / Argument	Author	Frequencies	Notes	Origin	Target
Hypertension 4	XTRA	6,7.83,9.18,15,20,95,304,324,528,727,787,880,10000,	As mentioned above	High	Pressure
Hypertension Portal	EDTFL	30,400,780,1000,2500,33390,75790,185580,425790,719340	High blood pressure in portal venous system (liver).	High	Pressure
Arterial Hypertension	BIOM	3.3		High	Pressure
Arterial pressure too high	BIOM	62.5; 65.0; 67.5; 96.0; 96.5		High	Pressure
Systolic Hypertension	BIOM	62.5; 65.0; 67.5; 96.0; 96.5		High	Pressure
Diastolic Hypertension	BIOM	9.19; 6		High	Pressure
Essential Hypertension	BIOM	3.3; 6.0; 9.19; 9.44; 9.5		High	Pressure
Hypertension, Malignant	EDTFL	30,400,780,1000,2500,33390,75790,185580,425790,719340	High blood pressure with acute impairment of organ systems (especially the CNS, cardiovascular system and/or the renal system) that can result in irreversible organ damage.	High	Pressure
Cruveilhier-Baumgarten Syndrome	EDTFL	30,240,620,950,7900,25750,87500,480000,525290,825000,		High	Pressure
Hypertension Pulmonary	EDTFL	30,400,780,1000,2500,33390,75790,185580,425790,719340	High blood pressure in lung vasculature, causing dizziness, shortness of breath, faints, and swollen leg.	High	Pressure
Ayerza's Syndrome [Pulmonary]	EDTFL	50,230,950,13390,121590,285430,325510,472500,612500,930000,	As mentioned above	High	Pressure
Hypertension Renin Induced	CAFL	9.19,6	RED high, diastolic high pressure. Use Kidney sets. See Blood Pressure High sets.	High	Pressure
Blood Pressure High Renin Induced	XTRA	6,9.18	Kidney renin high.	High	Pressure
Hypertension Spastic	CAFL	95	See Blood Pressure High sets. Use Kidney sets.	High	Pressure
Spastic Hypertension	BIOM	9.44; 9.5	As mentioned above	High	Pressure
Eclampsia	EDTFL	30,120,940,2500,22500,51330,328950,356720,426160,567700	As mentioned above	High	Pressure
Cerebral Hypertension	BIOM	1.2; 6.3		High	Pressure
HELLP Syndrome	EDTFL	50,440,700,970,2750,7500,15310,67500,122540,177030	Hypertensive disorder of pregnancy. Also see Hypertension.	High	Pressure
Blood Pressure Low	CAFL	20,727,787,880		Low	Pressure
Blood Hypotention	XTRA	20,471.5,660,690,727.5,787,880,	Low blood pressure.	Low	Pressure
Blood Pressure, Low [Hypotension]	EDTFL	70,180,750,830,2500,7500,326050,379930,425680,932000,		Low	Pressure
Hypotension	EDTFL	70,180,750,830,2500,7500,326050,379930,425680,932000		Low	Pressure
Hypotensive Effect	BIOM	3.3; 6.0; 9.25; 9.44; 9.5		Low	Pressure
Arterial pressure too low	BIOM	48; 48.5; 49; 49.5; 20		Low	Pressure
Idiopathic Orthostatic Hypotension	EDTFL	70,180,750,830,2500,7500,326050,379930,425680,932000,	Excessive drop in blood pressure when standing upright.	Low	Pressure
Orthostatic Hypotension	EDTFL	70,180,750,830,2500,7500,326050,379930,425680,932000,		Low	Pressure
Fainting	CAFL	20		Low	Pressure

4e - Heart

Subject / Argument	Author	Frequencies	Notes	Origin	Target
Heart	XTRA	10.5, 6			Heart
Heart General	CAFL	20,81,162,5000	Note: cardiac conditions are inherently unstable.		Heart
Center of heart	BIOM	98.5			Heart
Heart, ventricles	BIOM	41.0; 41.5; 43			Heart
Heart, intersectum	BIOM	42			Heart
Heart Function Stimulate Normal	XTRA	696			Heart
Cardiac center - Pilot frequencies	BIOM	7.5; 15; 40; 78.5; 2.5; 5; 100; 10; 12.5; 4; 42.5; 45; 99.75; 77.5; 80; 82.5; 99			Heart
Heart Tonic	CAFL	80,160,20,73,3.9,3000,880,787,727,465,162,125,95,20,1.2,	Note: cardiac conditions are inherently unstable. Lab animals only. See Chlamydia, Staphylacoccus, Circulatory Stasis, and Kidney sets.		Heart
Heart Function Normalize	XTRA	1.19,3.89,20,73,80,95,125,160,250,465,660,690,696,727.5,787,880,3000,			Heart
Normalization of Heart Function	BIOM	80; 160; 20; 73; 3.9; 3000; 880; 787; 727; 465; 162; 125; 95; 20; 1.2			Heart
Heart- Regulation	BIOM	41.0; 41.5			Heart
Heart- Regulation	BIOM	1.2; 3.8; 8; 9.44; 41; 43; 43.5; 97			Heart
Heart function activation	BIOM	7.5; 15; 78.5; 97			Heart
Heart Supply-2	BIOM	40.5; 47.5			Heart
Cardiovascular Diseases	EDTFL	170,250,20000,125160,377910,414170,515170,683000,712000,993410			Heart

Subject / Argument	Author	Frequencies	Notes	Origin	Target
Heart Failure	EDTFL	110,220,730,970,2750,52600,63500,194500,412500,673130			Heart
Cardiac insufficiency	BIOM	39; 39.5; 99.75			Heart
Congestive Heart Failure	XTRA	9.18,9.19	Inability of heart to pump blood efficiently enough to meet the body's needs.		Heart
Heart Decompensation	EDTFL	70,410,700,970,5290,30000,142500,350000,422060,775290			Heart
Heart Disease	HC	381000			Heart
Heartaches - Pilot frequencies	BIOM	85; 87.5; 90; 98; 94.5; 91.5; 92.5; 62; 62.5			Heart
Auriculo-Ventricular Dissociation	EDTFL	80,240,630,7820,32250,67500,307650,391020,415700,726070,			Heart
Heart Disorder	XTRA	727,787,880,5000			Heart
Heart Defects, Congenital	EDTFL	70,410,700,970,10530,105910,242500,391280,425520,815290			Heart
Holt-Oram Syndrome	EDTFL	50,440,680,930,7500,20000,86000,342060,635310,833000			Heart
Heart Abnormalities Heart Disease Heart Disease & COPD (Chronic Obstructive Pulmonary Disease) Comprehensive	EDTFL	70,410,700,970,2750,7500,15310,67500,115700,356720			Heart
Heart Valve Diseases	EDTFL	140,220,330,970,2750,117500,345230,567500,625870,775580,			Heart
Heart Block	EDTFL	130,230,900,8530,17500,72530,327050,334250,425000,805290			Heart
Heart Blockage	XTRA	59,60,61			Heart
Heart Catheterization	EDTFL	40,500,700,970,5760,7500,37500,96500,225910,425370			Heart
Heart Septal Defects	EDTFL	140,220,330,970,2750,50000,325560,334250,425000,805290			Heart
Angina	CAFL	787,776,727,465,428,660,	Chest pain indicative of cardiac problems.	Angina	Heart
Cardiac Angina	BIOM	5000; 2720; 2170; 1865; 1800; 1600; 1500; 880; 832; 787; 776; 727; 660; 465; 444; 120; 125; 20; 14; 7.83; 3	As mentioned above	Angina	Heart
Cardiac Angina-2	BIOM	9.44; 43.5; 95.5	As mentioned above	Angina	Heart
Angina Pectoris	CAFL	3,230,2720,2170,1800,1600,1500,880,832,787,776,727,465,444,1865,125,95,72,20,660,7.83,	As mentioned above	Angina	Heart
Angina Pectoris Angina, Microvascular	EDTFL	60,230,850,35230,63020,125030,235680,396500,575610,751770	As mentioned above	Angina	Heart
Angina Pectoris	BIOM	62; 62.5; 85; 87.5; 90; 91.5; 92.5; 94.5; 98	As mentioned above	Angina	Heart
Stenocardia [Angina pectoris]	EDTFL	60,230,850,35230,63020,125030,235680,396500,575610,751770,	As mentioned above	Angina	Heart
Heart Angina Pectoris	XTRA	5000	As mentioned above	Angina	Heart
Cardiac rhythm	BIOM	15; 37.5; 38; 38.5			Heart
Arrhythmia Cardiac	EDTFL	90,780,830,7500,8000,225330,510250,689930,750000,936420,	Irregular heartbeat, including tachycardia and bradycardia.	Arrhythmia	Heart
Arrhythmia	BIOM	1.2; 3.8; 7.84; 8; 9.45; 38; 38.5; 41; 43; 43.5; 95; 97; 696		Arrhythmia	Heart
Rhytm Abnormality	BIOM	38.0; 38.5; 95.0; 95.5; 97.0		Arrhythmia	Heart
Antirhytmical effect	BIOM	1.2		Arrhythmia	Heart
Cardiac Conduction Disorder	BIOM	59; 60; 61			Heart
Right Ventricular Dysplasia, Arrhythmogenic	EDTFL	80,240,630,7820,32250,67500,307650,391020,415700,726070	Cardiac arrhythmia caused by heart muscle genetic defects.	Arrhythmia	Heart
Ventricular Dysplasia [General]	EDTFL	80,240,630,7820,32250,67500,307650,391020,415700,726070,	As mentioned above		Heart
Arrhythmogenic Cardiomyopathy	EDTFL	50,400,850,2750,5000,55160,269710,555300,707000,825500,	As mentioned above		Heart
Atrial Fibrillation	EDTFL	80,730,970,5750,37500,85080,96500,125160,325000,377910,	Abnormal heart rhythm.		Heart
Auricular Fibrillation	EDTFL	70,180,1650,7930,102530,165500,320530,693500,875310,915930,			Heart
Ventricular Fibrillation	EDTFL	80,730,970,5750,37500,85080,96500,125160,325000,377910,	Uncoordinated contraction of the ventricular heart muscles, usually leading to cardiac arrest - see Myocardial Infarction, and use caution.		Heart
Bradycardia [Slow Heart Rate]	EDTFL	40,120,17330,57500,250000,451170,515110,689410,712000,995380,	Abnormally slow heart rate, usually under 60bpm in adult.	Bradycardia	Heart

Subject / Argument	Author	Frequencies	Notes	Origin	Target
Heart Bradycardia	XTRA	5000		Bradycardia	Heart
Bradyarrhythmia [Bradycardia]	EDTFL	40,120,17330,57500,250000,451170,515110,689410,712000,995380,		Bradycardia	Heart
Heart Fast Palpitations	XTRA	727,787,880,10000		Tachycardia	Heart
Cardiac Neurosis	BIOM	727.0; 787.0; 880.0; 5000.0; 10000.0		Tachycardia	Heart
Extrasystole	BIOM	6.0		Tachycardia	Heart
Tachycardia, extrosystolia	BIOM	1.2; 6		Tachycardia	Heart
Tachycardia	CAFL	1.2	Rapid heartbeat. Note: it is not recommended that this set be used on humans. See Heart tonic, and Relaxation to produce sets.	Tachycardia	Heart
Tachycardia	EDTFL	130,5120,7000,32300,95750,175000,522530,682030,759840,900000	As mentioned above	Tachycardia	Heart
Tachyarrhythmia [Tachycardia]	EDTFL	130,5120,7000,32299,95750,175000,522530,682030,759840,900000,		Tachycardia	Heart
Wolff Periodic Disease [Tachycardia SVT]	EDTFL	130,5120,7000,32299,95750,175000,522530,682030,759840,900000,		Tachycardia	Heart
Wolff-Parkinson-White [Tachycardia SVT]	EDTFL	130,5120,7000,32299,95750,175000,522530,682030,759840,900000,	Disorder of heart's electrical system, causing episodes of Tachycardia (see sets), with palpitations, dizziness, shortness of breath, or faints. See Heart Fast Palpitations, Dizziness, Giddiness, Dyspnea, and Fainting sets.	Tachycardia	Heart
Calcium on Heart Valve	XTRA	6004	Most commonly aortic valve. See Aortic Valve Stenosis, Mitral Stenosis, and Heart Stenosis.		Heart
Cardiac Edema	CAFL	9.19	Fluid retention due to congestive heart failure. Note: cardiac conditions are inherently unstable.		Heart
Asymmetric Septal Hypertrophy	EDTFL	130,260,900,125000,376290,404370,515160,687620,712810,992000		Hypertrophy	Heart
Cardiac Hypertrophy	EDTFL	140,400,720,800,2300,122850,329950,487500,725790,915700,		Hypertrophy	Heart
Left Ventricular Hypertrophy	EDTFL	40,400,780,1210,52780,122850,329950,487500,725790,915700,		Hypertrophy	Heart
Right Ventricular Hypertrophy	EDTFL	140,400,720,800,2300,122850,329950,487500,725790,915700,		Hypertrophy	Heart
Cardiomegaly [Enlarged Heart]	EDTFL	130,250,730,820,5120,7230,32500,90000,175750,434530			Heart
Enlarged Heart	EDTFL	50,420,410,820,10590,32500,62180,322330,353700,396170	Thickening of ventricular walls of heart.		Heart
Heart Stenosis	XTRA	5000	Narrowing of blood vessels. Note: cardiac conditions are inherently unstable.	Stenosis	Heart
Valvular Heart Diseases	EDTFL	140,220,330,970,2750,117500,345230,567500,625870,775580,		Stenosis	Heart
Aortic Valve Stenosis	EDTFL	130,230,750,800,5250,7250,35000,95400,759830,926700	Narrowing of aortic valve of the heart.	Stenosis	Heart
Idiopathic Hypertrophic Subaortic Stenosis	EDTFL	30,180,650,770,33520,72500,270960,321800,505670,715280	Also called Obstructive Hypertrophic Cardiomyopathy.	Stenosis	Heart
Idiopathic Hypertrophic Subvalvular Stenosis	EDTFL	120,550,950,5870,25000,42500,62500,90000,92600,515700,		Stenosis	Heart
Mitral Stenosis / Mitral Valve Stenosis	EDTFL	70,500,970,9000,12330,32500,142900,320000,425870,525560,	Narrowing of the heart's mitral valve. Use with caution.	Stenosis	Heart
Mitral Valve Prolapse	EDTFL	140,900,5620,93500,222700,425000,522549,689950,752630,923700,	Displacement of abnormally thick mitral valve leaflet into left atrium during systole.		Heart
Floppy Mitral Valve	EDTFL	140,900,5620,93500,222700,425000,522550,689950,752630,923700	As mentioned above		Heart
Mitral Click-Murmur	EDTFL	130,240,750,900,213540,335580,413980,635000,795220,826320	As mentioned above		Heart
Cardiomyopathy Congestive	EDTFL	180,220,850,5290,7250,50000,323540,334250,425000,805290	Now called Dilated Cardiomyopathy (DCM). Enlargement of heart affecting pump function.Can be caused by Coxsackie B virus.		Heart
Cardiomyopathy Dilated	EDTFL	130,260,23800,135600,390000,404370,515160,687630,712810,992000	As mentioned above		Heart
Cardiomyopathy [Hypertrophic Obstructive]	EDTFL	30,180,5530,20000,93500,175750,323350,527000,667000,749000	Thickening of myocardium which can cause sudden death.		Heart
Cardiomyopathy [Restrictive]	EDTFL	30,180,5530,20000,93500,404370,515159,687630,712810,992000,	Stiffening of walls of heart's chambers.		Heart
Ebstein Anomaly [Congenital Heart Defect]	EDTFL	150,230,620,950,7500,212850,455950,557500,796500,891500,	Congenital heart defect in tricuspid valve.		Heart
Heart Endocarditis	XTRA	5000	It can be caused by bacteria such as Staphylococcus and Streptococcus.		Heart
Endocarditis	XTRA	333,377,471,523,626,628,634,714,724,744,768,786,2162,	Inflammation of heart's inner tissues.		Heart
Endomyocarditis	BIOM	393			Heart

Subject / Argument	Author	Frequencies	Notes	Origin	Target
Endocarditis Bacterial	EDTFL	50,370,950,2500,3750,73400,95750,175820,269710,355080	Also called Infective Endocarditis. Pathogenic inflammation of heart's inner tissues.	Bacteria	Heart
Pericardial Tamponade [Heart Compression]	EDTFL	70,410,700,970,2750,7500,15310,67500,115700,356720,	Pressure on heart's sac due to build-up of fluid.		Heart
Cardiac Tamponade [pericardial]	EDTFL	170,490,920,112950,295870,347500,427500,695280,750000,875950,	Pressure on heart's sac due to build-up of fluid.		Heart
Eisenmenger Complex Eisenmenger Syndrome	EDTFL	30,400,780,1000,2500,33390,75790,185580,425790,719340,	Cyanotic heart defect in which blood flow is reversed, causing serious complications in pregnancy.		Heart
Left Heart Syndrome, Hypoplastic	EDTFL	150,230,650,930,7500,11090,52500,172510,383700,516520	Rare congenital defect where the left side of the heart is underdeveloped.		Heart
Long QT Syndrome	EDTFL	80,240,690,900,2500,27500,55910,119340,393500,536420	Rare heart disease which increases risk of irregular heartbeats originating from ventricles.		Heart
Romano-Ward Syndrome [congenital Long QT]	EDTFL	80,240,690,900,2500,27500,55910,119340,393500,536420,	As mentioned above		Heart
Systolic Click-Murmur Syndrome	EDTFL	130,240,750,900,213540,335580,413980,635000,795220,826320,			Heart
Postcommissurotomy Syndrome	EDTFL	170,350,8850,57500,117500,237520,357500,691020,810500,915700	Set of distressing symptoms arising after mitral valve surgeries.		Heart
Coronary heart disease		*Can be caused by Herpes Simplex virus 1 and the bacterium Chlamydia pneumoniae.*			
Microvascular Angina	EDTFL	60,230,850,35230,63020,125030,235680,396500,575610,751770,	Type of coronary heart disease that affects the arterioles and capillaries.		Heart
Cardiac Syndrome X	EDTFL	110,340,7250,45760,96500,325000,519370,655200,750000,922530,			Heart
Myocardial Infarction	EDTFL	180,320,950,7500,25750,52500,425170,571000,841000,932000	Commonly known as a heart attack. Can be caused by Chlamydia pneumoniae, Cytomegalovirus, Coxsackie B virus and Escherichia Coli.		Heart
Myocardial infarction	BIOM	43.5; 44; 95.5; 789			Heart
Ischemic Heart Disease	EDTFL	70,410,700,970,2750,50000,326570,334250,425000,805290			Heart
Myocardial Ischemia	EDTFL	470,520,2500,40000,366290,476500,527000,665340,752700,987230,	Also called coronary artery disease. Includes Angina (see sets), and Myocardial Infarction (see set). Usually due to Atherosclerosis (see set).		Heart
Carditis	EDTFL	70,410,700,970,2750,7500,15310,67500,115700,356720,	Infection and inflammation of heart muscle, usually due to viruses such as Parvovirus B19, or to bacteria like Borrelial Burgdorferi (see sets), or parasites like Trypanosoma Cruzi (see sets).		Heart
Heart Myocarditis	XTRA	5000		Myocarditis	Heart
Myocarditis	EDTFL	180,320,950,7500,25750,52500,425170,571000,841000,932000		Myocarditis	Heart
Myocarditis	BIOM	2720; 2170; 1600; 1550; 880; 802; 787; 761; 727; 625; 279; 125; 95; 72; 20		Myocarditis	Heart
Myocarditis Narbe	CAFL	279,761	.	Myocarditis	Heart
Pericardial Effusion [Septal]	EDTFL	140,220,330,970,2750,50000,325560,334250,425000,805290,	Abnormal accumulation of fluid around the heart.		Heart
Hemopericardium	EDTFL	20,120,5160,62500,110250,332410,517500,684810,712230,992000,			Heart
Chylopericardium	EDTFL	70,120,720,800,2500,22200,72500,434390,739100,905310	Is a rare condition in which lymphatic fluid leaks into the space around the heart.		Heart
Pericardio	BIOM	39			Heart
Pericarditis	CAFL	2720,2170,1600,880,1550,802,787,727,625,125,95,72,20,	Inflammation of pericardium, the sac that surrounds the heart. Note: cardiac conditions are inherently unstable. This set was developed for animal research only.	Pericarditis	Heart
Pericarditis	EDTFL	170,490,920,112950,295870,347500,427500,695280,750000,875950	Inflammation of pericardium, the sac that surrounds the heart. Note: cardiac conditions are inherently unstable.	Pericarditis	Heart
Pericarditis	BIOM	2720; 2170; 1600; 880; 1550; 802; 787; 727; 625; 279; 125; 95; 72; 33; 20		Pericarditis	Heart
Scimitar Syndrome	EDTFL	50,350,620,970,2500,177000,337200,439500,521700,568270	Rare congenital heart defect with anomalous venous return from right lung.		Heart
Tricuspid Atresia Tricuspid Valve Atresia	EDTFL	170,620,2750,15750,42500,62500,97500,357300,712230,997870	Congenital heart disease with complete absence of tricuspid valve.		Heart
Ulcer Ventricular	BIO	232,1000	Ulcers involving heart chamber.	Ulcer	Heart
Ulcer Ventricular	CAFL	769,760	As mentioned above	Ulcer	Heart
Ulcer Ventricular	CAFL	142,566,676,232,1000,	As mentioned above	Ulcer	Heart
Heart perfusion; arterialization	BIOM	40.5; 47.5; 50.5			Heart

Subject / Argument	Author	Frequencies	Notes	Origin	Target

5 - Lymphatic System

It plays the important role of draining tissues from liquids and waste substances and blocking the spread of pathogens. It is a system consisting of primary (**thymus** and **bone marrow**) and secondary lymphatic organs including the **spleen**, **lymph nodes**, lymphoid tissue associated with the mucous membranes (MALT: **tonsils**, Peyer plaques, cecal appendage and other lymphocyte groupings scattered in the mucous membranes) , connected together by a network of thin lymphatic vessels. Lymph contains **white blood** cells (**T and B lymphocytes**).

Subject / Argument	Author	Frequencies	Notes	Origin	Target
Detoxification			See Section **2c - Detox**		Lymphatic S.
Thymus	XTRA	10.5	It brings to fruition the various types of lymphocytes, finalizing to destroy intracellular pathogens (T lymphocytes)	Thymus	Lymphatic S.
Thymus	BIOM	69; 79		Thymus	Lymphatic S.
Thymus - Pilot frequencies	BIOM	17; 38; 38.5; 56; 25; 63.5; 69; 74.5; 79		Thymus	Lymphatic S.
Thymus Gland Stimulant	XTRA	20,727,787,880,5000,		Thymus	Lymphatic S.
Thymus Stimulation	CAFL	20		Thymus	Lymphatic S.
Lymph 4	XTRA	146,346,428,596,767,982,1078,3176,5443,8846,			Lymphatic S.
Lymph Glands	XTRA	10,440,727,787,880,5000,			Lymphatic S.
Lymph - Pilot frequencies	BIOM	15.5; 25; 27.5; 30; 70; 72.5; 75; 77.5; 80; 92.5; 94; 95; 95.5; 99.5			Lymphatic S.
Lymph System Normalize Stimulate	XTRA	676			Lymphatic S.
Lymphatic system, regulation control	BIOM	77.5; 80; 82.5; 99; 95.5; 92.5; 25; 25.5; 27; 27.5; 30; 94; 70; 72.5; 75; 15.5			Lymphatic S.
Regulation and cleaning of lymphatic system	BIOM	1.6; 1.7; 2.5; 25.5; 27; 75; 79; 95.5			Lymphatic S.
Lymph Support	CAFL	15.05,10.36,3176			Lymphatic S.
Lymph Glands Stimulate	XTRA	2.5,465,10000			Lymphatic S.
Lymph Stasis	CAFL	3176	See Lymphangitis set. Body massager must be used during this treatment.		Lymphatic S.
Lymph Stasis Secondary	CAFL	2.5,6.3,10,146,148,440,444,465,522,727,787,880,10000,	See Lymphangitis set.		Lymphatic S.
Lymph Stasis 1	XTRA	6.29,146,148,440,444,522,727,787,880,	See Lymphangitis set.		Lymphatic S.
Lymphostasis	BIOM	880; 787; 727; 522; 444; 440; 148; 146; 6			Lymphatic S.
Lymphostasis	BIOM	2.5; 6.3; 146; 148; 317; 440; 444; 522; 444; 440; 727; 787; 880; 3176			Lymphatic S.
Lymph Circulation Stimulate Increased	XTRA	15			Lymphatic S.
Lymph System Circulation Stimulate	XTRA	15.19			Lymphatic S.
Lymph Stimulation	BIOM	15.05; 10.36; 3176.0			Lymphatic S.
Lymph Drain Circulation	XTRA	1.5,3.6,6.3,8,10,10.36,15,15.05,15.33,20,20.5,66,146,148,324,428,440,444,465,522,528,660,676,690,727.5,743,787,880,1000,1865,2112,3176,5000,10000,			Lymphatic S.
Lymph Drain	XTRA	146,522			Lymphatic S.
Lymph drainage	BIOM	6.3; 7.84			Lymphatic S.
	BIOM	1.6; 1.7			Lymphatic S.
Lymphatic Diseases	EDTFL	140,350,930,11950,25540,35670,87500,93500,234250,527810			Lymphatic S.
Status Lymphaticus	EDTFL	50,900,1520,55150,375030,479930,527000,662710,789000,984230			Lymphatic S.
Lymphatism	EDTFL	190,350,930,7110,27500,35670,87500,93500,223010,515700			Lymphatic S.
Lymphadenopathy	EDTFL	650,2300,7500,25230,25540,35670,95670,378950,523010,682020			Lymphatic S.
Lymph Leukemia	VEGA	833	Also see appropriate Cancer Leukemia sets.		Lymphatic S.
Lymph Mover	XTRA	12500			Lymphatic S.
Lymph Plaque	CAFL	596,346	Lymphatic system blocked.		Lymphatic S.
Edema			See Section **1 - Various Conditions**		Lymphatic S.
Lymphedema	EDTFL	140,350,930,11950,25540,145850,262500,397500,633910,825170,	Localized fluid retention and tissue swelling in lymphatic system. Frequently caused by conventional cancer treatments or parasite infections.		Lymphatic S.
Milroy's Disease	EDTFL	130,230,970,5250,32500,475190,527000,661730,742000,988900			Lymphatic S.
Lymphedema	XTRA	6.29,20,24.3,146,148,440,444,465,522,660,690,727.5,787,880,1865,3000,5000,	As mentioned above		Lymphatic S.
Adenitis	EDTFL	120,210,930,7560,25540,35640,87500,93500,215700,533690,	Swollen or enlarged lymph nodes. See appropriate Lymph sets.		Lymphatic S.

Subject / Argument	Author	Frequencies	Notes	Origin	Target
Lymphadenitis	EDTFL	120,210,930,7560,25540,35640,87500,93500,215700,533690,	As mentioned above		Lymphatic S.
Lymphadenitis 1	XTRA	574,778,880,1078,1120,3176,	As mentioned above		Lymphatic S.
Lymphadenitis 2	XTRA	574,778,1078,1120,3176,	As mentioned above		Lymphatic S.
Lymphadenitis 3 Lymphangitis	XTRA	574	As mentioned above		Lymphatic S.
Lymphangitis	CAFL	880,574,778,1120,1078,3176,	Lymphatic vessel inflammation of humans and horses most commonly caused by Streptococcus but also by other bacteria, yeast Fungus, and cancer. See Streptococcus General.		Lymphatic S.
Lymphangitis	BIOM	10; 345; 440; 574; 596; 778; 880; 1078; 1120			Lymphatic S.
Lymphatic glands, inflammation	BIOM	10; 36; 53; 53.5; 62; 62.5; 68.5; 75; 75.5; 85; 86; 87.5; 90; 91.5; 94.5; 98			Lymphatic S.
Lymphangioleiomyomatosis	EDTFL	40,500,700,970,25540,35670,37500,96500,225910,425380	Rare, progressive, systemic disease that typically results in cystic lung destruction.		Lymphatic S.
Lymphangioma	EDTFL	170,240,700,830,2500,17500,432500,555910,625280,775520,			Lymphatic S.
Lymphangioma, Cavernous	EDTFL	170,240,700,830,2500,17500,432500,555910,625280,775520,	Malformations of lymphatic system with large or microscopic cysts.		Lymphatic S.
Lymphangioendothelioma	EDTFL	650,2500,7100,25230,25540,35670,87500,93500,523010,682020			Lymphatic S.
Lymphatic Depressant	XTRA	727,787,880,5000			Lymphatic S.
Lymphogranuloma	CAFL	552,1522	Abnormal lymphatic growths due to Chlamydia Trachomatis - see sets, and use Blood Cleanser.	Bacteria	Lymphatic S.
Lymphogranuloma 1	XTRA	263.11,334,552,1552,1566.4,1675,2008,2127,2385,2521,2655,2663,2787.5,3324,5013,5013.5,5020,5278,5318.8,5388.5,5575,6687.3,7037.5,7356,8020,8368.2,8610,8836.89,10025,10026,10027,	See Cancer Hodgkins disease, and Hodgkins disease.	Bacteria	Lymphatic S.
Lymphogranuloma Inguinale Lymphogranuloma Venereum	EDTFL	190,350,930,7110,27500,35670,87500,93500,223010,515700	Lymphatic system disease caused by Chlamydia Trachomatis - see sets.	Bacteria	Lymphatic S.
Lymphogranuloma Venereum LGV 1	XTRA	430,552,555.7,620,624,840,866,1111.4,1522,2213,2222,	As mentioned above	Bacteria	Lymphatic S.
Lymphogranuloma Venereum LGV 2	XTRA	479,620,940.1,942.89,1880.09,1885,9,3760.3,3771.69,4710.5,7520.5,7543.39,	As mentioned above	Bacteria	Lymphatic S.
Lymphogranuloma Venereum LGV 3	XTRA	430,479,552,555.7,620,624,940.1,942.89,1522,1880.09,1885.9,3760.3,3771.69,4710.5,7520.5,7543.39,	As mentioned above	Bacteria	Lymphatic S.
Lymphogranuloma, Malignant	EDTFL	190,350,930,7110,25540,35670,87500,93500,234250,527810	Tightly-packed collection of macrophages imprisoning foreign organisms or other materials which cannot be eliminated by the immune system.		Lymphatic S.
X-Linked Lymphoproliferative Syndrome	EDTFL	120,350,930,7500,17500,35000,87500,93500,224950,497610,	Several conditions where excess lymphocytes are produced - a sign of immune system compromise.		Lymphatic S.
Duncan's Syndrome	EDTFL	600,1000,5000,240600,365800,454370,515120,689410,712000,997870			Lymphatic S.
Elephantiasis	CAFL	623,824,865,710,	Caused by obstruction of the lymphatic vessels	Bacteria	Lymphatic S.
Elephantiasis 2	XTRA	112,120,623,710,824,865,	Massive swelling of parts of the body due to Lymphangitis, Filariasis, Lymphogranuloma Venereum, or Proteus Syndrome - see sets.	Bacteria	Lymphatic S.
Ganglionitis	XTRA	574,1557	Inflammation of nerve or lymphatic ganglions.		Lymphatic S.
Angiofollicular Lymphoid Hyperplasia	EDTFL	40,500,700,970,5750,7600,37500,96500,223910,425370,	Also called Castleman's or Castleman Disease. Single or multi site lymph node condition.		Lymphatic S.
Castleman Disease	EDTFL	40,280,3240,14200,23160,55500,208320,314370,563190,875960	As mentioned above		Lymphatic S.
Castleman's Tumor	EDTFL	20,240,2750,17500,35190,97500,269710,314370,563190,875960	As mentioned above		Lymphatic S.
Lymph Node Diseases (General)	EDTFL	140,350,930,11950,25540,35670,87500,93500,234250,527810			Lymphatic S.
Giant Lymph Node Hyperplasia	EDTFL	180,250,700,1160,2760,14550,33500,92500,356750,425520,			Lymphatic S.
Kimura Disease [Chronic inflammatory disorder]	EDTFL	70,120,850,9500,88000,141200,297500,425950,675310,827000,	Chronic inflammatory disease. Its main symptoms are skin lesions of the neck or head or painful unilateral adenomegaly of the cervical lymph nodes.		Lymphatic S.
Mucocutaneous Lymph Node	EDTFL	120,5810,25000,87500,224000,458500,522370,683000,712230,992000	Also called Kawasaki Disease. Autoimmune disease, mainly in children, with inflammation and vasculitis in medium-sized blood vessels.		Lymphatic S.
Kawasaki Disease	EDTFL	120,500,850,5500,32500,35000,75850,92500,125620,519340	As mentioned above		Lymphatic S.
Glands	XTRA	15136.71		Glands	Lymphatic S.
Glands General Normalize	XTRA	537		Glands	Lymphatic S.

Subject / Argument	Author	Frequencies	Notes	Origin	Target
Lymph Glands	XTRA	10,440,727,787,880,5000,		Glands	Lymphatic S.
Lymph Glands Stimulate	XTRA	2.5,465,10000		Glands	Lymphatic S.
Glands Enlarged	XTRA	20,727,787,880,10000,		Glands	Lymphatic S.
Swollen Glands	CAFL	152,242,642,674,922	See Mumps sets, and Angina Throat. Use Lymph set(s).	Glands	Lymphatic S.
Glandular Fever			See Mononucleosis in Section 17d - Virus	Glands	Lymphatic S.
Throat and Lymph Nodes	XTRA	20,146,380,440,522,660,690,727.5,760,776,784, 802,1550,880,1600,		Glands	Lymphatic S.
Lymph Nodes in Neck Swollen	XTRA	465	Also see Angina Throat.	Glands	Lymphatic S.
Cervic Gland Lumps	XTRA	320,727,787,880,5000,10000,	Swollen lymph nodes in the neck	Glands	Lymphatic S.
Leg Swelling -1	BIOM	44.5			Lymphatic S.
Leg Swelling	BIOM	20; 465; 727; 787; 880; 5000; 10000			Lymphatic S.
Parasites in Lymphatic System	BIOM	10000; 157			Lymphatic S.
Tonsillitis			See Section 12e - Throat	Throat	Lymphatic S.

5a - Spleen

Subject / Argument	Author	Frequencies	Notes	Origin	Target
Spleen	XTRA	4.6,147			Spleen
Spleen 1	XTRA	20			Spleen
Spleen 2	XTRA	492			Spleen
Spleen	BIOM	11.5			Spleen
Spleen Enlarged	CAFL	35,787,3176			Spleen
Spleen Enlarged 1	XTRA	20,27.44,35,465,660,690,727.5,787,802,880,155 0,1800,2170,2720,3176,10000,			Spleen
Spleen Secondary	CAFL	10000,2720,2170,1800,1550,880,802,727,465,2 0,			Spleen
Splenic Diseases	EDTFL	40,350,2500,7250,60000,125000,300000,47520 0,527000,752700,			Spleen
Splenic Rupture	EDTFL	180,320,25000,52500,134250,175750,426900,5 71000,843000,937410,			Spleen
Banti's Syndrome	BIO	1778	Chronic congestive enlargement of spleen, causing premature destruction of red blood cells.		Spleen

6 - Immune System

Subject / Argument	Author	Frequencies	Notes	Origin	Target
Immune system	BIOM	1.7; 1.75; 8.1; 9.4; 9.6			Immune s.
Immune System Improve	XTRA	3	Normalize. Also see Leukocytogenesis Stimulate.		Immune s.
Immunostimulating Effect	BIOM	9.4			Immune s.
Strengthening of host defenses	BIOM	26; 58; 11.5; 84.5; 97.5; 68			Immune s.
Immune system activation	BIOM	1.6; 1.7; 1.75; 8.1; 9.4; 9.6; 10; 12.5			Immune s.
Immune System Stabilization	XTRA	30,330,727,740,787,835,880,1234,1550,5000,73 44,10000,	As mentioned above		Immune s.
Immune System Stabilization	BIOM	330; 787; 1234; 7344; 10000			Immune s.
Immune System Stimulation 1	XTRA	8,432,835,1862,2008,2128,2180,2791,2855,286 7,2929,3347,3448,4014,5611,	As mentioned above		Immune s.
Immune System Stimulation 2	XTRA	40.39,40.5,40.6,40.7,40.79,	As mentioned above		Immune s.
Immune System Stimulation 3	PROV	8,20,120,304,432,464,665,728,800,880,1488,18 62,2008,2128,2180,2489,2720,2791,2855,2867, 2929,3176,3347,3448,4014,5000,5611,10000,	As mentioned above. NB: minimum of 5 treatments.		Immune s.
Immune System Stimulation 4	XTRA	8,20,120,304,432,464,665,728,787,800,880,148 8,1862,2008,2128,2180,2489,2720,2791,2855,2 867,2929,3176,3347,3448,4014,5000,5611,1000 0,	As mentioned above		Immune s.
Immune System Stimulation 5	XTRA	1434	As mentioned above		Immune s.
Immune System Stimulate Normalize	XTRA	835	As mentioned above. This set has been successfully used for unidentified airborne allergens.		Immune s.
Immune Support Sweep	XTRA	6-12	Based on research by Dr. G.J. Schummer, M. Crane, L. Wong.		Immune s.
Immune System Stabilization	BIOM	330.0; 10000.0; 7344.0; 5000.0; 1550.0; 1234.0; 740.0; 880.0; 835.0; 787.0; 727.0; 160.0; 500.0; 1600.0; 30.0			Immune s.
Immune System Stabilization 1	BIOM	5000.0; 2489.0; 1600.0; 1550.0; 1500.0; 880.0; 802.0; 787.0; 727.0; 660.0; 650.0; 465.0; 440.0; 428.0			Immune s.

Subject / Argument	Author	Frequencies	Notes	Origin	Target
Immune System Stabilization 2	BIOM	10000.0; 5610.5; 5000.0; 4014.0; 3448.0; 3347.0; 3176.0; 2929.0; 2867.0; 2855.0; 2791.0; 2720.0; 2489.0; 2180.0; 2128.0; 2008.0; 1862.0; 1488.0; 880.0; 800.0; 787.0; 728.0; 665.0; 464.0; 432.0; 304.0; 120.0; 20.0; 8.0			Immune s.
Immune System Balance	XTRA	1.19,3,7.69,7.7,9.39,9.4,9.59,20,28,146,230,250, 465,522,600,625,650,660,690,727.5,776,787,80 2,835,880,1550,1850,10000,			Immune s.
Immunity Restoration	BIOM	5610.5; 4014.0; 3448.0; 3347.0; 3176.0; 2929.0; 2867.0; 2855.0; 2791.0; 2720.0; 2489.0; 2180.0; 2128.0; 2008.0; 1862.0; 1488.0; 880.0; 800.0; 787.0; 728.0; 665.0; 464.0; 432.0; 304.0; 120.0; 20.0; 8.0			Immune s.
Immunoreconstitution	BIOM	4014; 3448; 3347; 2929; 2867; 2855; 2791; 2128; 1488; 800; 787; 728; 432; 304; 120; 8			Immune s.
Defense center	BIOM	26			Immune s.
Proactive Defence	BIOM	2.2; 10.0; 12.5; 15.0; 19.5; 26.0; 92.5			Immune s.
Body Defenses-1	BIOM	11.5; 19.5; 26.0; 58.0; 69.0; 79.0; 84.5; 97.5			Immune s.
Body Defenses-2	BIOM	60.5; 64.5; 67.0			Immune s.
Body Weakening	BIOM	19			Immune s.
Weakening of Body Defenses	BIOM	11; 26; 84.5; 97.5			Immune s.
Active protection	BIOM	2.2; 10; 12.5; 15; 19.5; 26; 55; 92.5			Immune s.
Immune Complex Diseases Immune System Diseases	EDTFL	150,240,680,810,32500,197500,332500,555370, 696500,875520,	Genetic and acquired. Autoimmunities include chronic Lyme, scleroderma, lupus, vasculitis, Graves disease, and some anemias and myopathies.		Immune s.
Interleukin			See Section 2d - Cells, Amino acids, Enzymes, etc.		Immune s.
Lysine			See Section 2d - Cells, Amino acids, Enzymes, etc.		Immune s.
Eosinophilia Eosinophilia, Tropical Eosinophilia-Myalgia	EDTFL	190,490,730,940,96500,174330,326050,528000, 663000,752200	Condition where count of eosinophil white blood cells is abnormally high, usually indicating parasites or allergic reaction.		Immune s.
Eosinophilia	XTRA	20,120,950,12330,82500,152000,362020,60400 0,713340,823580,	As mentioned above		Immune s.
Neutropenia [Low White Blood Cells]	EDTFL	180,550,850,2500,5500,27500,37500,123010,32 7250,533690,	Abnormally low concentration of neutrophils (type of white blood cell).		Immune s.
IgA Deficiency	EDTFL	60,490,680,7200,102500,231700,472500,62569 0,705700,857100	Lack of immunoglobulin A, an antibody that protects mouth, airways, and digestive tract mucous membranes from infection. Genetic.	Genetic disorder	Immune s.
Mastocytosis	EDTFL	40,240,920,1000,12050,177760,234000,591000, 683160,849340	Rare mast cell disease in adults and children caused by cell and precursor proliferation, causing itching, hives, and anaphylactic shock.		Immune s.
Mast cell activation syndrome (MCAS) Mast-Cell Disease	EDTFL	180,190,900,55750,322060,477500,527000,662 710,742000,988900			Immune s.
Histiocytosis Histiocytosis X	EDTFL	120,350,850,7500,117500,142500,267500,3959 10,625700,796010	Disorder with excessive numbers of histiocytes (tissue macrophages - immune system components).		Immune s.
Histiocytosis, Langerhans-Cell	EDTFL	20,450,900,2750,5870,15560,267500,395910,62 5700,796010,			Immune s.
Histiocytosis, Non-Langerhansl	EDTFL	120,350,850,7500,117500,142500,267500,3959 10,625700,796010,			Immune s.
Autoimmune Diseases		Truly the human body does not attack itself. It is the pathogens that are responsible (especially EBV). Can be caused by Enteroviruses such as Coxsackie B virus, Epstein-Barr virus, Cytomegalovirus, Parvovirus B19, HIV, and by the bacterium Mycobacterium tuberculosis.			
Autoimmune Diseases	EDTFL	50,260,570,2500,13390,85390,250000,456000,7 84000,927000	See Nanobacter and Human T Lymphocyte Virus 1.	Autoimmune Diseases	Immune s.
AutoImmune Disorders	CAFL	3,7.7,9.4,9.6,20,28,156,250,522,600,625,650,72 7,776,787,802,808,1550,10000,	As mentioned above	Autoimm. D.	Immune s.
Autoimmune Disease	BIOM	0.1; 1.2		Autoimm. D.	
Acquired Immunodeficiency Syndrome - AIS	EDTFL	150,900,5580,30000,47500,360590,365000,388 900,434000,456110		Autoimm. D.	Immune s.
Immunodeficiency AIS Immunodeficiency, Severe Immunologic Deficiency Syndromes	EDTFL	150,240,680,810,32500,197500,332500,555370, 696500,875520	Immunodeficiencies, mostly acquired, leading to immunosuppression.	Autoimm. D.	Immune s.
Common Variable immunodeficiency	EDTFL	110,700,5520,26330,41200,309420,361550,342 100,414000,416610		Autoimm. D.	Immune s.

Subject / Argument	Author	Frequencies	Notes	Origin	Target
Severe Combined Immunodeficiency	EDTFL	170,430,7200,13970,132460,275750,512330,651000,753040,926700		Autoimm. D.	Immune s.
Bare lymphocyte Syndrome	EDTFL	70,240,35110,150000,375000,477500,527000,662700,749000,969670,	Genetic disorder with disturbed development of functional T cells and B cells, caused by numerous genetic mutations.	Autoimm. D.	Immune s.
SCID (Severe Combined Immunodeficiency Disease)	EDTFL	140,420,730,3950,17510,7500,122500,306500,425520,624370	As mentioned above	Autoimm. D.	Immune s.
Omenn Syndrome	EDTFL	20,570,9000,12860,45000,92500,175750,450000,515160,689410	As mentioned above	Autoimm. D.	Immune s.
Immunodepressive effect	BIOM	1.6			
Autoimmune I - II, Polyglandular	EDTF	50,260,570,2500,13390,85390,157500,525830,757770,975340		Autoimm. D.	Immune s.
Polyglandular Type I Autoimmune Syndrome Polyglandular Type II Autoimmune Syndrome	EDTF	40,120,950,19300,121440,201330,323450,653020,807500,973340		Autoimm. D.	Immune s.
Autoimmune Polyendocrinopathy Candidiasis Ectodermal Dystrophy	EDTF	50,260,570,2500,13390,85340,157500,525500,757670,975340		Autoimm. D.	Immune s.
Acute Inflammatory polyneuropathy	EDTF	40,320,930,5970,35250,112730,296000,392970,701660,933500,	Autoimmune process that is characterized by progressive areflexic weakness and mild sensory changes		Immune s.
Agammaglobulinemia	EDTF	120,800,22500,90000,175000,451170,517700,683000,712230,992000,	Primary immune deficiency disease. Synonymous with Hypogammaglobulinemia.		Immune s.
Hypogammaglobulinemia	EDTF	140,530,930,5230,117500,162500,217500,393500,677910,797600	As mentioned above		Immune s.
AIDS 0	CAFL	727,787,880,2489,3175,3275,3375,3475,5000,	Acquired immune deficiency. See HIV. Use Human T Lymphocyte virus3.	AIDS	Immune s.
AIDS 1	CAFL	2489,465,727,787,880,1500,1.2,31000,31750,34750,	As mentioned above	AIDS	Immune s.
AIDS 2	CAFL	1.44,1550,1500,249,418,727,787,880,2489,3100,3175,3475,	As mentioned above	AIDS	Immune s.
AIDS 3	CAFL	2.88,249,418,727,787,880,1500,1550,2489,3100,3175,3475,	As mentioned above	AIDS	Immune s.
AIDS Kaposi's Sarcoma	BIO	249,418	Acquired immune deficiency. Skin cancer common in AIDS.	AIDS	Immune s.
AIDS Secondary	CAFL	1113=720,2128=960,6121=1260,33=60,1113=720,2128=960,6121=1260,		AIDS	Immune s.
AIDS	EDTFL	170,900,5580,30000,47500,360590,365000,388900,434000,456110		AIDS	Immune s.
AIDS/HIV	EDTFL	180,240,22000,30000,47500,162820,365000,388900,434000,456110,	Acquired immune deficiency.	AIDS	Immune s.
Anti-Glomerular Basement Membrane	EDTFL	170,950,2500,10530,125090,375170,525710,650000,752630,923700,	Autoimmune disease of lungs and kidneys.		Immune s.
Goodpasture Syndrome	EDTFL	40,250,570,870,2250,2500,226320,321560,515700,682020,	As mentioned above		Immune s.
Churg-Strauss Syndrome	EDTFL	40,230,730,850,5870,73250,324530,342500,596500,875270	Autoimmune respiratory vascular condition.		Immune s.
Evans Syndrome	EDTFL	120,180,650,970,7500,11980,40000,150000,525940,689930,	Autoimmune disease where antibodies attack red blood cells and platelets.		Immune s.
Guillain-Barre Syndrome		Can be caused by the bacterium *Campylobacter jejuni* , and with the viruses *Cytomegalovirus* and *Enterovirus* .			
AIDP [Acute Inflammatory Demyelinating Poly.]		190,350,13320,90000,329000,355080,475160,667000,789000,986220,	Guillain-Barré Syndrome	Guillain-Barre	Immune s.
Landry-Guillain-Barre [GBS]	EDTFL	80,250,570,7600,10530,12600,40000,313350,320000,615000,	Serious autoimmune disorder with rapid-onset muscle weakness, pain, and sensation changes like numbness and/or tingling.	Guillain-Barre	Immune s.
Guillain-Barre Syndrome [GBV, GBS]	EDTFL	80,250,570,7600,10530,12600,40000,313350,320000,615000,	As mentioned above	Guillain-Barre	Immune s.
Guillain-Barre Syndrome	XTRA	20.87,30,41.75,82.59,165,330,727,740,787,880,1234,1550,2600,2650,2900,2950,4412,5000,7344,10000,	As mentioned above	Guillain-Barre	Immune s.
Autoimmune neuropathy (Guillain-Barre syndrome)	BIOM	20.9; 41.8; 82.6; 165; 330; 740; 2600; 2650; 2900; 2950; 7344		Guillain-Barre	Immune s.
Fisher Syndrome [Miller Fisher, also use Guillain-Barré]	EDTFL	20,5250,25150,125750,275030,325750,477500,667000,749000,987230,	Subtype of Guillain-Barre Syndrome, usually without limb weakness.		Immune s.
Miller Fisher Syndrome	EDTFL	20,5250,25150,125750,275030,325750,477500,667000,749000,987230,			Immune s.
GBS Miller Fisher Variant	EDTFL	20,5250,25150,125750,275030,325750,477500,667000,749000,987230			Immune s.

Subject / Argument	Author	Frequencies	Notes	Origin	Target
Ophthalmoplegia, Ataxia and Areflexia Syndrome	EDTFL	70,370,12740,47500,97700,225750,377900,519340,691270,753070	As mentioned above		Immune s.
Lupus General	CAFL	3612=240,2489,2125=240,2010,2008,2006,942,802=480,800,798,702,633=300,632,442,386,243,	Can be caused by the viruses Parvovirus B19, Epstein-Barr virus,Cytomegalovirus and Enterococcus gallinarum.	Lupus	Immune s.
Lupus	BIO	205,243,244,352,386,633,921,942,993,1333,1464,	Autoimmune disease involving joints, skin, kidneys, blood cells, heart, and lungs. Use Nanobacter and Parasites Flukes sets.	Lupus	Immune s.
Lupus	VEGA	243,352,386,921,942,993,1333,1464,	As mentioned above	Lupus	Immune s.
Lupus	XTRA	8020	As mentioned above	Lupus	Immune s.
Lupus 1	XTRA	205,243,244,352,386,633,921,942,993,1333,1464,	As mentioned above	Lupus	Immune s.
Lupus 2	XTRA	243,352,386,921,942,993,1333,1464,	As mentioned above	Lupus	Immune s.
Systemic lupus erythematosus, basic	BIOM	3612; 2489; 2125; 2010; 2008; 2006; 1464; 1333; 993; 942; 921; 802; 800; 798; 702; 633; 632; 442; 386; 352; 243		Lupus	Immune s.
Systemic lupus erythematosus, secondary	BIOM	205; 244; 304; 352; 481; 633; 664; 678; 771; 784; 847; 880; 1552; 2128; 2180; 7864.5		Lupus	Immune s.
Lupus General Secondary	CAFL	205,244,352,633,771,847,921,993,1333,1464,7865,	As mentioned above	Lupus	Immune s.
Lupus Erythematosus 1	XTRA	243,244,352,386,442,633,660,690,702,727.5,776,787,802,880,921,942,993,1333,1464,1550,1850,2008=480,2125=240,2489,3612=240,	As mentioned above	Lupus	Immune s.
Lupus Erythematosus 2	XTRA	205,304,481,664,678,771,784,842,847,921,1552,2128,2180,7865,	As mentioned above	Lupus	Immune s.
Lupus Erythematosus 3	XTRA	727,776,787,880,1850,	As mentioned above	Lupus	Immune s.
Lupus Erythematosus, Cutaneous Lupus Erythematosus, Systemic	EDTFL	50,520,620,10890,32570,479500,527000,662710,752700,985670,	As mentioned above	Lupus	Immune s.
Lupus Erythematosus, [Subacute]	EDTFL	50,520,620,10890,32570,479500,527000,662710,752700,985670,		Lupus	Immune s.
Lupus Erythematosus, Cutaneous Subacute	EDTFL	50,520,620,10890,32570,479500,527000,662710,752700,985670,		Lupus	Immune s.
Lupus Erythematosus Disseminatus	EDTFL	50,520,620,10890,32570,479500,527000,662710,752700,985670,		Lupus	Immune s.
Libman-Sacks Disease	EDTFL	60,260,650,5710,7000,42500,92800,478500,527000,667000		Lupus	Immune s.
Lupus Systemic Erythematosis SLE	XTRA	633,702,802,2008,2125,2489,3612,	As mentioned above	Lupus	Immune s.
Lupus SLE Secondary	CAFL	304,386,481,664,678,784,880,1552,2008,2128,2180,	As mentioned above	Lupus	Immune s.
Lupus Vulgaris 1	XTRA	727,776,787,800,880,1550,	Lupus Vulgaris is a common form that manifests disfigurement and destruction of skin and cartilage of face. Use Nanobacter and Parasites Flukes sets.	Lupus	Immune s.
Lupus Vulgaris 2	XTRA	800,2489,10000	As mentioned above	Lupus	Immune s.
Polyendocrinopathies, Autoimmune	EDTFL	40,120,950,19300,121440,201330,322550,653020,807500,973340	Heterogeneous group of rare diseases with autoimmune activity against more than one endocrine organ, although other organs can be affected.		Immune s.
Schmidt's Syndrome	EDTFL	190,500,570,950,52300,112500,342500,567500,796500,825270			Immune s.
Polyradiculoneuropathy, Acute Inflammatory	EDTFL	130,520,6750,71250,105150,347500,572500,690000,775870,826900	Autoimmune process that is characterized by progressive areflexic weakness and mild sensory changes		Immune s.
Sjogren's Syndrome	EDTFL	90,540,650,930,5750,87400,255310,525290,675310,878500,	Chronic autoimmune disease where white blood cells destroy moisture producing glands. It can cause profound fatigue, chronic pain, and other problems.		Immune s.
Sicca Syndrome	EDTFL	90,540,650,930,5750,87400,255310,525290,675310,878500	As mentioned above		Immune s.
Granulomatous, Chronic	EDTFL	30,500,700,970,88000,370500,547500,656400,725370,825520			Immune s.
Allergic Granulomatous Angiitis	EDTFL	190,520,750,1780,13930,110530,380000,447500,728980,825270,	Type of vasculitis which destroys blood vessels by inflammation.	b.vessels	Immune s.

Subject / Argument	Author	Frequencies	Notes	Origin	Target

Subject / Argument	Author	Frequencies	Notes	Origin	Target
Hypersensitivity	EDTFL	100,570,950,12850,20000,37100,95790,96500,2 25920,425370	Undesirable immune system reactions like autoimmunity and allergies.		Immune s.
Hypersensitivity	XTRA	33	As mentioned above		Immune s.
Hypersensitivity, Atopic	EDTFL	100,570,950,12850,20000,37100,95790,250000, 475580,527000	Also called Type I hypersensitivity. Type of allergic response.		Immune s.
Hypersensitivity, Immediate	EDTFL	100,570,950,12850,20000,37100,95790,285400, 325110,813320			Immune s.
Hypersensitivity of mucous membranes	BIOM	20; 100; 120; 666; 690; 727; 2008; 2127; 10000			Immune s.
Hypersensitivity, Type I	EDTFL	100,570,950,12850,20000,37100,95790,192500, 375790,926060	Hypersensitivity, Immediate		Immune s.
Hypersensitivity, Type III	EDTFL	100,570,950,12850,20000,37100,95790,321260, 669710,823010	Occurs when antigen-antibody complexes are not completely cleared, causing inflammatory response.		Immune s.
Type III Hypersensitivity	EDTFL	100,570,950,12850,20000,37100,95790,321260, 669710,823010,			Immune s.
Immune Complex Diseases Immune System Diseases	EDTFL	150,240,680,810,32500,197500,332500,555370, 696500,875520,	As mentioned above		Immune s.
IgE-Mediated Hypersensitivity	EDTFL	70,410,710,42500,97500,325170,515700,65000 0,750000,927100			Immune s.
Allergy (General)	EDTFL	40,370,570,850,2500,27500,52500,95750,37579 0,871000,			Allergy
Allergies 1	CAFL	2.3,72,300,333,444,522,555.1,727,787,880,5000 ,10000,	See Pullularia Pullulans and Sorghum Smut sets.		Allergy
Allergies 2	CAFL	3,330,727,740,787,880,1234,1550,5000,7344,10 000,	See Pullularia Pullulans, and Sorghum Smut sets.		Allergy
Allergy	BIOM	0.7; 0.9; 1.7; 2.5; 2.9; 3.8; 7; 7.5; 8.1; 9.25; 9.4; 19.6; 28; 35.5; 36; 37.5; 36.5; 52; 64; 80.5; 87.5; 90; 97; 98			Allergy
Allergoses	BIOM	23; 30; 160; 3; 330; 727; 740; 787; 835; 880; 1234; 1550; 5000; 7344; 10000			Allergy
Antihistaminic effect	BIOM	0.7; 0.9; 1.75; 2.5; 2.9			Allergy
Effetto antiserotoninico	BIOM	9.6			Allergy
Anaphylaxis	CAFL	10000	Serious rapid allergic reaction.		Allergy
Anaphylaxis	EDTFL	120,750,2500,65000,87300,236420,327650,561 930,714820,978050,	As mentioned above		Allergy
Anaphylactic Reaction	EDTFL	120,750,2500,65000,87300,236420,327850,561 930,714820,978050,			Allergy
Shock, Anaphylactic	EDTFL	120,750,2500,65000,87300,236420,327850,561 930,714820,978050,			Allergy
Allergic diseases	BIOM	15.5; 25; 27.5; 30; 70; 72.5; 75; 77.5; 80; 92.5; 94; 95.5; 99			Allergy
Allergic reactions pilot frequencies	BIOM	0.7; 1.7; 1.75; 8.1; 9.4; 9.6			Allergy
Basic allergy	BIOM	10000; 880; 787; 727; 465; 3; 330; 5000			Allergy
Lymph in allergy - Pilot frequencies	BIOM	15.5; 25; 27.5; 30; 70; 72.5; 75; 77.5; 80; 92.5; 94; 95.5; 99			Allergy
Allergy (Drug)	EDTFL	40,420,610,920,2560,27800,52500,95790,37579 0,871000,			Allergy
Allergy Pollen	XTRA	14514.12,14882.62,14930.22,		Pollen	Allergy
Allergy (Pollen)	EDTFL	40,370,570,850,2500,27500,52500,95750,37579 0,871000,		Pollen	Allergy
Hay Fever	CAFL	880,787,727,20	Only some types.	Pollen	Allergy
Hay Fever	EDTFL	40,370,570,850,2500,27500,52500,95750,37579 0,871000		Pollen	Allergy
Pollen allergy (hay fever)	BIOM	20; 727; 787; 880; 83.5; 80		Pollen	Allergy
Allergic Rhinitis	EDTFL	40,480,780,7500,118000,215430,362510,42206 0,608410,751200,		Pollen	Allergy
Allergic bronchitis	BIOM	0.5; 14; 20; 72; 95; 125; 146; 444; 522; 555; 660; 727; 787; 880; 10000			Allergy
Dust allergy	BIOM	36.5			Allergy
Infection Allergies	XTRA	10000	Use for infection OR allergies.		Allergy
Allergy (Includes Pets, Insect, Bites)	EDTFL	40,460,520,980,3300,22100,83400,95300,37579 0,871000,			Allergy
Cat fur allergy	BIOM	77; 77.5			Allergy
Allergy (Mold Related, Moulds) RDPV3 Group 18	EDTFL	77000,126000,133000,177000,181000,188000,2 32000,242000,277000,288000			Allergy
Injection Allergic Reaction	CAFL	10000	Post-vaccination.		Allergy

Subject / Argument	Author	Frequencies	Notes	Origin	Target
Multiple Chemical Sensitivity	EDTFL	200,250,690,2500,3000,7500,96500,326160,534250,652430	Associated with Morgellons Disease. Also see Chemical Sensitivity Reduce and Chemical Sensitivity.		Allergy
Idiopathic Environmental Allergy	EDTFL	200,250,620,2500,3000,7500,96500,208190,534250,652430			Allergy
Allergy (Food Allergy General)	EDTFL	40,370,570,850,2500,27500,52500,95750,375790,871000,		Food	Allergy
Food Allergies 1	XTRA	10000,880,787,727,3,330,5000		Food	Allergy
Food Allergies 2	XTRA	465,440,380,1600,20522,146		Food	Allergy
Alimentary allergy	BIOM	37.5		Food	Allergy
Baker's Yeast Allergy	CAFL	775,843	Homeopathy preparation.	Food	Allergy
Baker's Yeast	VEGA	775		Food	Allergy
Allergy Dairy (Lactose Related)	EDTFL	40,420,610,920,2560,27800,52500,95790,375790,871000,		Lactose	Allergy
Lactose Intolerance	EDTFL	120,550,850,5500,22500,35690,321000,544100,631170,705000		Lactose	Allergy
Lactose Malabsorption	EDTFL	120,550,850,5500,22500,35690,73300,92500,125240,527810		Lactose	Allergy
Dermal allergy	BIOM	35.5; 36; 36.5; 3; 330; 10000		Skin	Allergy
Allergic dermatitis	BIOM	0.7; 1.7; 8.1; 9.6		Skin	Allergy
Latex Allergy Latex Hypersensitivity	EDTFL	70,370,950,7500,82000,193930,236500,487500,706210,946500,	Latex allergies, with one type potentially life-threatening.	Skin	Allergy
Rubber Allergy	EDTFL	70,370,950,7500,82000,193930,236500,487500,706210,946500		Skin	Allergy
Caeliacia	CAFL	674	It can be caused by the T1L reovirus.	Gluten	Intolerances
Coeliacs disease (gluten-sensitive enteropathy)	BIOM	154; 594; 656; 586; 668; 787; 7958; 665; 674; 7344; 4412; 1550; 1234; 740; 880; 787; 727; 330; 10000; 5000; 30; 5.13; 4.18; 3; 2		Gluten	Intolerances
Celiac Disease	EDTFL	110,550,850,72490,125750,375190,477500,521000,666000,752700		Gluten	Intolerances
Gluten Enteropathy [Celiac Disease]	EDTFL	110,550,850,72490,125750,375190,477500,521000,666000,752700,	Autoimmune disorder of small intestine due to gluten proteins.	Gluten	Intolerances
Sprue, Celiac	EDTFL	110,550,850,72490,125750,375190,477500,521000,666000,752700,		Gluten	Intolerances
Celiac Disease	XTRA	2,3,4.17,5.12,39	As mentioned above	Gluten	Intolerances
Coeliacia	BIO	154,594,656	As mentioned above	Gluten	Intolerances
Coeliacia	VEGA	594,656	As mentioned above	Gluten	Intolerances
Coeliacia	XTRA	154,586,584,656,665,668,674,787,7958,	As mentioned above	Gluten	Intolerances
Stings [Allergy]	EDTFL	40,460,520,980,3330,22100,83400,95300,375790,871000,		Insect	Allergy
Bites and Stings	EDTFL	40,460,520,980,3330,22100,83400,95300,375790,871000,		Insect	Allergy
Sun Allergy	CAFL	3,330,10000	Examine prescription drugs, such as Psoralen, for photo-sensitisation properties. Also called Polymorphic Light Eruption.	Sun	Allergy
Sun Allergy	XTRA	1000	Also called Polymorphic Light Eruption.	Sun	Allergy
Fever Sunstroke	CAFL	20,440,880		Sun	Allergy
Sunstroke	CAFL	444,440,190,3000,95,522,146,880,20,10000,	Drink lots of water and take an electrolyte solution. Use Electrolyte Levels to improve set.	Sun	Allergy
Sunstroke	XTRA	444,1000		Sun	Allergy
Sun stroke (heliosis)	BIOM	10000; 3000; 522; 444; 440; 190; 146		Sun	Allergy
Airsickness Altitude Sickness	EDTF	90,10570,30420,88320,109500,257680,344200,346260,572000,792330,	A sensation which is induced by air travel and altitudes.	Air	Cinetosi
Mountain Sickness [Altitude sickness]	EDTF	90,10570,30420,88310,109500,257680,344600,346270,572000,792330,		Air	Cinetosi
Seasickness	EDTF	30,1830,3230,11860,82360,95300,155260,325140,423200,760020		Sea	Cinetosi

Subject / Argument	Author	Frequencies	Notes	Origin	Target

It is a system that includes the glands, tissues and cells that produce **hormones**. The major endocrine organs are: the **pituitary gland**, the **pineal gland**, **thyroid**, **parathyroid**, **thymus**, the **endocrine pancreas** (alpha and beta cells, delta cells), the **adrenal glands**, **gonads** (ovary and testis).

Subject / Argument	Author	Frequencies	Notes	Origin	Target
Endocrine Systems	BIOM	**4.0; 4.9; 5.5; 9.4**			Endocrine S.
Sympathoadrenal System	BIOM	**1.75**			Endocrine S.
Endocrine System Balance	XTRA	1537			Endocrine S.
Endocrine System Function Normalize	XTRA	537			Endocrine S.
Regulation of Endocrine System	BIOM	662.0; 662.0; 1725.0; 1342.0; 1534.0; 1413.0; 1351.0; 635.0; 635.0; 763.0; 1335.0; 645.0; 1725.0; 1342.0; 645.0			Endocrine S.
Endocrine system, regulation	BIOM	1.2; 2.6; 4; 4.9; 5.5; 9.4; 62; 98			Endocrine S.
Neuroendocrine system, regulation	BIOM	**4; 4.9; 5.5; 9.4**			Endocrine S.
Endocrine system, stimulation	BIOM	662; 1725; 1342; 1534; 1413; 1351; 635; 763; 1335; 645; 10000			Endocrine S.
High Endocrine Production Stimulate	XTRA	645,1342,1725			Endocrine S.
Endocrine Glands Control Frequencies	BIOM	**85; 87.5; 90; 98**			Endocrine S.
Endocrine RX	XTRA	635,645,662,763,1335,1342,1351,1413,1534,1725,10000,			Endocrine S.
Hypothalamus	BIOM	**7.5; 15; 100**		Hypothalamus	Endocrine S.
Hypothalamus Balance	XTRA	15.42,537	Part of brain which links the nervous system with the endocrine system.	Hypothalamus	Endocrine S.
Hypothalamus Stimulate Normal Function	XTRA	1534,1413,1351	As mentioned above	Hypothalamus	Endocrine S.
Hormonal Imbalances	CAFL	5.5	Also use Circulation and/or Circulatory set(s).		Endocrine S.
Hormonal Disorders General	EDTFL	150,230,650,930,37500,130720,326600,525790, 693300,712500			Endocrine S.
Epiphysis	BIOM	2.5; 7.5; 20; 96; 100		Epiphysis	Endocrine S.
Pineal Gland Stimulate	XTRA	20		Pineal G,	Endocrine S.
Pineal Function Normalize Stimulate	XTRA	480		Pineal G,	Endocrine S.
Pineal Function Stimulate Normalize	XTRA	662,480		Pineal G,	Endocrine S.
Pineal Gland Balance	XTRA	20,537,662	The pineal gland produces melatonin, a serotonin-derived hormone which modulates sleep patterns in both circadian and seasonal cycles.	Pineal G,	Endocrine S.
Pineal Gland Fever	XTRA	20,10000		Pineal G,	Endocrine S.
Circadian Rhythm Resynchronization	XTRA	10	Re-establish normal sleep/waking cycles.	Pineal G,	Endocrine S.
Melatonin	XTRA	3716.512	Experimental - based on molar weight. Hormone regulating circadian rhythms, especially sleep.	Pineal G,	Endocrine S.
Pituitary Gland	XTRA	1.05		Pituitary G.	Endocrine S.
Pituitary Gland	BIOM	2.5; 7.5; 10; 91.5; 94.5; 96; 98		Pituitary G.	Endocrine S.
Pituitary	XTRA	13		Pituitary G.	Endocrine S.
Pituitary gland, anterior	BIOM	**91.5; 94.5; 98**		Pituitary G.	Endocrine S.
Pituitary gland, posterior	BIOM	**92.5; 95.5; 99**		Pituitary G.	Endocrine S.
Hypothalamus-Pituitary Gland	BIOM	**4.0; 4.9; 9.4**		Pituitary G.	Endocrine S.
Pituitary Gland Stimulate	CAFL	4	See Hypophyseal disturbances set.	Pituitary G.	Endocrine S.
Pituitary Function Normalize	XTRA	635	Also see Hypophyseal Disturbances.	Pituitary G.	Endocrine S.
Pituitary HGH Production Stimulate	XTRA	645,1342,1725	Also see Hypophyseal Disturbances.	Pituitary G.	Endocrine S.
Adenohypophyseal Diseases	EDTFL	320,970,2750,15030,71500,196900,275870,419340,612740,858570		Pituitary G.	Endocrine S.
Neurohypophyseal Diseases	EDTFL	80,250,650,2500,8000,77500,196500,315700,524940,660410		Pituitary G.	Endocrine S.
Pituitary Gland Dysfunction	CAFL	1.5,6,8,20	Also see Hypophyseal Disturbances.	Pituitary G.	Endocrine S.
Pituitary Diseases	EDTFL	130,570,6750,71210,101150,347500,579500,690000,775870,816900	Disorders of pituitary gland including Hypothyroidism, Hyperpituitarism, Diabetes Insipidus, tumors, and adenomas. See sets.	Pituitary G.	Endocrine S.
Hypophyseal Disorders	EDTFL	30,550,870,10720,27500,127500,329850,525610,826320,919550		Pituitary G.	Endocrine S.
Hypophyseal Disturbances	CAFL	4	Disruption in creation and transport of pituitary hormones.	Pituitary G.	Endocrine S.

Subject / Argument	Author	Frequencies	Notes	Origin	Target
Empty Sella Syndrome Empty Sella Primary Empty Sella Secondary	EDTFL	90,370,910,128500,236500,302220,491610,651020,708570,879210	Shrinkage or deformation of pituitary gland.	Pituitary G.	Endocrine S.
Hyperpituitarism [Overactive Pituitary]	EDTFL	130,570,6750,71210,101150,347500,579500,690000,775870,816900,	Production of excess pituitary hormones, usually due to pituitary adenoma. Also see Adenoma, and Cancer Adenoma sets.	Pituitary G.	Endocrine S.
Anterior Pituitary Hormone [Adenoma]	EDTFL	130,570,6750,71210,101150,347500,579500,690000,775870,816900,		Pituitary G.	Endocrine S.
Luteinizing Hormone	EDTFL	180,410,580,920,15630,128330,262430,381210,703440,798220		Pituitary G.	Endocrine S.
Inappropriate LH Secretion [Stein-Leventhal Syndrome] Inappropriate [Luteinizing Hormone]	EDTFL	180,410,580,920,15630,128330,262430,381210,703440,798220,	The pituitary gonadotropins FSH and LH are the main regulators of ovarian function.	Pituitary G.	Endocrine S.
Hypopituitarism	EDTFL	70,120,750,830,32750,107500,320450,350000,476290,605680		Pituitary G.	Endocrine S.
Panhypopituitarism	EDTFL	60,500,47500,150000,210500,219340,322350,434500,515160,688290		Pituitary G.	Endocrine S.
Sheehan Syndrome [Raynaud]	EDTFL	570,780,900,5250,7000,115710,255830,485430,691500,825000,		Pituitary G.	Endocrine S.
Simmonds Disease	EDTFL	230,850,7500,24500,32500,151640,312500,434500,705670,869340	Underactive pituitary gland. See Pituitary sets.	Pituitary G.	Endocrine S.
Adenohypophyseal Hyposecretion	EDTF	130,570,6750,71210,101150,347500,579500,690000,775870,816900,		Pituitary G.	Endocrine S.
Parathyroid glands, regulation	BIOM	4.59; 9.5; 9.6; 62.5		Parathyroid	Endocrine S.
Parathyroid Diseases	EDTFL	80,220,730,2700,5710,50000,322530,415700,566410,707260,	Disorders of parathyroid gland's function, usually causing Hyperparathyroidism - see set.	Parathyroid	Endocrine S.
Hyperparathyroidism	CAFL	4.6,9.5,9.6	Overactivity of parathyroid glands resulting in excess of parathyroid hormone.	Parathyroid	Endocrine S.
Hypoparathyroidism	EDTFL	80,220,730,2700,5710,50000,322530,415700,566410,707260		Parathyroid	Endocrine S.
Thyroid	XTRA	12		Thyroid	Endocrine S.
Thyroid Support	XTRA	160		Thyroid	Endocrine S.
Thyroid Function Stimulate Normalize	XTRA	763		Thyroid	Endocrine S.
Thyroid gland, regulation	BIOM	9.5; 12; 85; 87.5; 90; 98		Thyroid	Endocrine S.
Inappropriate Thyroid Stimulating Hormone [TSH]	EDTFL	170,520,750,950,2500,7500,325950,682020,759810,927100,		Thyroid	Endocrine S.
Inappropriate TSH Secretion	EDTFL	170,520,750,950,2500,7500,325950,682020,759810,927100,		Thyroid	Endocrine S.
Thyroid Balance and Normalize 1	XTRA	160,763,660,690,727.5,		Thyroid	Endocrine S.
Thyroid Balance and Normalize 2	XTRA	20,537,1570,10000,16000,		Thyroid	Endocrine S.
Hyperthyroid 1	CAFL	3,0.5	Excess production of thyroid hormone, leading to Thyrotoxicosis.	Thyroid	Endocrine S.
Hyperthyroid 2	XTRA	0.5,3,20,160	As mentioned above	Thyroid	Endocrine S.
Hyperthyroidism	EDTFL	70,410,780,3210,88520,109690,215230,505790,615580,725790	As mentioned above	Thyroid	Endocrine S.
Thyroid gland, hyperthyroidism	BIOM	3; 62		Thyroid	Endocrine S.
Hypothyroid 1	CAFL	2,12,35,16000,10000,160,80,20,	Underproduction of thyroid hormone, mainly caused by lack of iodine in the diet, or by Hashimoto's. See Goiter, and Struma sets.	Thyroid	Endocrine S.
Hypothyroid 2	XTRA	2,12,20,35,80,160,10000,16000,		Thyroid	Endocrine S.
Hypothyroid 3	XTRA	7.7,12,20,35,160,740,802,1550,16000,		Thyroid	Endocrine S.
Hypothyroidism	EDTFL	80,220,730,2700,5710,50000,322530,415700,566410,707260	Underproduction of thyroid hormone, mainly caused by lack of iodine in the diet, or by Hashimoto's. See Goiter, and Struma sets.	Thyroid	Endocrine S.
Congenital Hypothyroidism	EDTFL	80,220,730,2700,5710,50000,322530,415700,566410,707260,	Underactive thyroid from birth. Cretinism or congenital iodine deficiency syndrome is a condition in which there is permanent mental and physical deficiency and is usually caused by hypothyroidism.	Thyroid	Endocrine S.
Thyroid gland, hypothyroidism	BIOM	2; 12; 35; 1600; 10000; 200; 160; 80; 20		Thyroid	Endocrine S.
Cretinism	EDTFL	170,350,12800,89300,125680,243000,470000,532500,615230,762010		Thyroid	Endocrine S.

Subject / Argument	Author	Frequencies	Notes	Origin	Target
Endocrine Diseases [Thyroid Set]	EDTFL	190,950,2500,7500,15000,33000,426900,571000,836000,932000,		Thyroid	Endocrine S.
Thyroid Disease	EDTFL	190,950,2500,7500,15000,33000,426900,571000,836000,932000,		Thyroid	Endocrine S.
Thyroid Nodule	EDTFL	180,490,750,950,2500,7500,112360,325950,754370,815680	Abnormal growths of thyroid tissue, few of which are cancerous.	Thyroid	Endocrine S.
Thyroid Gland Fever	XTRA	20,160,660,690,727.5,1570,10000,16000,		Thyroid	Endocrine S.
Thyroiditis Thyroiditis, Lymphomatous Thyroiditis, Subacute	EDTFL	190,950,2500,7500,15000,33000,426900,571000,836000,932000	Inflammation of thyroid gland. Can be caused by drugs or radiation. Includes Hashimoto's. Also see Hypothyroid, and Hypothyroidism sets.	Thyroid	Endocrine S.
Autoimmune Thyroiditis	EDTFL	190,950,2500,7500,15000,33000,426900,571000,836000,932000,		Thyroid	Endocrine S.
Allergic thyroiditis	BIOM	20; 727; 787; 880; 3; 0.5		Thyroid	Endocrine S.
Thyroiditis, Lymphocytic	EDTFL	120,140,650,2500,32500,97500,225110,422530,707260,985900		Thyroid	Endocrine S.
De Quervain Thyroiditis	EDTFL	190,950,2500,7500,15000,33000,426900,571000,836000,932000,		Thyroid	Endocrine S.
Thyroid Stimulating Hormone	EDTFL	170,520,750,950,2500,7500,325950,682020,759810,927100		Thyroid	Endocrine S.
Thyroid Hormone Resistance Syndrome	EDTFL	10,220,32500,52500,150000,175110,479930,667000,789000,987230	Rare condition where thyroid hormone levels are elevated but the thyroid stimulating hormone (TSH) level is not suppressed.	Thyroid	Endocrine S.
Refetoff [Thyroid Hormone Resistance]	EDTFL	100,220,32500,52500,150000,175110,479930,667000,789000,987230,	As mentioned above	Thyroid	Endocrine S.
Struma	CAFL	105,121,122,321,361,517,531,532,576,651,714,756,5311,	Swelling of neck or larynx due to enlargement of dysfunctional thyroid gland, usually because of iodine deficiency. Also see Struma sets.	Goiter	Endocrine S.
Goiter 1	CAFL	105,121,122,321,361,517,531,532,576,651,714,756,5311,	As mentioned above	Goiter	Endocrine S.
Goiter 2	XTRA	20,727,787,880,5000,16000,	As mentioned above	Goiter	Endocrine S.
Goiter 3	XTRA	20,160,660,690,727.5,787,880,16000,	As mentioned above	Goiter	Endocrine S.
Goiter, diffuse-toxic	BIOM	20; 121; 576; 727; 787; 880; 5000		Goiter	Endocrine S.
Goiter Struma Cystica	XTRA	361,531,756,5311		Goiter	Endocrine S.
Struma Cystica	BIO	5311	Use if swelling involves cysts.	Goiter	Endocrine S.
Goiter, cystic	BIOM	5310.5; 531; 756; 517; 532; 651; 714; 576; 361; 321; 105; 122; 121		Goiter	Endocrine S.
Goiter Struma Nodosa	XTRA	105,122,321,517,532,651,714,	Use if condition is multi-nodular.	Goiter	Endocrine S.
Struma Nodosa	CAFL	105,122,321,517,532,651,714,	As mentioned above	Goiter	Endocrine S.
Struma Nodosa	VEGA	122,321,517,532,651,	As mentioned above	Goiter	Endocrine S.
Goiter, nodular	BIOM	105; 122; 321; 517; 532; 651; 714	As mentioned above	Goiter	Endocrine S.
Goiter Struma Parenchyma	XTRA	121,576	Use if swelling involves kidneys.	Goiter	Endocrine S.
Struma Parenchyma	BIO	121	As mentioned above	Goiter	Endocrine S.
Graves Disease and Goiter	XTRA	20,727,787,880	Autoimmune disorder affecting thyroid gland, often causing Hyperthyroidism (see sets) and enlargement. Also see Hyperthyroid.	Goiter	Endocrine S.
Basedow's Disease	EDTFL	80,430,55610,119870,232220,308290,455520,585370,697500,825910,	As mentioned above	Goiter	Endocrine S.
Graves Disease [Toxic Diffuse Goiter]	EDTFL	40,1520,14750,71870,152250,217500,320550,492500,675540,775350	Can be caused by EBV infection	Goiter	Endocrine S.
Exophthalmic Goiter	EDTFL	120,550,950,5290,95520,142500,362500,402500,590000,822530,	As mentioned above	Goiter	Endocrine S.
Thymus	XTRA	10.5	It brings to fruition the various types of lymphocytes, finalizing to destroy intracellular pathogens (T lymphocytes)	Thymus	Endocrine S.
Thymus	BIOM	69; 79		Thymus	Endocrine S.
Thymus - Pilot frequencies	BIOM	17; 38; 38.5; 56; 25; 63.5; 69; 74.5; 79		Thymus	Endocrine S.
Thymus Gland Stimulant	XTRA	20,727,787,880,5000,		Thymus	Endocrine S.
Thymus Stimulation	CAFL	20		Thymus	Endocrine S.
Adrenal Glands-2	BIOM	52.75; 53.0; 53.5		Adrenals	Endocrine S.
Adrenal Cortex	BIOM	1.2; 2.6		Adrenals	
Adrenal Gland Stimulant 1	CAFL	10,20,2250		Adrenals	Endocrine S.
Adrenal Gland Stimulant 2	CAFL	10,20=360,72,95=360,125,428,440,444,450,522,600,625,650,660,666,685,690,700,727,760,787,832,880,1500,1600,1865,1800,1865,2127,2170,2720,3000,		Adrenals	Endocrine S.

Subject / Argument	Author	Frequencies	Notes	Origin	Target
Adrenal Gland Stimulant 3	XTRA	10,20,72,95,125,428,440,444,450,522,600,625,6 50,660,666,685,690,700,727,760,776,787,832,8 80,1500,1550,1600,1800,1865,2008,2127,2170, 2720,3000,		Adrenals	Endocrine S.
Adrenal Function Normalize	XTRA	1335		Adrenals	Endocrine S.
Adrenal Gland Balance	XTRA	20,537,1335,2250,10000,12000,		Adrenals	Endocrine S.
Adrenal Gland Diseases	EDTFL KHZ	70,5500,73300,134250,357300,454370,519680, 689410,712230,993410,		Adrenals	Endocrine S.
Adrenal Gland Disorders	BIOM	9.44		Adrenals	Endocrine S.
Adrenal Gland Hypofunction	BIOM	53.0		Adrenals	Endocrine S.
Adrenal Hyperplasia	EDTFL KHZ	220,970,52500,93500,236420,376290,426900,5 71000,813000,932000,	Congenital. May cause vomiting and sexual development problems.	Adrenals	Endocrine S.
Detox Adrenal Gland	XTRA	20,10000,12000		Adrenals	Endocrine S.
Adrenalin, stimulation of production	BIOM	465; 40; 10; 2250		Adrenals	Endocrine S.
Nelson Syndrome	EDTFL	20,540,620,890,113500,142530,285020,412030, 528230,775560	Rare disorder which only occurs in those who have had both adrenals surgically removed.	Adrenals	Endocrine S.
Addison's Disease	EDTFL	190,750,900,7500,27500,222700,425710,56319 0,642910,978050,	Chronic adrenal insufficiency. See Adrenal sets.	Adrenals	Endocrine S.
Luteosterone	BIOM	3.5		Woman	Endocrine S.
Women's hormonal balance	BIOM	2.5; 3.5; 4.0; 4.9; 9.4; 9.5		Woman	Endocrine S.
Women's sexual glands	BIOM	3.5; 4.9; 98; 98.5; 98.75		Woman	Endocrine S.
Mammary gland	BIOM	2.5; 2.6; 3; 4; 4.9; 5.5; 9.4; 14.5; 20; 22; 25.5; 42; 49; 64; 63; 79.5; 85.5; 98; 91.5		Woman	Endocrine S.
Mammary gland, regulation	BIOM	91.5; 14.5; 3		Woman	Endocrine S.
Men's hormonal balance	BIOM	3.5; 5.5		Men	Endocrine S.
Hormonal Imbalances Male	XTRA	50.5,537,	Also use Circulation and/or Circulatory set(s).	Men	Endocrine S.
Men's sexual glands	BIOM	3.5; 51; 51.5; 57		Men	Endocrine S.
Gynecomastia	EDTFL	160,570,800,51710,195310,352500,595900,619 350,797610,891270	Endocrine system disorder with non-cancerous development of breasts in males. May also be caused by certain medications.	Men	Endocrine S.
Follicle Stimulating Hormone	EDTFL	30,120,930,7500,132310,247550,362540,59652 0,695610,819340			Endocrine S.
Inappropriate Follicle Stimulating Hormone Secretion	EDTFL	30,120,930,7480,132310,247550,362540,59652 0,695610,819340,			Endocrine S.
Inappropriate FSH Secretion	EDTFL	20,300,850,32880,234510,425680,571000,6627 10,879000,938000			Endocrine S.
Normalize Estrogen Production Male and Female	XTRA	1351			Endocrine S.
Hyperestrogen Hormonal Disorders Hyperestrogen Hormonal Disorder Oestrogen	EDTFL	150,230,650,2270,34200,123420,286330,52579 0,693300,712500			Endocrine S.
Progesterone Normalize Level	XTRA	763,1446,1443	Female hormone.	Woman	Endocrine S.
Hormone Disorders Testosterone	EDTFL	30,500,850,7500,8000,127500,326600,525790,7 25000,825790		Men	Endocrine S.
Testosterone Female Normalize Level	XTRA	1445		Woman	Endocrine S.
Testosterone Male Normalize Level	XTRA	1444		Men	Endocrine S.
Cells of Leydig	CAFL	2500	Testosterone-producing cells in testicles.	Testicle	Endocrine S.
Growth	XTRA	183.58			Endocrine S.
Growth Hormone	XTRA	1.05	Also called HGH.		Endocrine S.
Inappropriate Growth Hormone [GHD]	EDTFL	180,410,580,920,15630,128330,262430,381210, 703440,798220,			Endocrine S.
Growth, regulation	BIOM	2.5			Endocrine S.
Growth, stimulation	BIOM	47			Endocrine S.
Somatotropin Hypersecretion	EDTFL	2690,4220,5500,33500,42540,55820,191090,32 4930,662710,749000	Skull/brow/jaw expansion and soft tissue/organ swelling. Due to excess pituitary growth hormone production.		Endocrine S.
Aldosteronism	EDTFL	80,260,780,2500,17500,255870,321550,405000, 645870,723580,	Excess aldosterone produced by the adrenal glands - can lead to low blood potassium levels (hypokalemia).		Endocrine S.

Subject / Argument	Author	Frequencies	Notes	Origin	Target
Hyperaldosteronism	EDTFL	200,250,750,2530,3400,5580,95870,175910,425 870,571400	As mentioned above		Endocrine S.

8 - Nervous System

8a - Mind, Psyche and Soul

Subject / Argument	Author	Frequencies	Notes	Origin	Target
Brain alpha rhythm	BIOM	7.84			Mind
Brain beta rhythm	BIOM	15; 13; 18			Mind
Brain delta rhythm	BIOM	5; 1.8; 3.5			Mind
Brain theta rhythm	BIOM	4; 5.5; 7			Mind
Detox Mental Disorders	XTRA	4.9,20,72,95,125,146,428,522,550,802,10000,			Mind
Schizophrenia		*Can be caused by Bornavirus, Chlamydia trachomatis, Borrelia and neonatal infection by Coxsackie B virus (an enterovirus). The influenza virus in the first trimester of pregnancy increases the risk of schizophrenia by 7-fold.*			
Schizophrenia	EDTFL	250,780,930,7500,10890,95900,323510,415700, 562910,742060			Mind
Schizophrenic Disorders	EDTFL	250,780,930,7500,10890,95900,323510,415700, 714820,978050			Mind
Schizophreniform Disorders	EDTFL	250,780,930,7500,10890,137250,545750,68750 0,895270,976290			Mind
Multiple Personality [schizophrenia]	EDTFL	250,780,930,7500,10890,95900,323510,415700, 562910,742060,			Mind
Schizophrenia Paranoid 1	CAFL	802,1500,1550	Use Tuberculosis sets.		Mind
Schizoaffective [Schizophrenia & Mood]	EDTFL	50,460,900,7500,10890,95900,323510,415700,5 62910,742060,			Mind
Psychoses	EDTFL	60,490,680,7100,102500,231700,472500,62569 0,705200,857200			Mind
Psychosis, Brief Reactive	EDTFL	160,350,950,5500,27800,47500,350000,425310, 571000,859000			Mind
Psychosis, Manic-Depressive	EDTFL	160,350,950,5120,27150,52500,127500,234250, 842000,937440			Mind
Psychotropic	BIOM	2.2			Mind
Psychotic Disorders	EDTFL	160,350,950,5500,27800,47500,350000,415700, 562910,742060			Mind
Mental Disorders	CAFL	522,146,10000,125,95,72,20,4.9,428,550,802,	General aid, especially if toxins are the cause. Use a good mineral supplement.		Mind
Minimal Brain Dysfunction	EDTFL	150,180,2320,63770,72300,132200,220300,587 300,722520,915200			Mind
Hysterical Symptoms	XTRA	20,727,787,880,5000,			Mind
Munchausen Syndrome	KHZ	10,240,750,4850,182510,219290,412110,50529 0,881000,905090,	Factitious disorder where sufferers feign disease, illness, or psychological trauma to fain attention, sympathy, or reassurance.		Mind
Capgras Syndrome	EDTFL	150,930,2500,41500,71500,97500,125750,4340 00,642910,983170	Belief that someone known has been replaced by an impostor. Thought to be due to neuroanatomical damage.		Mind
Dysmorphophobia	EDTFL	180,390,630,7300,72500,97500,160180,202000, 390000,779730	Symptoms suggesting physical illness or injury that cannot be explained by a medical condition or the direct effect of a substance, and not attributable to another mental disorder.		Mind
Pain Disorder	EDTFL	160,350,950,5260,14500,17500,72500,215700,4 56500,517500	As mentioned above		Mind
Somatization Disorder	EDTFL	950,2250,32500,67500,97500,322060,375170,4 97610,653690,750000	As mentioned above		Mind
Somatoform [Briquet Syndrome]	EDTFL	40,250,970,9000,73890,123400,257510,302580, 592480,875430,	As mentioned above		Mind
Briquet Syndrome	EDTFL	40,250,970,9000,73890,123400,257510,302580, 592480,875430	As mentioned above		Mind
Unconscious Mind	XTRA	211.44			Mind
Personality Disorder, Borderline	EDTFL	70,240,3500,5210,8600,53000,275360,561510,6 98100,812770	Pattern of abnormal behavior with impulsivity, unstable emotions, inconsistent relationships, and poor self-image.		Mind
Personality Disorder, Dependent	EDTFL	70,220,730,1700,5300,53000,275360,561510,69 8100,812770,			Mind
Dissociative Disorders Dissociative Identity Disorder	EDTFL	260,650,5150,10530,42500,65310,95900,22583 0,455820,805330	Disruptions or breakdowns of memory, awareness, identity, or perception.		Mind
Dissociation	EDTFL	260,650,5150,10530,42500,65310,95900,22583 0,455820,805330,			Mind
Fugue	EDTFL	130,570,780,970,2560,87500,323980,665400,82 2700,906070			Mind
Hysteria, Dissociative	EDTFL	70,220,620,2500,7500,41010,119340,475690,52 4000,667000			Mind
Puerperal Disorders	EDTFL	100,260,680,7500,11020,45000,325430,515700, 682450,755460	Disorders arising during the postnatal period (about six weeks).		Mind

Subject / Argument	Author	Frequencies	Notes	Origin	Target
Anankastic Personality Disorder	EDTFL	190,750,1420,5250,25510,42570,326700,49283 0,671510,808530,	Also called Obsessive Compulsive Personality Disorder (OCPD).Can be caused by **Streptococcus** and **Borrelia**.		Mind
Hallucinations 1	CAFL	10000,880,787,727,20,			Mind
Hallucinations 2	XTRA	20,660,690,727.5,787,880,10000,			Mind
Hallucinations	EDTFL	80,220,730,2800,5710,50000,322560,415700,56 6410,707260			Mind
Charles Bonnet Syndrome	EDTFL	60,320,830,12330,225170,322650,452590,6830 00,712230,993410			Mind
Imagination	XTRA	211.44			Mind
Mental Contact	XTRA	3,582,295			Mind
Cleverness	XTRA	141.27			Mind
Center of thinking	BIOM	47.5			Mind
Mental Function Improve	XTRA	20.8	Schumann frequency.		Mind
Mental Function Stimulate	XTRA	35,			Mind
Intellectual Ability	XTRA	15.4			Mind
Intelligence and Clarity of Thought	CAFL	20,10000			Mind
Mental Clarity Stimulate	XTRA	12			Mind
Clarity of Thought/Mental Function Stimulate	XTRA	35			Mind
Intuition Awakening	XTRA	741	Solfeggio Frequency.		Mind
Center of intuition	BIOM	7.5			Mind
Center of creativity	BIOM	57.5; 99; 100			Mind
Creative Thought	XTRA	7.5			Mind
Creative Visualization	XTRA	6,10			Mind
Creativity	XTRA	8.22,183.58			Mind
Child Disorders	XTRA	20,727,787,880			Mind
Confused Thinking	XTRA	7.5			Mind
Dyslexia	XTRA	1.45		Dyslexia	Mind
Dyslexia	BIOM	7.5; 42.5; 47.5; 56.5		Dyslexia	Mind
Dyslexia Symptoms	EDTFL	150,230,620,950,7500,212850,455980,557400,7 96500,891500		Dyslexia	Mind
Reading Disability Reading Disorder	EDTFL	180,550,1000,7500,30000,42500,72500,90000,9 5750,519340			Mind
Attention deficit hyperactivity disorder		*Are associated with the bacteria **Borrelia burgdorferi** and **Streptococcus**, and with **HIV** and **Enterovirus 71**. Febrile seizures due to **Human Herpesvirus 6** or **Influenza A** are a risk factor for ADHD.*			
Attention Deficit Disorder	CAFL	428,444,450,465,470,471,621,660,727,760,762, 769,770,787,802,832,880,940.1,942.9,1550,188 0,1885.9,3760.3,3771.7,5000,7520.5,	Probably important to avoid preservatives, aspartame, dyes, and other potential toxins.	ADD	Mind
Ability to concentrate attention	BIOM	80; 81		ADD	Mind
Lack of attention	BIOM	7.8; 8		ADD	Mind
Attention Deficit Disorder with Hyperactivity	KHZ	10,250,460,320,520,750,42500,87500,132410,3 76290,	Also called ADHD. May be important to avoid preservatives, aspartame, dyes, and other toxins.	ADD	Mind
Attention Deficit Disorder ADD with Hyperactivity	EDTFL	40,250,460,320,520,750,42500,87500,132410,3 76290,		ADD	Mind
Counting problems	BIOM	37.5		ADD	Mind
Hyperkinetic Syndrome	EDTFL	170,180,840,7590,87330,132510,345030,65750 0,792500,925790		ADD	Mind
Attention Deficit Disorder	XTRA	10	ADD/hyperactivity.	ADD	Mind
Absentmindedness	CAFL	5.8		ADD	Mind
Nonverbal Learning Disorder	EDTFL	160,320,950,7500,32500,47500,95290,376290,6 75290,727000	Neurological disorder characterized by verbal strengths and visual-spatial, motor, and social skills difficulties.	ADD	Mind
Communication Disorders	EDTFL	120,240,700,1970,112750,217500,435270,6574 00,895000,925270			Mind
Dyscalculia [Learning Disability]	EDTFL	150,230,620,950,7500,212850,455980,557400,7 96500,891500,			Mind
Communication	XTRA	141.27			Mind
Center of speech	BIOM	67.5			Mind
Aprosodia	EDTFL	180,1070,4820,15250,58210,109420,324600,38 7020,434270,611050,	Neurological language/speech disorder.		Mind
Speech Disorders	EDTFL	60,320,900,32500,67500,97500,325450,519340, 691270,754190	As mentioned above		Mind
Stuttering	EDTFL	30,460,830,37500,62500,150000,225750,51934 0,652430,927100	As mentioned above		Mind

Subject / Argument	Author	Frequencies	Notes	Origin	Target
Stuttering	BIOM	7.83; 62.5; 10000			Mind
Dysphasia [Speech Impairment]	EDTFL	150,230,620,950,7500,212850,455980,557400,7 96500,891500,	Speech disorder consisting of the inability to order words according to a logical pattern.		Mind
Mutism	EDTF	170,1220,3720,17270,63230,119420,293240,40 3030,435000,711170	Inability to speak often caused by speech disorder, hearing loss, or surgery.		Mind
Anomia	EDTFL	560,800,920,37000,175330,275000,379930,450 000,519680,883000	Language disorder - problems recalling words or names		Mind
Color Anomia	EDTFL	280,750,810,980,107410,128310,317300,51710 0,609420,717210			Mind
Dysnomia [Memory & Learning Disorder]	EDTFL	150,230,620,950,7500,212850,455980,557400,7 96500,891500,			Mind
Aphasia Aphasia Acquired Aphasia, Amnesic Aphasia, Anomic Aphasia, Nominal	EDTFL	140,620,850,5070,12850,327450,453720,68481 0,712810,993410,	Language/speech disorders.		Mind
Aphasia, Acquired Epileptic	EDTFL	150,250,8620,17220,82500,115870,325000,491 580,673350,874540,			Mind
Landau-Kleffner Syndrome [epileptic aphasia]	EDTFL	150,250,8620,17220,82500,115870,325000,491 580,673350,874540,	Rare neurological disorder where children suddenly or gradually lose understanding and use of language.		Mind
Knowing Non-linear	XTRA	741	Solfeggio Frequency.		Mind
Language Accelerated Retention	XTRA	3.5			Mind
Information Processing Heighten	XTRA	40			Mind
Perception Heighten	XTRA	40			Mind
Accelerate Learning	XTRA	6.3			Mind
Learning Advanced	XTRA	7.83	Schumann frequency.		Mind
Mental Concentration	CAFL	10000,7.82			Mind
Concentration and Creative Thinking	XTRA	27.3			Mind
Concentration Improve	XTRA	5.79,7.83,20,35,10000,			Mind
Concentration	CAFL	7.82,10000			Mind
Concentration	XTRA	147.85			Mind
Concentration	BIOM	80; 81			Mind
Study Aid	XTRA	14.3	Schumann frequency.		Mind
Teaching	XTRA	6.79			Mind
Speech	XTRA	8.22			Mind
Speech Center	XTRA	141.27			Mind
Formal Concepts	XTRA	10.7			Mind
Amnesia	EDTFL	70,2250,87500,92500,275000,432410,564280,6 40000,690280,978050,	Memory loss.	Memory	Mind
Test-taking Improve	XTRA	398		Memory	Mind
Memory Centre	BIOM	90		Memory	Mind
Memory	BIOM	10000; 20		Memory	Mind
Memory Increase Retention	XTRA	6.3		Memory	Mind
Memory Long-term	XTRA	6		Memory	Mind
Memory Reading Spelling Improve	XTRA	10,18		Memory	Mind
Agnosia	EDTF	130,900,5620,93500,222200,425000,522530,68 9930,752630,923700	Inability to process information from one sensory system, usually after brain injury or illness.	Agnosia	Mind
Auditory Agnosia	EDTFL	130,900,5620,93500,222200,425000,522530,68 9930,752630,923700,	As mentioned above	Agnosia	Mind
Finger Agnosia	EDTFL	130,570,780,900,2250,144900,323720,602530,6 03210,918280	As mentioned above	Agnosia	Mind
Sensory Agnosia	EDTFL	130,900,5620,93500,222200,425000,522530,68 9930,752630,923700,	As mentioned above	Agnosia	Mind
Tactile Agnosia	EDTFL	180,430,7500,13980,132470,275750,512380,65 5000,753050,926300,	As mentioned above	Agnosia	Mind
Visual Agnosia	EDTFL	130,900,5620,93500,222200,425000,522530,68 9930,752630,923700,	As mentioned above	Agnosia	Mind
Prosopagnosia	EDTFL	160,1220,3720,17290,63210,119420,293250,40 3030,435000,711170	Impairment of ability to recognize faces, including one's own.		Mind
Facial Recognition Agnosia [Visual Agnosia]	EDTFL	130,900,5620,93500,222200,425000,522530,68 9930,752630,923700,	As mentioned above		Mind

Subject / Argument	Author	Frequencies	Notes	Origin	Target
Antidepressive	XTRA	172.06		Depression	Mind
Antidepressant	BIOM	5.8; 9.6		Depression	Mind
Antidepressant	BIOM	3.0; 7.83		Depression	Mind
Non-drug antidepressant	BIOM	5.5; 17.5; 31.5; 32; 72.5; 91.5; 91.5; 94.5		Depression	Mind
Depression		Can be caused by *Cytomegalovirus, West Nile virus* and the protozoan *Toxoplasma gondii*. Major depressive disorder can be caused by *Borna virus*, *Bartonella* and *Borrelia* bacteria.			
Easily Depressed	XTRA	727,787,880,10000	Avoid starches, use a multivitamin and multi-mineral supplement. Drink pure water - minimum 2.5 litres daily.	Depression	Mind
Depression General	CAFL	1.1,3.5,7.83,35,73,787,800,3176,5000,10000,	As mentioned above	Depression	Mind
Depression General 2	XTRA	5000,9999,10000,20000,		Depression	Mind
Depression General 3	XTRA	73,787,800		Depression	Mind
Mental depression	BIOM	91.5; 92.5; 94.5; 99.5; 10000		Depression	Mind
Depression	BIOM	5.8; 9.6		Depression	Mind
Depression	BIOM	1000.0; 5000.0; 3176.0; 800.0; 787.0; 73.0; 35.0; 33.0; 26.0; 14.0; 7.83; 3.5		Depression	Mind
Depression of unclear aetiology	BIOM	1.2; 3.5; 5.8; 9.5; 9.6; 31.75; 84		Depression	Mind
Depressive Disorder	EDTFL	150,200,900,2750,5120,52500,102320,362570,601680,775620,	Also called Clinical Depression or Unipolar Disorder.	Depression	Mind
Depressive Syndrome	EDTFL	150,200,900,2750,5120,52500,235000,547500,725080,923000,		Depression	Mind
Depression, Endogenous	EDTFL	150,200,900,2750,5120,52500,472000,532500,695230,762020,		Depression	Mind
Depression, Neurotic	EDTFL	150,200,900,2750,5120,52500,96400,175870,350770,452570,		Depression	Mind
Depression Due to Outside Circumstances	CAFL	35,787	Avoid starches, use a multivitamin and multi-mineral supplement. Drink pure water - minimum 2.5 litres daily.	Depression	Mind
Depression, Postpartum	EDTFL	150,200,900,2750,5120,52500,231530,347050,402500,717530,		Depression	Mind
Unipolar Depression	EDTFL	160,200,850,7500,8250,52500,61000,65540,99500,322050,		Depression	Mind
Frustration	BIOM	32.5			Mind
Neurosis	CAFL	28		Neurosis	Mind
Neurosis	BIOM	28; 200; 664; 764; 1000		Neurosis	Mind
Hyperphrenia	BIOM	6.3		Neurosis	Mind
Neurosis, Depressive	EDTFL	160,350,950,5120,27150,52500,127500,234250,842000,937440,		Neurosis	Mind
Neurosis, Obsessive-Compulsve	EDTFL	130,230,620,6950,27500,85540,122710,453010,743540,836420,		Neurosis	Mind
Obsessive-Compulsive Disorder	EDTFL	130,230,620,6950,27500,85540,122710,453010,743540,836420		Neurosis	Mind
Neurosis, Hypochondriacal	EDTFL	80,620,950,5120,27250,42500,95950,727330,841120,903910		Neurosis	Mind
PTSD [Post-Traumatic Stress Disorder]	EDTFL	140,680,2500,60000,122530,300000,496010,655200,750000,912330,		PTSD	Mind
Neurosis, Post-Traumatic	EDTFL	140,680,2500,60000,122530,300000,496010,655200,750000,912330,		PTSD	Mind
War Neuroses [PTSD]	EDTFL	140,680,2500,60000,122530,300000,496010,655200,750000,912330,		PTSD	Mind
Combat Disorders [PTSD]	EDTFL	140,680,2500,60000,122530,300000,496010,655200,750000,912330,	High stress situations.	PTSD	Mind
Seasonal Affective Disorder	EDTFL	50,330,3500,8830,42370,115380,240000,373220,741000,835320	Mental state and sometimes behavioral changes in response to seasonal patterns. Can be caused by *Epstein-Barr virus*.	Neurosis	Mind
Manic-Depressive Psychosis	EDTFL	150,370,900,2750,5120,52500,127500,234250,842000,937440			Mind
Psychosomatosis	BIOM	764; 664			Mind
Depression Manic	XTRA	263,1,304,802,6000,6130,	Also called Bipolar Disorder and Depression Bipolar - see sets.		Mind
Bipolar Disorder		Can be caused by *Borna virus, Herpes Simplex virus 1, HHV-6A* and by *Borrelia* species bacteria.			
Bipolar Disorder	EDTF	160,2500,10530,45160,62500,293830,425000,571000,833000,932000	Disorder with pronounced transitions between depression and elevation.		Mind
Bipolar Disorder	XTRA	263.1,304,802,6000,6130=300,			Mind
Depression, Bipolar	EDTF	160,200,10530,45160,62500,293830,425000,571000,833000,932000,	Also called Bipolar Disorder - see sets.		Mind
Affective Psychosis , Bipolar	EDTF	160,2500,10530,45160,62500,293830,425000,571000,833000,932000,			Mind

Subject / Argument	Author	Frequencies	Notes	Origin	Target
Sorrow	XTRA	147.85		Mood	Mind
Melancholia [Depression]	EDTFL	160,200,850,7500,8250,52500,61000,65540,99500,322050,		Mood	Mind
Hypochondria	XTRA	1,488,588,	The worry that one may have a serious illness. Also see Hypochondriasis.	Mood	Mind
Hypochondria [Neurosis]	EDTFL	80,620,950,5120,27250,42500,95950,727330,841120,903910,	As mentioned above	Mood	Mind
Exhaustion	XTRA	4		Mood	Mind
Cyclothymic Disorder Cyclothymic Personality	EDTFL	70,200,860,900,5690,7250,30000,55540,93500,322060,	Also called Cyclothymia. Chronic mood disorder less severe than Bipolar Disorder.	Mood	Mind
Dysthymic Disorder	EDTFL	80,120,17850,57710,122020,241400,485830,597540,725380,851170	Mood disorder also called Neurotic or Chronic Depression.	Mood	Mind
Serotonin	XTRA	2.5,10,80,160,	Neurotransmitter involved in regulating mood	Mood	Mind
Mood Elevator	XTRA	10		Mood	Mind
Mood Heighten	XTRA	40		Mood	Mind
Humor	XTRA	144.72		Mood	Mind
Joy Centre	BIOM	17.5		Mood	Mind
Vivacity, joviality	BIOM	77.5; 92.5		Mood	Mind
Joy	XTRA	360		Mood	Mind
Joy	XTRA	1126,1927,3127		Mood	Mind
Fear	XTRA	5.8		Fear	Mind
Fear 1	XTRA	1.1,5.79,73		Fear	Mind
Fears	CAFL	727,787,880,10000		Fear	Mind
Fear and Guilt Liberate	XTRA	396	Solfeggio Frequency.	Fear	Mind
Guilt and Shame	XTRA	126.22			Mind
Fear control	BIOM	5.5; 19; 84; 92.5; 95.5; 98.5			Mind
Center of courage	BIOM	77.5			Mind
Phobias	BIOM	3.9; 6.3; 5.5; 7.8; 61.5; 77.5; 90	Anxiety disorders characterised by fear of objects or situations.	Phobia	Mind
Phobias	EDTFL	80,240,570,970,2500,237500,495000,734260,852590,915350		Phobia	Mind
Phobia, School	EDTFL	80,240,570,970,2500,103000,222500,345000,497500,725350		Phobia	Mind
Phobia, Social	EDTFL	80,240,570,970,2500,75850,275540,321350,475350,857770		Phobia	Mind
Counterphobic	BIOM	3.9		Phobia	Mind
Claustrophobia	EDTFL	80,550,570,7250,8300,12690,141000,363020,492530,912480		Phobia	Mind
Phobic Disorders	EDTFL	80,240,570,970,2500,13930,527000,663710,752700,985670		Phobia	Mind
Phobic Neuroses	EDTFL	80,240,570,970,2500,13930,250000,322520,425750,625000,		Phobia	Mind
Emetophobia	EDTFL	120,410,8000,30000,57530,125000,357780,689930,750000,934250	Fear of vomiting or phobia of vomiting	Phobia	Mind
Crisis	XTRA	140.25			Mind
Anxiety disorder		Can be caused by Cytomegalovirus, Epstein-Barr Virus, by the bacterium Helicobacter pylori and by the protozoan Toxoplasma gondii.			
Depression Anxiety Trembling Weakness	CAFL	3.5,800	Avoid starches, use a multivitamin and multi-mineral supplement. Drink pure water - minimum 2.5 litres daily.	Anxiety	Mind
Anxiety	XTRA	40-60=1800,304,6130,		Anxiety	Mind
Anxiety 1	CAFL	1.5,6.8=300,7.8=300,95,10000=300,	General anxiety disorder.	Anxiety	Mind
Anxiety Disorders	EDTFL KHZ	80,620,870,5810,225000,423070,572000,727330,841120,903910,		Anxiety	Mind
Neuroses, Anxiety	EDTFL	80,620,870,5810,225000,423070,572000,727330,841120,903930,		Anxiety	Mind
Anxiety, ailment	BIOM	7.8; 8.5; 10		Anxiety	Mind
Apprehension	BIOM	1.5; 6.8; 7.8; 95; 10000		Anxiety	Mind
Disquietude, uneasiness	BIOM	24.5; 27.5; 98.5		Anxiety	Mind
Disquietude, tension	BIOM	0.5; 1; 1.2; 1.5; 2.5; 3.5; 5.8		Anxiety	Mind
Inner Anxiety-1	BIOM	24.5; 27.5; 98.5		Anxiety	Mind
Anxiety-Relaxation	BIOM	2720; 6000; 320; 250; 240; 160; 125; 80; 40; 20; 10; 5.8; 3.5; 2.5; 1.5; 1.2; 1; 0.5		Anxiety	Mind
Agitation	XTRA	3,7.83	Mental tension and anxiety.	Anxiety	Mind
Unsociable Behavior	CAFL	3.9		Irritability	Mind
Irritability and Whining	XTRA	3.6,3.89,6.29		Irritability	Mind
Irritability	XTRA	5000		Irritability	Mind

Subject / Argument	Author	Frequencies	Notes	Origin	Target
Anger and Irritability	CAFL	3.6,6.3		Irritability	Mind
Annoyance	BIOM	20.0; 727.0; 787.0; 880.0; 10000.0		Irritability	Mind
Antistress	BIOM	2.5; 3.6; 3.9; 5; 6.3; 8.1; 34; 92		Stress	Mind
Stress (General)	EDTFL	140,680,2500,60000,122530,300000,496010,65 5200,750000,912330	Disorder due to metabolic reaction to stress produced by events, substances, activities, worries, or the like.	Stress	Mind
Stress	BIOM	43.5; 88		Stress	Mind
Stress	BIOM	242.0; 253.0; 254.0; 255.0; 312.0; 442.0; 551.0; 573.0; 624.0; 671.0; 712.0; 760.0; 940.0; 950.0; 1269.0; 1950.0; 8566.5; 660.0		Stress	Mind
Stress Increase Tolerance	XTRA	7.83,	Schumann frequency.	Stress	Mind
Stress (Dr. Williams Alternate Set)	EDTFL	140,680,2500,60000,122530,372500,496010,65 5200,755000,805150		Stress	Mind
Calming	CAFL	6000		Relax	Mind
Calming 1	XTRA	2.5,7.83,10,80,304,6000,		Relax	Mind
Calming 4	XTRA	1.9,3.9,5.2,6.8,7.3,9.2,11.9,13.96,15.96,17.3,20. 4,		Relax	Mind
Meditation Induce	XTRA	4.9		Relax	Mind
Meditation	XTRA	7.5		Relax	Mind
Deep Meditation	XTRA	4		Relax	Mind
Peace and Relaxation	XTRA	1-3		Relax	Mind
Relaxation Enhance	XTRA	8		Relax	Mind
Relaxation Induce	XTRA	4.9		Relax	Mind
Relaxation State Of	XTRA	10.6		Relax	Mind
Relaxation to Produce	CAFL	6000,10,7.83		Relax	Mind
Relaxation, pain control	BIOM	304; 6000		Relax	Mind
Relaxation/Mood/Sleep	XTRA	10	Good for relaxation, mood, and stabilized sleep rhythms.	Relax	Mind
Emotion Abnormal Behaviour	CAFL	664,764,6000		Emotions	Mind
Emotional Ties to Diseases	CAFL	764,664		Emotions	Mind
Emotions	XTRA	9.19		Emotions	Mind
Emotions General Aid	XTRA	4.9,20,72,95,125,146,428,522,802,1550,10000,		Emotions	Mind
Emotional Acceptance	XTRA	5.14		Emotions	Mind
Emotional Balance 1	XTRA	15,644,764		Emotions	Mind
Emotional Balance 2	XTRA	360		Emotions	Mind
Emotional Impulse	XTRA	4.6		Emotions	Mind
Emotional Patterns Break	XTRA	417	Solfeggio Frequency.	Emotions	Mind
Emotional Patterns Release	XTRA	396	Solfeggio Frequency.	Emotions	Mind
Emotional Spectrum	XTRA	72		Emotions	Mind
Emotional Trauma Balance	XTRA	15	Clear energy blocks.	Emotions	Mind
Emotions and Sleep 1	XTRA	11,12,13,14,16,17,18,19,20,21,22,23,24,25,26,2 7,28,29,30,31,32,33,		Sleep	Mind
Emotions and Sleep 2	XTRA	32,33,34,35,36,37,38,39,40,41,42,43,44,45,46		Sleep	Mind
Emotions and Sleep 3	XTRA	47,48,49,50,51,52,53,54,55,56,57,58,59,60,61		Sleep	Mind
Paroxysmal [Sleep]	EDTFL	40,550,780,970,5870,15750,232500,492500,826 070,925950,		Sleep	Mind
Sleep, regulation	BIOM	5; 92.5		Sleep	Mind
Sleep, disfunction	BIOM	2.5; 3.6; 3.9; 5; 8.1; 92.5		Sleep	Mind
Sleep, sleep-onset insomnia	BIOM	3.9; 34		Sleep	Mind
Sleep, deep profound	BIOM	92		Sleep	Mind
Sleep Induce Deeper	XTRA	4.9		Sleep	Mind
Sleep to Induce	XTRA	1,3,3-1=300,		Sleep	Mind
Sleep Restorative	XTRA	1-3,		Sleep	Mind
Sleep Sound	XTRA	3.4		Sleep	Mind
Night Terror [Sleep Disorder]	EDTFL	190,370,7250,45750,120500,401000,409310,55 2200,751000,922530,		Sleep	Mind
Insomnia	CAFL	3.59,3,7.83,10,1550,1500,880,802,6000,304,	Use Parasites general set.	Sleep	Mind
Insomnia	CUST	2.7, 21.9, 42.7, 48.9 modulated on 27 MHz carrier	A combination of the four most commonly identified frequencies in patients with insomnia.	Sleep	Mind
Insomnia, basic	BIOM	2.5; 3.5; 3.6; 3.9; 5; 6.3; 8.1; 8.5; 24.5; 34; 43.5; 88; 92.5; 94; 97.5		Sleep	Mind
Insomnia, complex	BIOM	3.59; 3; 1550; 1500; 880; 802; 10000; 1550; 880; 3.9; 802		Sleep	Mind

Subject / Argument	Author	Frequencies	Notes	Origin	Target
Sleep Disorder [Insomnia]	EDTFL	150,900,5580,30000,47500,360000,360590,388900,434000,456110,		Sleep	Mind
Insomnia	EDTFL	150,900,5580,30000,47500,360000,360590,388900,434000,456110		Sleep	Mind
Insomnia	XTRA	2.5,		Sleep	Mind
Insomnia 1	XTRA	3,3.58,3.6,3.89,7.83,10,230,304,800,802,880,1500,1550,6000,		Sleep	Mind
Insomnia 3	XTRA	304,306.5,6000,		Sleep	Mind
Fatal Familial Insomnia	EDTFL	150,900,5580,30000,47500,360000,360590,388900,434000,456110,	Extremely rare and usually inherited prion disease of the brain with progressively worsening insomnia.	Sleep	Mind
Insomnia Secondary/Hypoglycemia	XTRA	2.5,0.512,31.32,0.512	Experimental. Wave=sine. Start 30 mins before bedtime.	Sleep	Mind
Sleeping Sickness	CAFL	120,20	Parasitic disease due to Trypanosoma Brucei (see sets) protozoa. Also see African Trypanosomiasis, Parasites Trypanosoma Brucei, and Trypanosomiasis.	Sleep	Mind
Hypersomnia, Periodic	EDTFL	40,240,900,1920,30720,57500,155010,321260,669730,823010	Excessive daytime sleep or sleepiness, or abnormally prolonged nighttime sleep.	Sleep	Mind
Hypersomnia [Sleeping Disorder]	EDTFL	190,370,7250,45750,120500,401000,409310,552200,751000,922530,		Sleep	Mind
Kleine-Levin Syndrome	EDTFL	180,240,900,5500,17500,32500,72500,127000,356500,624370	Rare sleep disorder with hypersomnia and cognitive/mood changes.	Sleep	Mind
Narcolepsy	EDTFL	50,310,1590,5030,7290,125440,322570,625910,732500,815030	Neurological disorder with loss of brain's ability to regulate sleep-wake cycles, leading to inappropriate sleep times/places, and daytime tiredness.	Sleep	Mind
Narcolepsy-Cataplexy Syndrome	EDTFL	50,310,1590,5030,7290,125440,175110,322570,475110,527000	Disorder characterized both by excessive daytime sleepiness, with short bouts of irresistible and sudden sleep, and by complete loss of muscle tone (cataplexy) following emotional shocks.	Sleep	Mind
Gelineau Syndrome [Narcolepsy]	EDTFL	50,310,1590,5030,7290,125440,322570,625910,732500,815030,	As mentioned above	Sleep	Mind
Center of dream	BIOM	97.5		Sleep	Mind
Dreams	XTRA	20,727,787,880,5000,10000,		Sleep	Mind
Rhythms of Life	XTRA	135.08,188.29,110.96	Order: body, mind, spirit.	Vitality	Mind
Activity Increase	XTRA	144.72		Vitality	Mind
Energy Vitality 1	XTRA	15,528,1056=300,2003=300,9999=300,		Vitality	Mind
Energy Vitality 2	XTRA	5000,9999,10000,20000,		Vitality	Mind
Energy Vitality 3	XTRA	10000		Vitality	Mind
Energy Vitality	CAFL	9999		Vitality	Mind
Vital Energy	BIOM	12.5; 36		Vitality	Mind
Energy	XTRA	144.72		Vitality	Mind
Energy Blocks Stimulate Clearing	XTRA	15		Vitality	Mind
Lack of Vivacity	BIOM	77.5; 92.5		Vitality	Mind
Vitality and Energy	XTRA	9999		Vitality	Mind
Vitality	XTRA	6.88		Vitality	Mind
Vitalisation	BIOM	528.0; 15.0; 35.0; 9998.5; 1725.0; 1342.0; 645.0; 150.0		Vitality	Mind
Vitalisation 1	BIOM	45.45; 49.65; 49.75; 56.65; 56.75; 59.5; 59.8; 62.0		Vitality	Mind
Vitalisation 2	BIOM	40.29; 42.7; 43.5; 43.7		Vitality	Mind
Energizing effect	BIOM	2.2		Vitality	Mind
Alertness Increase	XTRA	10		Vitality	Mind
Personal Growth	BIOM	20.0; 60.0; 95.0; 125.0; 225.0; 427.0; 440.0; 660.0; 727.0; 787.0; 800.0; 880.0; 5000.0; 10000.0		Vitality	Mind
Will, desire	BIOM	84		Vitality	Mind
Feel Good Overall	XTRA	90		Vitality	Mind
Well-being Sense of	XTRA	10,90		Vitality	Mind
Wellness	CAFL	6.8,7.83	The state or condition of being in good physical and mental health.	Vitality	Mind
Balance	XTRA	90	Mental and emotional balance.	Balance	Mind
Balance	XTRA	360	Mental and emotional balance.	Balance	Mind
Center of equilibrium	BIOM	30; 97.5		Balance	Mind
Balancing of Body	XTRA	33,1130,1131	Mental and emotional balance.	Balance	Mind
Environmental Balancing	XTRA	728		Balance	Mind
Alignment of Individual	KHZ	50,750,2250,72500,110250,379930,424370,561930,642060,978050,	May be respiratory, metabolic, or combined.	Balance	Mind

Subject / Argument	Author	Frequencies	Notes	Origin	Target
Harmony	XTRA	1			Mind
Harmony and Love	XTRA	221.23		Love	Mind
Love of Life	XTRA	10.5		Love	Mind
Love Unconditional	XTRA	852	Solfeggio Frequency.	Love	Mind
Love	XTRA	528	Solfeggio Frequency.	Love	Mind
Spiritual Love	XTRA	211.44		Love	Spirit
Spiritual Order Return To	XTRA	852	Solfeggio Frequency.		Spirit
Spiritual Well-being Stimulate Balance	XTRA	1565			Spirit
Spiritual Wisdom	XTRA	10			Spirit
Spirituality	XTRA	183.58			Spirit
Clarity of Spirit	XTRA	172.06			Spirit
Inner Guidance Connect To	XTRA	5.5			Mind
Aura Builder	XTRA	20			Spirit
Aura	XTRA	2675			Spirit
Aura	EDTFL	70,180,870,900,5710,7200,22500,97500,375350,500000			Spirit
Aura restoration	BIOM	20; 5000; 10000			Spirit
Soul/Anima	XTRA	420.82			Spirit
Secrets	XTRA	211.44			Mind
Compassion	XTRA	40			Mind
Forgiveness	XTRA	706			Mind
Conflict Resolution	XTRA	9.19			Mind
Problem-solving 1	XTRA	40	Use in fearful situations.		Mind
Problem-solving 2	XTRA	5			Mind
Situations Undo	XTRA	417	Solfeggio Frequency.		Mind
Change Facilitating	XTRA	417	Solfeggio Frequency.		Mind
Changes	XTRA	140.25			Mind
Relationships 1	XTRA	639	Solfeggio Frequency.		Mind
Relationships 2	XTRA	9			Mind
Control of Events	XTRA	942,161,942			Mind
Security	XTRA	90			Mind
Self Respect	XTRA	5,078,621			Mind
Self-confidence	BIOM	27.5; 2.5; 3			Mind
Success	XTRA	183.58,			Mind
Stability	XTRA	6.88,194.71			Mind
Freedom	XTRA	82.5			Mind
Egoism	BIOM	144.72			Mind
Independence	XTRA	207.36			Mind
Immunity	XTRA	10.5			Mind
Power	XTRA	140.25			Mind
Strength	XTRA	7.69			Mind
Dullness	XTRA	727,787,880,5000			Mind
Mobility	XTRA	141.27			Mind
Social Self	XTRA	12			Mind
Inner Self	XTRA	420.82			Mind
Originality	XTRA	207.36			
Spontaneity	XTRA	207.36			
Stimulate	XTRA	14.3	Schumann frequency.		
Beauty	XTRA	221.23			
Sensuality	XTRA	221.23			
Transformation	XTRA	528			
Expression	XTRA	12			
Receptivity	XTRA	3.5			
Separation	XTRA	147.85			
Banal	VEGA	1778			
Uplifting	XTRA	20.8	Schumann frequency.		

Subject / Argument	Author	Frequencies	Notes	Origin	Target
Brain	XTRA	315.8			Brain
Brain Normalize	XTRA	17578.13	Brain balance.		Brain
Cortex	XTRA	15.4			Brain
Brain Frontal Lobe	XTRA	6.5			Brain
Limbic Centre	BIOM	27.5			Brain
Whole-brain Interconnectedness	XTRA	639	Solfeggio Frequency.		Brain
Interconnectedness Whole-brain	XTRA	369			Brain
Brain Beta Stimulate	XTRA	7.83,19.5,22			Brain
Brain Cell Energise	XTRA	5000			Brain
Neutrophilic Effect	BIOM	5.8			Brain
Adrenergic effect	BIOM	1.75			Brain
Dopaminergic effect	BIOM	3.5			Brain
Cholinergic effect	BIOM	5.8			Brain
Brain Concussion	EDTFL	100,830,2500,10890,52500,87500,95190,21435 0,552540,719680	Head injury with temporary loss of brain function.		Brain
Brain Abscess	KHZ	10,50,7500,25750,87500,325110,375000,51934 0,682020,759830,	May be due to Aspergillus, Zygomycota, or Fusarium molds.		Brain
Brain Abscess	EDTFL	150,570,15160,52500,119340,357300,424370,5 61930,642910,930120	As mentioned above		Brain
Cerebral edema	BIOM	2.5; 2.6; 8; 9.19; 10			Brain
Brain Hypoxia	EDTFL	30,460,600,850,2500,5250,17500,405790,42970 0,539000,	Reduced oxygen supply to the brain.		Brain
Cerebral Anoxia	EDTFL	120,230,7200,13610,96500,175000,327750,682 450,753070,927100	Extreme form of Hypoxia.		Brain
Brain Dysfunction, Minimal Brain Disorders + Brain Diseases	EDTF	40,250,650,750,42500,87500,132410,376290,49 7610,689930,	As mentioned above		Brain
Brain Diseases	EDTFL	40,250,2750,17500,57500,92500,132410,37629 0,497610,689930			Brain
Diencephalic syndrome	BIOM	20.5			Brain
Brain Disorders (General) (Dr. Williams Alternative Set)	EDTFL	100,900,2500,20000,37500,97500,325000,4193 40,561930,823960			Brain
Intracranial Central Nervous System Disorders	EDTFL	50,520,780,7500,8000,32500,62500,125680,250 000,376290			Brain
Cerebral Blood Flow-1	BIOM	19.5; 19.64; 19.75; 50.0			Brain
Liquor-Dynamics	BIOM	1.2; 6.3			Brain
Apoplexy	CAFL	20,40,72,333,428,522,555.1,600,625,727,787,88 0,1800,1865,	Strokeparalysis. See Stroke Follow Up.	Apoplexy	Brain
Apoplexy	EDTFL	90,120,900,15170,96500,225000,425170,57100 0,841000,937410,		Apoplexy	Brain
Apoplexy	BIOM	40; 20; 1800; 880; 787; 727; 650; 625; 600; 125; 95; 72; 20; 1865; 5322; 465		Apoplexy	Brain
Apoplectic attack	BIOM	10000; 1865; 1800; 880; 787; 727; 650; 625; 522; 465; 125; 95; 72; 40; 20		Apoplexy	Brain
Apoplectic attack, rehabilitation	BIOM	10000; 2720; 2112; 1800; 880; 787; 727; 650; 625; 600; 125; 95; 72; 1865; 522; 428; 203; 20; 3		Apoplexy	Brain
Cerebral Ischemia, Transient	EDTFL	80,240,570,7500,10720,36210,142500,301330,4 15700,775680	Insufficient blood flow to brain causing vision, movement, and speech problems.	Ischemia	Brain
Brain Ischemia	EDTFL	80,240,570,7500,10720,36210,142500,301330,4 15700,775680,	As mentioned above	Ischemia	Brain
Brain Stem Ischemia, Transient	EDTFL	80,240,570,7500,10720,36210,142500,301330,4 15700,775680,	As mentioned above	Ischemia	Brain
Ischemic Encephalopathy	EDTFL	140,220,730,5290,7250,50000,326570,334250,4 25000,805290		Ischemia	Brain
Crescendo Transient Ischemic Attacks Ischemic Attack, Transient	EDTFL	70,410,700,970,2750,50000,326570,334250,425 000,805290,		TIA	Brain
Transient Ischemic Attack	EDTFL	70,410,700,970,2750,50000,326570,334250,425 000,805290,		TIA	Brain
Progressive Intracranial Occlusive Arteropathy	EDTFL	420,910,17000,38000,87000,96200,150000,433 000,592000,850000	Arterial constrictions in brain causing risk of hemorrhage, aneurysm, or thrombosis.	Cerebral arteries	Brain

Subject / Argument	Author	Frequencies	Notes	Origin	Target
Brain Vascular Disorders	EDTFL	160,570,780,930,2750,7500,22500,40000,12500 0,433770,	As mentioned above	Cerebral arteries	Brain
Intracranial Vascular Disorders	EDTFL	160,570,780,930,2750,7500,22500,40000,12500 0,433770,		Cerebral arteries	Brain
Cerebrovascular Disorders	EDTFL	40,250,650,750,42500,87500,132410,376290,49 7610,689930,		Cerebral arteries	Brain
Cerebrovascular Accident	EDTFL	100,830,2500,10890,52500,87500,95190,21435 0,552540,719680,		Cerebral arteries	Brain
Cerebrovascular Moyamoya	EDTFL	70,370,950,2520,28100,123920,407910,627280, 736220,816610	Rare cerebrovascular disease characterized by progressive occlusion of the arteries	Cerebral arteries	Brain
Moyamoya Disease [Cerebrovascular Disorder]	EDTFL	70,370,950,2520,28100,123920,407910,627280, 736220,816610,	As mentioned above	Cerebral arteries	Brain
Stroke		*Can be caused by the bacteria **Chlamydia pneumoniae, Helicobacter pylori, Mycobacterium tuberculosis, and Mycoplasma pneumoniae**, as well as the virus **Varicella Zoster virus** and the **Fungus Histoplasma**.*			
Stroke	EDTFL	50,350,2750,30930,75810,187500,325520,7150 00,803510,905320	Insufficient blood flow to brain resulting in cell death.	Stroke	Brain
Cerebral Stroke	EDTFL	80,240,570,7500,10720,36210,142500,301330,4 15700,775680		Stroke	Brain
Stroke [Transient Ischemic]	EDTFL	70,410,700,970,2750,50000,326570,334250,425 000,805290,		Stroke	Brain
Stroke [Vasculitis, Hemorrhagic]	EDTFL	80,350,5500,35170,62500,93500,225000,49609 0,682450,753070,		Stroke	Brain
Stroke 1	XTRA	230,3	As mentioned above	Stroke	Brain
Stroke Recovery	XTRA	2642	As mentioned above	Stroke	Brain
Stroke Follow Up	CAFL	2112,3,203,1800,880,787,727,650,625,600,125, 95,72,20,1865,522,428,10000,20,2720,	Should be run once a month as maintenance.	Stroke	Brain
Brain Hemorrhage [Cerebral]	EDTFL	60,230,970,7000,175200,212960,321510,47121 0,647070,815560,		Hemorrhage	Brain
Hemorrhage, Cranial Epidural	EDTFL	60,230,970,7000,175200,212960,325430,51570 0,682450,755480	Traumatic brain injury with build-up of blood between brain and skull.	Hemorrhage	Brain
Cerebral Parenchymal Hemorrhage	EDTFL	60,230,970,7000,175200,212960,321510,47121 0,647070,815560,		Hemorrhage	Brain
Intracerebral Hemorrhage	EDTFL	50,520,600,930,12690,125000,269710,434430,5 73000,839000		Hemorrhage	Brain
Alzheimers		*Can be caused by **Fungal infections**, the bacteria **Chlamydia Pneumoniae,Helicobacter pylori, Mycoplasma Fermentans**, **Porphyriomonas gengivalis**, a type of spiral-shaped bacteria called **Spirochaetes** and by the protozoan **Toxoplasma gondii**. Is associated with **Herpes simplex virus 1**, in individuals who possess the APOE-4 form of the APOE gene (APOE-4 enables the herpes virus to enter the brain), **HVS-1**, **Hhv-6a** and **Hhv-7**.*			
Alzheimers	CAFL	430,620,624,840,866,5148,2213,19180.5,742.4, 303,23.2,	See ALS sets. Also called Alzheimer. Chronic neurodegenerative illness.	Alzheimers	Brain
Alzheimers Disease and other Dementias Comprehensive	EDTFL KHZ	110,7500,67500,92500,377910,453720,515160, 688290,712000,995380,	As mentioned above	Alzheimers	Brain
Alzheimers	XTRA	1.45	As mentioned above	Alzheimers	Brain
Alzheimer's disease	BIOM	23.2; 303; 430; 470.9; 471.66; 484; 610; 620; 624; 742.4; 840; 864; 943; 986; 1918; 2213; 2900; 5148; 8430; 866; 3767.3; 3777.3		Alzheimers	Brain
Alzheimers 1	XTRA	23.19,303,430,470.89,471.66,620,624,742.39,84 0,866,941.79,943.29,2213,3767.3,3773.3,5148,1 9180.5,	As mentioned above	Alzheimers	Brain
Alzheimers 2	XTRA	430,620,624,840,866,2213,5148,19180.5,	As mentioned above	Alzheimers	Brain
Alzheimers 3	XTRA	2213,5148,19180.5,	As mentioned above	Alzheimers	Brain
Alzheimers 4	XTRA	6,23.19,30,33,254,303,430,470,484,610,620,624 ,644,690,742.39,790,864,866,986,1918,2213,29 00,5148,	As mentioned above	Alzheimers	Brain
Senile Dementia Alzheimer	EDTFL	110,7500,67500,92500,377910,453720,515159, 688290,712000,995380,		Alzheimers	Brain
Anencephaly	EDTFL	170,490,1000,2240,31000,97500,325710,34206 0,750000,934250,	Developmental disorder - absence of major portions of brain, skull, and scalp.		Brain
Aprosencephaly	EDTFL	160,490,1000,2290,30000,97300,325710,34206 0,750000,934250,			Brain
Apraxias	EDTFL	600,1000,5000,246200,365800,454340,515160, 689410,712000,997870,	Motor disorder due to brain damage.		Brain
Dressing Apraxia	EDTFL	600,1000,5000,246200,365800,454340,515159, 689410,712000,997870,	As mentioned above		Brain
Ideational Apraxia	EDTFL	130,490,970,17300,29540,422500,602800,7153 10,803500,924370	As mentioned above		Brain
Dyspraxia	EDTFL	150,180,930,2750,137530,263020,402500,5711 50,796530,825340			Brain
Cerebral atrophy	BIOM	10; 34.5			Brain

Subject / Argument	Author	Frequencies	Notes	Origin	Target
Aprosodia	EDTFL	180,1070,4820,15250,58210,109420,324600,387020,434270,611050,	Neurological language/speech disorder.		Brain
Speech Disorders	EDTFL	60,320,900,32500,67500,97500,325450,519340,691270,754190	As mentioned above		Brain
Stuttering	EDTFL	30,460,830,37500,62500,150000,225750,519340,652430,927100	As mentioned above		Brain
Dysarthria	BIOM	24; 62.5	Speech disorders due to brain lesions or the nerves that go to the tongue and lips.		Brain
Asperger Syndrome	EDTFL KHZ	40,400,2500,10530,47500,210250,518920,688290,712230,916000,	Autism spectrum disorder.	Autism	Brain
Kanners [Autism Infantile]	EDTFL	30,230,900,930,7500,13520,95000,322530,454370,517500,	As mentioned above	Autism	Brain
Autism		*Can be associated with* **Rubella virus, Cytomegalovirus, XMRV, Clostridia** *bacterial.*			
Autism	XTRA	47,48,49,75,214,317,342,443,467,521,552,712,725,727,745,747,757,763,783,787,880,962,1489,1902,4202.3,5333.69,9887,14164.1,15952.79,19007.15,19007.2,19169.38,19516.29,21822.15,		Autism	Brain
Autistic Disorder	EDTFL	30,250,900,980,7500,13520,95000,322530,454370,517500,		Autism	Brain
Autism, Infantile	EDTFL	30,230,900,930,7500,13520,95000,322530,454370,517500,		Autism	Brain
Autism-Dementia	EDTFL	110,7500,67500,92500,377910,453720,515159,688290,712000,995380,		Autism	Brain
Cerebro Spinal Trouble	XTRA	727,787,880,10000			Brain
Cerebrospinal Conditions	CAFL	10000			Brain
Dandy-Walker Syndrome Dandy-Walker Malformation	EDTFL	40,460,800,2230,113450,232500,335650,587500,822000,872290	Congenital brain malformations.		Brain
Dementia		*Can be caused by* **Herpes simplex virus type 1, Herpes simplex virus type 2, Cytomegalovirus, West Nile virus, Borna virus, HIV**, *the helminth* **Taenia solium** *(pork tapeworm), and by* **Borrelia** *species bacteria. Can be associated with* **Chlorovirus ATCV-1.**			
Senile Paranoid Dementia	EDTFL	490,950,67500,152300,275190,519380,682450,711210,859830,922530	Greater decrease in ability to think and remember than would be expected of simple aging.	Dementia	Brain
Frontotemporal Lobar Degeneration	EDTFL	160,490,710,960,5260,7250,92500,275000,327580,425430		Dementia	Brain
Pick's Disease {Degenerative Dementia]	EDTFL	110,7500,67500,92500,377910,453720,515159,688290,712000,995380,		Dementia	Brain
Dementia	EDTFL	70,220,620,2750,5500,40000,100000,522530,682450,754170		Dementia	Brain
Dementia Praecox	EDTFL	70,200,620,2750,5500,40000,100000,522530,682450,754170,		Dementia	Brain
Dementia, Alzheimer Type	EDTFL	110,7500,67500,92500,377910,453720,515159,688290,712000,995380,		Dementia	Brain
Dementia Lewy Body	EDTFL	70,200,660,2750,5500,40000,100000,522530,682450,754170,	Dementia closely associated with Parkinson's Disease - see sets.	Dementia	Brain
Dementia Senile	EDTFL	110,7500,67500,92500,377910,453720,515159,688290,712000,995380,	As mentioned above	Dementia	Brain
Dementia, Vascular	EDTFL	70,200,620,2750,5500,40000,100000,522580,682450,754170,	As mentioned above	Dementia	Brain
Vascular Dementia	EDTFL	110,7500,67500,92500,377910,453720,515159,688290,712000,995380,	As mentioned above	Dementia	Brain
Arteriosclerotic Dementia	EDTFL	110,7500,67500,92500,377910,453720,515159,688290,712000,995380,	Dementia due to brain blood supply problems or a series of minor strokes.	Dementia	Brain
Binswanger Disease [leukoencephalopathy]	EDTFL	150,230,900,950,7500,150890,455340,527500,896500,917200,	As mentioned above	Dementia	Brain
Leukoencephalopathy Subcortical	EDTFL	20,500,850,2500,7500,15690,125000,225690,321450,377910	As mentioned above	Dementia	Brain
Subcortical Arteriosclerotic Encephalopathy	EDTFL	60,250,950,65170,92500,210500,525710,650000,759830,912330	It is a rare variant of small vessel disease dementia associated with severe, poorly controlled hypertension and systemic vascular disease.	Dementia	Brain
Dementias Transmissible	EDTFL	70,200,620,2750,5500,40000,100000,522530,681930,754170,		Dementia	Brain
Retardation, Mental (Symptoms Only)	EDTFL	60,520,15170,42900,125710,376290,514350,682430,759830,918500		Dementia	Brain
Seizures, Convulsions, Spasms			See Section 9a - Neuromuscular Diseases		Brain
Cerebral dystonia	BIOM	97.5			Brain
Epilepsy		*Can be caused by* *the B variant of* **Human Herpesvirus 6 virus (HHV-6B)** *and* **Human Papillomavirus** *infection of the brain.*			

Subject / Argument	Author	Frequencies	Notes	Origin	Target
Epilepsy	CAFL	10000,880,802,787,727,700,650,600,210,633,125,20,		Epilepsy	Brain
Epilepsy	BIOM	12; 37; 90		Epilepsy	Brain
Epilepsy Epileptic Seizures Grand Mal Seizures Tonic–clonic seizures (grand mal)	EDTFL	150,250,8620,17220,82500,115870,325000,491580,673350,874540	See also Seizures	Epilepsy	Brain
Epilepsy 2	XTRA	20,21,125,210,600,625,633,650,660,690,700,727.5,787,802,880,1550,10000,		Epilepsy	Brain
Epilepsy Fits	XTRA	20,120,727,787,880,	Epileptic seizures.	Epilepsy	Brain
Epileptic attack	BIOM	33.5; 33		Epilepsy	Brain
Epileptic seizure	BIOM	10000; 880; 802; 787; 727; 700; 650; 329; 226; 125; 20		Epilepsy	Brain
Lennox-Gastaut Syndrome	EDTFL	850,900,980,17570,213220,321220,423610,597500,862500,915540		Epilepsy	Brain
Awakening Epilepsy	EDTFL	150,250,8620,17220,82500,115870,325000,491580,673350,874540,		Epilepsy	Brain
Alobar Holoprosencephaly	EDTFL	40,350,700,59000,150000,322500,479500,527000,662710,749000,	Failure of embryonic forebrain to full develop into two hemispheres, causing brain and facial defects.		Brain
Arhinencephaly	EDTFL	80,240,650,900,2500,27500,55910,119340,393500,536430,	Failure of embryonic forebrain to full develop into two hemispheres, causing brain and facial defects.		Brain
Holoprosencephaly [cephalic disorder]	EDTFL	40,350,700,59000,150000,322500,479500,527000,662710,749000,	As mentioned above		Brain
Lobar Holoprosencephaly	EDTFL	40,350,700,59000,150000,322500,479500,527000,662710,749000	As mentioned above		Brain
Semilobar Holoprosencephaly	EDTFL	40,350,700,59000,150000,322500,479500,527000,662710,749000,	As mentioned above		Brain
Hydrocephalus	EDTFL	20,180,25300,125150,269710,323200,475030,667000,761850,986220	Brain malfunction caused by decreased absorption of cerebrospinal fluid.	Hydrocephalus	Brain
Hydrocephalus, Normal	EDTFL	20,180,25300,125150,269710,323200,475030,625300,853000,915090	As mentioned above	Hydrocephalus	Brain
Normal Pressure Hydrocephalus	EDTFL	20,180,25300,125150,269710,323200,475030,667000,761850,986220,	As mentioned above	Hydrocephalus	Brain
Communicating Hydrocephalus	EDTFL	20,180,25300,125150,269710,323200,475030,667000,761850,986220,	Dilatazione dei ventricoli cerebrali	Hydrocephalus	Brain
Congenital Hydrocephalus [Birth Disorder]	EDTFL	20,180,25300,125150,269710,323200,475030,667000,761850,986220,	Abnormal accumulation of cerebrospinal fluid in the brain, causing increased intracranial pressure.	Hydrocephalus	Brain
Obstructive Hydrocephalus	EDTFL	20,180,25300,125150,269710,323200,475030,667000,761850,986220,		Hydrocephalus	Brain
Hakim Syndrome	EDTFL	20,420,4830,15230,17250,21050,25120,77010,351290,501710		Hydrocephalus	Brain
Agyria	EDTFL	120,220,690,2530,10720,124000,321150,421200,505520,632020	Rare brain formation disorder with lack of lobe folding.		Brain
Lissencephaly	EDTFL	870,2500,7510,32500,97500,250000,325200,527000,789000,987230	As mentioned above		Brain
Pachygyria	EDTFL	60,400,830,5250,85470,132200,328520,530200,618200,880300	Congenital malformation of the cerebral cortex.		Brain
Microcephaly	EDTFL	110,490,570,7500,12330,190830,431330,501200,653800,825610			Brain
Microlissencephaly [Brain]	EDTFL	870,2500,7510,32500,97500,250000,325200,527000,789000,987230,	Neurodevelopmental disorder where a child's skull growth fails to keep up with the rest of the skeleton, with many different causes.		Brain
Poliodystrophia Cerebri	EDTFL	50,240,970,970,7500,42500,172500,493020,622530,819340	Degenerative disease of the cerebral gray matter.		Brain
Parkinson's disease		*Can be caused by Xenotropic Murine Leukemia Virus (XMRV), Influenza A virus, Toxoplasma gondii, Mycoplasma Fermentans, Chlamydia Pneumoniae, and Nocardia Asteroides.*			
Paralysis Agitans	EDTFL	70,330,800,900,5250,72500,135470,203000,486100,535910	It has long been synonymous with Parkinson's disease.	Parkinson	Nervous S.
Morbus Parkinson	CAFL	33,693,813,5000,	As mentioned above	Parkinson	Nervous S.
Parkinson's Disease	CAFL	470,693,813,1.1,5000,1131,33=1800,	As mentioned above	Parkinson	Nervous S.
Idiopathic Parkinson Disease	EDTFL	680,900,2500,5500,13930,295560,484500,605720,723820,935420,	Degenerative CNS disorder mainly involving the motor system. ('Idiopathic' = unknown cause).	Parkinson	Nervous S.
Morbus Parkinson	BIO	813,	Slowly progressive, degenerative, neurologic disorder.	Parkinson	Nervous S.
Parkinson's Disease	EDTFL	680,900,2500,5500,13930,93500,386400,442350,447000,450000	As mentioned above	Parkinson	Nervous S.
Parkinson Disease	KHZ	80,350,650,830,9500,115710,255830,485430,692500,825000,	As mentioned above	Parkinson	Nervous S.

Subject / Argument	Author	Frequencies	Notes	Origin	Target
Parkinson's disease	BIOM	134; 172; 309.9; 314; 442; 470; 524; 531; 569; 577; 611; 658; 693; 733; 742; 744; 813; 827; 840; 1432; 4324; 6000		Parkinson	Nervous S.
Parkinson's Tremor Temporary Relief	CAFL	6000=600,130,169	As mentioned above	Parkinson	Nervous S.
Parkinson's V	CAFL	577,742,134,611,310,827,442,871,314,1422,733 ,569,531,813,744,840,658,524,4334,172,	As mentioned above	Parkinson	Nervous S.
Parkinsonism	EDTFL	680,900,2500,5500,13930,295560,484500,6057 20,723820,935420	As mentioned above	Parkinson	Nervous S.
Parkinsonism	BIOM	3.5; 88.5; 95.5; 96.5; 100		Parkinson	Nervous S.
Parkinsonian Disorders	EDTFL	680,900,2500,5500,13930,310320,481510,5208 30,622500,701520		Parkinson	Nervous S.
Parkinsonian Syndrome	EDTFL	680,900,2500,5500,13930,82500,142500,39560 0,619340,632610,	As mentioned above	Parkinson	Nervous S.
Familial Juvenile Parkinsonism	EDTFL	680,900,2500,5500,13930,295560,484500,6057 20,723820,935420,		Parkinson	Nervous S.
Parkinsonism, Juvenile	EDTFL	680,900,2500,5500,13930,93300,575710,65032 0,759830,924340	As mentioned above	Parkinson	Nervous S.
Parkinsonism, Experimental	EDTFL	680,900,2500,5500,13930,153300,351300,5324 10,613320,709800		Parkinson	Nervous S.
Lewy Body Parkinson Disease	EDTFL	680,900,2500,5500,13930,93500,386400,44235 0,447000,450000,		Parkinson	Nervous S.
Lewy Body Disease	EDTFL	680,900,2500,5500,13930,93500,386400,44235 0,447000,450000,		Parkinson	Nervous S.
Diffuse Lewy Body Disease	EDTFL	680,900,2500,5500,13930,93500,386400,44235 0,447000,450000,		Parkinson	Nervous S.
Dementia Lewy Body	EDTFL	70,200,660,2750,5500,40000,100000,522530,68 2450,754170,	Dementia closely associated with Parkinson's Disease - see sets.	Parkinson	Nervous S.
Pantothenate Kinase-Neurodegeneration	EDTFL	30,520,680,2750,7500,55910,324370,519340,65 3690,756530	Degenerative brain with iron accumulation disease leading to Parkinson's Disease, dementia, dystonia, and death.	Parkinson	Nervous S.
Schizencephaly	EDTFL	70,350,700,5580,17250,22500,150400,413020,5 50000,719340	Rare birth defect with abnormal brain clefts causing symptoms including epilepsy, motor deficits, and psychomotor retardation.		Brain
Synesthesia	EDTFL	20,450,650,2210,6150,10230,15910,30280,7780 0,327110	Neurological phenomenon where stimulation of one sense leads to automatic, involuntary experiences in a second sense.		Brain
Thalamus	BIOM	97; 98; 91		Thalamus	Brain
Thalamus Stimulant	CAFL	20		Thalamus	Brain
Thalamic Diseases	EDTFL	40,550,7250,50000,97500,222700,434540,5175 00,687620,718000	Includes post-stroke thalamic syndrome, thalamic infarction, akinetic mutism, thalamocortical dysrhythmia, Korsakoff's syndrome, and Fatal Familial Insomnia (see set).	Thalamus	Brain
Dejerine-Roussy Syndrome	EDTFL	160,200,790,950,2800,7500,112330,327550,376 290,534250,	As mentioned above	Thalamus	Brain
Hypothalamus Balance	XTRA	15.42,537	Part of brain which links the nervous system with the endocrine system.	Hypothalamus	Brain
Hypothalamus Stimulate Normal Function	XTRA	1534,1413,1351	As mentioned above	Hypothalamus	Brain
Hypothalamic Disease	EDTFL	130,570,6750,71210,101150,347500,579500,69 0000,775870,816900		Hypothalamus	Brain

					Inflammation

Subject / Argument	Author	Frequencies	Notes	Origin	Target
Arachnoiditis	EDTFL KHZ	160,600,850,2500,7500,35000,87500,479500,52 7000,665340,	Inflammation of arachnoid membrane, one of the meninges protecting brain and spine.	Meninges	Brain
Arachnoiditis	BIOM	4.9; 5.9; 7.7; 9.19; 9.35		Meninges	Brain
Encephalocele	EDTFL	160,230,900,950,7500,150890,455340,527500,8 96500,917200	Neural tube defect with sac-like protrusions of the brain and its membranes through openings in the skull.		Brain
Frontal Encephalocele	EDTFL	160,230,900,950,7500,150890,455340,527500,8 96500,917200,	As mentioned above		Brain
Occipital Encephalocele	EDTFL	160,230,900,950,7500,150890,455340,527500,8 96500,917200,	As mentioned above		Brain
Hernia, Cerebral	EDTFL	20,500,970,7500,22500,42500,125220,275560,3 22060,326160	As mentioned above		Brain
Inflammation, Brain	EDTFL	100,570,680,870,35580,141200,297500,425950, 675310,903740		Encephalitis	Brain
Encephalomyelitis Encephalomyelitis, Myalgic	EDTFL	50,960,5830,7500,12330,113230,425000,57100 0,865830,937410	Inflammation of the brain and spinal cord.		Brain
Encephalomyelitis, Subacute Necrotizing	EDTFL	50,960,5830,7500,12330,113230,425000,57100 0,865830,937410,			Brain
Myeloencephalitis [encephalomyelitis]	EDTFL	50,960,5830,7500,12330,113230,425000,57100 0,865830,937410,			Brain
Encephalitis	CAFL	841	Inflammation of the tissue of the brain and spinal cord.	Encephalitis	Brain

Subject / Argument	Author	Frequencies	Notes	Origin	Target
Encephalitis Encephalitis Periaxialis Encephalitis, Epidemic Encephalitis, Japanese Encephalitis, Saint Louis	EDTFL	120,9550,55850,102500,192500,247500,472500,525330,650000,974500	As mentioned above	Encephalitis	Brain
Encephalitis, Arbovirus	EDTFL	70,680,2330,35000,87500,476500,527000,667000,753230,987230,		Encephalitis	Brain
Encephalitis Herpes Simplex	EDTFL	110,7550,50800,97150,151340,252500,472500,525330,650000,974500		Encephalitis	Brain
Herpetic Acute Necrotizing Encephalitis	EDTFL	110,7550,50800,97150,151340,252500,472500,525330,650000,974500,		Encephalitis	Brain
Meningoencephalitis [Herpes]	EDTFL	110,7550,50800,97150,151340,252500,472500,525330,650000,974500,	Inflammation of the tissue of brain and spinal cord due to Herpes Simplex - see sets.	Encephalitis	Brain
Rasmussen Syndrome	EDTFL	250,500,2750,65350,105310,328210,357000,405150,424650,575200	Inflammation of the tissue of the brain and spinal cord.	Encephalitis	Brain
Arthropod-Borne Encephalitis	EDTFL	120,9550,55850,102500,192500,247500,472500,525330,650000,974500,		Encephalitis	Brain
Mosquito-Borne Encephalitis	EDTFL	120,9550,55850,102500,192500,247500,472500,525330,650000,974500,		Encephalitis	Brain
Encephalopathy Encephalopathy, Binswanger Encephalopathy, Hypoxic Encephalopathy, Wernicke	EDTFL	150,230,900,950,7500,150890,455340,527500,896500,917200	Brain disease, including metabolic, toxic, infectious, neoplastic and degenerative diseases of the brain.	Encephalopathy	Brain
Encephalopathy	BIOM	1.2; 3.6; 6.3			Brain
Wernicke Encephalopathy	EDTFL	150,230,900,950,7500,150890,455340,527500,896500,917200,		Encephalopathy	Brain
Anoxic Encephalopathy	EDTFL	150,180,800,5500,17500,32500,151270,257460,413910,692270,	Low oxygen in the brain.	Encephalopathy	Brain
Hypoxic Encephalopathy [Infant Brain]	EDTFL	30,460,600,850,2500,5250,17500,405790,429700,539000,	Low oxygen in the brain.	Encephalopathy	Brain
Ischemic Encephalopathy	EDTFL	140,220,730,5290,7250,50000,326570,334250,425000,805290		Encephalopathy	Brain
Leigh Disease	EDTFL	70,180,750,830,2500,7500,328510,379930,425680,932000	Subacute necrotizing encephalopathy.	Encephalopathy	Brain
Hyperammonemia Encephalopathy	EDTFL	150,5120,7000,32600,95750,173000,522560,682020,759830,901000	Presence of ammonia in the blood leading to hepatic encephalopathy.	Encephalopathy	Brain
Bilirubin Encephalopathy	EDTFL	150,180,800,5500,33200,172300,471200,557850,603440,921880	Bilirubin-induced brain dysfunction. Also see Bilirubinemia and Hyperbilirubinemia Hereditary.	Encephalopathy	Brain
Hyperbilirubinemic Encephalopathy	EDTFL	150,180,800,5500,33200,172300,471200,557850,603440,921880,	As mentioned above	Encephalopathy	Brain
Kuru Encephalopathy	EDTFL	130,280,520,1730,7250,27500,37500,123040,327230,533690	Transmissible spongiform encephalopathy caused by a prion. See Creutzfeldt-Jakob and Prions sets.	Encephalopathy	Brain
Spongiform Encephalopathies	EDTFL	40,350,2500,7250,60000,125000,300000,475170,527000,752700		Encephalopathy	Brain
Spongiform Encephalopathy, Subacute	EDTFL	130,250,620,5750,17250,37300,129560,345430,415700,682020,	Neurodegenerative disease due to Prions.	Encephalopathy	Brain
Reye Syndrome	EDTFL	70,340,460,620,2750,132240,265000,533630,657770,834250	Very rare rapidly progressive encephalopathy usually beginning shortly after recovery from acute viral illness, especially influenza and varicella, with rash, vomiting, and liver damage.	Encephalopathy	Brain
Morvan Disease [Fibrillary Chorea]	EDTFL	60,250,830,96500,375190,450000,517500,687620,712000,992000,	Rare and fatal acquired neurological disease characterized by neuromyotonia, dysautonomia, and encephalopathy with severe insomnia.		Brain
Leukoencephalitis	CAFL	324,572,776,934,1079,1111,1333,	Inflammation of brain's white matter, usually in infants and children, but also found in horses as a result of forage poisoning.		Brain
Leucoencephalitis	VEGA	572,932,1111	As mentioned above		Brain
Leukoencephalitis 2	XTRA	324,2720,47,266,2720,338,572,712,713,715,776,783,832,934,1035,1079,1111,1160,1244,1333,1630,	As mentioned above		Brain
Leukoencephalitis 3	XTRA	324,572,932,1035,1079,1111,1160,1333,1630	As mentioned above		Brain
Leucoencephalitis	BIOM	324; 572; 766; 934; 1079; 1111; 1333	As mentioned above		Brain
Leukoencephalitis Secondary	CAFL	338,783,932,1035,1160,1630,712,713,715,1244,	As mentioned above		Brain
Leukoencephalitis, Subacute Sclerosing	EDTFL	70,120,600,800,2500,22500,72500,421390,739100,905310			Brain

Subject / Argument	Author	Frequencies	Notes	Origin	Target

Subject / Argument	Author	Frequencies	Notes	Origin	Target
Cerebral Spinal Fluid Bacterial Infection	EDTFL	180,320,950,7500,25750,52400,425160,691270, 753070,912330			Brain
Meningitis		*Inflammation of membranes that envelop the brain and spinal cord. Bacterial infection - use S treptococcus pneumoniae, Influenza haemophilus type B , and see Listeriose and Leptospirosis sets. Viral infection - use Echo, Coxsackie , and Meningococcus sets.*			
Meningitis	CAFL	5000,1422,1044,822,764,733,720,517,423,322,20,	As mentioned above	Meningitis	Brain
Meningitis	VEGA	322,822,1044,1422	As mentioned above	Meningitis	Brain
Meningitis	BIOM	5000; 1865; 1865; 1550; 1422; 1043.9; 880; 832; 822; 802; 787; 727; 660; 650; 625; 600; 465; 465; 444; 428; 322; 125; 95; 72; 20		Meningitis	Brain
Meningitis 1	XTRA	130,322,423,465,507,517,660,676,677,690,727. 5,733,764,822,832,1044,1422,13343.75,	As mentioned above	Meningitis	Brain
Meningitis 2	XTRA	20,72,95,125,428,444,787,802,880,1550,1865,1 3343.75,	As mentioned above	Meningitis	Brain
Meningitis 3	XTRA	20,72,95,125,428,444,465,600,625,650,660,727, 787,802,832,880,1550,1865,	As mentioned above	Meningitis	Brain
Meningitis 5	XTRA	322,733,822,1044,1422,	As mentioned above	Meningitis	Brain
Meningitis 6	XTRA	720	As mentioned above	Meningitis	Brain
Bacterial Meningitis	EDTFL	110,260,970,2500,12800,35340,470000,592500, 625230,723010,		Meningitis	Brain
Viral Meningitis	EDTFL	50,260,970,2500,12800,35340,57500,96500,322 060,475870,	Acute inflammation of meningeal membranes, due to virus. Use Echo, Coxsackie, and Meningococcus sets.	Meningitis	Brain
Meningitis Echo Virus	XTRA	461,514,600,620,625,650,722,765,788,922,	Acute inflammation of meningeal membranes, due to Echo Virus (see sets).	Meningitis	Brain
Meningitis Secondary	CAFL	130,676,677,507,	Acute inflammation of meningeal membranes, due to viral, bacterial (including Lyme spirochetes), or other organisms.	Meningitis	Brain
Meningitis Tertiary	CAFL	1550,802,880,832,787,727,650,625,600,465,444 ,1865,125,95,72,20,428,660,		Meningitis	Brain
Spinal Meningitis	Rife	427000	Acute inflammation of protective membranes covering spinal cord (and brain).	Meningitis	Brain
Cysticercosis	EDTFL	30,200,700,7500,12330,325500,440000,672500, 797500,925950,	Infection of brain by Taenia solium, a pork tapeworm.	Parasites	Brain
Cysticercosis, Brain	EDTFL	30,200,700,7500,12330,18300,155030,517500,6 96500,893000,	As mentioned above	Parasites	Brain
Cysticercosis, Nerves	EDTFL	30,500,850,5250,77250,112780,321100,511880, 725370,825000,	As mentioned above	Parasites	Brain
Central Nervous System Cysticercosis	EDTFL	30,500,850,5250,77250,112780,321100,511880, 725370,825000	As mentioned above	Parasites	Brain
Neurocysticercosis	EDTFL	30,200,700,7500,12330,18300,155030,517500,6 96500,893000,	As mentioned above	Parasites	Brain
Panencephalitis, Subacute Sclerosing	EDTFL	40,240,910,48180,132790,209280,332300,5925 00,775280,819300,	Rare chronic form of progressive brain inflammation caused by persistent infection with Measles virus.		Brain
SSPE [panencephalitis]	EDTFL	40,240,910,48180,132790,209280,332300,5925 00,775280,819300,	Subacute sclerosing panencephalitis (SSPE)		Brain
Measles Body Encephalitis	EDTFL	110,890,1700,6970,12890,331000,337300,4080 00,409700,435850	As mentioned above		Brain
Van Bogaert's Leukoencephalitis	EDTFL	70,120,600,800,2500,22500,72500,421390,7391 00,905310,	As mentioned above		Brain
Brain Fungus 1	XTRA	2608	May be Mucormycosis, Aspergillus, or Fusarium.	Fungus	Brain
Brain Fungus 2	XTRA	469,633,855	As mentioned above	Fungus	Brain

8c - Central and peripheral nervous system

Subject / Argument	Author	Frequencies	Notes	Origin	Target
Nervous System Central	XTRA	6000	Stimulate		Nervous S.
Central Nervous System	BIOM	6.3			Nervous S.
Central nervous system, basic	BIOM	1.2; 2.2; 2.5; 3.5; 3.6; 4.9; 5.8; 6.3; 7.7; 8.1; 8.25; 8.5; 9.2; 9.35; 9.4; 9.45; 9.5; 9.6			Nervous S.
Central nervous system, regulation	BIOM	3.5; 3.6; 5.8; 7.7; 8.1; 8.25; 8.5; 9.2; 9.4			Nervous S.
Autonomic Nervous System	EDTFL	130,370,780,900,213520,335530,413980,63500 0,795220,826320,			Nervous S.
Autonomic Nervous System	BIOM	95.5			Nervous S.
Vegetative Disturbance	BIOM	2.5			Nervous S.
Sympathetic nervous system	BIOM	1.75; 2.5; 65; 92.5; 99			Nervous S.
Sympathotonic effect	BIOM	3.8; 5.5; 8; 9.44			Nervous S.
Sympathetic Nervous System Disorders	BIOM	65.0			Nervous S.

Subject / Argument	Author	Frequencies	Notes	Origin	Target
Parasympathetic system	BIOM	6			Nervous S.
Sympathetic Nervous System Diseases	EDTFL	130,370,780,900,213520,335530,413980,63500 0,795220,826320,			Nervous S.
Parasympathetic Nervous System Diseases	EDTFL	130,370,780,900,213520,335530,413980,63500 0,795220,826320,			Nervous S.
Autonomic Failure	EDTFL	70,3000,70000,95190,175160,325170,515700,6 50000,750000,927100	Degeneration of nerve cells in specific areas of brain, causing problems with movement, balance, and autonomic functions.	Muscle	Nervous S.
Central Autonomic Nervous System Diseases	EDTFL	900,920,32730,293700,329030,415840,423470, 472140,512140,629900	The ANS controls involuntary body functions.		Nervous S.
Peripheral Autonomic Nervous System Diseases	EDTFL	130,370,780,900,213520,335530,413980,63500 0,795220,826320,			Nervous S.
Peripheral nervous system	BIOM	5.9			Nervous S.
Peripheral nervous system - basic	BIOM	1.75; 3.9; 5.9; 7.7; 8.25; 9.2; 9.3; 9.35; 9.4; 9.7			Nervous S.
Spinal Cord	BIOM	16.5; 64.5			Nervous S.
Spinal Cord Disorder	BIOM	16.5; 100.0			Nervous S.
Spinal Cord Diseases Spinal Diseases	EDTFL	180,320,950,7500,25750,52400,425160,571000, 841000,932000			Nervous S.
Spinal Cord Inflammation Spinal Cord Infection	EDTFL	180,320,950,7500,25750,52400,425160,691270, 753070,912330			Nervous S.
Spinal Cord Injuries	EDTFL	180,320,950,7500,25750,52500,425160,691270, 753070,912330			Nervous S.
Nerves	BIOM	25; 78.5			Nervous S.
Cerebral nerves	BIOM	3.8; 3.9; 7.5			Nervous S.
Nerve center	BIOM	10; 25; 78.5; 93.5			Nervous S.
Nerves - Pilot frequencies	BIOM	12.5; 15; 4; 25; 27.5; 39; 94; 77.5; 80; 82.5; 99; 95.5; 92.5			Nervous S.
Nerves Treatment	BIOM	200; 467; 200; 467; 10; 7.64			Nervous S.
Nerve problems	BIOM	5.5; 10; 19; 24.5; 27.5; 43.5; 61.5; 73.5; 75.5; 77.5; 78.5; 79.5; 84; 88; 90; 92.5; 93.5; 94			Nervous S.
Nerves, restoration	BIOM	7.64; 10; 12.5; 15; 4; 25; 27.5; 39; 94; 77.5; 80; 82.5; 99; 95.5; 92.5			Nervous S.
Nervous System Function Stimulate Normal	XTRA	764			Nervous S.
Stimulate Repair Nerve Damage	XTRA	2,578,657,764,5000,10000,			Nervous S.
Nerve Healing	XTRA	2,657,5000,10000			Nervous S.
Nerve Healing 2	XTRA	7.63,10,200			Nervous S.
Nerves Stimulate Healing	XTRA	2			Nervous S.
Peripheral Neuropathies	EDTFL	140,570,920,5250,37250,132500,237700,52253 0,675430,819340,			Nervous S.
Nerve Disorders and Neuropathy	CAFL	95,72,20,440,660,2489,2720,3176,10000,	Peripheral nerves disorder.		Nervous S.
Nerve Disorders and Neuropathy	CAFL	10000,2720,2489,2112,2170,1800,1600,1550,80 2,880,787,727,650,625,600,125,3,7.83,20,72,95, 125,440,600,625,650,660,727,787,802,880,1550 ,1600,1800,2112,2170,	Peripheral nerves disorder.		Nervous S.
Nerve Pain	XTRA	968=1200,2720,	Nerve pain. See Nerve sets.	Pain	Nervous S.
Nerve Pain	EDTFL	30,370,780,900,7500,20000,322060,377300,425 710,568430		Pain	Nervous S.
Neuralgia	CAFL	833,3.9,10000		Pain	Nervous S.
Neuralgia	EDTFL	80,250,650,2500,8000,77500,196500,315700,52 4940,660410		Pain	Nervous S.
Neuralgia	BIOM	3.9; 73.5; 75.5; 79.5; 92.5		Pain	Nervous S.
Neurodynia	EDTFL	240,350,410,2100,18110,26010,42500,62210,10 1200,218310,	Neuralgia	Pain	Nervous S.
Neuralgia 2	XTRA	3.9,10000		Pain	Nervous S.
Neuralgia General	XTRA	3.89,802,1550,833,2720,10000,		Pain	Nervous S.
Nerve Inflammation	XTRA	727,787,880,10000		Pain	Nervous S.
Nerves, inflammation	BIOM	73.5; 75.5; 79.5; 92		Pain	Nervous S.
Paroxysmal Nerve Pain	EDTFL	30,370,780,900,7500,10720,40000,157500,3925 00,575560,	Rare genetic neurological disease.	Pain	Nervous S.
Causalgia	EDTFL	120,580,800,5110,15000,226210,512330,65369 0,753070,919340,	Severe pain, swelling, and skin changes in parts or all of the body.	Pain	Nervous S.

Subject / Argument	Author	Frequencies	Notes	Origin	Target
Central Pain Syndrome	EDTFL	100,500,87500,95000,225170,450000,522390,688290,712230,993410,		Pain	Nervous S.
Nerve Compression Syndromes	EDTFL	30,370,780,900,7500,10720,40000,157500,392500,575560	Commonly called trapped nerve.		Nervous S.
Nerve Entrapments Entrapment Neuropathies [Nerve]	EDTFL	30,370,780,900,7500,10720,40000,157500,392500,575560,			Nervous S.
Entrapment Neuropathy	EDTFL	190,220,730,5580,13390,150000,475850,736420,819350,915700,	As mentioned above		Nervous S.
Nervous System Diseases	EDTFL	130,370,780,900,213520,335530,413980,635000,795220,826320	Diseases which damage or impair nerves in the central or peripheral nervous systems.		Nervous S.
Neurologic Disorders	EDTFL	160,550,960,7500,22500,42500,125220,275560,533630,652430			Nervous S.
Central Nervous System Diseases	EDTFL	150,230,850,5250,77250,112780,321100,511880,527000,667000			Nervous S.
Central Nervous System Infections	EDTFL	30,500,850,5250,77250,112780,250000,320510,425750,625000			Nervous S.
Peripheral Nerve Diseases Peripheral Nervous System Diseases	EDTFL	130,370,780,900,213520,335530,413980,635000,795220,826320,	Disorders affecting nerves which may impair sensation, movement, gland or organ function.		Nervous S.
Nerve Disorders 1	XTRA	20,72,95,125,440,600,625,650,660,727,787,802,880,1550,1600,1800,2170,2489,2720,10000,			Nervous S.
Nerve Disorders 2	XTRA	3.89,802,10000,			Nervous S.
Nerves Motor Depressant Fatigued	XTRA	727,787,880,5000,	Motor nerves weakened functions.		Nervous S.
Cranial Nerve II Diseases	EDTFL	40,200,700,880,5780,364000,366100,475290,527000,667000,	As mentioned above	Cranial Nerve	Nervous S.
Cranial Nerve Diseases Cranial Nerve III Diseases Cranial Nerve VII Diseases Cranial Nerve IX Diseases	EDTFL	40,200,700,880,5780,32500,181930,621690,705530,815700,	Impaired functioning of one of the 12 cranial nerves.	Cranial Nerve	Nervous S.
Cranial Neuropathies Cranial Neuropathies, Multiple	EDTFL	40,200,700,880,5780,32500,181930,621690,705530,815700,	As mentioned above	Cranial Nerve	Nervous S.
Neuropathies, Cranial	EDTFL	50,570,600,2250,5290,37500,367650,475290,527000,831900	As mentioned above	Cranial Nerve	Nervous S.
Craniorachischisis [Rachischisis]	EDTFL	160,460,950,5850,62500,107500,217500,496500,855720,915310,	Very rare congenital malformation of the central nervous system.		Nervous S.
Neuralgia, Amyotrophic	EDTFL	80,250,650,2500,8000,77500,324530,326160,475560,527000			Nervous S.
Neuralgic Amyotrophy	EDTFL	80,250,650,2500,8000,77500,196500,315700,524940,660410			Nervous S.
Neuralgia, Diabetic	EDTFL	50,370,650,2500,8000,77500,95020,175160,274000,357300			Nervous S.
Foster-Kennedy Syndrome	EDTFL	130,350,370,850,5790,77250,133500,296500,625580,915700			Nervous S.
Facial nerve - irritation	BIOM	89.5			Nervous S.
Trifacial nerve	BIOM	10; 30; 87.5; 25; 78.5; 93.5; 12.5; 15; 4; 27.5; 39; 94; 77.5; 80; 82.5; 99; 95.5; 92.5		Trigeminal	Nervous S.
Neuralgia Trigeminal	CAFL	880	Intensely painful neuropathic chronic disorder affecting the face's trigeminal nerve.	Trigeminal	Nervous S.
Trigeminal Neuralgia	CAFL	2720,2489,2170,1800,1600,1550,802,7.5,880,832,787,776,760,727,650,146,7.82,27.5,428,	As mentioned above	Trigeminal	Nervous S.
Trigeminal Neuralgia	EDTFL	80,350,750,7400,32580,174500,407500,635000,723540,885540	As mentioned above	Trigeminal	Nervous S.
Trifacial nerve neuralgia	BIOM	5000; 2720; 2489; 1600; 1550; 802; 787; 776; 760; 725; 650; 428; 146; 7.5		Trigeminal	Nervous S.
Neuralgia Arms	XTRA	20,727,787,880,10000,	Nerve pain in arms. See Nerve sets.	Arms	Nervous S.
Shoulder-Girdle Neuropathy [Group 21]	EDTFL	240,920,1770,18320,28230,32119,48900,54300,109730,328500,			Nervous S.
Neuralgia Intercostal	CAFL	802	Nerve pain in rib musculature.	Ribs	Nervous S.
Intercostal Neuralgia	CAFL	3000,1550,880,802,787,776,727,125,20,1865,444,	Pain in rib musculature. See Neuralgia Intercostal set.	Ribs	Nervous S.
Intercostal Neuralgia	BIOM	3040; 1550; 880; 802; 787; 776; 727; 125; 20; 1865; 444		Ribs	Nervous S.
Intercostal Neuralgia 1	XTRA	20,125,444,660,690,727.5,776,787,802,880,1550,1865,2720,3000,	Pain in rib musculature. See Neuralgia Intercostal set.	Ribs	Nervous S.

Subject / Argument	Author	Frequencies	Notes	Origin	Target
Neuritis Nerve Inflammation	XTRA	727,787,880,10000,	Causes can be injury, infection (including Lyme), chemo, radiation, and certain underlying conditions like cancer.		Nervous S.
Seizures, Convulsions, Spasms			*See Section 9a - Neuromuscular Diseases*		
Amyotrophy, Neuralgic	EDTFL	20,2500,60000,95000,225330,479500,527000,667000,742000,985670	Rare disease of the peripheral nervous system, with sudden onset of pain in the upper limbs.		Nervous S.
Angelman Syndrome	EDTFL	200,7500,27500,95330,375160,419340,567700,642060,808230,980000,	Neuro-genetic disorder with intellectual and developmental disabilities.	Genetic disorder	Nervous S.
Puppet Children	EDTFL	70,240,570,87500,175160,307250,322060,667000,742000,985670	As mentioned above		Nervous S.
Brown Sequard Syndrome	EDTFL	30,400,830,71500,95750,175150,275150,357300,749000,987230,	Damage to one side of spinal cord, causing paralysis and loss of proprioception on that side, and loss of pain and temperature sensation on the other.		Nervous S.
Hemispinal Cord Syndrome	EDTFL	180,320,950,7500,25750,52400,412740,582650,835200,932000	As mentioned above		Nervous S.
Spastic Spinal Monoplegia	EDTFL	180,320,950,7500,25750,92500,325750,519340,841000,932000	As mentioned above		Nervous S.
Bulbospinal Neuropathy	EDTFL	180,320,950,7500,25750,52400,412740,532040,843550,937000	Damage to nerves in the medulla oblongata.		Nervous S.
Central Cord Syndrome	EDTFL	180,500,850,5120,7250,13930,72500,125170,379930,475190	Most common form of cervical spine injury.		Nervous S.
Corticobasal (CorticoBasal Ganglionic Degeneration)	EDTFL	40,210,9630,36850,172500,202000,412500,592300,775270,819310	Rare progressive neurodegenerative condition with marked movement disorders and cognitive dysfunction		Nervous S.
Lateral Bulbar Syndrome [Wallenbergs]	EDTFL	190,520,780,970,7500,116720,205540,325000,422500,925690,			Nervous S.
Lateral Medullary Syndrome	EDTFL	190,520,780,970,7500,116720,205540,325000,422500,925690			Nervous S.
Wallenberg Syndrome	EDTFL	190,520,780,970,7500,116720,205540,325000,422500,925690,	Collection of diverse neuro symptoms due to injury to lateral part of medulla oblongata.		Nervous S.
Vertebral artery syndrome	BIOM	9.6; 95			Nervous S.
Pica Syndrome [Lateral medullary syndrome]	EDTFL	190,520,780,970,7500,116720,205540,325000,422500,925690,	Also known as "Wallenberg syndrome," it is an occlusion or the posteroinferior cerebellar artery (PICA)		Nervous S.
Neural Tube Defects	EDTFL	30,240,930,970,7500,13520,95000,322540,454370,517500			Nervous S.
Developmental Defects, Neural [DCD]	EDTFL	30,180,930,940,7500,13520,95000,322590,454370,517500,	Conditions in which an opening in spinal cord or brain from early in fetal development remains.		Nervous S.
Exencephaly	EDTFL	150,490,1000,2250,32000,97400,325710,342060,750000,934250	Central nervous system malformation.		Nervous S.
Neuroleptic Malignant Syndrome	EDTFL	110,490,5570,62750,145180,246710,361030,435290,693500,787000	Life-threatening nerological disorder most commonly caused by neuroleptic/antipsychotic drugs.		Nervous S.
Batten Disease [Nervous System Disorders]	EDTFL	130,370,780,900,213520,335530,413980,635000,795220,826320,			Nervous S.
Jansky-Bielschowsky Disease	EDTFL	100,570,670,870,35580,127500,337500,638620,715230,903740			Nervous S.
Kufs Disease	EDTFL	200,410,2500,7500,30500,96500,222700,527000,749000,903220			Nervous S.
Santavuori-Haltia Disease	EDTFL	170,550,950,75000,125280,237500,362500,597500,775950,915700			Nervous S.
Spielmeyer-Vogt [Batten Disease]	EDTFL	130,370,780,900,213520,335530,413980,635000,795220,826320,			Nervous S.
Polyneuropathies	EDTFL	140,550,970,5710,13930,137500,262500,497500,626070,822530	Damage or disease affecting peripheral nerves in roughly the same areas on both sides of body, with weakness, numbness, 'pins and needles,' and burning pain.		Nervous S.
Polyneuropathy	BIOM	20.87; 82.6; 165			Nervous S.
Polyneuropathy, Acquired	EDTFL	140,550,970,5710,13930,137500,262500,523110,604220,625790			Nervous S.
Radiculitis	BIOM	212; 240; 464			Nervous S.
Radicular syndrome	BIOM	10000; 120; 20; 727; 787; 880; 120			Nervous S.
Polyradiculitis [GBV, GBS]	EDTFL	80,250,570,7600,10530,12600,40000,313350,320000,615000,	Injury or damage to nerve roots near spinal cord.		Nervous S.
Polyradiculopathy	EDTFL	130,520,6750,71250,95900,105150,225830,347500,455890,805310,	As mentioned above		Nervous S.
Polyradiculopathy, Abdominal	EDTFL	130,520,6750,71250,105150,347500,561930,709830,842500,985900			Nervous S.
Cauda Equina Syndrome	EDTFL	970,1120,17740,51200,131020,217500,517500,653000,772290,956030			Nervous S.
Radiculopathy	XTRA	5,481,321	Compression of nerves in the spine that can cause pain, numbness, tingling, weakness along the nerve		Nervous S.

Subject / Argument	Author	Frequencies	Notes	Origin	Target
POEMS Syndrome [Paraneoplastic]	EDTFL	20,220,900,7500,22700,85370,155470,355350,368000,398400,	Rare syndrome with plasma-cell proliferative disorder (usually myeloma), polyneuropathy, and effects on many other organ systems. See Myeloproliferative Disorders and Polyneuropathies.	Genetic disorder	Nervous S.
Crow-Fukase Syndrome	EDTFL	160,230,9850,87500,162500,212500,452500,597500,650000,726070,	As mentioned above		Nervous S.
Takatsuki's Syndrome	EDTFL	20,520,1180,2250,17500,72500,320350,688290,712000,995380	As mentioned above	Rare dis.	Nervous S.
Rett Syndrome	EDTFL	40,120,950,13390,13930,50000,165800,493200,722800,905310	Rare genetic postnatal neurological disorder of grey matter of brain almost exclusively affecting females, with small hands and feet and slow rate of head growth.	Genetic disorder	Nervous S.
Cerebroatrophic Hyperammonemia	EDTFL	150,550,950,7500,22500,42500,125220,275560,533630,652430,			Nervous S.
Dermal Sinus	EDTFL	130,400,57500,92500,175190,479920,527000,667000,742000,988900,	Uncommon form of cranial or spinal dysraphism.		Nervous S.
Spina Bifida	EDTFL	180,320,950,7500,25750,52500,105100,485000,697500,856720			Nervous S.
Spina Bifida Occulta	EDTFL	180,320,950,7500,25750,52500,105100,485000,697500,856720	Mildest form of spina bifida. Also see Spinal Dysraphism.		Nervous S.
Spinal Bifida, Closed	EDTFL	180,320,950,7500,25750,52860,107500,485000,697500,856720	As mentioned above		Nervous S.
Tethered Cord Syndrome	EDTFL	180,320,950,7500,25750,52400,425180,571000,841000,932000	As mentioned above		Nervous S.
Spinal Dysraphism	EDTFL	180,320,950,7500,25750,52400,425180,571000,841000,932000			Nervous S.
Status Dysraphicus	EDTFL	190,2120,20000,45150,73400,96500,125000,375750,434330,563190			Nervous S.
Rachischisis	EDTFL	160,460,950,5850,62500,107500,217500,496500,855720,915310			Nervous S.
Spinal Stenosis	EDTFL	180,320,950,7500,25750,52400,425180,571000,841000,932000	Abnormal narrowing of spinal canal causing neurological deficit.		Nervous S.

8d - Diseases of the myelin sheath

Subject / Argument	Author	Frequencies	Notes	Origin	Target
Medullary sheath, restoration	BIOM	4.4; 8; 9.4; 9.5; 9.8; 12.6; 13.3; 14.2; 14.4; 14.8			Nervous S.
Myelitis	EDTFL	180,560,5780,66830,132500,205780,472500,507500,782200,932100	Infection and/or inflammation of spinal cord, leading to multiple problems. Can be caused by Varicella Zoster virus, Herpes Simplex ", Cytomegalovirus, Epstein-Barr virus, HIV, Echovirus, hepatitis A, rubella.	Myelin	Nervous S.
Myelopathy	EDTFL	270,780,930,7500,10890,95900,322530,416700,562910,742060		Myelin	Nervous S.
Myelopathy, Inflammatory	EDTFL	270,780,930,7500,10890,50000,150000,350000,475870,523000		Myelin	Nervous S.
Myelopathy, Traumatic	EDTFL	270,780,930,7500,10890,50000,96500,315700,419340,562960		Myelin	Nervous S.
Demyelinating Diseases	EDTFL	190,350,13320,90000,329000,355080,475160,667000,789000,986220,	Destruction of nerve neurons' myelin sheath. Causes may be genetic, infectious, autoimmune, pesticides, insecticides, or herbicides.	Myelin	Nervous S.
Lysosomal storage disease			See Section 2d - Cells, Amino acids, Enzymes, etc.	Myelin	Nervous S.
Arylsulfatase A Deficiency	EDTFL	140,550,820,7160,32500,35540,317560,376290,515700,689980	Lysosomal storage disease affecting the growth and development of myelin nerve sheath. See Lysosomal Storage Diseases.	Myelin	Nervous S.
Leukodystrophy Metachromatic	EDTFL	70,220,620,2600,7500,41010,119340,475690,527000,665000	As mentioned above	Myelin	Nervous S.
Leukodystrophy, Spongiform	EDTFL	30,260,780,7500,11950,55540,97500,515700,652430,758780	Degenerative genetic cerebral disease involving neuronic myelin damage.	Myelin	Nervous S.
Spongy Disease	EDTFL	50,370,900,2500,3000,73300,93750,175000,269710,355080,	As mentioned above	Myelin	Nervous S.
Canavan Disease	EDTFL	50,370,900,2500,3000,73300,93750,175000,269710,355080	As mentioned above	Myelin	Nervous S.
Canavan-V Bogaert [Spongy]	EDTFL	50,370,900,2500,3000,73300,93750,175000,269710,355080,	As mentioned above	Myelin	Nervous S.
Amyotrophic Lateral Sclerosis		Can be caused by Mycoplasma Fermentans, Echo Virus, Coxsackie, Herpes 6, Bartonella, Xenotropic Murine Leukemia Virus (XMRV).			
ALS 1	CAFL	2900=1800,864,790,690,610,470,484,986,644,254,	Amyotrophic lateral sclerosis. Potential causative viruses. See Multiple sclerosis and Lyme sets.	ALS	Nervous S.
ALS 2	CAFL	5000,3636,2632,1850,1500,1488,1422,1189,1044,922,868,845,822,788,776,766,742,733,721,676,654,625,620,607,608,609,610,611,612,613,595,515,487,461,435,423,380,322,283,232,144,136,20,	As mentioned above	ALS	Nervous S.
ALS 3	CAFL	2900	As mentioned above	ALS	Nervous S.

Subject / Argument	Author	Frequencies	Notes	Origin	Target
ALS 4	CAFL	10000,5000,2900,2750,2700,2145,938,862,841, 777,766,741,739,688,682,660,572,532,520,477, 442,433,344,343,342,338,324,322,253,242,112,	As mentioned above	ALS	Nervous S.
Amyotrophic lateral sclerosis ALS 1 (*bacterial infection*)	BIOM	242; 253; 254; 324; 342; 442; 620; 644; 692; 741; 766		ALS	Nervous S.
Amyotrophic lateral sclerosis ALS 2 (*virus infection*)	BIOM	136; 144; 283; 380; 435; 477; 487; 607; 608; 610; 611; 612; 613; 676; 688; 721; 728; 739; 742; 788; 845; 862		ALS	Nervous S.
Amyotrophic lateral sclerosis ALS 3 (*herpetic infection*)	BIOM	322; 343; 484; 520; 532; 572; 654; 682; 733; 2145		ALS	Nervous S.
Amyotrophic lateral sclerosis ALS 4 (*uncertain aetiology*)	BIOM	254; 338; 477; 595; 938; 1500; 2632; 2700; 2750		ALS	Nervous S.
Amyotrophic Lateral Sclerosis	CAFL	254,484,610,644,690,790,864,986,	As mentioned above	ALS	Nervous S.
ALS [Amyotrophic Lateral Sclerosis]	EDTFL	20,2500,60000,95000,225330,479500,527000,6 67000,742000,985670,	As mentioned above	ALS	Nervous S.
Amyotrophic Lateral Sclerosis	XTRA	254,484,610,692,980,644,660,690,727.5,790,86 4,986,2900,	As mentioned above	ALS	Nervous S.
Lou Gehrig [amyotrophic lateral sclerosis (ALS)]	EDTFL	20,2500,60000,95000,225330,479500,527000,6 67000,742000,985670,		ALS	Nervous S.
Sclerosis Lateral	CAFL	254	Degeneration of spinal cord resulting in spastic paraplegia. See Lateral Sclerose, ALS, and Spastic Paresis sets.	ALS	Nervous S.
Lateral Sclerosis	EDTFL	200,250,760,2500,3000,5580,175540,325400,42 5690,571000,	As mentioned above	ALS	Nervous S.
Anterior Horn Cell Disease	EDTFL	190,320,940,5510,32450,47510,162210,215700, 397700,475870,	Also called Motor Neurone Disease, and ALS - see sets. Causes neuron destruction leading to muscular disorders.	ALS	Nervous S.
Familial Motor Neuron Disease	EDTFL	900,920,32750,293700,329090,415840,423470, 472120,512140,629900,	Also spelled 'neurone.' Systemic atrophy primarily affecting central nervous system.		Nervous S.
Motor Neuron Disease	EDTFL	900,920,32750,293700,329090,415840,423470, 682050,759840,900000,	As mentioned above		Nervous S.
Motor Neuron Disease, Lower	EDTFL	900,920,32750,293700,329090,415840,423470, 682050,759840,900000,	As mentioned above		Nervous S.
Motor Neuron Disease, Upper	EDTFL	900,920,32750,293700,329090,415840,423470, 726070,802060,923200,	As mentioned above		Nervous S.
Multiple Sclerosis		It can be caused by **Epstein-Barr virus, Human Herpesvirus 6, Varicella Zoster virus, Xenotropic Murine Leukemia Virus (XMRV)** and **Chlamydia pneumoniae** bacteria. Also use **Blastocystis Hominis, Parasites Flukes, Shigella, Nocardia**, and **Herpes Zoster** sets.			
Multiple Sclerosis 1	CAFL	20,80.9,143,166,218,224,235,241.68,253,275,30 4.6,317,421,430,464,470,524,620,624,660,690,7 28,784,787,802,1550,840,854,880,1331,1875,18 83,2088.59,2189,2213,2252.8,23570.5,2466.9,2 720,3056.9,3767,4992,5000=1800,	Demyelinating disease. Aspartame, mercury, benzene, lead, and toluene can cause same symptoms.	Sclerosis	Nervous S.
Multiple Sclerosis 2	CAFL	20,80.9,241.68,304.6,660,690,728,787,880,2088 .59,2252.8,23570.5,2466.9,3056.9,5000,	As mentioned above	Sclerosis	Nervous S.
Multiple Sclerosis 3	CAFL	2253,2467,2357,2358,242,305,2089,3057,81,50 00,1550,802,880,787,728,690,660,20,	As mentioned above	Sclerosis	Nervous S.
Multiple Sclerosis 4	CAFL	3040,5000,2720,10000,470,120,240,300,328,72 8,880,2005,2006,2007,2008,2009,2010,2011,20,	As mentioned above	Sclerosis	Nervous S.
Multiple Sclerosis 5	CAFL	5000=1800,728,166,224,317,727,787,880,218,	As mentioned above	Sclerosis	Nervous S.
Multiple Sclerosis 6	CAFL	10000,6000,5000=600,3176,2489,3057,2008,23 58,1488,2467,3040,880,787,800,728,665,464,24 2,224,304,166,120,20,	As mentioned above	Sclerosis	Nervous S.
Multiple Sclerosis V	CAFL	2145,938,862,841,741,739,682,660,572,532,520 ,477,442,433,344,343,342,338,324,322,253,242, 112,	As mentioned above	Sclerosis	Nervous S.
Sclerosi multipla (infezione virale)	BIOM	218; 224; 240; 304; 305; 328; 620; 1488; 2005; 2006; 2007; 2253; 2357; 2358; 2489; 3040		Sclerosis	Nervous S.
Multilocular sclerosis (virus-herpetic-bacterial infection)	BIOM	140; 166; 235; 242; 253; 300; 317; 322; 342; 421; 430; 470; 524; 532; 682; 739; 741; 784; 802; 862; 1550; 2213		Sclerosis	Nervous S.
Multilocular sclerosis (bacterial infection)	BIOM	2.8; 5.1; 6.7; 7.2; 11.3; 20; 80.9; 166; 169; 190; 199; 218; 259; 280; 304.6; 315.77; 324; 338; 464; 477; 520; 660; 665; 787; 841; 880; 938; 1331; 1875; 1883; 2008; 2089; 2145; 2467; 2489; 3040; 3057; 3767; 4992		Sclerosis	Nervous S.

Subject / Argument	Author	Frequencies	Notes	Origin	Target
Multilocular sclerosis (mycotic infection)	BIOM	112; 143; 158; 275; 344; 430; 442; 572; 624; 728; 840; 854		Sclerosis	Nervous S.
Multiple Sclerosis	EDTFL	90,10570,30420,88340,109500,257660,344200,346270,572000,792330,		Sclerosis	Nervous S.
Sclerosis, Disseminated	EDTFL	80,350,5190,55000,72500,92500,377550,475270,827000,967000	As mentioned above	Sclerosis	Nervous S.
Multiple Sclerosis Complications	XTRA	1550,802,880,787,727,20,	As mentioned above	Sclerosis	Nervous S.
Multiple Sclerosis Myelin Sheath Repair	XTRA	4.4,8,9.4,9.5,90.8,12,13.3,14.19,14.4,14.8,225,259,380,	As mentioned above	Sclerosis	Nervous S.
Multiple Sclerosis Secondary	CAFL	20,143,275,430,470,524,620,624,802,840,854,1550,2213,5000,728,784,880,464,	As mentioned above	Sclerosis	Nervous S.
Multiple Sclerosis Stiff Legs	CAFL	315.77	As mentioned above	Sclerosis	Nervous S.
Multiple Sclerosis Tremor Or Twitch	CAFL	470	As mentioned above	Sclerosis	Nervous S.
Schilder Disease	EDTFL	160,190,750,5160,30000,229320,323400,564280,714820,978050,	Progressive and fatal disease of the central nervous system due to widespread demyelination of the cerebral hemispheres	Sclerosis	Nervous S.
Diffuse Cerebral Sclerosis of Schilder	KHZ	250,780,930,10890,7500,95900,322530,415700,562910,742060,	Also called Diffuse Myelinoclastic Sclerosis. Rare, with tumor-mimicking demyelinating lesions.	Sclerosis	Nervous S.
Diffuse Cerebral Sclerosis	EDTFL	160,550,950,17500,93980,137200,396500,575830,824370,963190,		Sclerosis	Nervous S.
Balo Concentric Sclerosis	EDTFL	240,780,930,7500,10890,95900,322530,412700,562910,742060	Demyelinating inflammation similar to multiple sclerosis	Sclerosis	Nervous S.
Cerebral Sclerosis, Diffuse	EDTFL	160,550,950,17500,93980,137200,396500,575830,824370,963190,	As mentioned above	Sclerosis	Nervous S.
Pseudosclerosis	EDTFL	160,550,950,17500,93980,137200,396500,575830,824370,963190		Sclerosis	Nervous S.
Cerebral Pseudosclerosis	EDTFL	160,550,950,17500,93980,137200,396500,575830,824370,963190,	As mentioned above	Sclerosis	Nervous S.
Encephalitis Periaxialis	EDTFL	120,9550,55850,102500,192500,247500,472500,525330,650000,974500	As mentioned above	Sclerosis	Nervous S.
Myelinoclastic Diffuse Sclerosis	EDTFL	130,320,25000,52500,134250,175750,426900,572000,843000,937410	As mentioned above	Sclerosis	Nervous S.
Sclerosis, Hereditary Spinal	EDTFL	80,350,5190,55000,72500,92500,377550,475270,827000,967000	Genetic disease causing progressive nervous system damage. Can lead to Scoliosis (see set), heart disease, and diabetes.	Sclerosis	Nervous S.
Sclerosis, Systemic	EDTFL	80,350,5190,55000,72500,92500,377550,475270,827000,967000		Sclerosis	Nervous S.
Tuberous Sclerosis	EDTFL	80,350,5190,55000,72500,92500,377550,475270,827000,967000,	Multisystem genetic disease causing benign tumors in brain, kidneys, heart, eyes, lungs, and skin.	Sclerosis	Nervous S.
Bourneville Disease	EDTFL	150,490,620,800,5130,125000,426900,571000,838000,932000	As mentioned above	Sclerosis	Nervous S.
Phakomatosis, Bourneville	EDTFL	150,490,620,800,5130,125000,426900,571000,838000,932000,	As mentioned above	Sclerosis	Nervous S.
Phakomatosis, Sturge-Weber [SWS]	EDTFL	110,250,870,7500,8000,13940,85680,225230,475680,527000,	As mentioned above	Sclerosis	Nervous S.
Epiloia	EDTFL	50,440,22500,57500,325160,476600,527000,667000,749000,986220	As mentioned above	Sclerosis	Nervous S.
Neuromuscular Diseases			See Section 9a - Neuromuscular Diseases		Nervous S.

Subject / Argument	Author	Frequencies	Notes	Origin	Target
Palsy General	CAFL	10000	Various types of paralysis, often with weakness, shaking, and uncontrolled movements.		Paralysis
Paralysis	EDTFL	170,400,800,900,5250,72500,135470,296500,556720,879930	Loss of function in one or more muscles which may be accompanied by sensory loss.		Paralysis
Palsy	EDTFL	40,200,650,85750,90000,320150,325000,497610,689930,753070,			Paralysis
Paresis	CAFL	9.4	Partial loss, weakness, or impairment of movement.		Paralysis
Spastic Paresis	CAFL	30.87,48	Weakness of voluntary movement, or partial loss of voluntary movement, or impaired movement.		Paralysis
Paresthesia	CAFL	5.5	Tingling, tickling, prickling, or burning skin sensation with no apparent cause.		Paralysis
Infantile Paralysis 2	XTRA	727,776,787,880,1500,10000,	Also called Polio - see sets.		Paralysis
Infantile Paralysis	CAFL	1500,880,787,727,776,5000,10000,	Also called Polio - see sets.		Paralysis
Languorous Paralysis	XTRA	8.25,9.18,9.19,20,72,95,125,444,600,625,650,660,690,727.5,776,787,880,1865,10000,	May refer to hypotonia, an intense muscle weakness. Also see Amyotonia Congenita.		Paralysis
Paralyses, Familial Periodic	EDTFL	170,400,800,900,5250,60000,72500,90000,325360,863640	Group of rare genetic diseases leading to weakness/paralysis from cold, heat, high carbohydrate food, not eating, stress, or excitement and physical activity.	Genetic disorder	Paralysis
Normokalemic Periodic Paralysis	EDTFL	350,930,12330,25230,35680,87500,93500,233650,434000,519340			Paralysis

Subject / Argument	Author	Frequencies	Notes	Origin	Target
Paralysis from Stroke	CAFL	20,40,72,95,125,146,333,428,522,535.1,600,625,650,727,787,880,1800,1865,	Also see Stroke sets.		Paralysis
Paralysis Nonspastic	CAFL	10000,880,787,776,727,650,625,600,444,1865,125,95,72,20,9.19,8.25,	Muscle weakness/paralysis not caused by excessive muscle contraction.		Paralysis
Paralysis Spastic	CAFL	10000,880,787,776,727,650,625,600,444,1865,125,95,72,20,7.69,	Excessive muscle contraction leading to movement problems.		Paralysis
Flaccid paralysis	BIOM	10000; 880; 787; 776; 727; 650; 625; 600; 444; 1865; 125; 95; 72; 48; 31; 20; 9.19; 8.25			Paralysis
Cerebral Palsy	CAFL	880,787,727,522,146,	Group of movement disorders in early childhood with poor coordination, stiff/weak muscles, tremors, and possibly sensory problems.	Brain	Paralysis
Cerebral Palsy	EDTFL	40,200,650,85750,90000,320150,325000,497610,689930,753070	As mentioned above	Brain	Paralysis
Palsy Cerebral	XTRA	146,522,660,690,727.5,787,880,1000,	As mentioned above	Brain	Paralysis
Facial Paralysis	CAFL	10000,880,787,727,		Face	Paralysis
Facial nerve - paresis	BIOM	2.4; 3; 3.9; 7.83; 20; 27.57; 33; 35; 40; 47.5; 57.5; 72; 90.88; 110; 125; 194; 222; 304; 393.5; 464; 565.5; 600; 625; 650; 727; 776; 787; 833; 880; 932.5; 1250		Face	Paralysis
Facial Myokymia	EDTFL	30,230,700,730,5170,12690,32700,73500,175000,526070		Face	Paralysis
Geniculate Ganglionitis		170,520,750,950,2250,17500,135370,385910,593000,722530		Face	Paralysis
Facial Paralysis 1	XTRA	727,787,880,5000,10000,		Face	Paralysis
Facial Paralysis 2	XTRA	660,690,727.5,787,880,10000,		Face	Paralysis
Facial Palsy Facial Paralysis	EDTFL	80,320,610,2270,44250,115710,255550,485000,697500,856720		Face	Paralysis
Hemifacial Paralysis [Facial Paralysis/Spasm]	EDTFL	80,320,610,2270,44250,115710,255550,485000,697500,856720,		Face	Paralysis
Facial Nerve Diseases	EDTFL	80,320,610,2270,44250,115710,255550,485000,697500,856720,		Face	Paralysis
Herpetic Facial Paralysis	EDTFL	80,320,610,2270,44250,115710,255550,485000,697500,856720,		Face	Paralysis
Bell's Palsy	EDTFL	110,550,47500,92500,375750,475180,527000,667000,752700,987230	As mentioned above	Face	Paralysis
Bell's Palsy	CAFL	2.4,3,3.9,7.83,20,27.57,33,35,40,47.5,57.5,72,90.88,110,125,194,222,304,393.5,464,565.5,600,625,650,727,776,787,833,880,932.5,1250,	As mentioned above	Face	Paralysis
Bell's Palsy 1	XTRA	2.39,3,3.89,7.83,20,27.57,33,35,40,47.5,57.5,72,90.97,110,125,194,222,304,393.5,464,565.5,600,625,650,727,776,787,833,880,932.5,1250,	As mentioned above	Face	Paralysis
Bell's Palsy 2	XTRA	2.39,3,3.89,7.83,20,27.5,33,35,40,72,90.87,110,125,194,220,222,304,410,464,470.5,570.5,600,625,650,660,690,727.5,776,787,833,880,1250,3930.5,5650.5,9320.5,	As mentioned above	Face	Paralysis
Bell's Palsy 3	XTRA	2.39,3,3.89,7.83,20,27.57,33,35,40,47.5,57.5,72,90.87,110,125,194,222,304,393.5,464,565.5,600,625,650,727,776,787,833,880,932.5,1250,	As mentioned above	Face	Paralysis
Oculomotor Nerve Diseases	EDTFL	170,320,950,5500,32500,47500,162120,232030,397500,679930		Eyes	Paralysis
Oculomotor Paralysis	EDTFL	170,320,950,5500,32500,330000,537500,605830,754030,825310		Eyes	Paralysis
Supranuclear Palsy, Progressive	EDTFL	200,250,770,2500,3000,5580,175540,326500,425690,571000			Paralysis
Third-Nerve Palsy	EDTFL	20,220,25000,55750,125000,229360,450000,515160,712810,993410			Paralysis
Bulbar Palsy Progressive	EDTFL	80,400,750,890,2500,32500,305050,431200,632590,723010	Type of motor neuron(e) disease that attacks nerves of bulbar muscles. May be related to ALS.		Paralysis
Paralysis, Bulbar [Palsy]	EDTFL	80,400,750,890,2500,32500,305050,431200,632590,723010,			Paralysis
Fazio-Londe Syndrome {Bulbar Palsy]	EDTFL	80,400,750,890,2500,32500,305050,431200,632590,723010,			Paralysis
Vocal Cord Paralysis	EDTFL	50,730,2950,47500,222530,324530,452590,683000,712000,993410	Injury to laryngeal nerves, causing hoarseness, lack of vocal power, and severe shortness of breath.		Paralysis
Laryngeal Nerve Palsy [Vocal Cord Paralysis] Laryngeal Paralysis	EDTFL	50,730,2950,47500,222530,324530,452590,683000,712000,993410,			Paralysis
Erb Paralysis [Palsy Arm]	EDTFL	170,400,800,900,5250,72500,135470,296500,556720,879930,	Neonatal paralysis of the brachial plexus.		Paralysis

Subject / Argument	Author	Frequencies	Notes	Origin	Target
Klumpke Paralysis	EDTFL	40,520,5090,35000,175330,323750,432410,714820,823000,987230	As mentioned above		Paralysis
Plegia [Paralysis]	EDTFL	170,400,800,900,5250,72500,135470,296500,556720,879930,	Paralysis		Paralysis
Paraplegia	EDTFL	130,490,700,970,3500,14350,54500,226730,308150,427900			Paralysis
Moebius Syndrome	EDTFL	40,240,63230,135000,235510,323570,340040,592520,654320,706220			Paralysis
Monoplegic Cerebral Palsy	EDTFL	40,200,650,85750,90000,320150,325000,497610,689930,753070,			Paralysis
Hemiplegia	EDTFL	120,580,730,2570,5780,145910,372520,428010,511190,605590	Paralysis of one side of the body.		Paralysis
Hemiparesis	BIOM	5.7; 16.5; 22.5; 33.5; 39.9; 72; 80; 89.5; 91			Paralysis
Monoplegia	EDTFL	180,930,3740,42500,71500,96500,322400,434000,642910,983170	As mentioned above		Paralysis
Spastic Diplegia	EDTFL	140,220,730,5250,7250,52020,157510,290200,675350,821370	Group of movement, balance, and postural disorders that appears in early childhood.		Paralysis
Diplegic Infantile Cerebral Palsy	EDTFL	40,200,650,85750,90000,320150,325000,497610,689930,753070,			Paralysis
Little Disease Spastic Cerebral Palsy	EDTFL	20,500,870,172500,207300,315230,425620,691220,735540,962070,	Spastic diplegia		Paralysis
Tetraplegia [quadriplegia]	EDTFL	140,550,800,5190,151340,252400,562500,696600,797400,822530,	Paralysis from illness or injury with partial or total loss of use of all four limbs and tors.		Paralysis
Quadriplegia	EDTFL	140,550,800,5190,151340,252400,562500,696600,797400,822530			Paralysis
Spastic Quadriplegia	EDTFL	140,550,800,5190,151340,252400,562500,696600,797400,822530,			Paralysis
Quadriparesis [Quadriplegia]	EDTFL	140,550,800,5190,151340,252400,562500,696600,797400,822530,			Paralysis
Quadriplegic Infantile [Cerebral Palsy]	EDTFL	20,500,870,172500,207300,315230,425620,691220,735540,962070,			Paralysis
Locked-In Syndrome	EDTFL	160,550,950,5500,17500,37800,162500,383500,421000,645250			Paralysis
Tick Paralysis	EDTFL	140,250,600,2250,30500,112330,319340,525710,753070,900000			Paralysis

9 - Musculoskeletal System

9a - Neuromuscular Diseases

Subject / Argument	Author	Frequencies	Notes	Origin	Target
Antispastic effect	BIOM	3.8; 5; 7.7; 8.0; 9.4			Neuromuscular Diseases
Neuromuscular Diseases	EDTFL	130,400,620,900,5580,117250,442580,657510,722590,865870,	Diseases which affect muscles and/or their nervous system control.		Neuromuscular Diseases
Balance problem	BIOM	30; 53; 53.5; 62; 62.5; 70; 6; 6.8; 85; 90; 97; 98			Neuromuscular Diseases
Ataxia General	CAFL	20,72,444,600,625,650,727,776,787,806.5,814,880,1500,1600,1800,1865,2170,2720,	Incoordination of muscles. Slow results in some cases.	Ataxia	Neuromuscular Diseases
Ataxia	BIOM	2720; 2160; 1800; 1600; 1500; 880; 787; 727; 650; 625; 600; 444; 1865; 125; 95; 72; 20.5; 465		Ataxia	Neuromuscular Diseases
Ataxia Spastic	CAFL	9.19,8.25,7.69	Progressive stiffness and contraction (spasticity) in the lower limbs.	Ataxia	Neuromuscular Diseases
Cerebellar Ataxia	EDTFL	240,700,920,72500,97300,336420,475190,527000,662710,752700	Lack of coordination originating in the cerebellum.	Ataxia	Neuromuscular Diseases
Spinocerebellar Ataxia Type 3	EDTFL	190,1220,3720,17200,63210,119420,293240,403060,435000,711170		Ataxia	Neuromuscular Diseases
Cerebellar Dysmetria	EDTFL	170,550,990,7750,22500,42500,275520,387320,515700,650000		Ataxia	Neuromuscular Diseases
Locomotor Ataxia Muscle Failure	XTRA	727,787,880,10000		Ataxia	Neuromuscular Diseases
Striatonigral Degeneration, A.D	EDTFL	70,180,5630,37500,100000,275160,525710,655200,750000,926700		Ataxia	Neuromuscular Diseases
Ataxia Telangiectasia	EDTFL	160,5500,20000,37500,96500,312330,475150,527000,662710,789000,	Impairs movement/coordination, weakens immune system, and prevents DNA repair.	Ataxia	Neuromuscular Diseases
Senile ataxy	BIOM	465; 68; 60; 45; 27		Ataxia	Neuromuscular Diseases
Louis-Bar Syndrome	EDTFL	120,550,850,5800,32500,35540,71500,92500,125610,515700	As mentioned above	Ataxia	Neuromuscular Diseases
Friedreich's Ataxia	EDTFL	230,620,850,5500,7500,33980,295300,326300,375430,522530		Ataxia	Neuromuscular Diseases
Friedreich Disease	EDTFL	230,620,850,5500,7500,33980,95560,325870,473000,742060		Ataxia	Neuromuscular Diseases

Subject / Argument	Author	Frequencies	Notes	Origin	Target
Joseph Disease	EDTFL	180,190,650,9000,32390,119500,232500,72167 0,831000,925620	Rare inherited neurodegenerative disease that causes progressive cerebellar ataxia, leading to lack of muscle control.	Ataxia	Neuromuscular Diseases
Machado-Joseph Disease	EDTFL	180,190,650,9000,32390,119500,232500,72167 0,831000,925620,	As mentioned above	Ataxia	Neuromuscular Diseases
Azorean Disease	EDTFL	150,250,870,7500,8000,13930,85680,225230,47 5680,527000,	As mentioned above	Ataxia	Neuromuscular Diseases
Shy-Drager [Multiple system atrophy]	EDTFL	60,260,900,9000,10890,45910,125290,526180,6 52430,750000,	As mentioned above	Atrophy	Neuromuscular Diseases
Muscle atrophy	BIOM	5000; 880; 787; 727; 522; 146; 145; 45.5; 45		Atrophy	Neuromuscular Diseases
Progressive Muscular Atrophy	EDTFL	180,320,950,7500,25750,52400,425180,571000, 841000,932000,	Genetic disorder causing spinal motor neuron damage and systemic muscle wasting.	Atrophy	Neuromuscular Diseases
Olivopontocerebellar Atrophies Olivopontocerebellar Atrophy, Idiopathic	EDTFL	70,500,970,9000,12330,32500,142500,321000,4 25870,525560	Degeneration of neurons in cerebellum, pons, and inferior olives of brain, causing Ataxia. Associated with Prions, and present in Machado-Joseph Disease and Multiple System Atrophy - see appropriate sets.	Atrophy	Neuromuscular Diseases
Dejerine-Thomas Syndrome	EDTFL	160,200,790,950,2800,7500,112330,327550,376 290,534250,	As mentioned above	Atrophy	Neuromuscular Diseases
Muscular Atrophy, Spinal Muscular Atrophy, Spinal, Infantile	EDTFL	180,320,950,7500,25750,58300,423730,577630, 832450,935740		Atrophy	Neuromuscular Diseases
Oculopharyngeal Spinal Muscular Atrophy	EDTFL	180,320,950,7500,25750,52400,425180,571000, 841000,932000,		Atrophy	Neuromuscular Diseases
Muscular Atrophy, Postpoliomyelitis	EDTFL	130,300,830,2500,7500,22500,142020,251020,3 25580,471860	Condition where polio survivors develop muscular atrophy, muscles weakness and pain, and fatigue, very similar to Chronic Fatigue Syndrome (see sets).	Atrophy	Neuromuscular Diseases
Multiple System Atrophy	EDTFL	60,260,900,9000,10890,45910,125290,526180,6 52430,750000	Neurological disorder with degeneration of nerve cells in certain brain areas, leading to movement, balance, and autonomic function problems.	Atrophy	Neuromuscular Diseases
Juvenile Spinal Muscular Atrophy	EDTFL	180,320,950,7500,25750,58300,425790,582650, 835410,937550		Atrophy	Neuromuscular Diseases
Spinal Muscular Atrophy Spinal Muscular Atrophies of Childhood Spinal Muscular Atrophy, Infantile Spinal Muscular Atrophy, Juvenile	EDTFL	180,320,950,7500,25750,52400,425180,571000, 841000,932000	Genetic disorder with progressive muscle wasting and mobility impairment.	Atrophy	Neuromuscular Diseases
Peroneal Muscular Atrophy	EDTFL	40,460,620,1000,2750,15870,65000,219340,324 940,425870		Atrophy	Neuromuscular Diseases
Atrophy Muscular Peroneal	XTRA	190,1220,4330,17250,63210,119420,287210,40 3030,435000,711170,	Also called Charcot-Marie-Tooth disease (CMT). Progressive loss of muscle and touch sensation.	Atrophy	Neuromuscular Diseases
Charcot-Marie-Tooth Disease	EDTFL	220,700,980,72500,97500,336470,475190,5270 00,662710,752700	Progressive loss of muscle tissue and touch sensation.	Atrophy	Neuromuscular Diseases
Dejerine-Sottas Disease	EDTFL	160,200,790,950,2800,7500,112330,327550,376 290,534250,	Also called Charcot Marie Tooth disease type 3.	Atrophy	Neuromuscular Diseases
Kugelberg-Welander	EDTFL	190,680,10030,31230,127760,309600,436090,4 63970,502930,651820	Juvenile Spinal Muscular Atrophy, hereditary.	Atrophy	Neuromuscular Diseases
Parsonage-Turner Syndrome	EDTFL	130,300,830,2500,7500,22500,142020,251020,3 25550,471870	Form of neurological atrophy affecting the brachial plexus.	Atrophy	Neuromuscular Diseases
Chorea	EDTFL	60,250,830,96500,375190,450000,517500,6876 20,712000,992000	Abnormal involuntary movement disorder.	Chorea	Neuromuscular Diseases
Huntington Chorea	EDTFL	50,730,1550,13390,22500,247000,322510,5710 00,827000,937410	Genetic neurodegenerative disorder that affects muscle coordination and leads to mental decline and behavioral aberrations.	Chorea	Neuromuscular Diseases
Juvenile Huntington Disease	EDTFL	50,730,1550,13390,22500,247000,322510,3953 20,408220,526730,	As mentioned above	Chorea	Neuromuscular Diseases
Choreatic Disorders	EDTFL	60,250,830,96500,375190,450000,517500,6876 20,712000,992000,	Vedi sopra	Chorea	Neuromuscular Diseases
Choreiform Movement	EDTFL	40,230,22500,42500,62500,125190,150000,358 570,525710,655200	Vedi sopra	Chorea	Neuromuscular Diseases
Choreoathetosis	EDTFL	80,520,600,2250,11090,45750,222700,522530,6 91270,750000	Association of chorea (i.e. jerky, very rapid movements) and athetosis (very wide and, in explaining them, slow movements)	Chorea	Neuromuscular Diseases
Central Core Disease [muscle disorder]	EDTFL	130,400,620,900,5580,117250,442580,657510,7 22590,865870,	Congenital muscle disorder. Anesthesia may be contraindicated.		Neuromuscular Diseases
Amyotonia Congenita	EDTFL	40,350,2050,6790,115740,234250,342120,4725 00,551230,657710,	Also called Hypotonia, or Floppy Baby Syndrome. Due to low muscle tone/strength	Amyotonia	Neuromuscular Diseases
Myasthenia Gravis	KHZ	80,350,680,930,2500,5500,135580,333570,6135 40,705570,	Neuromuscular disease with cycles of muscle weakness and fatigue due to blocked acetylcholine receptors.	Myasthenia	Neuromuscular Diseases

Subject / Argument	Author	Frequencies	Notes	Origin	Target
Muscular Dystrophies	EDTFL	190,900,1220,17250,63210,119420,287210,403030,435000,711130	Inherited muscle disorders that weaken the body and hinder normal movement.	Dystrophy	Neuromuscular Diseases
Muscular Dystrophy 1	XTRA	1.19,3,7.69,7.7,9.39,9.4,19.6,20,28,153,230,250,660,690,727.5,787,880,2900,	As mentioned above	Dystrophy	Neuromuscular Diseases
Muscular Dystrophy 2	XTRA	146,333,465,522,523,555,600,625,650,768,776,786,802,1550,1850,10000,	As mentioned above	Dystrophy	Neuromuscular Diseases
Muscular Dystrophy 3	XTRA	146,153,522,727,787,880,5000,	As mentioned above	Dystrophy	Neuromuscular Diseases
Muscular Dystrophy 4	XTRA	153	As mentioned above	Dystrophy	Neuromuscular Diseases
Muscular Dystrophy 5	XTRA	2900	As mentioned above	Dystrophy	Neuromuscular Diseases
Muscular Dystrophy 6	XTRA	146,522,727,787,880,	As mentioned above	Dystrophy	Neuromuscular Diseases
Duchenne Muscular Dystrophy DMD	XTRA	146,153,522,727.5,787,880,5000,	Genetic form of Muscular Dystrophy - see sets.	Dystrophy	Neuromuscular Diseases
Hereditary Sensory and Autonomic Neuropathies	EDTFL	870,27500,45570,65290,95220,182500,320600,414550,418000,420800	Group of nerve diseases which inhibit sensation.	Neuropathy	Neuromuscular Diseases
Hereditary Sensory and Autonomic Neuropathies	XTRA	1000,5000	As mentioned above	Neuropathy	Neuromuscular Diseases
Neuropathies, Hereditary Motor and Sensory	EDTFL	70,500,970,7250,9000,12330,35000,95470,206320,422530	Hereditary Motor and Sensory Neuropathies. Also called Charcot-Marie-Tooth disease - see set. Also see Atrophy Muscular Peroneal.	Neuropathy	Neuromuscular Diseases
HSAN(Hereditary Sensory and Autonomic Neuropathy) Type I	EDTFL	70,500,970,9000,12330,33500,142500,320000,425870,525560	Hereditary Sensory and Autonomic Neuropathy. Type I has nerve abnormalities in hands and feet.	Neuropathy	Neuromuscular Diseases
HSAN(Hereditary Sensory and Autonomic Neuropathy) Type II	EDTFL	70,500,970,9000,12330,33500,142500,320000,425870,525560	Hereditary Sensory and Autonomic Neuropathy. Type II has sensory abnormalities involving pain, temperature, and touch.	Neuropathy	Neuromuscular Diseases
HSAN(Hereditary Sensory and Autonomic Neuropathy) Type III	EDTFL	70,500,970,7250,9000,12330,35000,95470,206320,422530	Disorder of autonomic nervous system affecting its development and that of sensory nervous system.	Neuropathy	Neuromuscular Diseases
HSAN(Hereditary Sensory and Autonomic Neuropathy) Type IV	EDTFL	70,500,970,7250,9000,12330,35000,95470,206320,422530	Hereditary Sensory and Autonomic Neuropathy. Type IV has insensitivity to pain, inability to sweat and intellectual disability.	Neuropathy	Neuromuscular Diseases
Neuropathy, Hereditary Motor and Sensory, Type IV	EDTFL	70,500,970,7250,9000,12330,35000,95470,206320,422530		Neuropathy	Neuromuscular Diseases
HSAN(Hereditary Sensory and Autonomic Neuropathy) Type V	EDTFL	70,500,970,7250,9000,12330,35000,672530,888030,937390	Hereditary Sensory and Autonomic Neuropathy. Type V has inability to feel deep pain or temperature changes.	Neuropathy	Neuromuscular Diseases
Dysautonomia Familial	EDTFL	200,460,600,2500,13000,35780,187500,235000,395690,805700	As mentioned above	Neuropathy	Neuromuscular Diseases
Riley-Day [familial dysautonomia]	EDTFL	200,460,600,2500,13000,35780,187500,235000,395690,805700,	As mentioned above	Neuropathy	Neuromuscular Diseases
HMN Proximal Type I	EDTFL	20,230,840,5710,55830,172500,325300,663500,725310,853020		Neuropathy	Neuromuscular Diseases
HMSN (Hereditary Motor and Sensory Neuropathy)	EDTFL	20,230,840,5710,12710,13930,55560,93500,375870,426900		Neuropathy	Neuromuscular Diseases
HMSN Type I	EDTFL	20,230,840,5710,55830,172500,409300,570400,832300,930440		Neuropathy	Neuromuscular Diseases
HMSN [Hereditary Motor and Sensory Neuropathy] Type II	EDTFL	20,230,840,5710,30000,47500,162820,365000,388900,456110,		Neuropathy	Neuromuscular Diseases
HMSN Type III	EDTFL	20,230,840,5710,55830,95090,172500,323950,375000,525710		Neuropathy	Neuromuscular Diseases
HMSN Type IV	EDTFL	20,230,840,5710,55830,172500,426900,571000,843000,937410		Neuropathy	Neuromuscular Diseases
HMSN Type VII	EDTFL	20,230,840,5710,55830,87500,172500,342060,615310,834450		Neuropathy	Neuromuscular Diseases
Roussy-Levy Syndrome	EDTFL	100,260,680,7500,11010,45000,325430,515700,682450,755420	Rare inherited demyelinating motor and sensory neuropathy.	Neuropathy	Neuromuscular Diseases
Joint Mobility	XTRA	18		Joints	Articular mob.
Anti-sclerotic	BIOM	3.3	Sclerosis is any process of hardening of an organ, or a considerable part of it, as a result of an increase in connective-fibrous tissue.		Articular mob.
Antitonic	BIOM	3.8; 5.9; 7.7	Decreased muscle or vascular tone		Articular mob.

Subject / Argument	Author	Frequencies	Notes	Origin	Target
Coordination Difficulties	XTRA	7.83,20,72,95,125,444,600,625,650,660,690,727.5,776,787,807,813,880,1500,1600,1800,1865,2170,2720,10000,			Neuromuscular Diseases
Motor Coordination Disorders	BIOM	10000.0; 880.0; 787.0; 776.0; 727.0; 650.0; 625.0; 600.0; 444.0; 1865.0; 125.0; 95.0; 72.0; 20.0			Neuromuscular Diseases
Dysmetria	EDTFL	80,410,9800,87500,202500,345000,607500,725830,850000,924370	Muscle coordination disorder, whereby there is too much or too little movement.	Dysmetria	Neuromuscular Diseases
Adiadochokinesis	EDTFL	70,830,2500,10890,52500,87500,103500,214350,552590,719680,	Inability to make certain movements in quick succession.		Neuromuscular Diseases
Alignment of Individual	XTRA	20,60,95,125,225,427,440,660,727,787,800,880,5000,10000,	Bring body into alignment. Also see Scoliosis.		Neuromuscular Diseases
Motor Disturbance	BIOM	1865.0; 880.0; 787.0; 776.0; 727.0; 650.0; 625.0; 600.0; 125.0; 95.0; 72.0; 20.0			Neuromuscular Diseases
Movement Disorder	EDTFL	120,320,960,5510,32450,47510,162210,215700,397500,475870	Includes tremors, palsy, choreas, akathisia, tardive dyskinesia, dystonias, RLS, tics, spasms, and others - also see appropriate sets.		Neuromuscular Diseases
Akathisia	XTRA	3,7.83,230	Movement disorder; motor restlessness; due to antipsychotic medication.	Akathisia	Neuromuscular Diseases
Nervousness Prozac Agitation	CAFL	3,7.83	Also see Akathisia, Movement Disorders, and Relaxation sets.		Neuromuscular Diseases
Stiff-Person Syndrome	EDTFL	40,500,970,2750,12850,20000,122530,320450,325870,840020,	Rare neurologic disorder with progressive rigidity and stiffness, primarily affecting truncal muscles and superimposed by spasms, resulting in postural deformities. Chronic pain, impaired mobility, and lumbar hyperlordosis are common.		Neuromuscular Diseases
Moersch-Woltmann Syndrome [Stiff P.]	EDTFL	40,500,970,2750,12850,20000,122530,320450,325870,840020,	As mentioned above		Neuromuscular Diseases
Fasciculation	EDTFL	580,780,900,5250,7000,115710,255830,485430,692500,825000	Involuntary muscle twitches.		Neuromuscular Diseases
Isaac's Syndrome	EDTFL	160,260,570,7800,12690,35350,322060,425710,564280,930120	Continuous activity of muscle fibers at rest, which causes muscle stiffness, cramps, myochemia and pseudomyotonia.		Neuromuscular Diseases
Contraction	XTRA	9.09,110,		Contraction	Neurom. D.
Contractions Arrests Discharges	XTRA	20,727,787,880,10000,		Contraction	Neuromuscular Diseases
Seizures	CAFL	226,329,953	Sudden attack of Convulsions and/or loss of consciousness, typical of Epilepsy (see sets) and other conditions like Hyperglycemia (see sets).	Seizures	Neuromuscular Diseases
Seizures Jackknife Seizures Jacksonian Seizure Salaam Seizures	EDTFL	150,250,8620,17220,82500,115870,325000,491580,673350,874540		Seizures	Neuromuscular Diseases
Seizures, Convulsive	EDTFL	150,250,8620,17220,82500,115870,275620,325000,523010,687450		Seizures	Neuromuscular Diseases
Anticonvulsive effect	BIOM	6; 6.8		Seizures	Neurom. D.
Anticonvulsive effect	BIOM	3.8; 5.0; 7.7; 8.0; 9.45		Seizures	Neurom. D.
Seizures, Generalized	EDTFL	150,250,8620,17220,82500,115870,325000,486500,706210,946500		Seizures	Neuromuscular Diseases
Seizures, Motor	EDTFL	150,250,8620,17220,82500,97500,115870,325000,375300,500000		Seizures	Neuromuscular Diseases
Seizures, Sensory	EDTFL	150,250,8620,17220,82500,115870,325000,491580,673350,874540,		Seizures	Neuromuscular Diseases
Convulsions	EDTFL	40,410,940,960,7500,125380,387500,682100,822000,925930	As mentioned above	Convulsions	Neuromuscular Diseases
Convulsions 1	XTRA	7.69,8.25,9.18,9.19,660,690,727.5,787,880,10000,	Rapid contraction and relaxation of muscles, leading to uncontrolled shaking.	Convulsions	Neuromuscular Diseases
Convulsions 2	XTRA	727,787,880,5000,10000,	As mentioned above	Convulsions	Neurom. D.
Convulsions General	CAFL	727,787,880,10000	As mentioned above	Convulsions	Neurom. D.
Locomotor Convulsions	XTRA	7.69,8.25,9.18	As mentioned above	Convulsions	Neurom. D.
Convulsions Spasticity	CAFL	9.19,8.25,7.69	As mentioned above	Convulsions	Neurom. D.
Convulsions with Spasticity	XTRA	7.69,8.25,9.18,9.19	As mentioned above	Convulsions	Neurom. D.
Clasp-Knife Spasticity	EDTFL	180,320,930,105500,210500,357550,475190,667000,742000,985610	As mentioned above	Convulsions	Neuromuscular Diseases
Spasm	EDTFL	170,550,950,35120,85310,137500,562800,697500,722530,920000		Spasms	Neuromuscular Diseases
Spasms	BIOM	10000; 880; 787; 727; 26; 25; 770; 5000		Spasms	Neurom. D.
Various Spasms	BIOM	3.8		Spasms	Neurom. D.
Spasm and Pain	BIOM	2.0; 2.2; 2.5; 2.7; 3.2; 3.5		Spasms	Neurom. D.
Spasms Muscle	CAFL	6.8	Sudden involuntary contraction of muscle.	Spasms	Neurom. D.
Myospasm	BIOM	212; 240; 300; 324; 328; 424; 515; 528; 728; 760; 946; 988; 6000		Spasms	Neuromuscular Diseases

Seizures

Neuromuscular

Subject / Argument	Author	Frequencies	Notes	Origin	Target
Myospasm (convulsion)	BIOM	6.8; 28; 28.5; 33.5; 33.5; 35; 54; 64; 70.5		Spasms	Neurom. D.
Spasmolytic effect	BIOM	3.8; 8; 9.45; 515		Spasms	Neurom. D.
Spasmolytic	BIOM	3.8; 8.0; 9.44		Spasms	Neurom. D.
Muscle Spasm Muscle Spasticity	EDTFL	90,410,15090,87500,122060,312390,532410,65 5200,752000,927200	Sudden involuntary contraction of muscle, a group of muscles, or a hollow organ such as the heart.	Spasms	Neuromuscular Diseases
Masseter Muscle Spasm	EDTFL	150,230,650,930,36290,211090,475680,527000, 665340,749000		Spasms	Neuromuscular Diseases
Trismus [Tetanus Lockjaw]	EDTFL	40,550,7250,50000,97500,222300,434590,5176 00,687620,717000,		Spasms	Neuromuscular Diseases
Neck Spasms	BIOM	5000; 880; 787; 727; 500; 49; 20; 9; 6; 5		Spasms	Neurom. D.
Pain in case of spasms	BIOM	120; 212; 240; 424; 465; 528; 760; 727; 787; 880; 1550; 2112; 5000; 10000		Spasms	Neuromuscular Diseases
Cryptogenic Infantile Spasms	EDTFL	70,550,950,35120,85310,137500,527000,66700 0,753200,986220,	Child epilepsy syndrome with unknown cause.	Spasms	Neuromuscular Diseases
Symptomatic Infantile Spasms	EDTFL	70,550,950,35120,85310,137500,527000,66700 0,753200,986220,		Spasms	Neuromuscular Diseases
Spasms, Infantile	EDTFL	70,550,950,35120,85310,137500,527000,66700 0,753200,986220	Sudden involuntary contraction of muscle, a group of muscles, or a hollow organ such as the heart.	Spasms	Neuromuscular Diseases
Spasmus Nutans	EDTFL	80,420,770,7940,31220,122740,255610,371330, 742800,955700	As mentioned above	Spasms	Neuromuscular Diseases
Nodding Spasm	EDTFL	130,400,620,42600,57500,92800,175000,47517 0,527000,667000	As mentioned above	Spasms	Neuromuscular Diseases
Hypsarrhythmia	EDTFL	190,320,980,117500,210500,367650,475190,66 7000,745000,985680	As mentioned above	Spasms	Neuromuscular Diseases
West Syndrome	EDTFL	80,490,650,6350,11980,17600,72100,416070,67 5550,870240	As mentioned above	Spasms	Neuromuscular Diseases
Dystonia [Movement Disorder]	EDTFL	150,180,930,2750,137530,263020,402500,5711 50,796530,825340,	Movement disorder with muscle contractions causing twisting and repetitive movements or abnormal postures.	Dystonia	Neuromuscular Diseases
Muscle Dystonia	EDTFL	40,240,950,1000,7250,12050,97500,229320,325 950,532410,	As mentioned above	Dystonia	Neuromuscular Diseases
Dystonia Osteitis	XTRA	2.64,20,660,690,724,727.5,736,743,770,787,880 ,3000,	Caused by bone inflammation.	Dystonia	Neuromuscular Diseases
Vegetative-Vascular Dystonia	BIOM	1.7; 4; 6; 9.4		Dystonia	Neurom. D.
Vegetative Dystonia	CAFL	40,	Involuntary muscle dysfunction.	Dystonia	Neurom. D.
Dystonia Vegetative	XTRA	20,40,120,240,	Unexplained disorder of functions and senses of the body.	Dystonia	Neurom. D.
Myoclonus	EDTFL	50,410,600,950,5780,30000,57500,97500,32587 0,675960	Brief, involuntary twitching of muscle or group of muscles.	Myoclonus	Neuromuscular Diseases
Myoclonus, Action	EDTFL	190,370,780,900,7500,121720,340000,457500,5 92500,775580	As mentioned above	Myoclonus	Neuromuscular Diseases
Myoclonus Cherry Red Spot	EDTFL	130,490,600,870,2250,5260,113980,545870,735 000,805070	As mentioned above	Myoclonus	Neuromuscular Diseases
Myoclonus, Nocturnal	EDTFL	190,370,780,900,7500,121720,345230,567500,6 25870,775580	As mentioned above	Myoclonus	Neuromuscular Diseases
Polymyoclonus [Body Tremor]	EDTFL	190,370,780,950,2250,5250,45000,65720,75263 0,924370,	As mentioned above	Myoclonus	Neuromuscular Diseases
Tourette Syndrome		Can be caused by the bacterium Streptococcus . Aggravating or contributory microbes may include the bacteria Mycoplasma pneumoniae, Chlamydia pneumoniae, Chlamydia trachomatis , and the protozoan Toxoplasma gondii .			
Tourette Syndrome	EDTFL	50,120,220,580,1380,5390,15250,30710,50110, 66210	Inherited disorder with multiple motor tics and at least one vocal tic.	Motor tics	Neuromuscular Diseases
Gilles de la Tourette's [Tourette Syndrome]	EDTFL	50,120,220,580,1380,5390,15250,30710,50110, 66210,	As mentioned above	Motor tics	Neuromuscular Diseases
Facial muscle paroxysm (habit spasms)	BIOM	304; 9; 880; 787; 727; 1131; 6000; 10000		Motor tics	Neuromuscular Diseases
Tardive Dyskinesia	EDTFL	140,250,850,5250,7260,325000,587500,745310, 815900,927000,	Disorder with involuntary repetitive movements. Caused by antipsychotic drug use for longer than three months in adults, and GI drugs in children and infants. See also Section 12b - Face	Motor tics	Neuromuscular Diseases
Ambulation Disorders, Neurogenic	EDTFL	130,250,620,2750,10890,25260,125370,245470, 393500,505400,	Deviations from normal walking patterns caused by neurological disorders.	Ambulation	Neuromuscular Diseases
Gait Disorders [Neurologic]	EDTFL	160,550,960,7500,22500,42500,125220,275560, 533630,652430,		Ambulation	Neuromuscular Diseases
Locomotor Dysfunction Incoordination	CAFL	10000,880,787,776,727,650,625,600,444,1865,1 25,95,72,20,	May be slow results. See Schumann Resonance set.	Ambulation	Neuromuscular Diseases
Locomotor Dysfunction Incoordination	XTRA	7.83,20,72,95,125,444,600,625,650,660,690,727 .5,776,787,807,813,880,1500,1600,1800,1865,2 170,2720,10000,		Ambulation	Neuromuscular Diseases
Intermittent Claudication	EDTFL	30,240,700,17500,35170,97500,314330,327570, 560000,707260	Muscle pain, cramp, or numbness, most often in calf, usually encountered while exercising.	Ambulation	Neuromuscular Diseases
Intermittent Claudication	CAFL	45,48	As mentioned above	Ambulation	Neurom. D.
Intermittent Claudication 2	XTRA	45,48,10000	As mentioned above	Ambulation	Neurom. D.

Subject / Argument	Author	Frequencies	Notes	Origin	Target
Intermittent lameness	BIOM	8.6; 45; 48		Ambulation	Neurom. D.
Tremor	EDTFL	190,370,780,950,2250,5250,45000,65720,75263 0,924370		Tremor	Neuromuscular Diseases
Intention Tremor	EDTFL	110,240,570,281830,301090,392420,431190,67 2530,703540,821690		Tremor	Neuromuscular Diseases
Resting Tremor	EDTFL	60,510,700,9870,74500,130000,317950,490000, 675290,879500	Involuntary muscle movement that may be rhythmic, mostly in hands.	Tremor	Neuromuscular Diseases
Benign Essential Tremor	EDTFL	190,370,780,950,2250,5250,45000,65720,75263 0,924370,	Most common movement disorder affecting finger, hands, arms, and sometimes other parts of the body. Cause unknown.	Tremor	Neuromuscular Diseases
Essential Tremor	EDTFL	130,230,620,9970,167330,325500,422500,6500 00,875950,919360	As mentioned above	Tremor	Neuromuscular Diseases
Familial Tremor	EDTFL	50,120,600,870,2250,45000,325430,515700,682 450,755490	As mentioned above	Tremor	Neuromuscular Diseases
Tremors Brain Tumors	XTRA	463,466		Tremor	Neurom. D.
Adynamia Geriatric	CAFL	60,27.5	Fatigue associated with age.		Neurom. D.
Adynamia Geriatric	CAFL	27,27.5,35,60	Fatigue associated with age.		Neurom. D.
Adynamia Geriatric	ODD	49,56	Fatigue associated with age.		Neurom. D.
Senile Adynamia	BIOM	27.5; 60; 100; 220; 410			Neurom. D.
Fatigue Geriatric	XTRA	27.5,60,100,220,410,	See Fatigue Adynamia and Adynamia Geriatric sets.		Neurom. D.
After-meal fatigue	BIOM	72.5			Neurom. D.
Back fatigue	BIOM	2.5; 9.6; 9.7; 68.5; 69; 84.5; 96; 100			Neurom. D.
Easily Fatigued	XTRA	727,787,880,5000		Fatigue	Neurom. D.
Lassitude Weak Exhausted	XTRA	20,727,787,880		Fatigue	Neurom. D.
Fatigue General	CAFL	428,424,664,660,464,125,120,95,72,20,444,186 5,10000,5000,		Fatigue	Neuromuscular Diseases
Fatigue, General	BIOM	428; 424; 664; 660; 464; 125; 120; 95; 72; 20; 444; 186; 10000; 5000		Fatigue	Neuromuscular Diseases
Fatigue	EDTFL	50,120,600,3870,72250,125430,352930,496010, 682450,755490		Fatigue	Neuromuscular Diseases
Fatigue	XTRA	120,428		Fatigue	Neurom. D.
Fatigue 1	XTRA	20,72,95,125,428,444,465,660,690,727.5,1865		Fatigue	Neuromuscular Diseases
Fatigue 2	XTRA	20,72,95,125,428,444,465,660,1865,		Fatigue	Neurom. D.
Fatigue 3	XTRA	20,72,95,120,125,424,428,444,464,660,664,186 5,5000,10000,		Fatigue	Neuromuscular Diseases
Fatigue of muscles	BIOM	4; 6; 10; 45; 70; 80		Fatigue	Neurom. D.
Fatigue Adynamia	XTRA	27.5,60,100,220,410,	Lack of strength or vigor often associated with neurological diseases.	Fatigue	Neuromuscular Diseases
Fatigue Easily Fatigued	XTRA	727,787,880,5000		Fatigue	Neurom. D.
Chronic Fatigue Syndrome		Can be caused by Enteroviruses (Coxsackie B virus), Epstein-Barr virus, Human Herpesvirus 6 variant A, Human Herpesvirus 7, Parvovirus B19, XMRV and bacteria Coxiella burnetii and Chlamydia pneumoniae.			
Chronic Fatigue	XTRA	1.5	Constant tiredness.	Fatigue	Neurom. D.
Chronic Fatigue Syndrome	CAFL	10000,660,2127,787,465,424,664,120,880,1550,	As mentioned above	Fatigue	Neuromuscular Diseases
Chronic Fatigue V	CAFL	1902,1000,959,649,568,243,922,2422,730,1522, 116,1489,962,172,1333,	Use EBV, Fatigue General, Parasites General, Roundworm, and Flukes sets. If no response, try Cancer Leukemia Hairy Cell.	Fatigue	Neuromuscular Diseases
Chronic Fatigue Syndrome	EDTFL	50,120,600,3870,72250,125430,387500,525910, 712500,825440,	CFS. Also see Chronic Fatigue Syndrome, and Chronic Fatigue sets.	Fatigue	Neuromuscular Diseases
Chronic Fatigue Syndrome	BIOM	10000; 2422; 2127; 1902; 1522; 1489; 1333; 1000; 962; 959; 922; 730; 727; 664; 660; 649; 568; 464; 444; 428; 424; 243; 172		Fatigue	Neuromuscular Diseases
Chronic Fatigue Syndrome 1	XTRA	1.1,4.9,6.29,20,27.5,35,72,73,105,120,148,172,2 20,253,274,410,424,428,465,660,663,664,667,6 69,690,727.5,738,744,776,778,787,825,880,101 3,1032,1920,2127.5,6618,8768,11640.62,11640. 62,11718.75,11875,18670.15,18919.09,	Use Chronic Fatigue V, EBV, Fatigue General, Parasites General, Roundworm, and Flukes sets. If no response, try Cancer Leukemia Hairy Cell.	Fatigue	Neuromuscular Diseases
Chronic Fatigue Syndrome 2	XTRA	95,125,330,444,788,802,1550,1800,1865,2720,1 0000,11640.62=1200,11718.75,11875,18670.15 ,18919.09,	As mentioned above	Fatigue	Neuromuscular Diseases
Chronic Fatigue Syndrome 3	XTRA	465,660,666,727,787,880,1550,2127,3902,6123,	As mentioned above	Fatigue	Neuromuscular Diseases
Chronic Fatigue Syndrome 5	XTRA	105,172,253,274,660,663,667,669,738,825,1013 ,1920,6618,8768,	As mentioned above	Fatigue	Neuromuscular Diseases
Chronic Fatigue Syndrome 6	XTRA	465,727,744,776,778,787,880,1032,1920,	As mentioned above	Fatigue	Neurom. D.
Chronic Fatigue Syndrome 7	XTRA	929.52,941.92,18670.15,18919.09,	As mentioned above	Fatigue	Neurom. D.
Chronic Feeling Tired	XTRA	727,787,880,10000		Fatigue	Neurom. D.
Dullness	XTRA	727,787,880,5000			Neurom. D.
Mobility	XTRA	141.27			Neurom. D.

Subject / Argument	Author	Frequencies	Notes	Origin	Target
Joint	BIOM	1.2; 1.6; 2.65; 9.19; 9.6; 9.7; 100			Joints
Joint Mobility	XTRA	18			Joints
Joint Diseases	EDTFL	80,320,20000,85030,150000,219340,307250,45 3720,515150,683000,			Joints
Joint Inflammation	CAFL	10000	See Arthritis sets.	Inflammation	Joints
Joint Inflammation	XTRA	727,787,880,10000		Inflammation	Joints
Joint Pain Basic	XTRA	160,324,500,528,1600,5000,		Pain	Joints
Joint Pains	XTRA	28,95,240,522,600,625,650,2900,		Pain	Joints
Basic pain in joints	BIOM	5000; 1600; 1550; 880; 802; 787; 727; 528; 524; 500; 324; 250; 160; 28; 20; 9.6; 9.39; 7.69; 3		Pain	Joints
Shoulder joint	BIOM	2; 46; 46.5			Joints
Arthritis General	CAFL	10000,5000,2720,1664,1550,962,880,802,800,7 87,776,766,727,688,683,650,625,600,120,20,	Use Streptococcus Pneumonia, and Mycoplasma General if needed. See Bursitis.	Arthritis	Joints
Arthritis 1	CAFL	120=1200,962,727,787,880,1550,802,1664,80,6 0,40,30,25,26,20,10,5000,10000,7.69,3,1.2,28,1. 5=600,	As mentioned above	Arthritis	Joints
Arthritis Secondary	CAFL	2720,1000,1500,770	As mentioned above	Arthritis	Joints
Arthritis	XTRA	1664	As mentioned above	Arthritis	Joints
Arthritis - Basic	BIOM	10000.0; 5000.0; 2720.0; 1664.0; 1550.0; 1500.0; 962.0; 880.0; 802.0; 800.0; 787.0; 776.0; 766.0; 727.0; 688.0; 683.0; 650.0; 625.0; 600.0; 120.0; 20.0; 9.6		Arthritis	Joints
Arthritis	XTRA	50,750,900,9000,11090,55330,398400,425710,6 42910,980000,	As mentioned above	Arthritis	Joints
Arthritis 2	XTRA	1.19,1.5,3,7,6.9,7.7,9.39,9.4,10,20,25,26,28,30,4 0,60,80,100,120,230,250,512,660,690,728,770,7 87,802,880,1500,1550,1664,2720,3000,3176,50 00,10000,	As mentioned above	Arthritis	Joints
Arthritis 1	BIOM	2.2; 10; 12.5; 19.5; 26; 49; 55; 92.5		Arthritis	Joints
Arthritis 2	BIOM	3.8; 4; 4.9; 5.5; 8; 9.4; 9.5; 9.6		Arthritis	Joints
Arthritis 3	BIOM	1.2; 1.6; 2.65; 6.8; 8.1; 9.19; 9.4; 9.6; 9.69; 46; 56; 64; 64.5; 69; 78; 88; 100		Arthritis	Joints
Arthritis 4	BIOM	7; 9.4; 19.5; 40.5; 46; 50		Arthritis	Joints
Arthritis 5	BIOM	2.8; 3.3; 8.1; 9.19; 54; 54.25; 54.5		Arthritis	Joints
Arthritis 6	BIOM	0.7; 0.9; 2.5; 3.3; 9.8; 56; 63.5; 74.5		Arthritis	Joints
Arthritis 7	BIOM	2.5; 3.6; 3.9; 5; 6.3; 8.1; 34; 92		Arthritis	Joints
Arthritis Specific Arthritis, Degenerative Arthritis, Juvenile Chronic Arthritis, Juvenile Idiopathic Arthritis, Postinfectious Arthritis, Reactive Arthritis, Rheumatic, Acute Arthritis, Rheumatism and Osteoporosis, includes Headaches, joint & neck pain Comprehensive	EDTFL	50,900,9000,11090,55330,225470,398400,4257 10,522530,642910	As mentioned above	Arthritis	Joints
Still's Disease, Juvenile	EDTFL	120,170,300,890,6910,79710,132820,206110,43 4540,513790	Systemic Juvenile Idiopathic Arthritis.	Arthritis	Joints
Arthritis Reactive	KHZ	60,650,800,5810,42500,275000,410000,571000, 828000,937410,	As mentioned above	Arthritis	Joints
Infectious-ethyology arthritis	BIOM	1.2; 7.8; 10; 28; 230; 250; 512; 660; 688; 727; 770; 787; 880; 1664; 3000; 10000		Arthritis	Joints
Arthritis Arthrosis and Parathyroid Disturbances Affecting Calcium Metabolism	CAFL	9.6,	As mentioned above	Arthritis	Joints
Arthritis in parathyroid gland disfunction	BIOM	9.6; 465		Arthritis	Joints
Arthritis / Arthrosis, basic	BIOM	1.2; 1.6; 2.65; 6.8; 8.1; 9.19; 9.4; 9.6; 9.69; 46; 56; 64; 64.5; 69; 78; 88; 100		Arthritis	Joints
Arthritis / arthrosis of hip joints (coxarthrosis)	BIOM	5000; 880; 727; 99; 88.5; 58.5; 20; 8.5		Arthritis	Joints

Subject / Argument	Author	Frequencies	Notes	Origin	Target
Arthrosis - neck	BIOM	64.5		Arthritis	Joints
Arthrosis	BIOM	465; 10		Arthritis	Joints
Arthrosis-1	BIOM	1.6; 9.19; 9.6; 56.0; 64.0; 64.5; 78.0; 88.0		Arthritis	Joints
Gout	CAFL	9.39,3000,10000,880,787,727,20,		Gout	Joints
Gout	BIOM	10000.0; 3040.0; 2720.0; 880.0; 787.0; 727.0; 465.0; 100.0; 20.0; 9.39; 1.0		Gout	Joints
Gout- 1	BIOM	9.19; 9.69; 38; 38.5; 74; 75.5; 89.5; 95.5		Gout	Joints
Gout	EDTFL	70,570,730,2500,50000,150000,427500,695280,750000,875950	It is caused by elevated uric acid levels. Also use Kidney Insufficiency.	Gout	Joints
Pseudogout [Gout]	EDTFL	70,570,730,2500,50000,150000,427500,695280,750000,875950,		Gout	Joints
Gout 1	XTRA	9.39,20,727,787,880,3000,5000,10000,		Gout	Joints
Gout 2	XTRA	9.39,9.4,20,465,660,690,727.5,784=600,787,880,1560=600,3000,10000,		Gout	Joints
Gout 3	XTRA	9.39,20,727,787,880,3000,10000,		Gout	Joints
Anti-gout effect	BIOM	9.4		Gout	Joints
Arthritis Arthralgia Due to Gout	CAFL	9.39	As mentioned above	Gout	Joints
Arthritis Gout	XTRA	9.39,9.4,20,660,690,727.5,787,880,3000,10000,	As mentioned above	Gout	Joints
Gouty arthritis	BIOM	10000; 3040; 2720; 880; 787; 727; 465; 100; 20; 9.39		Gout	Joints
Rheumatism-gout	BIOM	38; 38.5		Gout	Joints
Hypoxanthine-Phosphoribosyl-Transferase Deficiency Disease	EDTFL	20,240,850,39500,101320,221100,419340,562910,709830,976900	Also called juvenile gout. Hereditary disease of purine metabolism associated with an overproduction of uric acid.		Joints
Rheumatoid Arthritis		*Can be caused by the bacteria Proteus mirabilis, Chlamydia Pneumoniae, Prophyromonas gengivalis and Parvovirus B19.*			
Rheumatoid Arthritis	CAFL	2.4,250,262,600,625,650,727,776,787,	Use Arthritis rheumatoid set. See Rheumatism set.	R.Arthritis	Joints
Arthritis Rheumatoid	CAFL	2.4,250,262,600,625,650,727,751,	Muscles and tendons. Use General Antiseptic and Parasites General if no response. See Bursitis.	R.Arthritis	Joints
Arthritis Rheumatoid	XTRA	1.19,250,262,600,625,650,727,766,787,	As mentioned above	R.Arthritis	Joints
Rheumatoid Arthritis	BIOM	10000; 2720; 1550; 880; 802; 787; 766; 727; 650; 625; 600; 465; 262; 250; 120; 78; 64.5; 64; 28; 20; 9.7; 9.2; 1.6; 1.2	As mentioned above	R.Arthritis	Joints
Rheumatoid Arthritis of Mixed Type	BIOM	250; 1.2; 650; 625; 600; 787; 727; 262; 776; 766		R.Arthritis	Joints
Arthritis, Rheumatoid Arthritis, Juvenile Rheumatoid	EDTFL	50,900,9000,11090,55330,225470,398400,425710,522530,642910	As mentioned above	R.Arthritis	Joints
Juvenile arthritis	BIOM	10000; 5000; 3176; 1664; 1550; 962; 880; 802; 787; 727; 120; 100; 96; 93.9; 80; 76.9; 60; 40; 30; 28; 150; 9; 76.9; 26; 25		R.Arthritis	Joints
Felty Syndrome [R.A.]	EDTFL	50,900,9000,11090,55330,225470,398400,425710,522530,642910,	As mentioned above	R.Arthritis	Joints
Polyarthritis	CAFL	512	Any type of Arthritis involving five or more joints at the same time. See Arthritis sets.	Arthritis	Joints
Polyarthritis	EDTFL	200,250,650,2500,3000,25500,96500,326160,534250,651300,	As mentioned above	Arthritis	Joints
Chronic Poly-Arthritis	BIOM	64.0; 73.5		Arthritis	Joints
Polymyalgia Rheumatica	EDTFL	50,260,570,2500,13390,85340,157500,525830,757770,975340	Syndrome with pain or stiffness, usually in neck, shoulders, upper arms, and hips, but which may occur all over.		Joints
Pseudopolyarthritis, Rhizomelic	EDTFL	200,250,650,2500,3000,25500,96500,326160,534250,651300	Typical pathology of the elderly.		Joints
Forestier-Certonciny Syndrome	EDTFL	40,240,49710,132850,235510,321510,405620,592520,654320,779300	As mentioned above		Joints
Osteoarthritis	CAFL	962,1500,770	Joint disease resulting from breakdown of cartilage and bone. Use Arthritis sets, and try Yersinia Pestis sets.	Osteoarthritis	Joints
Osteoarthritis	BIOM	770; 962; 1550		Osteoarthritis	Joints
Osteoarthritis	EDTFL	50,900,9000,11090,55330,225470,398400,425710,522530,642910	As mentioned above	Osteoarthritis	Joints
Osteoarthrosis Osteoarthrosis Deformans	EDTFL	70,460,650,42400,97500,325170,398400,425710,522530,642910	As mentioned above	Osteoarthritis	Joints
Bouchard's Node	EDTFL	70,570,730,2600,50200,150000,475500,527000,663710,776500	As mentioned above	Osteoarthritis	Joints
Heberden's Node [Osteoarthritis, Hands]	EDTFL	50,900,9000,11090,55330,225470,398400,425710,522530,642910,	As mentioned above	Osteoarthritis	Joints

Subject / Argument	Author	Frequencies	Notes	Origin	Target
Alkaptonuria	EDTFL KHZ	70,400,7500,55000,96500,376290,426900,571000,822000,937410,	Also called Black Urine Disease. Asymptomatic in children, in adults it causes disabling joint pain.		Joints
Amyoplasia Congenita	EDTFL	140,570,830,20500,40000,90500,330410,470110,667000,702700	Congenital joint contractures in two or more body areas.		Joints
Arthrogryposis	EDTFL	190,570,830,2250,5090,67500,96500,325160,424370,566410,	As mentioned above		Joints
Arthromyodysplasia congenita	EDTFL	130,570,830,2250,5090,67500,96500,325160,424370,566410,	As mentioned above		Joints
Arthropathy Neurogenic	EDTFL	110,5380,7000,15800,125000,349700,425000,571000,828000,932000,	Rapidly destructive joint disease with impaired pain sensation.		Joints
Charcot's Joint	EDTFL	30,220,2920,40000,222700,325450,477500,667000,721000,988900	As mentioned above		Joints
Beals Syndrome [Contractural Arachnodactyly]	EDTFL KHZ	160,490,620,850,15730,105250,335500,432500,725000,933910,	Rare congenital disorder with multiple joint contractures.		Joints
Contractural Arachnodactyly	EDTFL	160,490,620,850,15730,105250,335500,432500,725000,933910	As mentioned above		Joints
Bursitis	CAFL	880,787,727	Inflammation affecting the joints.	Bursitis	Joints
Bursitis	EDTFL	50,570,850,52400,119340,375030,425710,568430,642910,985900	Can be caused by Staphylococcus Aureus.	Bursitis	Joints
Bursitis 2	XTRA	660,690,727.5,787,880,10000,		Bursitis	Joints
Bursitis, pain	BIOM	54.5; 1500; 880; 787; 727		Bursitis	Joints
Calcifications	XTRA	326	Abnormal deposition of calcium in soft tissue, causing hardening.		Joints
Rheumatic Disease	EDTF KHZ	170,230,620,9970,167110,325500,422500,650000,875950,919340	Conditions causing chronic pain, often intermittent, affecting joints and/or connective tissue. See Rheumatism, Joint, Joints, and Connective Tissue sets, as well as specific body part sets.	Rheumatism	Joints
Enthesopathy	EDTFL	30,410,620,950,7500,25720,87500,480000,525290,825000	As mentioned above	Rheumatism	Joints
Rheumatic Fever	EDTFL	170,230,620,9970,167110,325500,422500,591000,710500,835280		Rheumatism	Joints
Rheumatic Fever	XTRA	333,523,768,786,376,952,	As mentioned above	Rheumatism	Joints
Reumatic Disease-1	BIOM	9.69		Rheumatism	Joints
Rheumatism	BIOM	10000; 2720; 2170; 1550; 880; 820; 802; 787; 776; 766; 727; 660; 465; 444; 376; 333; 428; 262; 20		Rheumatism	Joints
Antirheumatic	BIOM	9.6; 9.69		Rheumatism	Joints
Rheumaticus	BIO	333,376		Rheumatism	Joints
Rheumaticus	VEGA	376		Rheumatism	Joints
Rheumaticus	XTRA	333,376,820		Rheumatism	Joints
Rheumatism	CAFL	10000,776,766,262	Use Arthritis rheumatoid set. See Rheumatoid arthritis set.	Rheumatism	Joints
Rheumatism Rheumatism, Articular, Acute Rheumatism, Peri-Articular Rheumatism, Muscular Rheumatism, Arthritis and Osteo	EDTFL	50,900,9000,11090,55330,225470,398400,425710,522530,642910	As mentioned above	Rheumatism	Joints

9c - Pain and Inflammation

Subject / Argument	Author	Frequencies	Notes	Origin	Target
Endorphin Release	XTRA	38	Pain-killing morphine-like neuropeptide produced by the CNS and pituitary gland.		
Pain General			See Section 1 - Various Conditions		Pain
Nerve Pain			See Section 8c - Central and peripheral nervous system		Neuralgia
Inflammation General			See Section 1 - Various Conditions		Inflammation
Ecchymosis	EDTFL	160,220,640,58350,215500,327750,442010,617500,869730,975340	Bruise-like tissue bleed not necessarily caused by trauma		Bruises
Bruises	CAFL	9.1,110,10000			Bruises
Bruises	XTRA	9.09,727,787,880,10000,			Bruises
Contusion Bruise	XTRA	9.09,110,2720			Bruises
Contusion	CAFL	9.1,110,2720	Bruise. See Bruises set.		Bruises
Brain contusion	BIOM	9.1; 110; 2720			Bruises
Distortion, Luxation	CAFL	9.1,110	Twisting of muscles, spine. See Scoliosis.		Bruises
Sprain	BIOM	65; 65.5; 66			Bruises
Subluxation Induced Disorders	CAFL	9.6	Problems due to spinal misalignment.		Bruises
Injuries (Specific to Fractures and Dislocations)	EDTFL	80,250,570,7500,10530,12500,40000,173300,329370,675000			Bruises

Subject / Argument	Author	Frequencies	Notes	Origin	Target
Dislocations	BIOM	9.1; 110			Bruises
Injuries	EDTFL	240,920,1770,18320,28230,32120,48900,54300, 109730,328500	Groin Pull, Knee, Hamstring, Hip Flexor strain, Patellofemoral, Sciatica, Shin Splints,Shoulder Injury, Tennis elbow (epicondylitis).		Bruises
Shock	EDTFL	120,450,900,5910,137500,372500,416600,4180 00,420200,824370			Shock
Trauma	CAFL	96,192,300,760,3000,			Trauma
Traumas	BIOM	3040; 3000; 880; 787; 760; 727; 465; 300; 192; 190; 96; 95			Trauma
Trauma - Rehabilitation	BIOM	10000.0; 5000.0; 2720.0; 1550.0; 880.0; 802.0; 787.0; 727.0; 380.0; 100.0; 25.0			Trauma
Trauma, aftertreatment	BIOM	1.2; 2.5; 3.6; 3.8; 3.9; 8.6; 92			Trauma
Bone Trauma	CAFL	380,1550,802,10000,880,787,727,2720,	Cuts, fractures.	Bone	Trauma
Iinjuries to Bones	BIOM	380.0; 1550.0; 802.0; 10000.0; 880.0; 787.0; 727.0; 2720.0		Bone	Trauma
Traumatic brain injury	BIOM	4.9; 5.8; 6.3; 83.5; 3000		Head	Trauma
Head Trauma Head Injuries	EDTFL	790,900,920,3500,5820,48000,97500,123010,46 8420,592260,		Head	Trauma
Head Injuries 1	XTRA	4.9,5.79,9.59,72,160,522,660,690,727.5,787,880 ,3000		Head	Trauma
Head Injuries 2	XTRA	4.9,5.79,9.59,72,522,727,787,880,3000,		Head	Trauma
Head Injury Follow-up	CAFL	9.6,3000,880,787,727,522,72,5.8,4.9,	Seek immediate medical attention for this injury.	Head	Trauma
Frontal Region Trauma [Head Trauma]	EDTFL	790,900,920,3500,5820,48000,97500,123010,46 8420,592260,		Head	Trauma
Occipital Region Trauma	EDTFL	50,370,850,7500,87000,193930,237500,487500, 706210,946500		Head	Trauma
Parietal Region Trauma [Head Trauma]	EDTFL	790,900,920,3500,5820,48000,97500,123010,46 8420,592260,		Head	Trauma
Temporal Region Trauma	EDTFL	350,930,12330,25230,35680,87500,93500,2336 30,434000,519360		Head	Trauma

Subject / Argument	Author	Frequencies	Notes	Origin	Target
Facial Neuralgia	EDTFL	380,950,1230,5500,32500,47500,162120,23203 0,397500,679930			Face
Facial Pain Syndromes	EDTFL	100,500,700,970,5830,17500,87500,157500,596 500,857770			Face
Sphenopalatine Neuralgia	EDTFL	150,460,950,5850,62500,107600,217500,49650 0,855720,915310			Face
Facial Neuropathy	EDTFL	70,220,730,2600,5250,50000,275360,536420,65 5200,755490			Face
Neuralgia Trigeminal			See Section 8c - Central and peripheral nervous system		Face
Stiff Neck	CAFL	4.9,6,9.19,			Neck
Wry neck	BIOM	9.19; 6; 54; 64			Neck
Neck Pain Neckache	EDTFL	20,520,750,830,112500,217500,328150,497500, 775280,825000			Neck
Neck Pain	KHZ	80,490,730,800,7500,142530,285020,412030,52 8230,775560,			Neck
Crick in the Neck	XTRA	727,787,880,5000			Neck
Torticollis	EDTFL	350,750,1720,15290,113250,245910,323200,45 2000,525520,779500	Dystonic neck muscle condition with abnormal, asymmetrical head or neck position.		Neck
Spasmodic Torticollis	EDTFL	350,750,1720,15290,113250,245910,323200,45 2000,525520,779500,			Neck
Wryneck [Torticollis]	EDTFL	350,750,1720,15290,113250,245910,323200,45 2000,525520,779500,			Neck
Cervical Pain [Neck]	EDTFL	20,520,750,830,112500,217500,328150,497500, 775280,825000,			Neck
Cervical Dystonia	EDTFL	150,550,810,7950,32500,35540,337570,376290, 515500,689930	Movement disorder with muscle contractions causing twisting and repetitive movements or abnormal postures.		Neck
Cervical Spondylolysis [Neck]	EDTFL	20,520,750,830,112500,217500,328150,497500, 775280,825000,			Neck
Cervical myositis	BIOM	70.5; 64			Neck
Whiplash	CAFL	20,2720,10000	Range of neck injuries caused by or related to sudden distortion, as in a traffic accident.		Neck
Whiplash	XTRA	20	As mentioned above		Neck
Whiplash Injuries	EDTFL	20,250,970,9000,13390,15000,67500,92200,317 800,569710	As mentioned above		Neck
Chest Pain [Group 13]	EDTFL	70,410,700,970,2750,7500,15310,67500,115700 ,356720,			Chest
Costalgia	CAFL	10000,880,787,727	Rib-cage pain.		Rib
Costalgia 1	XTRA	727,787,880,5000,10000,	Rib-cage pain.		Rib

Subject / Argument	Author	Frequencies	Notes	Origin	Target
Costalgia 2	XTRA	26,160,660,690,727.5,787,802,880,1500,1550,2720,3000,10000,	Rib-cage pain.		Rib
Neuralgia Intercostal			See Section 8c - Central and peripheral nervous system		Rib
Shoulders	XTRA	7.69			Shoulder
Shoulder Injury [RDPV3 Group 21]	EDTFL	240,920,1770,18320,28230,32119,48900,54300,109730,328500,			Shoulder
Shoulder joint	BIOM	2; 46; 46.5			Shoulder
Stiff Shoulder	CAFL	10000,727,766,20	See Rheumatism, Adhesive Capsulitis, and Frozen Shoulder sets. Hook thumb under armpit and draw a figure 8 lying on its side (infinity sign). Starting at front, go up and forward, down and up to back, down in line with body (1st repetition). Repeat 10 times.		Shoulder
Frozen Shoulder	CAFL	10000,880,802,787,766,727,	Use Streptococcus Pneumoniae and try Streptococcus Pyogenes and Streptococcus Mitis sets. See Stiff Shoulder, and Adhesive Capsulitis sets.		Shoulder
Scapulohumeral periarthritis (Duplay's disease)	BIOM	10000; 880; 802; 787; 766; 727			Shoulder
Sprengel's Deformity	EDTFL	130,190,900,55750,322060,477500,527000,662410,742000,988900	Rare congenital skeletal abnormality where one shoulder blade sits higher on the back than the other.		Shoulder
Adhesive Capsulitis	EDTFL	60,230,20000,62000,125750,150000,357700,532410,653690,759830,	See Frozen Shoulder and Stiff Shoulder. Use Streptococcus Pneumoniae, and also try S. Pyogenes and S. Mitis.		Shoulder
Collarbone	XTRA	6.88			Shoulder
Shoulder-Girdle Neuropathy [Group 21]	EDTFL	240,920,1770,18320,28230,32119,48900,54300,109730,328500,			Shoulder
Algodystrophy	EDTFL	90,520,650,930,5710,87500,255310,525230,675310,878500,	Chronic systemic disease with severe pain, swelling, and skin changes. Also called Complex Regional Pain Syndrome, and Causalgia - see sets.		Shoulder - Hands
Reflex Sympathetic Dystrophy	EDTFL	440,930,17000,33000,87000,96200,150000,434000,592000,850000			Shoulder - Hands
Shoulder-Hand Syndrome	EDTFL	180,220,55000,62500,132420,210500,475170,527000,667000,749000			Shoulder - Hands
Sudek Atrophy	EDTFL	50,900,1520,55150,375030,474930,527000,662710,789000,987230			Shoulder - Hands
Brachial Neuralgia	CAFL	0.5	Shoulder, arm, or neck pain due to brachial plexus damage.		Arms
Neuritis, Brachial Plexus	EDTFL	30,250,870,2500,5870,357300,424370,561930,642910,930120			Arms
Cervico-Brachial Neuralgia	EDTFL	80,250,700,850,7200,17500,185750,350000,425170,510500	Shoulder, arm, or neck pain due to brachial plexus damage.		Arms
Brachial Plexus Neuritis	EDTFL	30,250,870,2500,5870,357300,424370,561930,642910,930120,			Arms
Brachial Plexopathy Brachial Plexus Neuropathy	EDTFL	20,320,16550,85000,232410,357200,458500,687620,712420,992000,	As mentioned above		Arms
Cubital Tunnel Syndrome	EDTFL	30,220,7500,10530,95150,312330,455820,517500,688290,843500,	Also called Ulnar Nerve Entrapment.		Arms
Neuralgia Arms	XTRA	20,727,787,880,10000,	Nerve pain in arms.		Arms
Arm Injuries	EDTFL KHZ	180,900,5500,13930,55160,250000,425090,571000,827000,932000,	As mentioned above		Arms
Elbow Pain 1	XTRA	1.19,26,160,250,2720,3000,10000,			Elbow
Elbow Pain 2	XTRA	20,727,787,880,5000,			Elbow
Epicondylalgia	XTRA	1.2,26,160,250,2720,3000,10000,	Also called Tennis Elbow or (Lateral) Epicondylitis - see sets.		Elbow
Epicondylitis	XTRA	1.2,250,728,766,776,880,	Also called Tennis Elbow or (Lateral) Epicondylalgia - see sets.		Elbow
Epicondylitis	BIOM	1.2; 9.6; 20; 65.5; 250; 728; 766; 776; 880; 5000			Elbow
Tennis Elbow	CAFL	2.4,26,160,250,3040,	Also see Epicondylitis, Epicondylalgia, and Tendomyopathy sets.		Elbow
Tennis Elbow [Epicondylitis, Lateral]	EDTFL	240,920,1770,18320,28230,32119,48900,54300,109730,328500,	As mentioned above		Elbow
Epicondylitis, Lateral Humeral [RDPV3 Group 21]	EDTFL	240,920,1770,18320,28230,32119,48900,54300,109730,328500,	As mentioned above		Elbow
Ulnar Nerve Compression	EDTFL	30,370,780,900,7500,10720,40000,157500,392500,575560,	Trapped ulnar nerve, which runs through the elbow.		Elbow
Guyon Syndrome	EDTFL	190,570,830,2290,5110,67600,96500,325160,424370,566410	As mentioned above		Elbow
Hand Tremors	XTRA	470			Hands
Shoulder-arm syndrome	BIOM	2; 46; 64; 95; 100			Hands
Carpal Tunnel Secondary	CAFL	2008,666	Median nerve compression at wrist, causing pain, numbness, and tingling. Also use Arthritis.		Hands
Carpal Tunnel Syndrome	EDTFL	130,900,5580,30000,47500,360490,365000,388900,434000,456110,	As mentioned above		Hands

Subject / Argument	Author	Frequencies	Notes	Origin	Target
Tunnel syndrome	BIOM	**2008; 666**			Hands
Entrapment Neuropathy	EDTFL	190,220,730,5580,13390,150000,475850,73642 0,819350,915700			Hands
Compression Neuropathy, Carpal Tunnel	EDTFL	130,900,5580,30000,47500,360490,365000,388 900,434000,456110			Hands
Carpal Tunnel Syndrome 1	XTRA	465,660,666,784,787,800,880,960,1560,1840,19 98,	As mentioned above		Hands
Carpal Tunnel Syndrome 2	XTRA	6.29,15,20.5,146,148,444,465,522,600,625,650, 660,685,690,700,727,737,760,776,787,802,832, 880,1000,1500,1550,1865,2008,10000,	As mentioned above		Hands
Carpal Tunnel Syndrome 3	XTRA	**666,2008**	As mentioned above		Hands
Dupuytren's Contracture	CAFL	**1.2,250**	4th and 5th finger curling into palm, unable to straighten.		Hands
Dupuytren's Contracture	BIOM	**1.2; 65; 250**			Hands
Dupuytren's Contracture	EDTFL	1060,2260,5650,7170,8220,9430,17220,668000, 721000,987260	As mentioned above		Hands
Felon 1	CAFL	657,659,738,751,	Also called a Whitlow. Purulent infection of fingertips.		Hands
Felon 2	CAFL	663,665,720,722,	As mentioned above		Hands
Felon 3	XTRA	657,659,663,665,720,722,738,751,	As mentioned above		Hands
Panaritium	BIOM	657; 659; 663; 665; 720; 722; 723; 738; 751			Hands
Spine Problems A=432 Hz	XTRA	128.43,144.16,161.82,171.44,192.43,216,242.45 ,136.07,152.74,181.63,203.88,228.84,	See "The Spine Frequencies". Based on A=432Hz tuning. Waveform=square. Repeat Program=0.		Spine
Spine Problems A=440 Hz	XTRA	130.81,146.83,164.81,174.61,196,220.2,246.94, 138.57,155.56,185,207.65,233.08,	See "The Spine Frequencies". Based on A=440Hz tuning. Waveform=square. Repeat Program=0.		Spine
Vertebral column - total	BIOM	2.65; 4; 9.6; 9.69; 67.5; 76; 94; 96; 100			Spine
Spinal Column 2	BIOM	1.2; 2.5; 3.6; 3.8; 3.9; 7.5; 33.0; 79.0; 2.5; 9.6; 9.69; 68.5; 69.0; 84.5; 96.0; 100.0			Spine
Vertebral column degeneration	BIOM	**69; 84.5; 96**			Spine
Cervical spine	BIOM	2; 2.5; 3; 3.5; 9.0; 59; 60; 67.5; 95			Spine
Rachialgia	BIOM	3000.0; 95.0; 1550.0; 802.0; 880.0; 787.0; 776.0; 727.0; 650.0; 625.0; 600.0; 28.0; 10.0; 35.0; 28.0; 7.69; 1.2; 110.0; 100.0; 60.0; 428.0; 680.0; 326.0			Spine
Lordosis	EDTFL	50,350,750,930,5710,7500,345730,465340,5915 00,725000	Excessive inward curvature of lower back - the opposite to kyphosis.		Back
Lordosis	XTRA	150,230,620,930,7500,12690,52500,72500,9350 0,96500,	As mentioned above		Back
Scoliosis	EDTFL	20,320,630,950,124370,175000,337900,479500, 527000,667000	Abnormal lateral curvatures of spine, Also see Alignment of Individual, Distortion, and Lumbar Vertebrae Deformed.		Back
Central Cord Syndrome	EDTFL	180,500,850,5120,7250,13930,72500,125170,37 9930,475190	Most common form of cervical spine injury.		Spine
Spondylitis	XTRA	**28,**	Inflammation of the vertebra.	Spondylitis	Spine
Ankylosing Spondylitis	CAFL	3000,95,1550,802,880,787,776,727,650,625,600 ,28,10,35,28,7.69,2.4,110,100,60,428,680,	Chronic inflammatory disease of spinal and sacroiliac joints. Also see Ankylosing Spondylitis sets.	Spondylitis	Spine
Ankylosing Spondylitis	BIOM	3000; 1550; 802; 880; 787; 776; 727; 650; 625; 600; 428; 680; 326; 110; 100; 95; 77; 60; 35; 28; 10; 1.2			Spine
Ankylosing Spondylitis	EDTFL	140,320,970,7500,125710,175750,512330,6820 20,759830,927100,	Also see Ankylosing Spondylitis sets.	Spondylitis	Spine
Bechterew Disease [Rheumatic]	EDTFL	170,230,620,9970,167110,325500,422500,6500 00,875950,919340,	Also known as ankylosing spondylitis (AS)	Spondylitis	Spine
Bekhterev's disease	BIOM	**9.6**			Spine
Marie-Struempell Disease	EDTFL	30,500,870,10440,37110,87500,135230,225680, 397500,597500	As mentioned above	Spondylitis	Spine
Rheumatoid Spondylitis	EDTFL	50,900,9000,11090,55330,68500,232500,55110 0,779230,839430,		Spondylitis	Spine
Spondylarthritis Ankylopoietica	EDTFL	210,320,52500,110350,175130,475370,520090, 600790,740000,906220		Spondylitis	Spine
Psoriatic Ankylosing Spondylitis	BIOM	3000; 1550; 880; 802; 787; 776; 727; 680; 650; 625; 600; 428; 110; 100; 95; 60; 35; 28; 10		Spondylitis	Spine
Psoriasis Ankylosing Spondylitis	CAFL	3000,95,1550,802,880,787,776,727,650,625,600 ,28,1.2,10,35,28,7.69,110,100,60,428,680,	Chronic inflammatory disease of spinal and sacroiliac joints. Also see Ankylosing Spondylitis, and Spondylitis Ankylosing sets. Use Nanobacter set.	Spondylitis	Spine
Spondylolisthesis	EDTFL	120,250,870,7500,8300,13930,85680,225230,47 5680,527000	Forward displacement of a vertebra, especially the fifth lumbar vertebra, most commonly after fracture.	Spondylitis	Spine

Subject / Argument	Author	Frequencies	Notes	Origin	Target
Disc Herniated	CAFL	727,787,2720,10000,	As mentioned above	Hernia	Discs
Hernia Disc	CAFL	10000,787,727,2720,5000,	As mentioned above	Hernia	Discs
Disc Herniated 1	XTRA	15,25.39,324,660,690,727.5,787,2720,10000,	As mentioned above	Hernia	Discs
Intervertebral hernia	BIOM	727; 787; 2720; 10000			Discs
Slipped Discs	CAFL	125,880,787,727,95,72,20,	As mentioned above	Hernia	Discs
Disc Slipped	XTRA	20,26,57,72,95,125,146,333,523,555,660,690,727.5,768,786,787,880,	As mentioned above	Hernia	Discs
Disc Swelling	XTRA	15,25.39,326	As mentioned above	Hernia	Discs
Herniated Disc Reduce Swelling	XTRA	25.4,324,15	As mentioned above	Hernia	Discs
Intervertebral Disk [Herniated]	EDTFL	180,560,950,7500,22500,42500,125220,275560,533630,652430,		Hernia	Discs
Disk, Herniated	EDTFL	180,560,950,7500,22500,42500,125220,275560,533630,652430,		Hernia	Discs
Disk degeneration	BIOM	2.5; 67; 92; 96			Discs
Disk trauma	BIOM	68.5			Discs
Disk regeneration	BIOM	2.5; 96			Discs
Prolapsed Disk [Herniated Disc]	EDTFL	180,560,950,7500,22500,42500,125220,275560,533630,652430,			Discs
Slipped Disk [Herniated Disk]	EDTFL	180,560,950,7500,22500,42500,125220,275560,533630,652430,	As mentioned above		Discs
Backache 1	CAFL	10000,1550,880,802,787,760,727,305=360,212=360,41.2,33=300,	Can be caused by a spinal disc infection with anaerobic bacteria, especially the bacterium Propionibacterium acnes.		Back
Backache 2	CAFL	9.3,9.4,9.6,7.6,7.7,3,0.5,432,465,727,728,776,784,787,	Together with one of these sets, also use a Disc Herniated set and conclude with Muscles to Relax.		Back
Backache Chronic Lower 1	CAFL	728	As mentioned above		Back
Pain, Back Pain	EDTFL	160,350,950,5260,11900,17500,72500,215700,456500,517500			Back
Backache	BIOM	10000; 880; 787; 727; 125; 95; 72; 444; 1865; 432; 305; 212; 125; 9572; 41.2; 33; 9.6; 7.7; 9.4; 7.6; 9.3; 3			Back
Backache	EDTFL	140,400,7400,55000,96500,376290,425090,571000,833000,932000,	As mentioned above		Back
Low-back pain	BIOM	760; 1550; 802; 880; 787; 727; 10000; 465; 212; 412; 33			Back
Back Pain Generalized	XTRA	328	As mentioned above		Back
Muscle pain in back; trauma	BIOM	320; 305; 250; 240; 10; 80; 40; 41.2; 20; 10; 5.8; 2.5; 1.5; 1.2; 1.0; 0.5			Back
Back Pain Lower	XTRA	0.5	Lumbar back pain.		Back
Back Pain Reduce	XTRA	326			Back
Back Harm	XTRA	727,787,880,5000,10000,	Back and spine complaints		Back
Backache and Spasms 1	CAFL	120,212,240,424,465,528,760,727,787,880,1550,2112,5000,10000,	If no relief, use Kidney Insufficiency set, take magnesium and B6 supplements, drink plenty of water.		Back
Back Spasms	XTRA	26,33,41.2,120,146,160,212,240,305,326,333,424,464,465,466,522,523,528,555,660,690,727.5,760,768,784,786,787,789,800,802,880,1550,1552,2112,3000,5000,10000			Back
Lumbago	CAFL	10000,800,880,787,727,125,95,72,444,1865,9.19,8.25,7.69,300,	Also called low back pain. Also see Back sets, and Pain sets.	Lumbago	Back
Lumbago	XTRA	30,190	As mentioned above	Lumbago	Back
Lumbago	BIOM	10000; 880; 787; 727; 125; 95; 72; 444; 1865; 9.2; 8.25; 7.7		Lumbago	Back
Lumbago, lumbar myalgia	BIOM	62.5; 64.5; 67.5; 76.5		Lumbago	Back
Lumbago 1	XTRA	7.69,8.25,9.18,72,95,125,444,727,787,880,1865,10000,	As mentioned above	Lumbago	Back
Lumbago 2	XTRA	7.69,7.7,8.25,9.18,9.19,72,95,125,300,444,660,690,727.5,787,800,802,880,1550,1865,10000,	As mentioned above	Lumbago	Back
Lumbar Compression	XTRA	6110	See sets for Sciatica, and Disc.	Lumbago	Back
Lumbar Vertebrae Deformed	XTRA	727,787,880,10000,	Also see Alignment of Individual, Distortion, and Scoliosis.	Lumbago	Back
Sacroiliac Joint Dysfunction	EDTFL	60,260,750,2250,7500,52500,320550,371050,373010,687620	Pain in sacroiliac joint region caused by abnormal motion in the joint, usually causing inflammation.	Lumbago	Back
Sciatica 1	CAFL	254,464,465,866,15,25.4,	Can be caused by Propionibacterium acnes. Pain radiating down leg from lower back, usually due to spinal disc herniation. Also see Disc Herniated.		Sciatica
Sciatica Ischias	CAFL	1550,802,880,787,727,690,666,10,			Sciatica
Sciatica	EDTFL	240,730,880,7500,30520,57500,95870,97500,424980,562960			Sciatica

Subject / Argument	Author	Frequencies	Notes	Origin	Target
Sciatic Neuralgia	EDTFL	240,730,880,7500,30520,323000,502100,69009 0,722920,951000			Sciatica
Piriformis Syndrome	EDTFL	140,220,610,58550,215500,328950,442010,617 500,869710,975340	Neuromuscular disorder that occurs when the piriformis muscle, located in the gluteal region, compresses or irritates the sciatic nerve.		Sciatica
Hip joint	BIOM	13	See Arthritis sets.		Hip
Hip Pain	CAFL	880,787,727,20,	See Arthritis sets.		Hip
Hip Pain 1	XTRA	20,727,787,880,5000,			Hip
Hip Pain 2	XTRA	20,660,690,727.5,787,880,2720,10000,			Hip
Coxa Plana	EDTFL	60,320,730,850,10890,66300,185290,253040,73 5300,957500			Hip
Legg-Perthes Disease [Perthes]	EDTFL	50,370,870,2250,33500,75850,275540,320250,4 75350,857770,	Childhood hip disorder caused by disrupted blood supply to femoral head.		Hip
Perthes Disease	EDTFL	50,370,870,2250,33500,75850,275540,320250,4 75350,857770	Flattening of head of femur due to Osteochondrosis - also see this set.		Hip
Hip Joint Pain	XTRA	15.19,47.29,72.7,338,528,2422,2475,3255,4225, 4332,5754,7433,7938,8967,	See Arthritis sets.		Hip
Hip Ligaments Irritated	XTRA	5120			Hip
Hip Ligaments Tensions	XTRA	5403			Hip
Knee	BIOM	1.2; 1.6; 2.65; 9.19; 9.6			Knee
Knee Injury	EDTFL	240,920,1770,18320,28230,32119,48900,54300, 109730,328500,			Knee
Meniscus Tear (Knee)	EDTFL	100,410,870,5500,130090,255610,362000,4926 80,597500,654370			Knee
Knee Joint Pain	CAFL	1550,880,802,787,727,28,20,7.69,3,1.2,250,9.6, 9.39,	See Arthritis sets.		Knee
Knee Joint Pain 1	XTRA	1.19,3,7.69,9.39,9.59,20,28,250,727,787,802,88 0,1550,			Knee
Chondromalacia Patellae	EDTFL	120,250,960,5250,32500,475130,527000,66171 0,742000,988900	Inflammation of the back of the kneecap and softening of cartilage		Knee
Legs	XTRA	727,787,800,880,10000,			Legs
Legs; curvature	BIOM	46			Legs
Restless Legs Syndrome	EDTFL	40,550,570,870,7500,50190,140000,390000,624 370,819340	Neurological disorder with an irresistible urge to move the body to stop uncomfortable sensations, most commonly the legs.		Legs
Leg Ulcer	EDTFL	150,240,650,830,2500,127500,255470,387500,6 96500,825910,			Legs
Swelling Legs and Feet	XTRA	20,727,787,880,5000,10000,	Also see Kidney Insufficiency, and Lymph Stasis sets.		Legs
Plantar fasciitis	EDTFL	200,320,2880,5250,132500,237500,496500,626 070,875340,927000	Inflammation of the muscle band that lines the sole of the foot and is manifested by intense pain in the heel.		Bone
Plantaris	CAFL	2008	Plantaris muscle and tendon of leg.		Foot
Cavus Deformity [PES}	EDTFL	150,900,5620,93500,222700,425000,522530,68 9960,752630,923700,	Type of foot deformity.		Foot
Pes Cavus	EDTFL	150,900,5620,93500,222700,425000,522530,68 9960,752630,923700,			Foot
Flatfoot	BIOM	71; 71.5; 72; 89			Foot
Talipes Cavus	EDTFL	150,900,5620,93500,222700,425000,522530,68 9960,752630,923700			Foot
Foot Deformities	EDTFL	130,350,850,5430,17500,42500,236420,478500, 527000,667000			Foot
Metatarsal Deformity	EDTFL	150,230,720,1830,82530,137510,242100,40750 0,592520,693200			Foot
Freiberg's Disease	EDTFL	570,5000,32500,50000,90000,319350,522530,6 89930,752630,910250,	Metatarsal bone destruction caused by loss of blood supply.		Foot
Sever's Disease / Calcaneal Apophysitis	EDTFL	180,230,55000,62500,132410,210500,475170,5 27000,667000,749000	Painful inflammation of growth plate in heel of growing children, typically adolescents.		Foot
Metatarsus Primus Varus	EDTFL	130,520,2610,110390,211110,351020,405850,6 22280,753050,832630	Commonly called a bunion.		Foot
Trench Foot	EDTFL	170,400,620,850,2500,25000,109320,362580,62 1680,775670			Foot
Morton's Neuroma	EDTFL	60,500,900,2250,7500,32710,155610,397500,62 4940,815700	It is a neuropathy that consists of a swelling of a nerve in the foot that is located between the third and fourth toes		Foot
Hammertoes	EDTFL	70,240,650,5760,72260,123000,502500,622880, 713230,807730			Foot
Bunion Pain	CAFL	20		Big Toe	Foot
Bunions	XTRA	20,2720,10000		Big Toe	Foot
Bunion	EDTFL	50,240,72500,122530,342060,512330,682450,7 53070,802590,926700		Big Toe	Foot
Hallux Abductovalgus Hallux Valgus	EDTFL	190,570,1120,7500,27500,42700,96500,325430, 415700,562910		Big Toe	Foot

Subject / Argument	Author	Frequencies	Notes	Origin	Target
Feet Excessive Sweating	XTRA	148	Excessively sweaty feet.		Foot
Cold Feet and Hands	CAFL	20,125,146,200,727,787,880,5000,			Foot
Chilblains	CAFL	20,232,622,822,2112,4211,	See Perniosis set.		Hands Feet
Chilblains	EDTFL	200,250,650,2500,3000,7500,96500,327160,534 250,652480			Hands Feet
Frigorism	BIOM	10000; 8237.5; 7879.5; 7727.5; 7344; 5000; 4887.9; 2950; 2900; 2650; 2600; 2413; 1550; 1234; 880; 802; 787; 776; 766; 746; 740; 727			Hands Feet
Raynaud's Disease			See Section 4b - Blood vessels		Hands Feet
Phantom Limb	KHZ	160,550,950,17500,93980,137500,396500,5758 30,824370,963190,	Sensation that an amputated limb or removed organ is still present, usually painful.		
Phantom limb pains	BIOM	49.5; 29.5			
Pseudomelia	EDTFL	30,410,15190,87500,122060,312330,532410,65 5200,750000,927200	As mentioned above		

9d - Muscles

Subject / Argument	Author	Frequencies	Notes	Origin	Target
Muscles - Pilot frequencies	BIOM	3.8; 6.8; 10; 40; 42.5; 45; 45.5			Muscle
Musculature - Pilot frequencies	BIOM	77.5; 80; 82.5; 99; 95.5; 92.5			Muscle
Stimulate Muscle Healing	XTRA	13.5			Muscle
Muscle Growth and Repair	XTRA	25			Muscle
Muscle regeneration	BIOM	2.5; 9.4; 10; 45.5; 84; 84.5; 85; 99			Muscle
Muscles - laxity	BIOM	240; 304; 965; 6000			Muscle
Muscle Tonic	CAFL	20,120,240,300,304,328,728,880,5000,10000,			Muscle
Muscle Repair	XTRA	5000			Muscle
Muscles to Relax	CAFL	965,20,120,240,760,6.8,6000,304,	Important set to insert, together with specific ones, in case of back pain and the like.		Muscle
Muscular Diseases	EDTFL	130,400,620,900,5580,117250,442580,657510,7 22590,865870			Muscle
Stiff Muscles Secondary	CAFL	0.05,1,1.2,1.5,2.5,5.9,10,250,776,787,802,880,1 550,	See Muscles to Relax, and Stiff Muscles sets. Relax in a hot bath, liberally laced with epsom salt.		Muscle
Stiff Muscles	CAFL	320,328,304,300,240,160,776,728,1800,125,80, 40,20,6000,	As mentioned above		Muscle
Muscles Stiff	XTRA	304	As mentioned above		Muscle
Stiff muscles - basic	BIOM	320; 250; 240; 160; 125; 80; 40; 20; 10; 5.8; 2.5; 1.5; 1.2; 1; 0.5; 1800; 1550; 802; 880; 787; 727; 776; 727			Muscle
Stiff muscles - secondary	BIOM	6000; 5000; 1800; 1550; 802; 776; 728; 328; 320; 304; 300; 250; 240; 160; 125; 80; 40; 20; 10; 6; 3; 2			Muscle
Muscle pain	BIOM	6000; 2170; 324; 320; 250; 240; 10; 80; 40; 20; 10; 5.8; 2.5; 1.5; 1.2			Muscle
Muscular Pain and Injury	CAFL	2720,6000,320,250,240,160,125,80,40,20,10,5.8 ,2.5,1.5,1.2,1,0.5,	See Pain, and General antiseptic sets.		Muscle
Muscle Pain and Injury	XTRA	160	As mentioned above		Muscle
Limb Cramp	EDTFL	20,200,900,20000,55000,92500,224700,475110, 527000,987230,		Muscle	Muscle
Muscle Cramps/Spasms	XTRA	6.8		Muscle	Muscle
Muscle Cramp	KHZ	130,400,620,3830,35250,132250,282500,32750 0,522500,748000,			Muscle
Muscle fatigue accompanied with pain	BIOM	4; 6; 10; 45; 47.5; 50; 52.5; 70; 80; 99.5			Muscle
Muscle / Spasms			See Section 9a - Neuromuscular Diseases		Muscle
Neck muscles - stiffness	BIOM	20; 727; 787; 880; 10000; 4.9; 6; 9.19		Neck	Muscle
Neck muscles convulsion	BIOM	5; 6.8		Neck	Muscle
Back muscles	BIOM	1550; 880; 802; 787; 776; 727; 725; 625; 428; 110; 95; 60; 14; 10; 8		Back	Muscle
Body 1 (muscles of the Head)	BIOM	52; 58; 60; 62; 70; 98; 100; 102; 110; 112; 114; 118; 120; 122; 124; 126; 130; 132; 134; 136; 138; 140		Head	Muscle
Body 2 (Neck muscles)	BIOM	270; 272; 274; 276; 278; 282; 284; 286; 288; 290; 292; 294; 296; 298; 300; 302; 304; 306; 308; 314; 322; 326; 332; 334; 346; 350; 362; 370; 380; 394; 396		Neck	Muscle
Body 3 (the muscles of the Upper back)	BIOM	390; 392; 398; 400; 414; 416; 418; 420; 422; 424; 426; 428; 430; 432; 434; 436; 438; 440; 442		Upper back	Muscle

Subject / Argument	Author	Frequencies	Notes	Origin	Target
Body 4 (Chest muscles)	BIOM	402; 404; 406; 408; 410; 412; 460; 462; 464		Chest	Muscle
Body 5 (Shoulder muscles)	BIOM	444; 446; 448; 450; 452; 454; 456; 458; 466; 468; 470; 472; 474		Shoulder	Muscle
Body 6 (Forearm)	BIOM	476; 478; 480; 482; 484; 486; 488; 490; 492; 494; 496; 498; 500; 502; 504; 506; 508; 510; 512; 514; 516; 518; 520; 522; 524; 526; 528; 530; 532; 534; 536; 538; 540; 542; 544; 546; 548; 550; 552; 554; 556; 558; 560; 562		Forearm	Muscle
Body 7 (Hand muscles)	BIOM	564; 566; 568; 570; 572; 574; 576; 578; 580; 582; 584; 586; 588; 590; 592; 594; 596		Hand	Muscle
Body 8 (average muscle and Lower back)	BIOM	610; 612; 614; 618; 642; 648; 652; 656; 662; 690		Lower back	Muscle
Body 9 (Abdominal muscles)	BIOM	692; 694; 696; 698; 700; 702; 704; 706; 708; 710; 712; 714; 718		Abdominal	Muscle
Body 10 (muscles of the Buttocks and Pelvis)	BIOM	722; 724; 726; 728; 730; 732; 734; 736; 738; 740; 742; 744; 746; 752; 780; 782; 784; 786; 788; 848; 850; 852; 860; 862; 864		Buttocks and Pelvis	Muscle
Body 11 (Femoris)	BIOM	790; 792; 794; 796; 798; 800; 804; 806; 808; 810; 812; 814; 816; 818; 820; 822; 824; 826; 828; 830; 832; 834; 836; 838; 840		Femoris	Muscle
Body 12 (Calf muscle)	BIOM	842; 844; 846; 854; 856; 858; 870; 872; 874; 876; 878; 880; 882; 884; 886; 888; 890; 892; 894; 896; 898; 900; 902; 904; 906; 908; 910; 912; 914; 920; 922; 924; 926; 928; 930; 932; 934; 936; 938; 940; 942; 944		Calf	Muscle
Body 13 (the muscles of the Foot)	BIOM	946; 948; 950; 952; 954; 956; 958; 960; 962; 964; 966; 968; 970; 972; 974; 976		Foot	Muscle
Oppenheim Disease	EDTFL	70,400,900,16850,20140,67110,135520,325000, 475520,612560	Congenital hypotonia of skeletal muscle.		Muscle
Myopathies, Structural	EDTFL	80,320,1730,32900,67500,125230,328350,5390 00,832590,915580	Disease that damages the voluntary muscles.	Myopathy	Muscle
Congenital Fiber Type Disproportion	EDTFL	180,350,17600,37900,210500,327150,476500,6 65350,789000,987230	Muscular condition that may accompany some neurological disorders.	Myopathy	Muscle
Inflammatory Myopathy	EDTFL	80,350,600,700,141200,212030,297500,425950, 675310,826320	Weakness, inflammation, and sometimes pain in muscles.	Myopathy	Muscle
Centronuclear Myopathy	EDTFL	170,520,730,13610,125290,255560,434120,551 230,673290,713720		Myopathy	Muscle
Myositis	CAFL	120,122,125,129,1124,1169,762,	Involves progressive muscle weakness. Caused by autoimmune conditions and statin drugs.	Myositis	Muscle
Myositis	EDTFL	530,910,15750,62200,95000,250000,434000,52 4370,682020,753070		Myositis	Muscle
Myositis	BIO	120,122,125,129,1124,1169,	As mentioned above	Myositis	Muscle
Myositis	VEGA	122,1124,1169,	As mentioned above	Myositis	Muscle
Myositis	BIOM	1.2; 6.8; 64; 70.5; 72; 122; 129; 762; 1124; 1169		Myositis	Muscle
Cervical myositis	BIOM	70.5; 64		Myositis	Muscle
Polymyositis	EDTFL	180,550,1000,5250,27500,42500,72500,195890, 420020,719340	Chronic inflammation of the muscles (Inflammatory Myopathy - see set) related to Dermatomyositis (see set) and inclusion body Myositis (see sets).	Myositis	Muscle
Fibromyalgia			See Section 15 - Connective Tissue		

9e - Bones

Subject / Argument	Author	Frequencies	Notes	Origin	Target
Bone	XTRA	418.3	General bone program.		Bone
Bone structure	BIOM	4.5			Bone
Bony skeleton	BIOM	100			Bone
Bone Stimulate Healing	XTRA	7			Bone
Bones Stimulate Healing	XTRA	7,25,50			Bone
Bone Stimulation	XTRA	50			Bone
Bone Regeneration	CAFL	2720,10000			Bone
Bone Regeneration	BIOM	10000; 3176; 2720; 266; 148; 50.5; 47; 20.5; 2; 20.5; 3.9; 4; 6.3; 7			Bone
Bone tissue regeneration	BIOM	2; 7; 47; 50.5; 69; 6.8; 148; 266			Bone
Bone Regeneration 1	XTRA	7,424,465,660,690,727.5,784,787,880,1552,156 0,1577,2720,10000,			Bone
Bone Growth	XTRA	25,50			Bone
Bone Conduction	XTRA	4902	Bone enhancement.		Bone
Bone Trauma			See Section 9c - Pain and Inflammation	Trauma	Bone
Treatment of Bones	BIOM	82.5; 83.5; 85.5			Bone
Fracture	XTRA	124		Trauma	Bone

Subject / Argument	Author	Frequencies	Notes	Origin	Target
Bone Fractures	XTRA	3,220,230,380,660,690,727.5,787,802,880,1550,2720,10000,		Fractures	Bone
Bone fracture; healing	BIOM	220; 230; 380; 1550; 802; 10000; 880; 787; 727; 2720; 3176			Bone
Fracture - Fusion	BIOM	220.0; 230.0; 10000.0; 880.0; 787.0; 727.0			Bone
Bone Fracture Treatment	BIOM	92.0			Bone
Bone Fractures	EDTFL	80,250,570,7500,10530,12500,40000,173300,329370,675000,		Fractures	Bone
Fractures Bone 1	XTRA	220,230,727,787,880,10000,		Fractures	Bone
Fractures Bone 2	XTRA	1028	Use in Contact Mode on both sides of injury 3 times daily. Accelerates healing of broken bones and non-union joints.	Fractures	Bone
Fractures Healing	CAFL	220,230,10000,880,787,727,		Fractures	Bone
Fracture Healing	XTRA	25,50		Fractures	Bone
Injuries (Specific to Fractures and Dislocations)	EDTFL	80,250,570,7500,10530,12500,40000,173300,329370,675000		Fractures	Bone
Posttraumatic osteopathy	BIOM	82.5			Bone
Bone Pain and Inflammation	RL	40,783	From Dr. Richard Loyd.	Pain	Bone
Inflammation Bone	XTRA	724,736,743,770		Inflammation	Bone
Bone Diseases Bone Diseases, Metabolic	EDTFL	70,490,32500,125750,275000,329570,425000,721000,835750,937410			Bone
Osteopenia	EDTFL	180,200,620,112500,230890,412500,615000,752500,802500,925520			Bone
Infection Bone	XTRA	47,600,625,650,660,690,727.5,776,787,880,1600,1800,10000	Also see Osteomyelitis sets.	Infection	Bone
Bone and periosteal coverage diseases	BIOM	2720; 1800; 1600; 650; 625; 600; 880; 787; 776; 743; 736; 727; 444; 85.5; 83.5; 58; 47.5			Bone
Bone Disease and Periodontal	XTRA	47.5,600,625,650,728=900,776,787,880,1600,1800,		Oral Cavity	Bone
Bone Disease Periodontal Disease	CAFL	47.5,600,625,650,727,776,787,880,1600,1800,	See Bone regeneration, dental, and osteo sets.	Oral Cavity	Bone
Bone Spurs	CAFL	1.2,250	Excrescence of bone tissue localized on the articular surface of a bone	Osteophytes	Bone
Bone Spur 1	XTRA	1.19,3.39,250		Osteophytes	Bone
Bone Spur 2	XTRA	4931		Osteophytes	Bone
Osteophytosis, Spinal	EDTFL			Osteophytes	Bone
Spinal Osteophytosis	EDTFL	320,320,950,7500,25750,52400,425180,571000,753070,912330	Formation of Bone Spurs (see sets) in spine.	Osteophytes	Bone
Osteophytosis, Arthritis, Rheumatism	EDTFL	50,900,9000,11090,55330,225470,398400,425710,522530,642910		Osteophytes	Bone
Osteophytes	BIOM	120; 250		Osteophytes	Bone
Osteophytes (Bone Spurs)	EDTFL	160,230,7730,72250,105290,207000,332500,547500,750000,875000		Osteophytes	Bone
Heel Spurs	XTRA	1.19,120,250,	Bony projections called osteophytes that can build up at joint margins. Also see Bone Spurs.	Osteophytes	Bone
Heel Spur	EDTFL	110,220,730,3750,7050,51260,137500,236420,472290,851170	As mentioned above	Osteophytes	Bone
Eperon	BIOM	1.2; 120; 250		Osteophytes	Bone
Exostoses	EDTFL	100,500,680,5950,35710,87400,137500,357500,596500,742060	Formation of new bone on surface of existing bone due to excess calcium. Also see Calcium sets.		Bone
Fibrous Dysplasia of Bone	EDTFL	850,900,980,17530,213260,215470,362510,422060,608410,751200	Non-cancerous abnormal bone growth where normal bone is replaced with fibrous bone tissue.		Bone
Osteitis Fibrosa Disseminata	EDTFL	70,120,2540,6250,12750,106700,195330,338210,752630,923700	As mentioned above		Bone
Freiberg's Disease	EDTFL	570,5000,32500,50000,90000,319350,522530,689930,752630,910250,	Metatarsal bone destruction caused by loss of blood supply.		Bone
Bone Hypertrophy	EDTFL	70,500,850,7500,20000,37500,57500,661710,742000,988900	Excessive growth of bone.		Bone
Hyperostosis	EDTFL	40,250,460,520,750,900,42500,87500,132440,376290	As mentioned above		Bone
Cortical Hyperostosis, Congenital	EDTFL	30,220,6480,30850,95690,292500,313200,612500,674020,925950	As mentioned above		Bone
Hyperostosis, Cortical, Congenital	EDTFL	30,180,6480,30850,95690,292500,313200,612500,674020,925950,	As mentioned above		Bone
Caffey-De Toni-Silvermann Syndrome	EDTFL	40,410,30000,55150,67500,125000,350000,412330,563190,714820	Causes irritability, pain, tenderness, hyperaesthesia, swelling, and redness.		Bone
Hypophosphatasia	EDTFL	100,780,1500,2850,5580,67500,137500,285790,495800,726000,	Rare genetic metabolic bone disease.	Genetic disorder	Bone

Subject / Argument	Author	Frequencies	Notes	Origin	Target
Osteitis	BIO	770	Inflammation of bone - causes include bacteria, 'dry socket,' and Paget's Disease of Bone. Can be caused by **Staphylococcus aureus.**	Osteitis	Bone
Osteitis	CAFL	2.65	As mentioned above	Osteitis	Bone
Osteitis 2	CAFL	770,743,736,724	As mentioned above	Osteitis	Bone
Kieferosteitis	BIO	432,516	Type of bone inflammation marked by enlargement and pain.	Osteitis	Bone
Kieferosteitis	CAFL	432,516,384	As mentioned above	Osteitis	Bone
Osteitis Deformans	EDTFL	110,480,2540,6250,12750,106700,195330,3382 10,402230,592090	Also called Paget's Disease of Bone - see set. Condition with deranged bone remodelling, leading to enlarged and/or misshapen bones.	Osteitis	Bone
Paget's Disease	EDTFL	40,320,620,950,5000,22500,60000,90000,32536 0,863610	As mentioned above	Osteitis	Bone
Paget's Disease of Bone	EDTFL	30,320,620,950,5000,22500,90000,322060,3375 90,524940	As mentioned above	Osteitis	Bone
Osteochondritis	EDTFL	300,830,7500,8000,22500,40000,225370,47552 0,527000,667000	Inflammation of cartilage or bone in a joint. Also see Osteoarthritis sets.	Inflammation	Bone
Osteochondrosis	BIOM	787; 784; 776; 728; 727; 465; 432; 728; 96; 94; 93.0; 77; 76; 30; 50; 9.6; 9.4; 9.3; 7.7; 7.6; 3; 0.5			Bone
Disseminated osteochondrosis	BIOM	1.2; 1.6; 2; 2.65; 3; 9.19; 9.6; 9.69; 62.5; 64.5; 67.5; 76; 76.5; 95; 100			Bone
Blount's Disease	EDTFL	40,520,11090,55750,60000,125000,275160,571 000,834000,932000	As mentioned above	Inflammation	Bone
Osteogenesis Imperfecta	EDTFL	130,570,780,900,2250,144900,323720,527000,6 02530,918280	Congenital disorder with brittle bones prone to fracture, due to defective or no connective tissue production.		Bone
Fragilitas Ossium	EDTFL	130,550,960,5710,13930,137500,262500,49750 0,626070,822530			Bone
Lobstein Disease [Osteogenesis imperfecta]	EDTFL	130,570,780,900,2250,144900,323720,527000,6 02530,918280,			Bone
Osteomalacia	EDTFL	60,410,900,7500,8000,77500,187500,358810,72 1000,986220	Softening of bones usually due to low phosphate or calcium levels. Called Rickets in children - see sets.		Bone
Osteohalisteresis; bone softening	BIOM	44.5; 69.5; 80; 84; 88; 95; 96; 100			Bone
Osteomyelitis	CAFL	2720,2489,2170,2127,2008,1800,1600,1550,802 ,1500,880,832,787,776,727,690,666,	Infection and inflammation of bone and marrow. Usually caused by **Staphylococcus Aureus,** certain **Streptococcus** spp, **Enterobacter** spp, **Haemophilus Influenzae,** and **Salmonella** spp in Sickle Cell Anemia cases. See appropriate sets. Also see Infection Bone.		Bone
Osteomyelitis	BIOM	330; 666; 727; 776; 787; 802; 832; 880; 1500; 1600; 1800; 2127; 2170; 2489; 2720			Bone
Osteomyelitis [Bone Infection]	EDTFL	70,490,32500,125750,275000,329570,425000,7 21000,835750,937410,	As mentioned above		Bone
Osteomyelosclerosis	BIO	79,330,	Marrow replacement by bone in response to low-grade infection.		Bone
Osteomyelosclerosis	BIOM	330; 243; 327; 79; 47.5; 2.65; 1.2			Bone
Aseptic Necrosis of Bone	EDTFL	100,520,5500,7500,17500,32500,72500,127000, 356500,624370,	Bone cell death due to blood supply interruption. Also use appropriate blood circulation sets.	Necrosis	Bone
Avascular Necrosis of Bone	EDTFL	130,220,900,5500,17500,32500,72500,127000,3 56500,624370,	As mentioned above	Necrosis	Bone
Necrosis, Avascular, of Bone	EDTFL	130,220,900,5500,17500,32500,72500,127000,3 56500,624370,		Necrosis	Bone
Osteonecrosis [Avascular]	EDTFL	130,220,900,5500,17500,32500,72500,127000,3 56500,624370,	As mentioned above	Necrosis	Bone
Kienbock Disease	EDTFL	150,340,520,830,11230,13540,50700,72870,905 00,98500	As mentioned above	Necrosis	Bone
Albers-Schoenberg Disease (Osteopetrosis)	EDTFL	30,240,700,1770,12330,27500,135520,550000,7 25290,875000,	Very rare inherited disorder where bone becomes denser than normal.		Bone
Osteopetrosis	EDTFL	100,220,680,7250,39250,125370,220910,40537 0,593500,875520			Bone
Osteosclerosis Fragilis	EDTFL	110,320,52500,112330,175170,475000,528000, 662710,742000,986220	Very rare inherited disorder where bone becomes denser than normal.		Bone
Marble Bone Disease	EDTFL	50,250,970,9000,73860,123200,257500,302580, 592490,875430			Bone
Osteoporosis Osteoporosis, Age-Related Osteoporosis, Senile	EDTFL	50,900,9000,11090,55330,225470,398400,4257 10,522530,642910		Osteoporosis	Bone
Senile Osteoporosis	EDTFL	50,900,9000,11090,55330,225470,398400,4257 10,522530,642910,		Osteoporosis	Bone

Subject / Argument	Author	Frequencies	Notes	Origin	Target
Osteoporosis, Post-Traumatic	EDTFL	50,900,9000,11090,55330,78250,114700,125970,642910,855820		Osteoporosis	Bone
Bone Loss, Age-Related	EDTFL	70,490,32500,125750,275000,329570,425000,721000,835750,937410		Osteoporosis	Bone
Osteosinusitis Max	CAFL	243,327	Infection of maxillary sinuses (located in cheekbones).		Bone
Osteosinusitis Max	BIO	243	As mentioned above		Bone
Rachitis [Rickets]	EDTFL	190,1000,2580,17500,225000,323200,398400,682020,759830,932410,	As mentioned above	Rickets	Bone
Rickets 1	XTRA	129,521,523,549,607,632,720,726,943,1062,1357,2084,	Defective mineralization of bones due to vitamin D, phosphorus, or calcium deficiency.	Rickets	Bone
Rickets Vitamin D and Sunlight	XTRA	880,5000	As mentioned above	Rickets	Bone
Renal Osteodystrophy	EDTFL	60,500,890,12850,132600,347500,377650,591000,683560,825090	Changes in bone formation due to chronic kidney disease (CKD).	Rickets	Bone
Renal Rickets	EDTFL	190,1000,2580,17500,225000,323200,398400,682020,759830,932410,	As mentioned above	Rickets	Bone
Cleidocranial Dysostosis	EDTFL	110,570,950,5500,17500,37500,162500,383500,421000,645250,			Bone
Craniofacial Dysostosis	EDTFL	70,230,970,14030,32500,72910,326590,497500,675000,954370,			Bone
Scheuermann Disease	EDTFL	20,400,900,20000,55000,92500,222700,474110,527000,987230	Childhood skeletal disorder with uneven vertebral development, causing abnormal spinal curvature (kyphosis).		Bone
Klippel-Feil Syndrome	EDTFL	80,350,600,900,212030,305210,451270,565610,692000,826320	Congenital spinal deformity involving fusion of two or more cervical vertebrae.		Bone
Dystrophia Brevicollis Congenita	EDTFL	160,620,830,5080,12850,327650,453720,684810,712810,993410	As mentioned above		Bone
Synovitis	EDTFL	50,370,900,2750,3000,70000,95090,174160,275000,357300	Inflammation of synovial membrane lining joints which possess cavities.		Bone
Maffucci Syndrome [Cartilage Enchondromas]	EDTFL	20,240,2750,8330,72500,132000,302020,456720,604230,880000,	Disorder of development of bone and cartilage.		Spine

9f - Cartilages

Subject / Argument	Author	Frequencies	Notes	Origin	Target
Cartilage and Connective Tissue	XTRA	1028	Best in Contact Mode.		Cartilage
Cartilage formation in joints	BIOM	84.5			Cartilage
Cartilage Diseases	EDTFL	20,240,2750,8330,72500,132000,302020,456720,604230,880000			Cartilage
Cartilage Diseases	KHZ	60,520,27500,55750,125190,250000,453720,517500,683000,712420,			Cartilage
Chondromalacia	EDTFL	120,250,960,5250,32500,475130,527000,661710,742000,988900			Cartilage
Cartilages softening	BIOM	7.5			Cartilage
Polychondritis, [Chronic Chondritis] Polychondritis, [Relapsing Chondritis]	EDTFL	60,490,570,72500,225000,477500,527000,667000,749000,986220,	Multi-systemic condition with inflammation and deterioration of cartilage. Can cause joint deformity and be life-threatening if respiratory tract, heart valves, or blood vessels are involved.	Inflammation	Cartilage
Costal Chondritis Costochondritis	EDTFL	60,490,570,72500,225000,477500,527000,667000,749000,986220,	Painful inflammation and swelling of costal (rib) cartilages. Also see Intercostal Neuralgia, and Neuralgia Intercostal sets.	Inflammation	Cartilage
Tietze's Syndrome [Cartilage inflammation]	EDTFL	20,240,2750,8330,72500,132000,302020,456720,604230,880000,	As mentioned above		Cartilage
Meniscus	BIOM	47.5			Cartilage
Knee, cartilages	BIOM	7.5; 63			Cartilage
Meniscus Tear (Knee)	EDTFL	100,410,870,5500,130090,255610,362000,492680,597500,654370		Knee	Cartilage

Subject / Argument	Author	Frequencies	Notes	Origin	Target

Subject / Argument	Author	Frequencies	Notes	Origin	Target
Stimulate Ligaments Healing	XTRA	9.69			Ligament
Ligaments Stimulate Healing	XTRA	9.7			Ligament
Ligament Stimulate Healing	XTRA	9.69,50,120			Ligament
Tendons Repair	XTRA	120			Ligament
Tendinitis	EDTFL	130,230,750,800,5050,7250,35000,95470,22632 0,442530	Chronic tendon injury.		Ligament
Tendinosis	EDTFL	160,230,750,800,5050,7250,35000,95470,84120 0,997870			Ligament
Tendinopathy	EDTFL	180,230,750,800,5050,7250,35000,95470,43748 0,828570			Ligament
Tendomyopathy	CAFL	320,250,160,80,40,20,10,5.8,2.5,1.5,1.2,1,0.5,	Fibromyalgia - see sets. Chronic widespread pain and heightened response to pressure with pronounced fatigue, sleep disturbance, stiff joints, and other symptoms.	Ligament Muscle	Ligament
Tendonitis and Tibialis Posterior	XTRA	120,300,12710,50000,150000,358570,479500,5 27000,662710,749000,986220,20,727,787,880,5 000,2008	Also spelt Tendinitis. Inflammation or tears in posterior tibial tendon, leading to flatfoot. See Tendons Repair set.		Ligament
Tenosynovitis	EDTFL	120,550,870,5130,15030,47500,357550,458600, 712230,992000	Inflammation of sheath surrounding tendon, most commonly bacterial in origin. Try **Neisseria Gonorrheae** set.		Ligament
Tendovaginitis	BIOM	25; 66; 66.5; 88; 92.5			Ligament
De Quervain's Tendinitis	EDTFL	130,230,750,800,5050,7250,35000,95470,22632 0,442530,	As mentioned above		Ligament

10 - Connective Tissue

Subject / Argument	Author	Frequencies	Notes	Origin	Target
Connective tissue	BIOM	9.6; 17; 28; 75.5; 76; 85; 85.5; 87.5; 90; 98			Connective T.
Center of skin and connective tissue - Pilot frequencies	BIOM	85; 87.5; 90; 98			Connective T.
Mixed Connective Tissue	EDTFL	70,370,870,7500,8000,67500,195870,427020,57 3820,854000,	Autoimmune disease combining symptoms of scleroderma, myositis, systemic lupus erythematosus, rheumatoid arthritis, and possibly other conditions.		Connective T.
Connective Tissue Diseases	EDTFL	70,370,870,7500,8000,67500,195870,427020,57 3820,854000,			Connective T.
Dermatolysis [Skin Inflammatory Disease]	EDTFL	130,370,7250,45750,96500,325000,527000,667 000,742000,988900,	Connective tissue disorder where the skin loses elasticity and hangs loose.	Skin	Connective T.
Dermatomegaly [Newborn, Folding Hanging Skin]	EDTFL	30,410,900,950,7500,125310,387500,682100,82 2060,925930		Skin	Connective T.
Dermatomyositis [Skin Inflammation]	EDTFL	130,370,7250,45750,96500,325000,527000,667 000,742000,988900,	Connective tissue disease affecting skin, muscles, and possibly heart, lungs, esophagus, and joints.	Skin	Connective T.
Polymyositis-Dermatomyositis	EDTFL	180,550,1000,5250,27500,42500,72500,606000, 811520,903090	As mentioned above	Skin	Connective T.
Cutis Laxa [Pachydermatocele]	EDTFL	170,200,920,2700,15000,20000,45310,670000,7 25900,825830,		Skin	Connective T.
Cutis Elastica [Ehlers-Danlos Syndrome]	EDTFL	120,350,950,7500,127500,247500,465000,5965 00,655720,875340,		Skin	Connective T.
Ehlers-Danlos Syndrome	EDTFL	120,350,950,7500,127500,247500,465000,5965 00,655720,875340	Inherited connective tissue disorder with six different types.		Connective T.
Epidermolysis Bullosa	EDTFL	190,400,950,322850,323500,323900,342750,34 6000,349300,923010	Inherited connective tissue disease complex causing skin and mucous membranes to be damaged easily - young sufferers have been called 'Butterfly Children.'		Connective T.
Fascia	CAFL	20	Connective tissue bands or sheets surrounding or involved with muscles or internal organs. Also see Fibroid sets.		Connective T.
Fasciitis	EDTFL	120,570,950,5250,37270,132500,237500,52253 0,675430,819340	Inflammation of connective tissue surrounding muscle and internal organs. See Fascia sets.	Fasciitis	Connective T.
Fasciitis Necrotizing	EDTFL	120,570,950,5250,37270,42500,96500,325430,4 15700,562970	Commonly called Flesh-eating Disease. Also use **Streptococcus Pyogenes**, **Staphylococcus Aureus**, **Clostridium Perfringens**, and **Bacteroides Fragilis**. Also see Fournier Gangrene, and Gangrene.	Fasciitis	Connective T.
Fournier's Gangrene	EDTFL	120,230,830,5500,12710,375190,477600,52500 0,667000,752700	Type of necrotizing fasciitis, usually perineal. See Fasciitis Necrotizing, and Gangrene. Also use **Streptococcus Pyogenes**, **Staphylococcus Aureus**, **Clostridium Perfringens**, and **Bacteroides Fragilis**.	Fasciitis	Connective T.
Fournier Disease	EDTFL	120,230,830,5500,12710,83930,192500,475440, 624370,882450		Fasciitis	Connective T.
Diffuse Myofascial Pain Syndrome	EDTFL	200,460,2500,7400,37500,96700,222700,52700 0,749000,985670	Chronic pain in multiple myofascial trigger points ('knots') and fascial constrictions. See Fascia sets, and Fasciitis.		Connective T.
Fibrodysplasia Ossificans Progressiva	EDTFL	190,230,830,5450,12710,13930,92500,376290,5 19340,652430	Extremely rare disease where connective tissue ossifies spontaneously or when damaged. Also see Fascia sets.		Connective T.
Fibrosis	EDTFL	50,230,950,13390,121590,285430,325510,4725 00,612500,930000	Formation of excess fibrous connective tissue in organ or other tissue.	Fibrosis	Connective T.

Subject / Argument	Author	Frequencies	Notes	Origin	Target
General Fibrosis Syndrome	EDTFL	30,500,930,2500,119000,417500,545310,67330 0,796500,825000		Fibrosis	Connective T.
General fibrosis	BIOM	2950; 2189; 2128; 2127; 2008; 1744; 1552; 1550; 1488; 1384; 1234; 880; 802; 787; 776; 727; 690; 666; 465; 267		Fibrosis	Connective T.
Fibrositis	EDTFL	20,520,750,2750,5250,47500,275000,424370,56 0000,815960		Fibrosis	Connective T.
Fibromyalgia	CAFL	328,880,800,728,5000,2720,2180,2128,664,464, 304,120,20,	Chronic widespread pain and heightened response to pressure with pronounced fatigue, sleep disturbance, stiff joints, and other symptoms.Can be caused by Epstein Barr Virus, Xenotropic Murine Leukemia Virus (XMRV). Also see Chronic Fatigue Syndrome .	Fibromyalgia	Connective T.
Fibromyalgia 1	CAFL	120,140,304,464,728,800,880,2489,3176,5000,6 000,9000,	As mentioned above	Fibromyalgia	Connective T.
Fibromyalgia 2	CAFL	2008,2050,2080,2127,880,800,787,728,600,420, 320,120,3790,3792,3794,3796,3798,3800,3802, 3804,3806,3808,3810,	As mentioned above	Fibromyalgia	Connective T.
Fibromyalgia (mycotic-parasitic infection)	BIOM	2050; 3790; 3792; 3794; 3796; 3798; 3800; 3802; 3804; 3906	As mentioned above	Fibromyalgia	Connective T.
Fibromyalgia (virus-bacterial infection)	BIOM	40; 68; 120; 140; 200; 304; 321; 328; 384; 420; 464; 600; 664; 728; 760; 800; 965; 2128; 2180; 6000; 9000	As mentioned above	Fibromyalgia	Connective T.
Fibromyalgia	KHZ	40=720,490,780,7500,118000,215430,362510,4 22060,608410,751200,	As mentioned above	Fibromyalgia	Connective T.
Fibromyalgia	EDTFL	70,350,25400,51000,60000,150000,475110,527 000,667000,987230	As mentioned above	Fibromyalgia	Connective T.
Fibromyalgia	XTRA	328	As mentioned above	Fibromyalgia	Connective T.
Fibromyalgia 2	XTRA	28,95,240,522,600,625,650,2900,	As mentioned above	Fibromyalgia	Connective T.
Fibromyalgia 3	XTRA	120,140,304,464,728,800,880,2489,3176,5000,6 000,9000,	As mentioned above	Fibromyalgia	Connective T.
Fibromyalgia 4	XTRA	328,2720=1800,9000,	As mentioned above	Fibromyalgia	Connective T.
Fibromyalgia 5	XTRA	120,320,420,600,728,787,800,880,2008,2050,20 80,2127,3790,3792,3794,3796,3798,3800,3802, 3804,3806,3808,3810,	As mentioned above	Fibromyalgia	Connective T.
Marfan Syndrome	EDTFL	160,800,7500,30000,67500,125000,352930,563 190,642910,930130	Genetic disorder of connective tissue that may involve heart, lungs, eyes, spine, skeleton, and hard palate.	Genetic disorder	Connective T.
Pseudoxanthoma Elasticum	EDTFL	80,520,650,2500,10530,35830,323350,675870,7 27000,867000	Genetic disease causing fragmentation and mineralization of elastic fibers in some tissues.	Genetic disorder	Connective T.
Gronblad-Strandberg Syndrome	EDTFL	350,930,12330,25230,35680,87600,93500,2336 30,434000,519340	Hereditary connective tissue disease, mainly affecting the elastic tissue of the skin, retina and arterial walls.		Connective T.
Sarcoidosis		Disease with abnormal inflammatory cells forming lumps (Granulomas - see set), usually starting in lungs, skin, or lymph nodes, sometimes eyes, liver, heart, or brain. Any organ can be affected. Also see Cancer Lymphogranuloma, and Lymphogranuloma. Can be caused bybacteria Helicobacter pylori, Chlamydia trachomatis, Propionibacterium acnes, Borrelia burgdorferi, Mycoplasmas, Mycobacterium Tuberculosis, Rickettsie or Herpes virus, Epstein-Barr virus (EBV), Retrovirus.		
Sarcoidosis	CAFL	2167,2967,3289	As mentioned above	Sarcoidosis	Connective T.
Sarcoidosis	EDTFL	120,550,940,5150,13980,137500,362500,69750 0,775000,922530	As mentioned above	Sarcoidosis	Connective T.
Besnier-Boeck [Lung Fibrosis]	EDTFL	50,230,950,13390,121590,285430,325510,4725 00,612500,930000,	As mentioned above	Sarcoidosis	Connective T.
Boeck's Sarcoid	EDTFL	20,240,850,37100,101320,221100,419340,5629 10,709830,976100	As mentioned above	Sarcoidosis	Connective T.
Schaumann's Disease	EDTFL	60,520,15170,42700,125710,376290,514340,68 2450,759830,918500	As mentioned above	Sarcoidosis	Connective T.
Sarcoidosis Pulmonary	EDTFL	120,550,940,5150,13980,137500,362500,69750 0,775000,922530,	As mentioned above	Sarcoidosis	Connective T.
Sharp Syndrome	EDTFL	120,560,34210,53770,291240,381610,502360,5 81260,638190,708920	Rare connective tissue disease		Connective T.

11 - Integumentary System

Subject / Argument	Author	Frequencies	Notes	Origin	Target
Skin	BIOM	6.0; 26.5; 85.0			Skin
Skin	BIOM	0.7; 1.7; 2.2; 2.5; 9.2; 9.4			Skin
Skin barrier	BIOM	1.6; 1.7; 9.4			Skin
Skin regeneration	BIOM	69.5			Skin
Skin rejuvination	BIOM	0.7; 1.7; 2.6; 9.19; 9.4; 35.5; 36; 36.5; 1.6; 26.5; 52; 69.5; 85; 87.5; 97			Skin
Skin, function regulation	BIOM	52; 85; 87.5; 90; 91.5; 94.5; 98			Skin
Skin, regulation of immune functions and host defenses	BIOM	1.6; 1.7; 9.4			Skin
Skin Problems	BIOM	20.0; 727.0; 787.0; 880.0; 1500.0			Skin
Greasy Skin	BIOM	52.0; 85.0; 87.5; 90.0; 91.5; 94.5; 98.0			Skin
Skin aging	BIOM	97			Skin
Mucous Inflammation	BIOM	1550.0; 880.0; 802.0; 787.0; 727.0; 444.0; 20.0			Skin
Beauty	XTRA	221.23,	Complexion.		Skin
Skin Tonus	BIOM	727.0; 787.0; 880.0; 5000.0; 20.0			Skin
Facial Toning	XTRA	9.6		Face	Skin
Facial Toning 1	CAFL	1.2		Face	Skin
Facial Toning 2	CAFL	2.4,9.6		Face	Skin
Facial Toning 3	CAFL	1.2,250		Face	Skin
Skin + Facial Toning	XTRA	9.6,2.4,1.2		Face	Skin
Bad Complexion	XTRA	5000	Facial skin problems.		Skin
Skin – Collagen Building	ETDFL	120,370,7250,45670,45750,57500,92500,93500, 96500,325000,	Main structural protein in various connective tissues, including skin.		Skin
Rhytide Effacement	BIOM	1.2; 20.0; 727.0; 787.0; 800.0; 880.0; 5000.0; 10000.0			Skin
Cosmetology 3	BIOM	2.8; 3.3; 8.1; 9.19; 54.0; 54.25; 54.5			Skin
Cosmetology 4	BIOM	0.9; 2.5; 2.6; 3.3; 6.0; 8.5; 9.8; 56.0			Skin
Cosmetology 5	BIOM	2.5; 3.6; 3.9; 5.0; 6.3; 8.1; 34.0; 92.0			Skin
Pigmentation	BIOM	53.5			Skin
Injuries	EDTFL	240,920,1770,18320,28230,32120,48900,54300, 109730,328500	Groin Pull, Knee, Hamstring, Hip Flexor strain, Patellofemoral, Sciatica, Shin Splints,Shoulder Injury, Tennis elbow (epicondylitis).	Injuries	Skin
Injuries	XTRA	5000		Injuries	Skin
Injuries (Specific to Fractures and Dislocations)	EDTFL	80,250,570,7500,10530,12500,40000,173300,32 9370,675000		Injuries	Skin
Wounds and Injuries	EDTFL	240,920,1770,18320,28230,32119,48900,54300, 109730,328500,	Use General Antiseptic. See all Healing sets, and Jade Machine sets.	Injuries	Skin
Incised wound		880; 787; 727; 220; 190; 20		Wound	Skin
Wound Repair		2720.0; 880.0; 787.0; 727.0; 220.0; 190.0; 20.0; 40.0		Wound	Skin
Granulating wound		100; 220		Wound	Skin
Wound Healing	CAFL	2720,880,787,727,220,190,20,40,	As mentioned above	Wound	Skin
Wound Healing	XTRA	20,40	As mentioned above	Wound	Skin
Wounds Penetrating and Non-penetrating	KHZ	160,350,850,5810,17500,37500,229320,425160, 826000,932000,	As mentioned above	Wound	Skin
Wound edges inflammation	BIOM	31		Wound	Skin
Cuts	CAFL	20,		Wound	Skin
Bedsores 1	XTRA	1.1,1.19,20,73,250,465,660,690,727.5,784,787,8 02,880,1550,		Bedsores	Skin
Bedsores 3	XTRA	20,465,727,787,802,880,1550,		Bedsores	Skin
Bedsores	CAFL	880,1550,802,787,727,465,20,1.2,73,	Also called Pressure ulcers.	Bedsores	Skin
Bedsores	BIOM	1.2; 20; 73; 727; 728; 787; 802; 880; 1550		Bedsores	
Bedsores	EDTFL	150,850,282250,292000,293010,305500,434000 ,494220,734200,823370		Bedsores	Skin
Decubitus Ulcer	EDTFL	200,1060,5790,7810,12330,23000,255470,3875 00,696500,825910,		Bedsores	Skin
Pressure Ulcer	EDTFL	150,240,650,830,2500,127500,255470,387500,6 96500,825910,		Bedsores	Skin
Ulcers General			See Section 1 - Various Conditions	Ulcers	Skin

Subject / Argument	Author	Frequencies	Notes	Origin	Target
Ulcer Repair	BIOM	2489; 2170; 2127; 1800; 1600; 880; 832; 787; 776; 727; 1.2; 73		Ulcers	Skin
Diabetic Toe Ulcer 1	CAFL	786,2112,1050,1.2,5000,832,20,	Use Staphylococcus Aureus and General sets. Also use General Antiseptic, and Circulatory Stasis if no progress after 2nd treatment. Soak feet in strong epsom salts solution - hot as possible.	Ulcers	Skin
Diabetic Ulcers	XTRA	727,776,787,880	As mentioned above	Ulcers	Skin
Leg Ulcer	EDTFL	150,240,650,830,2500,127500,255470,387500,6 96500,825910,		Ulcers	Skin
Skin Ulcer	ETDFL	190,370,7250,45750,96500,325000,519340,655 200,750000,922530	Skin lesion exhibiting complete loss of epidermis and often portions of dermis and even subcutaneous fat.	Ulcers	Skin
Buruli Ulcer	ETDFL	150,240,650,830,2500,127500,255470,387500,6 96500,825910,		Ulcers	Skin
Ulcer, parasitic	BIOM	3; 3.5; 4; 6.8; 9.9		Ulcers	Skin
Fistula Ulcer	CAFL	880,832,787,727	Complication of fistula in GI tract, found in Crohn's Disease (see sets). Also use appropriate Staphylococcus set(s).	Fistula	Skin
Fistula, General	ETDFL	180,240,10530,27500,35000,57500,96500,3251 10,475160,527000,	Abnormal connection between two hollow organs, intestines, or blood vessels.	Fistula	Skin
Fistula	XTRA	660,690,727.5,787,832,880,	As mentioned above	Fistula	Skin
Burns	CAFL	190,10000,880,787,727,465,200,	Use in Contact Mode immediately to halt tissue damage and pain.	Burns	Skin
Burns	ETDFL	70,120,750,930,12330,22500,92500,225000,322 650,324370	As mentioned above	Burns	Skin
Burn injury	BIOM	190; 10000; 880; 787; 727; 465; 200		Burns	Skin
Burn injury blisters	BIOM	18		Burns	Skin
Radiation Burns 2	XTRA	190,200,465,660,690,727.5,787,880,10000,	Injuries caused by radiation for cancer care	Burns	Skin
Radiation Burns 3	XTRA	727,787,880,10000		Burns	Skin
Sun scald	BIOM	72.5		Burns	Skin
Skin and Connective Tissue Diseases	EDTFL	70,370,870,7500,8000,67500,195870,427020,57 3820,854000,		Connective T.	Skin
Skin Diseases	ETDFL	50,120,870,5000,27500,62500,193000,322530,4 75170,527000	Conditions of human integumentary system.		Skin
Skin Diseases, Inflammation	ETDFL	130,370,7250,45750,96500,325000,527000,667 000,742000,988900,			Skin
Skin Diseases, Infectious	ETDFL	130,370,7250,45750,96500,325000,527000,667 000,742000,988900,			Skin
Skin Diseases, Hardening Dermatoses	ETDFL	130,370,7250,45750,96500,325000,527000,667 000,742000,988900,			Skin
Skin Diseases, Bacterial	ETDFL	130,370,7250,45750,96500,325000,527000,667 000,742000,988900			Skin
Skin Diseases, Fungal	ETDFL	190,390,750,5820,47300,72500,102100,457240, 582330,726330			Skin
Skin Diseases, Parasitic	ETDFL	160,2120,21000,45250,73300,97500,125000,51 9340,655200,750000			Skin
Scar Tissue Diseases [General]	ETDFL	130,370,7250,45750,96500,325000,527000,667 000,742000,988900,			Skin
Skin – Scar Tissue healing	ETDFL	120,370,7250,45670,45750,57500,92500,93500, 96500,325000,			Skin
Cicatricial tissue, pressure	BIOM	93.5			Skin
Barotrauma	EDTFL KHZ	180,230,850,5810,20000,62500,150000,350000, 510250,653690,	Tissue injury caused by pressure differences between gas and liquid.		Skin
Sweat Gland Diseases	ETDFL	160,350,950,5260,27500,52500,225470,522530, 682090,750000		Glands	Skin
Miliaria	ETDFL	140,250,900,2500,57500,132500,365610,42616 0,675680,897000			Skin
Athletes Foot	CAFL	20,379,727,787,880,5000,644,766,464,802,1552 ,9999,20,379,727,787,880,5000,644,766,464,80 2,1552,9999,3176,304,	Also see Epidermophyton Floccinum, and Tinea sets. (mycosis caused by a Fungus). See Section 17b - Fungi	Feet Fungus	Skin
Athletes Foot	ETDFL	20,750,900,5950,8500,125690,262500,592600,7 58570,823440	As mentioned above	Feet Fungus	Skin
Tinea Pedis	EDTFL	140,260,600,2500,32500,37570,47500,60000,16 5820,368000	As mentioned above	Feet Fungus	Skin
Skin rash of unclear aetiology	BIOM	1800; 880; 787; 727; 522; 146; 4.9			Skin
Acne	ETDFL	50,370,830,2500,3000,73300,383750,387000,38 9000,393000,	Pimples, white/blackheads, greasy skin, possible scars. Also see Propionibacterium Acnes.	Acne	Skin
Acne	XTRA	727,787,880,5000,	As mentioned above	Acne	Skin
Acne 1	CAFL	2720,2170,1800,1600,1550,1552,1500,802,880, 787,727,564=360,778,760,741,660,564=360,46 5,450,444,428,	As mentioned above	Acne	Skin
Acne 2	CAFL	760,465,444,450,428,660,	As mentioned above	Acne	Skin

Subject / Argument	Author	Frequencies	Notes	Origin	Target
Acne Vulgaris	BIOM	1.7		Acne	Skin
Cutaneous Acne 1	BIOM	52.0; 53.0; 53.5; 75.0; 75.0; 86.0; 92.0; 93.0		Acne	Skin
Cutaneous Acne 2	BIOM	62.0; 62.5; 75.5; 85.0; 87.5; 90.0; 91.8; 94.5		Acne	Skin
Cutaneous Acne 3	BIOM	98.0		Acne	Skin
Purulent Pimples	BIOM	77.0		Acne	Skin
Acne Vulgaris Junior	XTRA	514,832,185,		Acne	Skin
Acne Vulgaris	CAFL	564,		Acne	Skin
Acne, blackheads	BIOM	5000; 2720; 2170; 1800; 1600; 1550; 1552; 1500; 802; 880; 778; 787; 760; 741; 727; 660; 564; 465; 450; 444; 428		Acne	Skin
Comedones Blackheads	CAFL	778	Commonly called Blackheads.	Acne	Skin
Skin comedoes	BIOM	75; 86; 92; 93; 52.75; 53; 53.5; 62; 62.5; 75.5; 85; 87.5; 90; 91.5; 94.5; 98		Acne	Skin
Angioedema	KHZ	120,520,800,5070,15000,90000,375050,410250, 564280,824960,	Rapid swelling of the mouth, throat, and facial tissue.		Skin
Angiofibroma	KHZ	160,620,7500,65330,175000,434250,563190,64 2910,930120,	Small papules over the side of the nose and on cheeks.		Skin
Abscesses			See Section 1 - Various conditions		Skin
Aplasia Cutis Congenita	EDTFL	130,520,900,8400,12530,145830,262500,39750 0,633910,825170	Rare specific form of genetic aplasia.	Genetic disorder	Skin
Blister	XTRA	465,660,690,727.5,787,880,10000,			Skin
Boils	CAFL	20,465,660,727,770,787,802,880,1550,	Usually due to Staphylococcus Aureus or Streptococcus Pyogenes - see sets. Also see Furunculosis sets.	Boils	Skin
Boils [Deep Folliculitis]	EDTFL	50,120,870,5000,27500,62500,193000,322530,4 75170,527000,	As mentioned above	Boils	Skin
Boils 1	XTRA	6.79,48,60,100,333,465,523,590,660,690,727.5, 768,786,787,802,880,1550,	Also called furuncles/Furunculosis.	Boils	Skin
Boils Carbuncles	XTRA	20,465,660,727,787,880,1550,5000,	Clusters of boils.	Boils	Skin
Boils Furunculosis	XTRA	20,116,200,465,660,727,728,770,784,787,802,8 80,1000,1550,	As mentioned above	Boils	Skin
Boils Open	XTRA	20	As mentioned above	Boils	Skin
Boils Pus	XTRA	5000	As mentioned above	Boils	Skin
Furunculosis	CAFL	880,1550,802,787,727,465,660,20,116,770,	See Boils, and Furunculosis sets. Also use Staphylococcus Aureus.	Furunculosis	Skin
Furunculosis [Skin Infection]	EDTFL	130,370,7250,45750,96500,325000,527000,667 000,742000,988900,	As mentioned above	Furunculosis	Skin
Furunculosis Secondary	XTRA	727,787	As mentioned above	Furunculosis	Skin
Furunculosis	BIOM	5000; 1550; 880; 802; 800; 787; 727; 660; 500; 465; 20; 9.4; 9.2; 4.9; 3.3; 1.7		Furunculosis	Skin
Furunculosis-herpes	BIOM	200; 1000; 1550; 802; 787; 727; 644		Furunculosis	Skin
Furunculosis Herpes	CAFL	200,1000,1550,802,787,727,	Also use Herpes Simplex (type1/i). See Herpes Furuncolosis, Boils, Furunculosis, and Herpes General sets.	Furunculosis	Skin
Furunculosis Herpes	XTRA	20,116,200,465,660,690,802,1000,1550,2000,	As mentioned above	Furunculosis	Skin
Furunculosis Herpes 2	XTRA	200,802,1000,1550	As mentioned above	Furunculosis	Skin
Carbuncles	CAFL	48,424,644,647,727,738,744,745,786,943,1050, 8697,	Cluster of boils. See Boils, Furunculosis, and Staphylococcus Aureus.	Carbuncles	Skin
Carbuncles	BIOM	622; 634; 639; 643; 644		Carbuncles	Skin
Carbuncles 2	XTRA	20,727,787,880,5000,	A severe abscess or multiple boil in the skin, typically infected with staphylococcus bacteria. Cluster of boils. See Boils, Furunculosis, and Staphylococcus Aureus.	Carbuncles	Skin
Carbuncles 3	XTRA	424,478,555,644,647,727,728,738,745,784,786, 787,824,943,999,1050,7270,8697,	Cluster of boils. See Boils, Furunculosis, and Staphylococcus Aureus.	Carbuncles	Skin
Carbuncles 4	XTRA	936.97,944.39,18819.5,18968.86,	Cluster of boils. See Boils, Furunculosis, and Staphylococcus Aureus.	Carbuncles	Skin
Cafe-au-Lait Spots	EDTFL	50,570,850,52100,119340,375040,425710,5684 30,642910,985900	Flat light-brown birthmarks.		Skin
Cellulitis Cellulitis, Orbital	EDTFL	140,490,790,12500,43000,122500,262500,5553 50,692500,819340	Bacterial deep skin infection, usually by Streptococci and Staphylococcus Aureus - see sets.	Cellulitis	Skin
Complex Regional Pain Syndrome Type I / II	EDTFL	140,550,850,7470,120000,315500,472500,7257 50,852000,975930	Severe pain, swelling, and skin changes in parts or all of the body. Also see Causalgia.		Skin
Condylomata	BIO	466	Usually venereal warts, caused by the Papilloma virus. Occurs near intersection of mucous membranes and skin. See Papilloma Virus and Warts Papilloma.	Condylomata	Skin
Condylomata Basic Set	CAFL	45,265,404,466,489,767,794,874,907=720,		Condylomata	Skin
Condylomata Advanced Set	CAFL	45,265,397.4,404,419.9,466=720,487,767,794.9 ,839.8,874,907=720,1011,1051,	See Condylomata Basic, Papilloma Virus, and Warts Papilloma.	Condylomata	Skin
Condylomata Acuminata	EDTFL	70,370,870,5520,17240,27500,180400,413080,5 51000,719380		Condylomata	Skin

Subject / Argument	Author	Frequencies	Notes	Origin	Target
Larva Migrans, Cutaneous [Hookworm Infection]	EDTFL	170,460,10880,55160,96500,350000,567000,692330,810200,982110,	Meandering bright red tracks in skin caused by Hookworm infection - see sets. Also see Ancylostoma sets.	Roundworm	Skin
Creeping Eruption	EDTFL	150,180,16750,81930,118850,282500,315950,523500,775290,954500,		Roundworm	Skin
Dermatolysis [Skin Inflammatory Disease]	EDTFL	130,370,7250,45750,96500,325000,527000,667000,742000,988900,	Connective tissue disorder where the skin loses elasticity and hangs loose.		Skin
Dermatomegaly [Newborn, Folding Hanging Skin]	EDTFL	30,410,900,950,7500,125310,387500,682100,822060,925930			Skin
Cutis Laxa [Pachydermatocele]	EDTFL	170,200,920,2700,15000,20000,45310,670000,725900,825830,			Skin
Cutis Elastica [Ehlers-Danlos Syndrome]	EDTFL	120,350,950,7500,127500,247500,465000,596500,655720,875340,		Connective T.	Skin
Dermatitis / Dermatitis Herpetiformis / Dermatitis, Actinic / Dermatitis, Contagious Pustular / Dermatitis, Exfoliative	EDTFL	140,200,620,7500,15500,41090,465690,597500,722700,875930,	Also called Eczema - see sets. Skin condition with itchy, weeping, crusting patches.	Dermatitis	Skin
Dermatitis	XTRA	9.18,9.19,9.39,9.4,20,120.415,660,664,690,707,727.5,770,787,802,916,1550,2127.5,2180,2720,5000,10000,	As mentioned above	Dermatitis	Skin
Dermatitis, Eczematous	EDTFL	150,830,7620,67920,197500,212850,405000,527500,716500,871200,		Dermatitis	Skin
Contagious Pustular Dermatitis	EDTFL	140,200,620,7500,15500,41090,465690,597500,722700,875930,		Dermatitis	Skin
Contact dermatitis	BIOM	7344; 4412; 1550; 1234; 740; 880; 787; 727; 10000; 5000; 30; 330		Dermatitis	Skin
Dermatoses [Skin disease,hardening]	EDTFL	130,370,7250,45750,96500,325000,527000,667000,742000,988900,		Dermatitis	Skin
Erythroderma	EDTFL	40,520,730,870,2250,17500,35830,65110,325540,533630		Dermatitis	Skin
Boils	EDTFL	40,520,730,870,2250,17500,35830,192500,675360,826900		Dermatitis	Skin
Dermatitis Herpetiformis	EDTFL	140,200,620,7500,15500,41090,465690,597500,722700,875930,	Chronic blistering skin condition. Manifestation of Celiac Disease - see sets. Unrelated to Herpes.	Dermatitis	Skin
Duhring's Disease	EDTFL	170,570,800,54730,195310,352500,595400,619340,797610,891270	As mentioned above	Dermatitis	Skin
Neurodermatitis (Atopic dermatitis)	BIOM	0.7; 1.7; 9.19; 9.4; 28			Skin
Neutrophilic Dermatosis	EDTFL	30,500,850,7500,8000,127500,328700,525790,725000,825790			Skin
Dermatomyositis [Skin Inflammation]	EDTFL	130,370,7250,45750,96500,325000,527000,667000,742000,988900,	Connective tissue disease affecting skin, muscles, and possibly heart, lungs, esophagus, and joints.		Skin
Polymyositis-Dermatomyositis	EDTFL	180,550,1000,5250,27500,42500,72500,606000,811520,903090	As mentioned above		Skin
Dermatophytoses [Ringworm]	EDTFL	40,120,950,14030,118520,251290,365280,590000,722700,977500,	Fungal infections of skin.	Fungus	Skin
Dermatophytoses	XTRA	1752.48,11046.87,	As mentioned above	Fungus	Skin
Dermatomycoses [Fungal Skin Disease]	EDTFL	190,390,750,5820,47300,72500,102100,457240,582330,726330,	As mentioned above	Fungus	Skin
Skin Diseases, Fungal	KHZ	20,750,2620,5950,8500,125690,262500,592500,758570,823440,	Fungal infections of skin.	Fungus	Skin
Ringworm	CAFL	422,442,732,5000,60,76,92,120,128,440,800,	Fungal skin infection in man and animals. See Microsporum Audouini, and Canis, Trichophyton, and/or Epidermophyton.	Fungus	Skin
Ringworm	EDTFL	40,120,950,14030,118520,251290,365280,590000,722700,977500	As mentioned above	Fungus	Skin
Tinea	EDTFL	140,260,600,2500,32500,37570,87500,175160,317350,323060	Superficial fungal infections (dermatophytosis) that affects the skin. Ringworm - see set. Also see Epidermophyton Floccosum, Microsporum Audouini, Nagel Trichophyton, and Fungus General sets.	Fungus	Skin
Epidermophytosis	EDTFL	80,7250,50000,62500,93500,322540,475030,527000,667000,987230	As mentioned above	Fungus	Skin
Trichophytosis	EDTFL	430,600,860,5090,7250,92500,357400,476500,527000,663710	As mentioned above	Fungus	Skin
Trichophytosis	BIOM	76; 92; 128; 422; 440; 442; 732; 800; 5000		Fungus	Skin
Tinea Cruris / Jock Itch	CAFL	345,465,644,766,784,	Dermatophyte fungal infection, also called Jock Itch - see set. Also see Tinea, Nagel Trichophyton, Epidermophyton Floccinum, Ringworm, and Dermatophytoses sets.	Fungus	Skin

Subject / Argument	Author	Frequencies	Notes	Origin	Target
Jock Itch [Tinea Cruris]	EDTFL	140,260,600,2500,32500,37570,87500,175160,3 17350,323060,		Fungus	Skin
Jock itch 2	XTRA	20,345,465,634,644,660,690,727.5,766,784,802, 880,1550,	As mentioned above	Fungus	Skin
Jock itch 3	XTRA	345,465,644,766,784,11053.5,	Also see Epidermophyton Floccosum CAFL set.	Fungus	Skin
Tinea Versicolor	CAFL	222,225,491,616,700,	Pale eruptions on skin of trunk, head, and tops of limbs caused by yeast. See Malassezia Furfur, Yeast General, Fungus General and other yeast sets.	Fungus	Skin
Tinea Versicolor	EDTFL	140,260,600,2500,32500,37570,325150,655200, 750000,926700	As mentioned above	Fungus	Skin
Dermoid Dermoid Cyst	EDTFL	20,200,900,5950,8500,125690,262500,592500,7 58520,823440,	Tumor, usually benign, that contains tissue types inconsistent with its location.		Skin
Eczema	CAFL	9.19,707,1550,802,787,727,10000,5000,2720,20 08,2180,2128,664,120,20,	Also called Dermatitis - see sets. Skin condition with itchy, weeping, crusting patches.	Eczema	Skin
Eczema	EDTFL	150,830,7620,67920,197500,212850,405000,52 7500,716500,871200	As mentioned above	Eczema	Skin
Dyshidrosis [Dermatitis]	EDTFL	140,200,620,7500,15500,41090,465690,597500, 722700,875930,		Eczema	Skin
Eczema 1	CAFL	770,916,415,	As mentioned above	Eczema	Skin
Eczema 2	CAFL	730.2,1550,802,787,690,	As mentioned above	Eczema	Skin
Eczema 2	XTRA	9.18,9.19,9.39,9.4,20,120,415,660,664,690,707, 727.5,770,787,802,916,1550,2127.5,2180,2720, 5000,10000,	As mentioned above	Eczema	Skin
Eczema 3	XTRA	415,770,916	As mentioned above	Eczema	Skin
Eczema Skin Trouble	CAFL	5000,	As mentioned above	Eczema	Skin
Bacterial eczema	BIOM	415; 730.2; 787; 802; 916; 1550		Eczema	Skin
Bacterial-herpetic eczema	BIOM	9.19; 20; 120; 664; 707; 727; 787; 802; 1550; 2008; 2128; 2180; 2720; 5000; 10000		Eczema	Skin
Neurogenic eczema	BIOM	28; 64		Eczema	Skin
Dry eczema	BIOM	0.7; 1.7; 2.5; 9.19; 9.4		Eczema	Skin
Eczema Vascular and Lung Disturbances	CAFL	9.39,	Also called Dermatitis - see sets. Skin condition with itchy, weeping, crusting patches. Can also cause blood vessel and lung problems.	Eczema	Skin
Eczema Vascular and Lung	CAFL	9.19,727,787,1550,	As mentioned above	Eczema	Skin
Eczema Vascular and Lung	XTRA	9.18,9.39,727,787,1550,	As mentioned above	Eczema	Skin
Edema - Swelling			See Section 1 - Various conditions		Skin
Epidermal Cyst Epidermoid Cyst	EDTFL	70,180,6750,40870,172690,201250,421500,597 500,835350,923070		Cyst	Skin
Sebaceous Cyst	EDTFL	170,2230,4300,7210,72740,165280,362500,414 700,734840,840150		Cyst	Skin
Erythema	CAFL	9.39,809,1618,3236,	Redness of skin or mucous membranes from injury, infection, or inflammation.	Erythema	Skin
Erythema	EDTFL	80,240,650,900,2500,27500,55360,492500,6755 40,775350	As mentioned above	Erythema	Skin
Erythema 2	XTRA	9.4	As mentioned above	Erythema	Skin
Erythema	BIOM	809; 1618; 3225			Skin
Erythema Infectiosum	EDTFL	80,240,650,900,2500,27500,55360,115700,3260 70,534250	Also called Fifth Disease, or Slapped Cheek Syndrome. Common childhood condition.	Erythema	Skin
Fifth Disease [Erythema infectiosum]	EDTFL	80,240,650,900,2500,27500,55360,115700,3260 70,534250,		Erythema	Skin
Fifth Disease	XTRA	809,1618,3236	Also called Erythema Infectiosum, or Slapped Cheek Syndrome. Common childhood condition.	Erythema	Skin
Erythema Infectiosum	XTRA	809,1618,3236	As mentioned above	Erythema	Skin
Erythema Nodosum	CAFL	9.39	Inflammation of fat cells under skin, leading to sore red lumps, usually on both shins.	Erythema	Skin
Fissures	CAFL	787,20,10000	Tears in skin or mucosa, usually in anus.	Fissures	Skin
Fissures	XTRA	20,727,787,880,10000,	Tears in skin or mucosa, usually in anus.	Fissures	Skin
Gangrene	EDTFL	120,230,830,5500,12710,83930,192500,475440, 624370,882450,	Tissue necrosis due to insufficient blood supply. Also see Clostridium, Circulatory Stasis, Infections General, and Bacterium Coli sets.	Gangrene	Skin
Gangrene	BIOM	20; 73; 880; 787; 727; 20		Gangrene	Skin
Gangrene	XTRA	20,73,727,787,880,	As mentioned above	Gangrene	Skin
Symmetric gangrene	BIOM	727; 20; 465		Gangrene	Skin
Gangrene General	CAFL	880,787,727,20,73,	As mentioned above	Gangrene	Skin
Granuloma	EDTFL	70,500,970,9000,12850,267000,320850,602210, 733630,925000	Tightly-packed collection of macrophages imprisoning foreign organisms or other materials which cannot be eliminated by the immune system.	Granuloma	Skin
Granuloma Annulare	EDTFL	70,500,970,9000,12850,32500,42500,190000,32 5370,425520	Chronic dermatological condition which presents as reddish bumps on skin arranged in a circle or ring - also try Granuloma.	Granuloma	Skin
Granuloma, Pseudopyogenic	EDTFL	70,500,970,9000,12850,370500,547500,656500, 725370,825520		Granuloma	Skin

Subject / Argument	Author	Frequencies	Notes	Origin	Target
Granuloma Inguinale	EDTFL	70,500,970,9000,12850,42500,190000,325370,795520,901030		Granuloma	Skin
Granuloma Venereum	EDTFL	70,500,970,9000,12850,32500,307250,435370,587500,795520	Ulcerative genital lesions due to Klebsiella granulomatis - also try Granuloma, and Klebsiella Infections sets.	Granuloma	Skin
Donovanosis	EDTFL	1260,2320,3900,65730,152000,213200,602500,715310,803200,924370		Granuloma	Skin
Hidradenitis Suppurativa	KHZ	150,9230,66730,185640,215250,537110,632220,781500,893000,952000,	Chronic skin disorder with abscesses in areas with sweat glands.		Skin
Dermatofibroma [Fibrous Histiocytoma]	EDTFL	150,520,9730,11640,12530,145830,262500,434500,633910,825170,			Skin
Hives	CAFL	4.9,146,522,727,787,880,1800,	Itchy bumps on skin. See Detox Urticaria, and Urticaria sets.	Hives	Skin
Hives 1	XTRA	4.9,6.29,95,125,146,148,444,522,660,690,727.5,787,880,1800,1865,	As mentioned above	Hives	Skin
Hives 2	XTRA	4.9,146,522,727,787,880,1800,5000,	As mentioned above	Hives	Skin
Urticaria	CAFL	1800,880,787,727,522,146,4.9,	Hives, often due to toxins.	Hives	Skin
Urticaria [Hives]	EDTFL	110,540,9790,11630,19520,135820,222350,414250,603910,805070,		Hives	Skin
Nettle rash	BIOM	4.9; 7.5; 9.4; 146; 522; 727; 787; 880; 1800;5000; 10000		Hives	Skin
Epifolliculitis	BIOM	174; 482; 5311			Skin
Folliculitis Hot Tub			Red pimples due to hair follicle infection. Use Pseudomonas Aeruginosa sets. See Section 17c - Bacteria and Diseases		Skin
Hyperhidrosis	EDTFL	80,410,950,2500,5500,15580,292500,329540,619340,815700	Abnormally increased sweating.	Sweat	Skin
Sudorrhea Excessive sweating	BIOM	40; 42.5; 92.5; 98.5; 99.75		Sweat	Skin
Anhidrosis	EDTFL	30,550,870,10720,27500,127500,328950,525610,826320,919550,	Inability to sweat given appropriate stimuli which can lead to heat stroke, exhaustion, and hyperthermia.	Sweat	Skin
Hypohidrosis	EDTFL	140,420,18110,89100,115180,220050,375000,532510,615200,713870	As mentioned above	Sweat	Skin
Ichthyosis	EDTFL	130,180,900,5500,17500,32500,151240,257460,413910,692270	Group of genetic cutaneous conditions with dry, thickened, scaly, or flaky skin.	Genetic disorder	Skin
Netherton Syndrome	EDTFL	20,240,850,2600,5250,72500,196500,375950,456720,880000	As mentioned above		Skin
Xeroderma [Dry Skin Disorder]	EDTFL	50,120,870,5000,27500,62500,193000,322530,475170,527000,			Skin
Xeroderma Pigmentosum	EDTFL	130,410,970,7500,10760,20000,57500,175870,415700,568430	Rare genetic disorder of DNA repair in which ability to repair damage caused by ultraviolet (UV) light is deficient.		Skin
Kaposi Disease	EDTFL	160,230,720,3830,52250,177270,318500,563190,642910,976900	As mentioned above	Genetic disorder	Skin
Impetigo	EDTFL	20,300,850,7500,12500,40000,162900,350000,433630,909210,	Infection caused by pyogenic germs that affect, above all in pediatric age, the superficial layers of the skin.	Bacteria	Skin
Impetigo, Contagiosa	EDTFL	20,300,850,7500,12500,40000,162900,350000,433630,909210	Contagious bacterial skin infection common among young children and certain contact sport athletes. Can be caused by Staphylococcus aureus and Streptococcus pyogene.	Bacteria	Skin
Incontinentia Pigmenti Incontinentia Pigmenti Achromians	EDTFL	130,350,700,850,5790,77250,130000,296500,625580,915700	Genetic disorder affecting skin (various types of lesions), hair, teeth, nails, and CNS.	Genetic disorder	Skin
Bloch-Sulzberger Syndrome	EDTFL	40,460,750,2750,7500,47500,96500,357300,834000,937410	As mentioned above		Skin
Ito Syndrome	EDTFL	180,400,620,850,2500,25000,109330,362570,621680,775670	As mentioned above		Skin
Schamberg's Disease	EDTFL	130,220,720,2560,193110,247590,385270,521680,657300,729340	As mentioned above		Skin
Keloid	EDTFL	30,190,500,850,7300,88400,151750,284000,635210,917020	Type of scar resulting from overgrowth of collagen at the site of a healed skin injury.		Skin
Keratosis [Actinic] (2023	EDTFL	150,350,620,930,7500,41090,465690,597500,722700,875930,	Potentially pre-cancerous patches of thick, scaly, or crusty skin caused by UV radiation.		Skin
Lentigo	EDTFL	60,120,850,7510,32520,43060,151180,225530,515760,659020	Harmless small pigmented spot with clearly-defined edge surrounded by normal-looking skin.	Lentigo	Skin
Lentigo, Malignant	EDTFL	60,120,850,7510,32520,43060,151180,225530,434620,659020		Lentigo	Skin
Lentiginosis	EDTFL	110,180,180,7750,47210,132580,327350,486900,530240,841690		Lentigo	Skin
Lentiginosis, Perioral	EDTFL	170,180,280,7650,47210,132580,337450,486900,530220,841630		Lentigo	Skin
Freckles	EDTFL	230,620,960,5500,7500,33980,295300,325200,375430,522530,		Lentigo	Skin
Hutchinson's Melanotic Freckle	EDTFL	70,880,9710,68830,102850,205280,323450,492500,675950,823370	Also called a lentigo. Harmless small flat pigmented spot on skin, similar to a freckle, but with different composition.	Lentigo	Skin
Melanotic Freckle	EDTFL	70,880,9710,68830,102850,205280,323450,492500,675950,823370,		Lentigo	Skin

Subject / Argument	Author	Frequencies	Notes	Origin	Target
Leprosy			See Section **17c - Bacteria and Diseases**	Leprosy	Skin
Lichen Planus Lichen Ruber Planus	EDTFL	170,220,650,2490,7500,40000,150000,326650,3 75680,519330	Skin and/or mucous membrane disease that resembles lichen. Can be caused by Herpesviruses including HHV-3, HHV-6, HHV-7 and in rare cases to infections with Hepatitis B and C.		Skin
Lichen ruber planus	BIOM	166; 224; 317; 330; 1234			Skin
Lichen Sclerosus [Labia, Penis Sclerosus]	EDTFL	30,460,2500,7200,17500,96500,355080,517500, 687670,712420,	Disorder with white patches of skin, mostly around genitals. Cause unknown.		Skin
Lipodystrophy	EDTFL	50,570,870,12330,42500,152500,287800,39231 0,810500,901040	Abnormal or degenerative conditions of the body's adipose (fat) tissue.		Skin
Mange	XTRA	90=1200,253,693=600,701,774,920,1436,1821. 88,2871,5742,11484,	Contagious dermatitis found in many mammals caused by Demodex mites living in the hair follicles. See Follicular Mange.	Mange	Skin
Mange Follicular	CAFL	90=600,110=600,253=600,693=600,920,1436,2 871,5742,	As mentioned above	Mange	Skin
Mange Follicular 1	XTRA	90,110,253,693,920,1436,2871,5742,	As mentioned above	Mange	Skin
Mange Follicular 2	XTRA	253,693	As mentioned above	Mange	Skin
Follicular Mange	CAFL	253,693,701,774	As mentioned above	Mange	Skin
Melanosis	EDTFL	70,480,700,830,2300,32500,305050,431200,632 590,723010	Form of hyperpigmentation associated with increased melanin.		Skin
Melasma	EDTFL	70,490,700,32800,102250,212750,326540,5456 80,795610,857770			Skin
Chloasma	EDTFL	50,240,72500,122530,342060,512330,616300,6 82450,753070,926700			Skin
Molluscum Contagiosum	CAFL	134.7,190.5,254,1524,3044.5,6096.1,	Also called water warts. Viral skin infection with domed pearly lesions.	Virus	Skin
Molluscum Contagiosum [Water Warts]	EDTFL	40,520,5090,35000,175330,324850,432410,714 820,823000,987230,	As mentioned above	Virus	Skin
Mycoses			See Section **17b - Fungi**	Fungus	Skin
Moles 1	CAFL	761.7=900,650,625,600,76.2,			Skin
Moles	BIOM	20; 120; 177; 600; 625; 626; 650; 659; 660; 728; 784; 880; 464			Skin
Skin Mole	EDTFL	20,750,900,5950,96500,325000,519340,592500, 758570,823440			Skin
Nevus	EDTFL	20,400,900,20000,55000,93500,222700,475110, 527000,987230	Commonly called Moles - see set. Also see Melanoma and HPV sets.		Skin
Nevus Flammeus	EDTFL	20,400,900,20000,55000,93500,222700,391500, 421220,515700	Birthmark, due to capillary malformation.		Skin
Hemangioma			See Section **16c - Tumor**		Skin
Panniculitis	EDTFL	80,400,830,5470,105000,215470,324050,63100 0,801910,931220	Group of diseases with inflammation of subcutaneous adipose tissue.		Skin
Panniculitis, Subacute Nodular	EDTFL	80,400,830,5470,105000,215470,324050,35750 0,596500,742060	As mentioned above		Skin
Weber-Christian Disease	EDTFL	80,2750,20000,62800,322060,410250,567700,6 42910,806000,930120	As mentioned above		Skin
Pemphigus	CAFL	694,893,665	Autoimmune skin disorder characterized by blisters in the outer layer of skin and mucous membranes.	Immune system	Skin
Pemphigus	VEGA	893	As mentioned above	Immune	Skin
Pemphigus Pemphigus Vulgaris	EDTFL	190,230,950,82500,192710,227500,452020,592 500,731310,815720,			Skin
Pemphigus, Benign Familial [Hailey]	EDTFL	50,660,1320,7500,15910,17500,151200,231200, 341000,525290,			Skin
Hailey-Hailey Disease	EDTFL	50,660,1320,7500,15910,17500,151200,231200, 341000,525290			Skin
Familial Chronic Pemphigus	EDTFL	80,220,730,2900,5710,50000,322530,415200,56 6410,707260			Skin
Pemphigoid Pemphigoid Bullous	EDTFL	130,230,730,800,5250,7250,35370,95950,21550 0,510000	Acute or chronic autoimmune skin disease, involving the formation of blisters.		Skin
Pityriasis [Rosea] Pityriasis Versicolor	EDTFL	70,520,750,3970,8500,13610,22500,265830,425 340,879500	Flaking or scaling of skin.		Skin
Poikiloderma of Civatte [Melanoderma, Melasma]	EDTFL	70,490,700,32800,102250,212750,326540,5456 80,795610,857770,	Reddish brown discoloration on sides of the neck, usually both, essentially due to dilation of blood vessels.		Skin
Parapsoriasis	EDTFL	150,550,980,5710,13930,137500,262500,49750 0,626070,822530,	Group of skin disorders characterized primarily by their resemblance to psoriasis.		Skin
Parapsoriasis en Plaques	EDTFL	150,550,980,5710,13930,137500,262500,49750 0,626070,822530,	As mentioned above		Skin
Parakeratosis Variegata [Keratosis]	EDTFL	150,350,620,930,7500,37500,131980,285000,62 4110,881190,	As mentioned above		Skin
Petechiae	EDTFL	170,220,720,125880,236710,336000,421040,57 1670,681530,702030	Small, flat, round skin spot caused by a small hemorrhage.		Skin

Subject / Argument	Author	Frequencies	Notes	Origin	Target
Psoriasis		*May be associated with a Helicobacter pylori trigger. See Parasites General, Ascaris and Roundworm set. Use Nanobacter set.*			
Psoriasis	CAFL	2180,2128,2008,2489,1552,880,800,786,728,664,304,96,112,100,60,104,64,152,2170,2720,	Autoimmune disease with patches of red, itchy, and scaly skin. Use Hypothyroid sets. Do ozone therapy every 2nd day for 30 days. Reduce dietary starch drastically.	Psoriasis	Skin
Psoriasis	EDTFL	150,550,980,5710,13930,137500,262500,497500,626070,822530	As mentioned above	Psoriasis	Skin
Psoriasis	XTRA	104	As mentioned above	Psoriasis	Skin
Psoriasis	BIOM	6; 65.5; 92.5; 85; 110; 100; 60		Psoriasis	Skin
Pustular Psoriasis of Palms and Soles	EDTFL	140,200,620,7500,15500,41090,465690,597500,722700,875930,		Psoriasis	Skin
Pustulosis of Palms and Soles Pustulosis Palmaris et Plantaris	EDTFL	40,500,600,9070,73500,283500,325050,635000,805310,975900,		Psoriasis	Skin
Psoriasis of parasitic aetiology	BIOM	2720; 2489; 2180; 2170; 2160; 2128; 2008; 1552; 893; 880; 800; 786; 787; 727; 728; 694; 664; 304; 152; 112; 104; 100; 96; 64; 60		Psoriasis	Skin
Psoric itch	BIOM	90; 94; 98; 102; 106; 253; 693; 774; 920; 5742		Psoriasis	Skin
Psorinum	BIO	786	Homeopathic nosode for psoriasis. Useful for persistent skin itch, especially post-scabies.	Psoriasis	Skin
Psorinum	CAFL	786,767	As mentioned above	Psoriasis	Skin
Psoriasis Ankylosing Spondylitis	CAFL	3000,95,1550,802,880,787,776,727,650,625,600,28,1.2,10,35,28,7.69,110,100,60,428,680,	Chronic inflammatory disease of spinal and sacroiliac joints. Also see Ankylosing Spondylitis, and Spondylitis Ankylosing sets. Use Nanobacter set.	Psoriasis	Skin
Purpura	EDTFL	100,350,52500,72000,97100,225150,450000,689410,712000,993410	Disease of skin and other organs most common in children. In skin, it causes palpable purpura (small hemorrhages); often with kidney problems, joint and abdominal pain.	Purpura	Skin
Allergic Purpura	EDTFL	150,230,650,18200,56500,108020,305310,606300,719940,822530	Red or purple spots on skin that do not blanch with manual pressure, caused by bleeding beneath skin.	Purpura	Skin
Anaphylactoid Purpura	EDTFL	140,230,650,18200,56500,108020,305310,606300,719940,822530	As mentioned above	Purpura	Skin
Rheumatoid Purpura	EDTFL	50,90,9000,11090,55330,68500,232500,551100,779230,839430	Known as Henoch-Schoenlein purpura (PSH) it is a systemic IgA vasculitis of the small vessels. It is characterized by purpura of the skin, arthritis, abdominal and / or renal impairment.	Purpura	Skin
Henoch Purpura [Vasculitis IgA] Henoch-Schoenlein Purpura [Vasculitis IgA]	EDTFL	80,350,5500,35170,62500,93500,225000,496090,682450,753070,	As mentioned above	Purpura	Skin
Purpura Hemorrhagica [Vasculitis IgA] Purpura, Nonthrombocytopenic [Vasculitis IgA]	EDTFL	80,350,5500,35170,62500,93500,225000,496090,682450,753070,		Purpura	Skin
Purpura, Thrombotic Thrombocytopenic	EDTFL	200,7500,27500,95330,375160,419340,567700,642060,780310,980000,	Rare disorder of blood coagulation, causing many microscopic clots to form in small blood vessels.	Purpura	Skin
Moschkowitz Disease	EDTFL	160,300,2500,5500,13950,93500,356720,451170,483520,680000		Purpura	Skin
Werlhof's Disease	BIO	690	Also called Immune Thrombocytopenic Purpura. Low platelet count with normal bone marrow, purpuric rash, and bleeding problems. See Purpura Thrombocytopenic, and Purpura Thrombotic Thrombocytopenic.	Purpura	Skin
Werlhof's Disease	CAFL	690,452	As mentioned above	Purpura	Skin
Pyoderma Gangrenosum	EDTFL	120,230,830,5500,12710,83930,192500,475440,624370,882450,	Rare skin disorder of unknown cause. Small pustules develop into large ulcers at various body sites. Use Parasites General, and General Antiseptic sets.		Skin
Pyoderma Gangrenosum	XTRA	123,132,663,967,974,1489,1556,	As mentioned above		Skin
Pyoderma	CAFL	123,132,967,974,1556,1489,663,	See Pyoderma gangrenosum. A rare skin disorder of unknown cause. Small pustules develop into large ulcers at various sites on the body. Use Parasites general, and General antiseptic sets.		Skin
Pyoderma	VEGA	123	As mentioned above		Skin
Pyodermatitis	BIOM	123; 132; 663; 967; 974; 1489; 1556			Skin
Red patches	BIOM	89.5			Skin
Rosacea	EDTFL	80,120,850,5130,20000,40000,85000,97500,355720,434500	Long term skin condition with facial redness, small dilated blood vessels on face, papules, pustules, and swelling. May be associated with Demodex Folliculorum mites - see sets.	Rosacea	Skin
Scabies	CAFL	90,110,253	Also see Parasites Scabies, and Sarcoptes Scabiei Itch. Also use Psorinum.	Scabies	Skin

Subject / Argument	Author	Frequencies	Notes	Origin	Target
Scabies	EDTFL	350,930,7200,17500,52500,70000,215700,3265 00,434000,523010	Contagious skin infection caused by the mite Sarcoptes scabiei.	Scabies	Skin
Sarcoptes Scabiei Itch	HC	735000,	Caused by scabies mites. See Scabies, and Parasites Scabies sets. Also use Psorinum.	Scabies	Skin
Sarcoptes Scabiei Itch	XTRA	11484.37,1821.88	As mentioned above	Scabies	Skin
Scleroderma V	CAFL	4334,42046,44178,49847,55687,67868,75969,3 5237,54778,44837,39703,31888,34112,36769,4 2938,38882,48686,30121,64734,44679,70542,4 8450,	Chronic systemic autoimmune disease with hardening of skin. A more severe form also affects internal organs. Also use Nanobacter sets.		Skin
Scleroderma, Systemic	EDTFL	190,500,970,970,14630,42500,196500,321200,4 52930,777500			Skin
Hidebound disease	BIOM	4334; 3000; 1550; 880; 802; 787; 776; 727; 680; 650; 625; 600; 428; 110; 100; 95; 60; 35; 28; 10			Skin
Shingles			See Section 17d - Virus e Malattie correlate		Skin
Shingles	CAFL	664,787,802,880,914,1500,1600,2170,3343,	Due to Herpes virus that causes Chicken Pox during childhood and Shingles in adulthood. See Herpes Zoster sets.	Virus	Skin
Shingles [Herpes Zoster]	EDTFL	120,550,950,291230,292000,293050,367500,62 5220,816720,824370,			Skin
Sweet Syndrome	EDTFL	70,460,600,970,11090,32500,367450,395830,61 9340,725540	Skin disease with sudden onset of fever, elevated white blood cell count, and tender, red, well-demarcated papules and plaques that show dense infiltrates by neutrophil granulocytes.		Skin
Verruca	CAFL	173,644,767,787,797,827,953,	As mentioned above	Warts	Skin
Verruca [Plantar Wart]	EDTFL	40,520,5090,35000,175330,324850,432410,714 820,823000,987230,		Warts	Skin
Verruca	BIO	644,767,953	A rough-surfaced, supposedly harmless, virus-caused skin wart. See Warts verruca set. Use General antiseptic set.	Warts	Skin
Warts	EDTFL	40,520,5090,35000,175330,324850,432410,714 820,823000,987230	Use Fungus Foot and General 1, and General Antiseptic sets. Also see Parasites General Flukes, and Roundworm sets.	Warts	Skin
Warts Verruca	CAFL	495,644,767,797,877,953,173,787,	A rough-surfaced, supposedly harmless, virus-caused skin wart. See Verruca set. Use General antiseptic set.	Warts	Skin
Warts General	XTRA	110	Use Fungus Foot and General 1, and General Antiseptic sets. Also see Parasites General Flukes, and Roundworm sets.	Warts	Skin
Warts General	CAFL	2720,2489,2170,2127,2008,1800,1600,1500,907 ,915,874,727,690,666,644,767,953,495,466,110,	As mentioned above	Warts	Skin
Warts	BIOM	26.5; 36; 85.5; 89.5		Warts	Skin
Warts, basic	BIOM	2720; 2489; 2160; 2127; 2008; 1800; 1600; 1500; 727.5; 727; 690; 666		Warts	Skin
Warts Plantar	CAFL	915,918	Use Fungus foot and general 1, and General antiseptic sets.	Warts	Skin
Warts Condyloma	CAFL	466,907	Venereal warts caused by the infectious Papilloma virus. See Condylomata, Papilloma HPV, and Papillomavirus sets.	Warts	Skin
Wart Human Papilloma Plantar	HC	404700-406750=3600,	Skin growth caused by Human Papilloma Virus - see sets. See Papilloma HPV, and Papillomavirus sets.	Warts	Skin
Wart Human Papilloma Virus	HC	402850-410700=3600,	Virus causing warts. See Papilloma HPV, and Papillomavirus sets.	Warts	Skin
Wart Papilloma Cervix Smear	HC	404050-404600=3600,	Virus responsible for pre-cancerous lesions in cervix, and cervical cancer. See Papilloma HPV, and Papillomavirus sets.	Warts	Skin
Katy Luce Finger Wart	VEGA	495	Fungus	Warts	Skin
Vitiligo	CAFL	440,600,650,2112,880,787,727,444,20,	Loss of pigmentation in areas of skin. Use with B Complex with extra PABA internally and PABA Cream topically. See E Coli, Parasites General, and Fungus sets if required.	Vitiligo	Skin
Vitiligo	BIOM	5000; 2112; 880; 787; 727; 650; 600; 500; 444; 440; 68; 86; 20	As mentioned above	Vitiligo	Skin
Vitiligo	EDTFL	50,410,1000,45000,97500,324370,326850,5664 10,709830,930120	As mentioned above	Vitiligo	Skin
Vitiligo	XTRA	20	As mentioned above	Vitiligo	Skin
Leukoderma Acquired	CAFL	20,440,444,600,650,727,787,880,2112,	Also called leukodermia. See Vitiligo set. - Non-pigmented		Skin
Stevens-Johnson Syndrome	EDTFL	150,220,3570,14810,57630,291130,522800,608 110,771420,795020	Life-threatening skin condition where cell death causes epidermis to separate from dermis. Commonly caused by drugs such as epilepsy medication Lamotrigine, infections, or (rarely) cancers.		Skin
Xanthoma	EDTFL	200,460,2500,7500,37400,96500,222700,52700 0,749000,985670	Is a skin lesion caused by the accumulation of fat in macrophage immune cells in the skin and more rarely in the layer of fat under the skin.		Skin
Xanthoma Disseminatum	EDTFL	200,460,2500,7500,37400,96500,222700,52700 0,564280,985900	Rare skin condition that preferably affects males during childhood, characterized by the insidious onset of newborns, papules and nodules.		Skin
Xanthomatosis [Xanthoma}	EDTFL	200,460,2500,7500,37400,96500,222700,52700 0,749000,985670,	As mentioned above		Skin
Xanthomatosis [Familial]	EDTFL	200,460,2500,7500,12710,35000,90000,410250, 642910,978050,	As mentioned above		Skin
Xanthomatosis [Wolmans]	EDTFL	200,460,2500,5590,7500,95870,175910,343920, 425870,571400,	As mentioned above		Skin
Reticulohistiocytoma	EDTFL	110,550,730,840,67200,172850,230000,434500, 675960,875260			Skin

Subject / Argument	Author	Frequencies	Notes	Origin	Target
Rosai-Dorfman Disease	EDTFL	30,500,850,7500,8000,27500,95000,95690,1256 90,320900			Skin
Langerhans-Cell Granulomatosis	EDTFL	30,500,700,970,88000,370500,547500,656400,7 25370,825520,	Rare disorder involving clonal proliferation of Langerhans cells, abnormal cells derived from bone marrow migrating from skin to lymph nodes.		Skin
Langerhans-Cell Histiocytosis	EDTFL	20,450,900,2750,5870,15560,267500,395910,62 5700,796010,	As mentioned above		Skin
Hand-Schuller-Christian Syndrome [histiocytosis X]	EDTFL	120,350,850,7500,117500,142500,267500,3959 10,625700,796010,			Skin
Itching	CAFL	880,787,727,444,125,95,72,20,1865,3176,	Pruritis. Have a hot bath and drink a cup of apple cider vinegar after. If chronic and no long-term relief, use Parasites sets including General and Blood Flukes.	Itching	Skin
Itching [Pruritus]	EDTFL	170,720,1650,16850,55250,127500,455870,565 000,752000,975310,		Itching	Skin
Itching 1	XTRA	1865		Itching	Skin
Itching 2	XTRA	20,72,95,125,444,727,787,880,1865,3176,		Itching	Skin
Swimmers Itch [Flatworm infection]	EDTFL	680,900,2500,5500,13930,93500,386400,42950 0,434000,436250,		Itching	Skin
Feet itch	BIOM	787; 880; 5000		Itching	Skin
Itching of Anus Toes Feet Blue	XTRA	727,787,880,5000		Itching	Skin
Pruritus Vulvae	EDTFL	170,720,1650,16850,55250,127500,455870,565 000,752000,975310,	Genital itch (vulval).	Itching	Skin
Anal Itching	CAFL	10000,880,787,760,727,465,125,120,95,72,444, 1865,20,773,826,827,835,4152,	Pruritis. Use Parasites enterobiasis, and see General set.	Itching	Skin
Callosity-blister	BIOM	36.5; 10000; 800; 787; 727; 465; 880			Skin
Callosities	BIOM	36.5; 289; 546; 1642			Skin
Corns Feet	XTRA	20,727,787,880,5000,10000,			Skin
Foot Blisters	CAFL	465,727,787,880,10000,			Skin

11b - Morgellons

Subject / Argument	Author	Frequencies	Notes	Origin	Target
Morgellons General	XTRA	888,751,			Morgellons
Morgellons Disease 1	XTRA	5858.25,5856.38,4271.25,4264,330,10000,7344, 5000,1550,1234,740,880,835,787,727,160,500,1 600,5611,4014,3448,3347,3176,2929,2867,2855 ,2791,2720,2489,2180,1862,1488,880,787,728,6 65,464,432,304,120,30,20,8,920,2016,625,			Morgellons
Morgellons Disease 2	XTRA	8,20,30,120,160,304,330,432,464,500,625,665,7 27.5,740,787,800,538,880,920,1234,1488,1550, 1600,1862,2016,2180,2489,2720,2791,2855,286 7,2929,3176,3347,3448,4014,4264,4271.25,500 0,5611,5856.38,5858.25,7344,10000,			Morgellons
Morgellons Chronic Lesions and Fibres	XTRA	5100,10880,10800,27860,31167,27320,39392,3 6900,39776,37500,	Apply=.02% Feathering.		Morgellons
Morgellons Chronic (Ruptures and Fibre growths)	EDTFL	110,490,780,2250,77500,102750,262500,45591 0,837500,910500			Morgellons
Morgellons Expeller	XTRA	2014,	Forces artefacts out of the skin. Apply=+- .05% Feathering. If no result, try Frequencies Directly.		Morgellons
Morgellons External Skin Parasite (Symptoms Surface Scratching, itching skin)	EDTFL	60,320,900,85750,150000,222700,225000,4545 00,515170,687620			Morgellons
Morgellons (Internal & External Skin Parasites)	EDTFL	180,780,2500,37500,85000,110250,175000,352 930,495000,921260			Morgellons
Morgellons Int and Ext	XTRA	2560,5100,35000,27500,27860,31167,36827,29 095,39776,37500,	Apply=.02% Feathering.		Morgellons
Morgellons (Internal Parasites)	EDTFL	130,400,800,900,5260,72500,135470,296500,55 6740,879930			Morgellons
Morgellons Internal	XTRA	2560,5100,10880,10800,35000,27500,27860,36 827,29095,39776,	Apply=.02% Feathering.		Morgellons
Morgellons Nancy DB	XTRA	200.2,520.2,941.6,6270.2,13254.6,32273.4,	Dowsed by Nancy Sliwa.		Morgellons
Morgellons Skin Itch	XTRA	37500,	Apply=.02% Feathering. Run for 1 hour, or as needed.		Morgellons
Delusionary Parasitosis	EDTFL	130,400,800,900,5260,72500,135470,296500,55 6740,879930,			Morgellons
Ekbom Syndrome {Psychological, Morgellons]	EDTFL	190,370,780,950,2250,5240,45000,65750,75263 0,924370			Morgellons

Subject / Argument	Author	Frequencies	Notes	Origin	Target

Subject / Argument	Author	Frequencies	Notes	Origin	Target
Hand nails	BIOM	42.5; 46.5			Nail
Toe nails	BIOM	46.5; 75.5			Nail
Nail Disease / Nail Fungus	EDTFL	70,350,700,45000,77250,114690,320000,63710 0,805870,973500			Nail
Onychomycosis	EDTFL	70,240,35160,150000,375000,477500,527000,6 62710,749540,969670	Infection of nail by mold, usually Trichophyton Rubrum, Trichophyton Nagel, Trichophyton Mentagrophytes, Trichophyton Tonsurans, Epidermophyton Floccosum, Candida Parapsilosis, and Ringworm (Microsporum gypseum) - see sets. Also see Dermatomycoses.		Nail
Onychomycosis	BIOM	20; 37; 53.5; 100; 465; 727; 802; 880; 923; 1489; 1550			Nail
Tinea Pedis	EDTFL	140,260,600,2500,32500,37570,47500,60000,16 5820,368000	As mentioned above		Nail
Tinea Unguium	EDTFL	140,260,600,2500,32500,37570,324250,655200, 750000,926700	As mentioned above		Nail
Paronychia	EDTFL	30,220,350,410,7500,12930,84540,93300,32781 0,405220	Painful fungal (usually Candida Albicans - see sets) or bacterial (usually Streptococcus Pyogenes - see sets) infection of finger where nail and skin meet.		Nail

Subject / Argument	Author	Frequencies	Notes	Origin	Target
Hair Human	BIO	646			Hair
Head Skin	BIOM	85			Hair
Hair Diseases	EDTFL	20,450,650,2210,6150,10230,15940,30280,7750 0,327110			Hair
Pseudofolliculitis Barbae	EDTFL	80,520,24500,30650,117300,335000,536420,61 1000,804280,941020			Hair
Hair Regain Color/Grow	XTRA	1.05			Hair
Hair, loss of color	BIOM	93.5; 97.5			Hair
Hair Losing	XTRA	20,800,10000,		Alopecia	Hair
Hair Loss 1	XTRA	3,20,28,95,146,330,465,660,690,727.5,787,800, 880,1552,2170,2720,4200,5000,10000,15000,		Alopecia	Hair
Hair Loss 2	XTRA	727,800,880,10000		Alopecia	Hair
Alopecia	CAFL	20,10000,880,787,727,465,146,800,1552,	Loss of hair.Can be caused by Herpes zoster and Epstein-Barr virus.	Alopecia	Hair
ALOPECIA Areata (Hair Loss) Baldness Hair Loss Hair Loss, BALDNESS Hair Loss Telogen Effluvium	EDTFL	60,5070,95000,127670,275070,455820,515160, 684810,712230,993410,	Use Dr Rife Culique IR Mat on Scalp	Alopecia	Hair
Pseudopelade [Alopecia]	EDTFL	60,5070,95000,127670,275070,455820,515159, 684810,712230,993410,		Alopecia	Hair
Calvities (hair loss)	BIOM	10000; 5000; 2720; 2170; 1552; 880; 800; 787; 727; 646; 465; 330; 146; 100; 95; 28; 20; 3		Alopecia	Hair
Alopecia	XTRA	60,5070,95000,127630,275050,455820,515160, 684810,712230,993410,		Alopecia	Hair
Alopecia 1	XTRA	3,20,28,95,146,330,465,727,787,800,880,1552,2 170,2720,5000,10000,15000,	Loss of hair.	Alopecia	Hair
Hair - regulation of loss	BIOM	45; 81.5; 85; 85.5			Hair
Hair excess (Women)	BIOM	81.5			Hair
Steely Hair Syndrome	EDTFL	190,350,940,11950,25540,35670,87500,93500,2 34250,527810			Hair
Kinky Hair Syndrome	EDTFL	130,180,650,970,7500,11950,40000,150000,524 940,689930			Hair
Dandruff	BIOM	85; 87.5; 90; 98; 222; 225; 491; 616; 700		Dandruff	Hair
Seborrhea	BIOM	5000; 500; 465		Dandruff	Hair
Dandruff-1	BIOM	85		Dandruff	Hair
Dandruff Scales	XTRA	20,727,787,880,5000,	Shedding of plentiful dead scalp cells.	Dandruff	Hair
Hirsutism	EDTFL	60,300,620,51250,117250,245560,367500,6252 20,816720,905000	Excessive hair growth in women in areas where terminal hair is normally absent or minimal.		Hair
Trichotillomania	EDTFL	100,520,870,2500,13390,325170,475000,52700 0,759000,985670	Obsessive-compulsive disorder with urge to pull out one's hair.		Hair

12 - Human body and Sense organs

Subject / Argument	Author	Frequencies	Notes	Origin	Target
Human Body	XTRA	15136.71			

12a - Head

Subject / Argument	Author	Frequencies	Notes	Origin	Target
Head Top Of	XTRA	1052			Head
Human Head Cavity	XTRA	17700.2			Head
Headache	EDTFL	150,520,7500,30000,226090,430150,527000,662710,749000,986220		Headache	Head
Hemicrania	EDTFL	180,650,25070,87500,125330,222530,479930,527000,667000,987230		Headache	Head
Cephalgia	EDTFL	80,900,820,15230,74230,102730,251300,310520,424730,855280		Headache	Head
Headaches	XTRA	10,1.2,304		Headache	Head
Headache - Pilot frequencies	BIOM	62.5; 65; 67.5; 7; 8; 10; 96; 96.6			Head
Migraine	CAFL	10	Also use Parasites Strongyloides, and Parasites General sets.	Headache	Head
Headaches 1	CAFL	144,160,1.2,520,10,10000,304,		Headache	Head
Headaches 2	XTRA	1.19,10,144,160,304,520,10000,		Headache	Head
Headache, Migraine Migraine Disorders Pain, Migraine	EDTFL	100,520,7500,30230,226500,430150,527000,662800,749000,986220		Headache	Head
Headache Migraine	XTRA	0.5		Headache	Head
Migrainous headache	BIOM	47.5; 50; 52.5; 66.5; 95; 99.5; 7; 19.5; 19.65; 19.75; 25.5; 40.5; 46; 50.5; 85.5		Headache	Head
Headache Rapid Relief	XTRA	160		Headache	Head
Status Migrainosus	EDTFL	50,410,800,5250,42500,87500,376270,378000,380850,381000		Headache	Head
Headaches Unknown Cause	CAFL	10,4,5.8,6.3,7.83,3000,650,625,600,		Headache	Head
Headache of uncertain aetiology	BIOM	9.6; 3040; 880; 787; 727; 522; 72; 5.8; 4.9; 4.5		Headache	Head
Headache caused by craniocerebral injury	BIOM	1.2; 3.6; 6.3		Headache	Head
Headache, frontal	BIOM	96; 7		Headache	Head
Headaches Biliary	XTRA	3.5,8.5		Headache	Head
Bilious headache	BIOM	32.5; 35; 37.5		Headache	Head
Headaches Comp	XTRA	1.19,4,4.9,5.79,6.29,7.83,9.39,9.59,10,20,73,95,125,144,146,160,304,520,522,600,625,650,727,787,880,3000,10000,		Headache	Head
Headache: eye disease	BIOM	3.6; 3.9; 4.9; 9.7		Headache	Head
Headache: tonsil disease	BIOM	9.39		Headache	Head
Headache, endocrine	BIOM	4; 4.9; 5.5; 9.4		Headache	Head
Headaches Due to Toxicity	CAFL	522,146,4.9,3000,880,787,727,20,		Headache	Head
Headaches Toxicity 1	XTRA	1.19,4.9,20,146,160,250,522,660,690,727.5,787,880,3000,		Headache	Head
Headaches Toxicity 2	XTRA	4.9,20,146,522,727,787,880,3000,		Headache	Head
Headache, toxic substances	BIOM	10; 6.3; 5.8; 3040; 650; 625; 600		Headache	Head
Headache caused by infection	BIOM	3040; 95; 880; 1550; 802; 787; 776; 727; 4.9		Headache	Head
Headache of parasitic aetiology	BIOM	3000		Headache	Head
Headaches Due to Parasites	CAFL	125,95,73,20,727,3000,	See Parasites strongyloides set.	Headache	Head
Headaches Parasites 1	XTRA	20,73,95,125,727,3000,		Headache	Head
Headaches Parasites 2	XTRA	1.1,1.19,20,72,73,95,125,160,250,660,690,727.5,3000,		Headache	Head
Headaches Urogenital 1	XTRA	1.19,9.39,9.4,160,250,333,523,555,768,786,3000,		Headache	Head
Headaches Urogenital 2	XTRA	9.39,3000		Headache	Head
Headache: urogenital	BIOM	9.39; 9.4; 3000; 3040		Headache	Head
Vertebrogenic headache	BIOM	10000; 3040; 3000; 10; 9.6		Headache	Head
Headaches Vertebral Misalignment	CAFL	9.6,3000	Not a substitute for chiropractic adjustment.	Headache	Head
Headaches Vertebral Misalignment	XTRA	1.19,9.59,160,250,3000,	Not a substitute for chiropractic adjustment.	Headache	Head
Head Pressure In	XTRA	20,727,787,880,5000,		Headache	Head

Subject / Argument	Author	Frequencies	Notes	Origin	Target
Acrocephalosyndactylia	EDTFL	140,1220,2620,12720,125780,158330,351300,5 32410,613320,709800	Incorrect fusing of skull and digits. Other use: Apert Syndrome, Pfeiffer Syndrome, Saethre-Chotzen Syndrome		Head
Pfeiffer Syndrome	EDTFL	900,920,32750,293700,329050,415840,423470, 474150,512140,629900,			Head
Saethre-Chotzen Syndrome	EDTFL	70,150,3500,67110,81500,109500,112020,3840 70,471000,551000			Head
Apert Syndrome	EDTFL	140,1220,2620,12720,125750,158330,351300,5 32410,613320,709800			Head
Acromegaly	EDTFL	80,420,770,7910,31210,122740,255610,371330, 742800,955200,	Skull/brow/jaw expansion and soft tissue/organ swelling. Due to excess pituitary growth hormone production.		Head
Angiolymphoid Hyperplasia	EDTFL	150,1000,5500,11330,45000,234510,475160,52 7000,752600,987230	Domed papules/nodules on head or neck.		Head
Kimura Disease	EDTFL	70,120,850,9500,88000,141200,297500,425950, 675310,827000,	Chronic inflammatory disease. Its main symptoms are skin lesions of the neck or head or painful unilateral adenomegaly of the cervical lymph nodes.		Head
Cleidocranial Dysostosis	EDTFL	110,570,950,5500,17500,37500,162500,383500, 421000,645250,			Head
Craniofacial Dysostosis	EDTFL	70,230,970,14030,32500,72910,326590,497500, 675000,954370,			Head
Crouzon's Disease	EDTFL	70,190,750,930,17500,29000,412000,515000,79 1500,995150,	As mentioned above		Head
Craniosynostoses	EDTFL	90,3500,12680,51890,110600,292500,452500,6 95750,825290,953720	Premature fusing of infant skull sutures, causing abnormal shape.		Head
Oxycephaly	EDTFL	70,550,900,22500,47500,434030,527000,66700 0,752700,988900			Head
Hematoma, intracranial posttraumatic	BIOM	83.5		Hematoma	Head
Cranial Epidural Hematoma	EDTFL	150,240,700,830,2500,17600,432500,555910,62 5290,775520,		Hematoma	Head
Subdural Hematoma	EDTFL	150,240,700,830,2500,17600,432500,555910,62 5290,775520,		Hematoma	Head
Hemorrhage, Cranial Epidural	EDTFL	60,230,970,7000,175200,212960,325430,51570 0,682450,755480	Traumatic brain injury with build-up of blood between brain and skull.		Head
Hemorrhage, Subdural	EDTFL	40,550,910,93500,210500,453720,515150,6830 00,712230,993410	Traumatic brain injury with build-up of blood between brain and dura mater.		Head
Plagiocephaly, Nonsynostotic	EDTFL	20,240,850,2700,5250,72500,196500,375910,45 6780,880000	Also called flat head syndrome. Asymmetrical in utero flattening of one side or back of skull.		Head
Pseudotumor Cerebri	EDTFL	60,230,8850,45250,115300,215310,437500,662 500,825340,917030	Neurological disorder with increased intracranial pressure in the absence of a tumor or other disorders.		Head
Benign Intracranial Hypertension	EDTFL	30,400,780,1000,2500,33390,75790,185580,425 790,719340,	As mentioned above		Head
Intracranial hypertension	BIOM	1.2; 6.3; 20; 727; 787; 880; 5000			Head
Idiopathic Intracranial Hypertension	EDTFL	30,400,780,1000,2500,33390,75790,185580,425 790,719340,			Head

12b - Face

Subject / Argument	Author	Frequencies	Notes	Origin	Target
Facial Skin			See Section 11a - Skin		Face
Facial Cramps	CAFL	10000,6000,304,1131,33,			Face
Facial Hemiatrophy	EDTFL	60,230,730,32500,90000,175000,323240,65369 0,753070,922530	Also called Romberg Disease - see set. Neurocutaneous disorder with tissue degeneration beneath skin, usually on one side of the face.		Face
Romberg Disease [Hemifacial Atrophy]	EDTFL	80,320,610,2270,44250,115710,255550,485000, 697500,856720,	Neurocutaneous disorder with tissue degeneration beneath skin, usually on one side of the face.		Face
Rosacea	EDTFL	80,120,850,5130,20000,40000,85000,97500,355 720,434500	Long term skin condition with facial redness, small dilated blood vessels on face, papules, pustules, and swelling. May be associated with Demodex Folliculorum mites - see sets.		Face
Rosacea 2	XTRA	20,4160,11680,9130,3500032500,34336,38750, 3000,36465	As mentioned above		Face
Facial Neuralgia			See Section 9c - Pain and Inflammation	Nerve	Face
Facial Paralysis			See Section 8e - Paralysis	Nerve	Face
Angioedema	EDTFL KHZ	120,520,800,5070,15000,90000,375050,410250, 564280,824960,	Rapid swelling of oral, throat, and facial tissues.	Skin	Face
Quincke's Edema	EDTFL	800,1120,9850,51710,75930,385690,412020,69 0000,812930,906420	As mentioned above	Skin	Face
Angiofibroma	EDTFL	160,620,7500,65330,175000,434250,563190,64 2910,764730,930120,	Small papules over the side of the nose and on cheeks.	Skin	Face
Cherubism	EDTFL	100,570,1000,7500,27500,37400,96500,342060, 515700,691270	Genetic disorder causing prominence of lower part of face.	Genetic disorder	Face
Mandibulofacial Dysostosis	EDTFL	150,280,830,5500,37400,62200,93500,97200,15 3000,468200	Congenital malformations of skull, jaw, face, and neck.	Genetic disorder	Face

Subject / Argument	Author	Frequencies	Notes	Origin	Target
Treacher Collins Syndrome	EDTFL	130,400,730,5620,7250,42500,90000,479300,52 7000,986220	As mentioned above	Genetic disorder	Face
Tardive Dyskinesia	EDTFL	140,250,850,5250,7260,325000,587500,745310, 815900,927000,	Disorder with involuntary repetitive movements. Caused by antipsychotic drug use for longer than three months in adults, and GI drugs in children and infants.		Face
Orofacial Dyskinesia	EDTFL	560,950,15750,62500,95000,250000,432000,52 4370,682020,753070	Orofacial or tardive dyskinesias are involuntary repetitive movements of the mouth and face.		Face
Idiopathic Orofacial Dyskinesia	EDTFL	140,250,850,5250,7260,325000,587500,745310, 815900,927000,	Dystonia with difficulties in mouth, jaw, tongue, and eyelid movements.		Face
Meige Syndrome Jaw Spasms [Dystonia]	EDTFL	40,240,950,1000,7250,12050,97500,229320,325 950,532410,	As mentioned above		Face
Brueghel Syndrome	EDTFL	40,370,830,2500,70000,95030,175000,269710,3 55720,755000	As mentioned above		Face
Lingual-Facial-Buccal Dyskinesia	EDTFL	150,180,800,5500,107500,372500,515540,6318 50,711120,907500			Face
Dyskinesia Syndromes	EDTFL	140,250,850,5250,7260,325000,587500,745310, 815900,927000			Face
Skew Deviation	EDTFL	110,550,850,16900,47560,376290,476500,5270 00,667000,742000			Face
Brown Tendon Sheath Syndrome	EDTFL	40,370,830,2500,3000,75850,95160,175030,269 710,350000			Face
Status Marmoratus	EDTFL	40,70,520,680,900,2740,5000,15360,325540,53 3630			Face
Etat Marbre	EDTFL	140,550,950,5260,25520,42800,162520,492570, 675510,828530	Tardive Dyskinesia		Face
Mumps			See section 17d - Virus	Virus	Face
Parotid gland	BIOM	29.5			Face

12c - Eyes - Sight

Subject / Argument	Author	Frequencies	Notes	Origin	Target
Eyes	XTRA	12.3			Eyes
Eyes-1		3.6; 4.9; 64.0; 72.5			Eyes
Eyes - Pilot frequencies	BIOM	15.5; 70; 72.5; 75			Eyes
Center of vision	BIOM	70			Eyes
Eyes General	CUST	5752,5581,2876,2790,1438,1395,718,698,359,3 45,180,174,	Frequencies provided by Paul Jones. They produced excellent sharpness results very quickly on many people who used them. Experimental		Eyes
Organ of sight	BIOM	3.6; 4.9; 15.5; 70; 72.5; 75.5			Eyes
Eyesight to Improve	CAFL	350,360,1830,	See Vision Poor, and Visual Acuity.		Eyes
Eyesight to Improve	XTRA	266,350,360,1830,			Eyes
Vision Acuity	CAFL	350,360,1802,1806,1810,1814,1818,1822,1826, 1830,1834,1838,1842,1846,1848,1852,1856,186 0,3176,	See Eye degeneration, Eyesight to improve, and Macular Degeneration and Visual Acuity sets.		Eyes
Sharpness of Vision		72.5			Eyes
Visualization	XTRA	12.3			Eyes
Eyesight, regulation	BIOM	3.6; 4.9; 31.5; 64; 72.5			Eyes
Eye General Ailments	XTRA	20,80,160,350,360,400,496,660,690,727.5,787,8 02,880,1335,1550,1552,1600,1830,2010,10000,			Eyes
Vision Disorders	EDTFL	190,260,570,9000,17200,35750,176090,355080, 642910,978050	See Eye Disorders, Eyesight to Improve, and Macular Degeneration and Visual Acuity sets.		Eyes
Eye Fatigue	BIOM	3.6; 4.9; 7.0; 46.0; 70.0; 70.5; 72.5; 95.0			Eyes
Visual impairments	BIOM	70; 70.5; 95			Eyes
Eye Disorders	CAFL	10000,2010,1831,1830,1829,1600,1552,1335,88 0,787,727,496,400,360,350,160,20,	Blurred vision, cataracts, crossed eyes, diplopia, infections, etc. Also use Macular Degeneration.		Eyes
Eye Disorders	XTRA	1600	As mentioned above		Eyes
Eye Abnormalities	EDTFL	60,500,870,12850,27500,32500,42500,190000,4 50000,856720	Use Retyne™ Light mat		Eyes
Vision Poor	CAFL	350,360,1830=900,	See Eye degeneration, Eyesight to improve, and Macular Degeneration and Visual Acuity sets.		Eyes
Myopia		*Can be associated with childhood febrile illnesses of Measles, Rubella, Pertussis and Mumps.*			
Myopia	BIOM	3.6; 4.9; 31.5; 58.0; 64.5; 72.5; 85.5			Eyes
Myopia Eye Myopia Eye Presbyopia	EDTFL	150,180,800,5500,33200,172300,471200,55782 0,603440,921880			Eyes
Eye Near and Farsighted	CAFL	727,787,880,5000,10000,			Eyes
Myopia and hypermetropia	BIOM	31.5; 727; 787; 880; 5000; 10000			Eyes
Hypermetropia	BIOM	31.5			Eyes
Hypermetropia	BIOM	3.6; 4.9; 31.5; 58.0; 64.5; 72.5; 85.5			Eyes

Subject / Argument	Author	Frequencies	Notes	Origin	Target
Hypermetropia Hyperopia	EDTFL	100,570,950,12850,20000,37700,95790,250000, 475580,527000	Commonly called farsightedness.		Eyes
Astigmatism	EDTFL KHZ	600,900,7500,12330,12710,55000,234510,3257 10,491000,667900,	Blurred vision due to corneal or lens defect.		Eyes
Macropsia	EDTFL	320,1390,2830,8130,13230,15630,57320,13320 0,321560,585700	Anomaly of vision, whereby objects are seen in larger than actual size.		Eyes
Micropsia	EDTFL	70,240,650,5750,72230,124000,502500,622880, 713230,807730			Eyes
Hemeralopia	EDTFL	70,250,570,870,2250,72500,226320,323510,526 160,682020			Eyes
Color Blindness	EDTFL	130,250,730,5750,7500,55500,122500,442500,6 25710,875270			Eyes
Color Vision Defects [Group 22]	EDTFL	150,180,800,5500,33200,172300,471200,55782 0,603440,921880,			Eyes
Monochromatopsia	EDTFL	110,350,800,35250,72500,142370,271500,5925 00,725680,836420			Eyes
Eye Arteriosclerosis	CAFL	20,727,787,880,10000,	Hardening of arteries and arterioles in the eyes, affecting vision.		Eyes
Eye Bifocal	CAFL	20,727,787,880,5000,			Eyes
Eye Discharge	XTRA	**436,595,775,952**			Eyes
Eye Hemorrhage	EDTFL	50,350,750,930,5710,7500,345730,465340,5925 00,725000	Use Retyne™ Light mat		Eyes
Hemophthalmos [Hyphema]	EDTFL	110,670,960,5250,28430,37560,262500,593500, 775790,808500,			Eyes
Eye Inflammation	CAFL	**1.2,80**	Use General antiseptic.		Eyes
Eye Inflammation 2	XTRA	**1.19,80,250**			Eyes
Eye Inflammation	EDTFL	60,500,870,12850,27500,141000,301230,45302 0,783400,825030,	Use Retyne™ Light mat		Eyes
Eye Night Blindness Eye Optic Nerve Disorders Eye Strain (General) Optic Disc Disorders Refractive errors	EDTFL	150,180,800,5500,33200,172300,471200,55782 0,603440,921880			Eyes
Eye Nerve Pain	CAFL	**727,787,10000**			Eyes
Eye Strain	CAFL	**727,787,880**			Eyes

		Diseases			
Eye diseases	BIOM	2010; 1831; 1830; 1829; 1600; 1552; 1335; 496; 400; 360; 350; 160			Eyes
Eye Infected	CAFL	727,787,880,5000,10000,		Infections	Eyes
Eye Infections	EDTFL	60,500,870,12850,27500,141000,301230,45302 0,783400,825030	Use Retyne™ Light mat	Infections	Eyes
Trachoma	CAFL	430,620,624,840,866,2213,	Painful and potentially blinding infectious eye disease caused by Chlamydia Trachomatis - see sets.	Infections	Eyes
Trachoma [Chlamydia trachomatis]	EDTFL	800,1270,7500,65000,125750,229320,415700,5 63190,709830,978850,	As mentioned above	Infections	Eyes
Egyptian Ophthalmia	EDTFL	140,230,730,5580,13390,150000,475850,73642 0,819340,915700,	As mentioned above	Infections	Eyes
Eye Fusarium General	XTRA	600,625,650,746,768,	Eye infection due to pathogenic plant Fungus. Bioweapon. See Fusarium Oxysporum, and Fusarium General.	Infections	Eyes
Adie Syndrome	EDTFL	170,480,10850,55160,96500,350000,567000,69 2330,810200,982110,	Neurological disorder causing dilation problems with eye pupils.	Nerve	Eyes
Amaurosis Fugax	EDTFL	180,780,2500,37500,85000,110250,175000,352 930,495000,552880	Transient loss of sight in one eye.		Eyes
Monocular Blindness, Transient	EDTFL	80,410,950,2750,5500,15650,192930,236420,32 2570,585700			Eyes
Leber's Congenital Amaurosis	EDTFL	30,240,660,880,189390,215620,334580,491600, 722550,823440			Eyes
Amblyopia	EDTFL	50,700,2500,67500,125050,322060,347350,655 200,752630,924370,	Lazy eye.		Eyes
Anisometropic Amblyopia	EDTFL	50,700,2500,67500,125050,322060,357350,655 200,752630,924370,	Lazy eye.		Eyes
Eye Amblyopia	EDTFL	90,1500,2830,4840,62300,88230,105430,21556 0,375220,485620			Eyes
Aniridia	EDTFL KHZ	70,240,680,830,2500,157000,357300,451170,51 7500,687620,	Absence of irises, usually in both eyes - can be congenital or due to injury.		Eyes
Anisocoria	EDTFL KHZ	120,570,830,2500,5330,65000,93500,325160,51 5050,884810,	Unequal size of pupils of eyes, normally harmless but sometimes due to life-threatening causes.		Eyes
Anophthalmos	EDTFL KHZ	120,970,5050,7000,40000,222700,425160,5710 00,824000,932000,	Developmental problem resulting in absence of one or both eyes.		Eyes
Eye Cataract	CAFL	727,787,880,5000,	Use also for Diplopia (double vision).	Cataract	Eyes

Subject / Argument	Author	Frequencies	Notes	Origin	Target
Eye Cataract 2	XTRA	6110		Cataract	Eyes
Cataract	CAFL	728,784,787,800,880,10000,	Clouding of lens of eye. Also see Eye and Eyes sets.	Cataract	Eyes
Cataract Cataract, Membranous Eye Cataract	EDTFL	970,5780,7500,37500,125190,250000,325650,5 17500,683000,712420	As mentioned above	Cataract	Eyes
Lens Opacities [Cataract]	EDTFL	970,5780,7500,37500,125190,250000,325650,5 17500,683000,712420,	[Retyne™ Light mat]	Cataract	Eyes
Cataract	ODD	20,160,350,360,400,666,727,728,740,784,790,8 80,1335,1552,1600,1654,2010,2110,2187,2195, 2211,5000,10000,	As mentioned above	Cataract	Eyes
Cataract	BIOM	12.5; 18.5; 23.0; 64.5; 72.5; 79.5; 85.5; 99.5		Cataract	Eyes
Cataract, basic	BIOM	10000; 2211; 2195; 2187; 2110; 2010; 1830; 1654; 1600; 1335; 1335; 880; 800; 787; 774; 496; 325		Cataract	Eyes
Cataract-1	BIOM	10000; 9998.5; 5000; 2211; 2195; 2187; 2110; 1830; 1654; 1600; 1552; 1335; 880; 787; 784; 774; 728; 496; 360; 350; 325; 292; 100; 30; 20; 9.1; 0.3		Cataract	Eyes
Cataract 1	CAFL	1830=600,1600,9999,1552,2110,1335,1654,218 7,2195,2211,	As mentioned above	Cataract	Eyes
Cataract 1	ODD	728,784,787,880,1335,1600,1654,1552,1830=6 00,2110,2187,2195,2211,	As mentioned above	Cataract	Eyes
Cataract 3	XTRA	0.29,9.09,30,292,1335,1552,1600,1654,1830=6 00,2110,2187,2195,2211,9999,	As mentioned above	Cataract	Eyes
Cataract General 1	CAFL	325,496,728,774,784,787,800,880,1335,1552,16 00,1654,1830,2010,2187,2195,2211,10000,	As mentioned above	Cataract	Eyes
Cataract Brunescent	CAFL	2010,1335,1830=600,	Clouding of lens of eye. Brown opacity in later life.	Cataract	Eyes
Cataract Brunescent	VEGA	1335	As mentioned above	Cataract	Eyes
Cataract, combined	BIOM	2010; 1830; 728; 784; 787; 800; 880; 10000		Cataract	Eyes
Cataract Complicated	BIOM	1830; 496; 325; 774		Cataract	Eyes
Cataract Complicated	BIO	496	Clouding of lens of eye. Secondary type caused by disease, degeneration, or surgery.	Cataract	Eyes
Cataract Complicated	XTRA	325,496,774,1830	As mentioned above	Cataract	Eyes
Chorioretinitis	EDTFL	80,550,50000,85750,95000,229320,475750,527 000,667000,721000	Inflammation of eye's vascular coat. Often due to Toxoplasmosis and Cytomegalovirus (CMV) - see these sets.		Eyes
Choroideremia [Retinal Degeneration]	EDTFL	150,180,800,5500,33200,172300,471200,55782 0,603440,921880,	Genetic disorder leading to blindness (cecità).	Genetic disorder	Eyes
Coloboma	EDTFL	130,230,620,1000,7500,155980,396500,415700, 575270,927000	A hole in one of the eye's structures.		Eyes
Conjunctival Diseases	EDTFL	80,220,630,840,215680,317240,532530,742540, 894500,970320	Use Chlamydia Trachomatis. See Bacillus Subtilis.	Conjunctivitis	Eyes
Conjunctivitis	CAFL	489,1550,880,802,787,727,20,80,432,722,822,1 246,1830,	As mentioned above	Conjunctivitis	Eyes
Conjunctivitis	XTRA	1246	As mentioned above	Conjunctivitis	Eyes
Conjunctivitis 2	XTRA	20,80,489,660,690,727.5,787,802,880,1550,160 0,1830,10000,	As mentioned above	Conjunctivitis	Eyes
Conjunctivitis 3	XTRA	20,80,727,787,802,880,1550,	As mentioned above	Conjunctivitis	Eyes
Conjunctivitis Conjunctivitis, Red Eye (Pink Eye)	EDTFL	50,410,830,105210,220500,347250,532500,742 500,896500,975980	Use Retyne™ Light mat	Conjunctivitis	Eyes
Conjunctivitis, of unclear aetiology	BIOM	11; 63.5; 66.5; 70; 75.5		Conjunctivitis	Eyes
Conjunctivitis, of infectious aetiology	BIOM	10000; 5000; 2025; 1830; 1552; 1550; 1246; 1205.9; 880; 822; 802; 787; 728; 727; 489; 432; 120; 80; 20; 1.2		Conjunctivitis	Eyes
Conjunctivitis Bacilius Subtilis	XTRA	432,722,822,1246	See also Chlamydia Trachomatis.	Conjunctivitis	Eyes
Conjunctivitis Chlamydia Trachomatis	XTRA	430,555.7,620,624,840,866,1111.4,2213,2222.8,	See also Bacillus Subtilis.	Conjunctivitis	Eyes
Conjunctivitis Eyelid	XTRA	727,787,800,880	Use Chlamydia Trachomatis. See Bacillus Subtilis.	Conjunctivitis	Eyes
Contagious Conjunctivitis	Rife	1206000,2025625,	As mentioned above	Conjunctivitis	Eyes
Contagious Conjunctivitis	XTRA	148,15825.2,18843.75	As mentioned above	Conjunctivitis	Eyes
Cornea	BIOM	18.5		Cornea	Eyes
Corneal Diseases Corneal Dystrophy Hereditary Corneal Edema Eye Corneal Disease	EDTFL	70,320,950,7500,84000,193930,237500,487500, 706210,946500	Swelling of cornea. May be indicated by seeing rainbows around lights, especially at night. Use Retyne™ Light mat	Cornea	Eyes

Subject / Argument	Author	Frequencies	Notes	Origin	Target
Granular Dystrophy (Corneal)	EDTFL	100,570,800,7500,15300,52500,95120,655200,750000,923700		Cornea	Eyes
Stromal Dystrophies, Corneal	EDTFL	70,320,950,7500,84000,193930,237500,487500,706210,946500,	Abnormal accumulation of extraneous material in corneas.	Cornea	Eyes
Corneal Ulcer	EDTFL	70,320,950,7500,84000,519340,682450,711210,850830,922530	Use Retyne™ Light mat	Cornea	Eyes
Corneal Ulcer	KHZ	40,240,9680,42850,172500,203000,412500,592500,775290,819340,	Also called Ulcerative Keratitis. Inflammatory or infective condition.	Cornea	Eyes
Corneal Ulcer	XTRA	959.27,5996.1,6046.89,19267.59,	As mentioned above	Cornea	Eyes
Keratitis Keratitis Ulcerative	EDTFL	150,180,800,5500,33200,172300,471200,557820,603440,921880,	Inflammation of the cornea of the eye, usually painful and 'gritty.'	Cornea	Eyes
Thygeson's SP Keratitis [Group 22]	EDTFL	150,180,800,5500,33200,172300,471200,557820,603440,921880,	Damage to corneal epithelium, with red eye, foreign body sensation, tearing, and burning.	Cornea	Eyes
Diabetic Retinopathy (Eye Disease)	EDTFL	150,890,1700,6970,12890,62300,421000,465000,895000,951302	Retinal damage due to diabetes which can cause blindness.		Eyes
Diplopia [Cerebal]	EDTFL	70,410,730,5860,72500,135000,367500,550300,725340,920320,	Eye muscle problem that causes double vision.		Eyes
Duane Retraction	EDTFL	1860,7270,7660,7870,8020,8450,17220,62220,131200,218310	Inability of an eye to turn outwards.		Eyes
Ocular Retraction Syndrome	EDTFL	110,230,870,7500,8040,87500,155290,396500,437400,828570	As mentioned above		Eyes
Endophthalmitis	EDTFL	280,620,810,2100,33000,47500,117500,396500,655720,825540	Inflammation of internal coats of eye, usually due to bacteria or fungi.		Eyes
Ophthalmia	EDTFL	140,230,730,5580,13390,150000,475850,736420,819340,915700	As mentioned above		Eyes
Eyes Crossed	CAFL	727,787,880,5000,10000,	Also see Esotropia, Exotropia, and Strabismus.	Strabismus	Eyes
Eyes Crossed	XTRA	20,80,160,350,360,400,496,660,690,727.5,787,802,880,1335,1550,1552,1600,1830,2010,10000,	As mentioned above	Strabismus	Eyes
Eye muscles, heterotropy	BIOM	88.5		Strabismus	Eyes
Squint	BIOM	25.5; 45.0; 45.0; 58.8; 72.5; 78.5; 88.5		Strabismus	Eyes
Strabismus	EDTFL	20,780,7500,40000,398400,476500,527000,665340,761850,987230	Eye squint, commonly called crossed eyes. Also see Esotropia set.	Strabismus	Eyes
Strabismus, Convergent	EDTFL	30,550,780,7250,50000,85160,210500,326560,752630,925710		Strabismus	Eyes
Strabismus, Divergent	EDTFL	50,550,780,7250,50000,85160,210500,326560,662740,789000		Strabismus	Eyes
Strabismus, Internal	EDTFL	180,550,780,7250,50000,85160,210500,326560,842000,937420		Strabismus	Eyes
Strabismus, Noncomitant	EDTFL	110,550,780,7250,50000,85160,210500,326560,821520,924370		Strabismus	Eyes
Hypertropia	EDTFL	100,230,830,5550,12710,13930,92500,376290,519340,652430			Eyes
Esotropia [Eye Muscle Disorder]	EDTFL	60,500,870,12850,27500,32500,42500,190000,450000,856720,	Inward eye squint, or Strabismus.		Eyes
Esophoria [Eye Muscle Disorder]	EDTFL	60,500,870,12850,27500,32500,42500,190000,450000,856720,	As mentioned above		Eyes
Exophoria [Eye]	EDTFL	60,500,870,12850,27500,32500,42500,190000,450000,856720,			Eyes
Exotropia	EDTFL	140,220,730,5580,13390,150000,475850,736420,819340,915800			Eyes
Exfoliation Syndrome	EDTFL	50,370,900,2500,3000,73300,94750,175000,269710,355080	Also called Pseudoexfoliation Syndrome, or PEX. Age-related systemic disease mainly manifesting in eyes with accumulation of protein fibres.		Eyes
Pseudoexfoliation Syndrome	EDTFL	20,230,850,5710,55830,172500,326400,663500,725310,853020	As mentioned above		Eyes
Glaucoma Capsulare	EDTFL	70,120,600,870,2250,22500,187500,396500,587500,790000	As mentioned above		Eyes
Floaters Eye Floaters	EDTFL	150,180,800,5500,33200,172300,471200,557820,603440,921880	Deposits in vitreous humour of eyes due to degeneration. Use Retyne™ Light mat		Eyes
Eye Floaters	XTRA	1830	As mentioned above		Eyes
Eye Glaucoma	CAFL	727,787,880,5000,1600,	Group of eye diseases that can cause optic nerve damage and vision loss. Also see Eye Glaucoma, and Eyes Glaucoma.	Glaucoma	Eyes
Eyes Glaucoma	CAFL	1600,1830,880,787,727,	As mentioned above	Glaucoma	Eyes
Glaucoma	BIOM	5000; 1600; 1830; 880; 787; 727; 98.5; 70		Glaucoma	Eyes
Glaucoma (special)	BIOM	3.6; 4.9; 12.5; 18.5; 23.0; 70; 72.5; 98.5		Glaucoma	Eyes
Glaucoma Eye Disorder Glaucoma	EDTFL	70,120,600,870,2250,22500,187500,396500,587500,696500	Use Retyne™ Light mat	Glaucoma	Eyes
Glaucoma 1	XTRA	660,690,727.5,787,880,1600,1830,	As mentioned above	Glaucoma	Eyes
Glaucoma 2	XTRA	3022	As mentioned above	Glaucoma	Eyes

Subject / Argument	Author	Frequencies	Notes	Origin	Target
Peter's Anomaly [Corneal Disorder]	EDTFL	70,320,950,7500,84000,193930,237500,487500,706210,946500,	Failure in normal development of part of the eye.		Eyes
Gyrate Atrophy	EDTFL	80,410,2830,15250,67250,221050,471020,597520,722300,822570	Also called Ornithine aminotransferase deficiency. Inherited disorder with poor night vision, leading to blindness.		Eyes
Hemianopsia [Visual Defect Blindness] 2023	EDTFL	110,320,910,3720,78300,122200,306500,401620,473290,517230,	Loss of vision or blindness in half the visual field, usually one side of the vertical midline.		Eyes
Hemianopsia, Binasal Hemianopsia, Bitemporal Hemianopsia, Homonymous	EDTFL	110,320,910,3720,78300,122200,306500,473290,401620,517230	As mentioned above		Eyes
Quadrantanopsia [Anopia vision disorder]	EDTFL	190,260,570,9000,17200,35750,176090,355080,642910,978050,	As mentioned above		Eyes
Hyphema	EDTFL	110,670,960,5250,28430,37560,262500,593500,775790,808500	Presence of blood in front chamber of eye, usually due to trauma.		Eyes
Keratoconus	KHZ	190,520,680,970,57500,119530,325620,634200,701500,881620,	Degenerative eye disorder with structural corneal changes.It can be caused by the Conidiophores of Aspergillus niger.		Eyes
Keratoconus [Conical Cornea]	EDTFL	70,320,950,7500,84000,193930,237500,487500,706210,946500,	[Retyne™ Light mat]		Eyes
Larva Migrans, Ocular [Hookworm Infection]	EDTFL	170,460,10880,55160,96500,350000,567000,692330,810200,982110,	See Ancylostoma Parasites.	Roundworm	Eyes
Macular Degeneration 1	XTRA	0.59,1.1,1.39,1.89,9.9,10,21,23.6,24,25.6,27.69,32,34.1,410,	Age-related diminution or blurring of center of visual field. Use with Cataract sets. Can be caused by Cytomegalovirus.	Macular D.	Eyes
Macular distrophy	BIOM	1830; 1832; 1834; 1836; 1838; 1840; 1842; 1844; 1846; 1848; 1850; 1852; 1854; 1856; 1858; 1860; 1830		Macular D.	Eyes
Macular Degeneration and Visual Acuity	CAFL	1828,1830,1832,1834,1836,1838,1840,1842,1844,1846,1848,1850,1852,1854,1856,1858,1860,	As mentioned above	Macular D.	Eyes
Macular Degeneration Visual Acuity	XTRA	8,1830,1832,1834,1836,1838,1840,1842,1844,1846,1848,1850,1852,1854,1856,1858,1860,	As mentioned above	Macular D.	Eyes
Macular Dystrophy, Corneal	EDTFL	150,180,800,5500,33200,15650,85680,225230,475680,527000		Macular D.	Eyes
Best Disease [Macular Degeneration]	EDTFL	150,180,800,5500,33200,172300,471200,557820,603440,921880,	As mentioned above	Macular D.	Eyes
Macular Degeneration Maculopathy, Age-Related Eye Macular Degeneration	EDTFL	150,180,800,5500,33200,172300,471200,557820,603440,921880	As mentioned above	Macular D.	Eyes
Stargardt Disease	EDTFL	160,550,850,2450,20000,47500,72400,125120,379930,475190	As mentioned above	Macular D.	Eyes
Microphthalmos	EDTFL	900,920,32750,293300,329050,415840,423470,472120,512140,629900	Developmental disorder where one or both eyes are abnormally small with anatomical malformations.		Eyes
Extraocular Muscles-1	BIOM	88.5			Eyes
Eye muscles regulation	BIOM	3.6; 4.9; 19.5; 45; 88.5			Eyes
Eye muscles, degeneration	BIOM	23.6; 25.6; 26.7; 34.1; 88.5; 410			Eyes
Eye muscles, fatigue and pain	BIOM	4; 6; 10; 45; 47.5; 50; 52.5; 70; 80; 99.5			Eyes
Eye muscles, spasms	BIOM	324; 328			Eyes
Nystagmus Pathologic	EDTFL	50,120,870,870,27500,62710,145470,262500,392500,591000	Often called 'dancing eyes.' Involuntary movement of eyes, due to congenital disorders, acquired or CNS disorders, toxicity, drugs, alcohol, or rotation.	Nystagmus	Eyes
Convergence Nystagmus	EDTFL	50,120,870,870,27500,62710,145470,262500,392500,591000,	As mentioned above	Nystagmus	Eyes
Convergence Insufficiency [Eye]	EDTFL	60,500,870,12850,27500,32500,42500,190000,450000,856720,	As mentioned above	Nystagmus	Eyes
Horizontal Nystagmus	EDTFL	50,120,870,870,27500,62710,145470,262500,392500,591000,	As mentioned above	Nystagmus	Eyes
Vertical Nystagmus	EDTFL	50,120,870,870,27500,62710,145470,262500,392500,591000,	As mentioned above	Nystagmus	Eyes
Jerk Nystagmus	EDTFL	50,120,870,870,27500,62710,145470,262500,392500,591000,	As mentioned above	Nystagmus	Eyes
Periodic Alternating Nystagmus	EDTFL	50,120,870,870,27500,62710,145470,262500,392500,591000,	As mentioned above	Nystagmus	Eyes
Rotary Nystagmus	EDTFL	50,120,870,870,27500,62710,145470,262500,392500,591000,	As mentioned above	Nystagmus	Eyes
Pendular Nystagmus	EDTFL	50,120,870,870,27500,62710,145470,262500,392500,591000,	As mentioned above	Nystagmus	Eyes
See-Saw Nystagmus	EDTFL	50,120,870,870,27500,62710,145470,262500,392500,591000,	As mentioned above	Nystagmus	Eyes
Eye Movement Disorders	EDTFL	60,500,870,12850,27500,32500,42500,190000,450000,856720	Use Retyne™ Light mat		Eyes

Subject / Argument	Author	Frequencies	Notes	Origin	Target
Ocular Motility Disorders	EDTFL	70,370,870,7500,8040,87500,323980,665700,82 2700,906040	Problems include Diplopia, Nystagmus, poor Vision Acuity, and Strabismus - see sets.		Eyes
Heterophoria [Eye Movement Disorder General]	EDTFL	60,500,870,12850,27500,32500,42500,190000,4 50000,856720,	Constant tendency of one or both eyes to deviate from the normal direction of gaze.		Eyes
Ocular Torticollis	EDTFL	190,370,910,3200,45200,52570,177320,281190, 398620,408200			Eyes
Smooth Pursuit Deficiency	EDTFL	190,370,750,45190,65000,96500,225750,51435 0,652430,759830			Eyes
Opsoclonus	EDTFL	70,460,600,950,10530,32500,347250,595540,73 2410,925350	Involuntary uncontrolled movements of the eyes, chaotic and multi-vector.		Eyes
Ophthalmoplegia Ophthalmoplegia, Ataxia and Areflexia Syndrome	EDTFL	70,370,12740,47500,97700,225750,377900,519 340,691270,753070	Weakness or paralysis of certain eye muscles.		Eyes
IInternuclear Ophthalmoplegia	EDTFL	70,370,12740,47500,97700,225750,377900,519 340,691270,753070,	Paresis of ipsilateral eye adduction in horizontal gaze.		Eyes
Ophthalmoplegia, Progressive Supranuclear	EDTFL	70,370,12740,47500,97700,224750,377900,519 340,691270,753070	Gradual deterioration and death of specific volumes of the brain, with many different symptoms.		Eyes
Steele-Richardson-Olszewski [supranuclear palsy]	EDTFL	200,250,770,2500,3000,5580,175540,326500,42 5690,571000,	As mentioned above		Eyes
Tolosa-Hunt Syndrome	EDTFL	50,410,600,850,323550,350000,479500,663710, 752700,987230	As mentioned above		Eyes
Optic Nerve	BIOM	94.5		Nerve	Eyes
Visual nerve regeneration	BIOM	3.6; 4.9; 20; 72.5; 80; 94.5		Nerve	Eyes
Oculomotor Paralysis	EDTFL	170,320,950,5500,32500,330000,537500,60583 0,754030,825310		Paralysis	Eyes
Oculomotor Nerve Diseases	EDTFL	170,320,950,5500,32500,47500,162120,232030, 397500,679930	Paralysis of nerve due to trauma, Demyelinating Diseases, high intracranial pressure, brain Cancer, Hemorrhage, or microvascular diseases such as Diabetes - see appropriate sets.	Paralysis	Eyes
Optic Atrophies, Hereditary	EDTFL	350,750,1750,15290,113250,245910,307100,45 2000,525520,779500	Progressive optic nerve damage with symmetric bilateral central visual loss.	Nerve	Eyes
Optic Nerve Diseases	EDTFL	40,350,6790,7200,115780,234250,342190,4725 00,551220,657540	Causes can include Glaucoma (see sets), Optic Neuritis (see set), tumors, trauma, and other eye problems.	Nerve	Eyes
Optic Neuropathy	EDTFL	80,410,950,2750,5500,15650,192930,236420,32 2570,585700	Use Retyne™ Light mat	Nerve	Eyes
Ischemic Optic Neuropathy	EDTFL	80,410,950,2750,5500,15650,192930,236420,32 2570,585700	Use Retyne™ Light mat	Nerve	Eyes
Optic Nerve Ischemia	EDTFL	50,780,8930,10400,29300,32430,342190,47250 0,551220,819340	Use Retyne™ Light mat	Nerve	Eyes
Optic Neuritis	EDTFL	70,570,600,11090,75290,137500,375520,45650 0,517500,687620	Demyelinating inflammation of optic nerve which can cause complete or partial blindness, most often due to Multiple Sclerosis, or Diabetes Mellitus (see sets).	Nerve	Eyes
Papillitis, Optic {Optic Neuritis]	EDTFL	70,570,600,11090,75290,137500,375520,45650 0,517500,687620,		Nerve	Eyes
Neuropapillitis [Optic Neuritis]	EDTFL	70,570,600,11090,75290,137500,375520,45650 0,517500,687620,		Nerve	Eyes
Retrobulbar Neuritis (Optic neuritis)	EDTFL	70,570,600,11090,75290,137500,375520,45650 0,517500,687620,		Nerve	Eyes
Neuromyelitis Optic	EDTFL	80,410,800,5200,5750,122900,287500,319340,4 72290,673510	Simultaneous inflammation and demyelination of optic nerve (Optic Neuritis - see set) and spinal cord (Myelitis - see set).	Nerve	Eyes
Optic Neuritis	BIOM	3.6; 4.9		Nerve	Eyes
Devic Disease [neuromyelitis optica, NMO]	EDTFL	80,410,800,5200,5750,122900,287500,319340,4 72290,673510,	As mentioned above	Nerve	Eyes
Parinaud Syndrome [Nystagmus]	EDTFL	50,120,870,870,27500,62710,145470,262500,39 2500,591000,	Paralysis of the gaze.	Paralysis	Eyes
Orbital Cellulitis	EDTFL	140,490,790,12500,43000,122500,262500,5553 50,692500,819340,	Inflammation and severe swelling due to infection of eye tissues, usually by Staphylococcus Aureus, Streptococcus Pneumoniae, or Beta Streptococcus.	Skin	Eyes
Papilledema [Optic Eye Swelling]	EDTFL	40,350,6790,7200,115780,234250,342190,4725 00,551220,657540,	Swelling in the eyeball due to increased intracranial pressure.		Eyes
Choked Disk	EDTFL	40,120,57500,92500,225170,324350,332410,51 7500,689410,712810			Eyes
Optic Disk Edema	EDTFL	80,410,950,2750,5500,15650,192930,236420,32 2570,585700	Use Retyne™ Light mat		Eyes
Optic Papilla Edema	EDTFL	40,180,700,10400,29300,32430,342190,425290, 572000,813000	Use Retyne™ Light mat		Eyes
Penqueculum	CAFL	746,755,1375,6965,626,948,	Possibly Pinguecula, a common type of conjunctival degeneration in the eye.		Eyes
Penqueculum	VEGA	746,755,6965	As mentioned above		Eyes
Light Sensitivity	EDTFL	110,490,790,2250,7500,30000,270280,333910,7 91030,905070			Eyes

Subject / Argument	Author	Frequencies	Notes	Origin	Target
Photosensitivity Disorders	KHZ	130,240,1700,34870,62250,102750,232500,425540,725350,869710,	Notable or increased reactivity to light that can result in serious discomfort, disease, or injury.		Eyes
Pterygium	EDTFL	570,680,870,2500,5710,32500,92500,322540,519340,653690	A Pinguecula is called a Pterygium if it invades the cornea of the eye.		Eyes
Afferent Pupillary Defect	EDTFL	20,240,900,9850,201750,365000,423010,697300,875930,979530	Injuries involving both the nucleus of the oculomotor nerve and its fascicle in its mesencephalic path.		Eyes
Efferent Pupillary Defect	EDTFL	230,2120,5940,7500,22500,51390,228950,557400,603920,725120	As mentioned above		Eyes
Marcus-Gunn Pupil [Pupil Eye Disorder]	EDTFL	350,410,710,970,7500,13420,205410,377800,476290,515700,	or afferent pupillary defect (APD)		Eyes
Pupil Disorders	EDTFL	350,410,710,970,7500,13420,205410,377800,476290,515700	Conditions of the pupil of the eye.		Eyes
Pupillary Functions, Abnormal	EDTFL	50,260,940,2500,12850,35340,5750,96500,322060,475870	.		Eyes
Ametropia	EDTFL	30,240,710,15830,29750,187500,324540,592500,820110,923530,	Light focussing error by eye, leading to reduced vision acuity. Also see appropriate Eye, Eyes, and Vision sets.		Eyes
Retina	BIOM	65.5; 74.5		Retina	Eyes
Retina Control	BIOM	65.5		Retina	Eyes
Retina regeneration	BIOM	3.6; 4.9; 19.5; 65.5; 70; 72.5; 74.5; 94.5		Retina	Eyes
Retina, regulation	BIOM	65.5; 74.5		Retina	Eyes
Retinal detachment	BIOM	47.5; 50; 52.5; 66.5; 95; 99.5; 7; 19.65; 19.75; 25.5; 40.5; 46; 50; 85.5		Retina	Eyes
Retinal Detachment	EDTFL	440,600,850,5090,7250,92500,337300,476500,527000,663710	Eye disorder due to fluid leaking behind the retina through physical damage, by traction, or by fluid exuding from the retina.	Retina	Eyes
Retina Detachment1	BIOM	5.7; 19.5; 47.5; 50.0; 52.5; 66.5; 95.0; 99.0		Retina	Eyes
Retina Detachment2	BIOM	19.64; 19.75; 25.5		Retina	Eyes
Retinal Pigment Epithelial Detachment	EDTFL	140,230,410,2370,4050,19500,175000,376300,407600,513060	Use Retyne™ Light mat	Retina	Eyes
Retinal disorders Eye Retinal disorders Retinal Vein Occlusion Retinitis Pigmentosa	EDTFL	150,180,800,5500,33200,172300,471200,557820,603440,921880	Use Retyne™ Light mat	Retina	Eyes
Tapetoretinal Degeneration	EDTFL	40,220,620,5700,13520,40000,175830,432410,565360,709830	Inherited degenerative eye disease with severe vision impairment due to degeneration of rod photoreceptor cells in retina.	Retina	Eyes
Retina dystrophy	BIOM	0.6; 1.4; 1.9; 9.9; 10; 23.6		Retina	Eyes
Rod-Cone Dystrophy	EDTFL	70,410,22500,57500,325180,476500,527000,667000,749000,986220		Retina	Eyes
Retinopathy of Prematurity	EDTFL	70,500,630,7400,17500,127500,335230,565750,725950,919340	Eye disease of premature babies, generally due to intensive oxygen therapy.Use Retyne™ Light mat	Retina	Eyes
Retrolental Fibroplasia	EDTFL	160,570,850,950,8500,95690,217520,491000,524370,892410		Retina	Eyes
Retinoschisis	EDTFL	80,460,1560,7500,217500,327500,347950,665750,796500,834250	Eye disease with abnormal splitting of retina's neurosensory layers, usually in the outer layer.	Retina	Eyes
Retinoschisis, Degenerative	EDTF KHZ	70,500,780,7500,17500,127200,335290,565750,725950,919340	Use Retyne™ Light mat	Retina	Eyes
Retinoschisis, Juvenile, X-Linked	EDTFL	70,500,830,7100,17500,127500,335290,525150,705220,813660	Use Retyne™ Light mat	Retina	Eyes
X-Linked Retinoschisis	EDTFL	80,460,1560,7500,217500,327500,347950,665750,796500,834250,			Eyes
Scleritis [Eye Inflammation]	EDTFL	60,500,870,12850,27500,141000,301230,453020,783400,825030,	Serious inflammatory disease that affects white outer coating of the eye.		Eyes
Episcleritis [Eye Inflammation]	EDTFL	60,500,870,12850,27500,141000,301230,453020,783400,825030,	As mentioned above		Eyes
Scotoma	EDTFL	80,240,730,3950,17510,125210,162520,391020,415700,726070	Area of partially or completely diminished visual acuity surrounded by field of normal vision.	Scotoma	Eyes
Scotoma, Arcuate	EDTFL	80,240,730,3950,17510,125210,162520,275870,523520,671220		Scotoma	Eyes
Scotoma, Bjerrum	EDTFL	80,240,730,3950,17510,125210,125210,162520,275000,425430		Scotoma	Eyes
Scotoma, Central	EDTFL	80,240,730,3950,17510,125210,162520,479500,527000,667000		Scotoma	Eyes
Scotoma, Centrocecal	EDTFL	80,240,730,3950,17510,125210,219340,422530,561930,987230		Scotoma	Eyes
Uveitis Eye Uveitis (infection)	EDTFL	40,240,10530,20000,124370,342060,527000,667000,742000,987230			Eyes
Iritis	EDTFL	80,240,500,7500,10720,36210,142500,321000,415700,775680	Also called Uveitis - see set. Inflammation of eye's uvea, lying between retina and sclera/cornea.		Eyes
Vitreous Disorders	EDTFL	140,520,2500,12850,35160,97500,200000,476900,665340,986220,	Disorders of vitreous body of eye. Also see Eye, Eyes, and Vision sets.		Eyes
Opacity of vitreous body	BIOM	64; 72.5			Eyes

Subject / Argument	Author	Frequencies	Notes	Origin	Target
Opacity of Vitreous Body	BIOM	72.5			Eyes
White Dot Syndrome	EDTFL	410,750,820,970,7500,19860,37530,125310,375930,519340,	Inflammatory eye disorders with white dots on the interior surface of eye causing blurred vision and visual field loss.		Eyes
Kearns Syndrome Kearns-Sayer Syndrome	EDTFL	30,210,930,950,7500,13520,95000,322530,454330,517500	Neuromuscular disorder of eyelids and eyes leading to ptosis and ophthalmoplegia.		Eyes
Eye Lacrimal	CAFL	727,787,880,5000	Secretion of tears.	Tears	Eyes
Scant tear secretion	BIOM	4; 10; 11; 12.5; 15			Eyes
Lacrimal Apparatus Diseases	EDTFL	120,320,25000,52400,134250,175750,426900,571000,843000,937410	Conditions of eye structures for producing and draining tears - see appropriate Eye sets.	Tears	Eyes
Epiphora	EDTFL	20,120,950,13610,52500,150000,463040,633250,723530,855350	As mentioned above	Tears	Eyes
Lacrimal Duct Obstruction	EDTFL	70,320,25000,52400,134250,213980,321650,426420,613010,719340		Tears	Eyes
Chalazion	EDTFL	20,240,850,37500,101330,221100,419340,562910,709830,976900	Cyst in eyelid due to blocked meibomian gland.		Eyelid
Meibomian Cyst	EDTFL	150,220,720,2580,193110,247590,385210,521680,652300,729340			Eyelid
Ectropion	EDTFL	30,500,850,5710,7250,13980,324300,450000,695830,895870	Eversion of the lower eyelid .		Eyelid
Entropion	EDTFL	280,750,830,980,107410,128310,307000,517100,609420,717210	Condition where eyelid folds inward, causing eyelash friction with cornea.		Eyelid
Distichiasis	EDTFL	130,720,920,9500,128000,302500,432700,597500,773910,901170	Growth of eyelashes from abnormal eyelid location.		Eyelid
Blepharitis	BIOM	8697; 7270; 999; 943; 824.4; 787; 784; 745; 738; 728; 727; 647; 644; 555; 478; 424; 7344; 4412; 1234; 740; 701; 330; 253	Chronic inflammation of eyelid at eyelash follicles. May involve Demodex follicular mites.		Eyelid
Blepharitis	EDTFL	30,550,780,7250,50000,85160,210500,325550,752630,925710			Eyelid
Blepharoptosis	EDTFL	40,240,950,1000,12050,177710,234000,591000,683160,849340	Eyelid droop. Also called Ptosis.		Eyelid
Ptosis, Eyelid	EDTFL	150,800,7500,30000,67500,125000,352930,563190,642910,930120	As mentioned above		Eyelid
Blepharospasm {Eye Disorder]	EDTFL	40,240,950,1000,7250,12050,97500,229320,325950,532410,	Uncontrolled eyelid twitch.		Eyelid
Eye Ptosis	CAFL	5000,10000	Drooping eyelid. See Eye Droop of Lid, and Ptosis sets.		Eyelid
Eye Droop of Lid	CAFL	727,787,880,5000,10000,	See Eye Ptosis, and Ptosis.		Eyelid
Ptosis	CAFL	10000	Eyelid droop. Use Parasites General, Ascaris, and Roundworm. See Eye Droop of Lid, and Eye Ptosis.		Eyelid
Eye Swollen Lid	CAFL	787			Eyelid
Stye	CAFL	10000,880,787,727,20,453,2600,	Staphylococci infection of sebaceous gland of eyelash. Use Staphylococci infection sets.	Stye	Eyelid
Hordeolum	CAFL	20,453,727,880,2600,10000,	See Stye set. Use Staphylococcus Infection set.	Stye	Eyelid
Sty (hordeolum)	BIOM	10000; 880; 787; 727; 20; 453; 2600		Stye	Eyelid
Stye [hordeolum]	EDTFL	70,240,620,900,2500,27500,55910,119340,393500,536420,	As mentioned above	Stye	Eyelid

12d - Ears - Hearing

Subject / Argument	Author	Frequencies	Notes	Origin	Target
Acoustic apparatus	BIOM	5.8; 6; 9.25; 9.8			Ear
Ears	XTRA	10.7,			Ear
Ears	BIOM	2.5; 6			Ear
Hearing center	BIOM	60			Ear
Auditory center - Pilot frequencies	BIOM	11; 55; 57.5; 60			Ear
Hearing function regulation	BIOM	2.5; 6; 8.8; 8.9; 9			Ear
Ear Conditions Various	CAFL	10000,880,787,727,776,766,688,683,652,645,542,535,440,410,340,201,158,20,9.19,	Discharges, tinnitus, itching and hearing loss. See Deafness, Otitis, and Ears sets.		Ear
Ear General Conditions	XTRA	9.19,9.2,20,158,201,340,410,440,535,542,645,652,660,683,690,727.5,787,880,10000,			Ear
Ear Conditions Various 2	XTRA	9.18,20,727,787,880,10000,			Ear
Ears Balance	CAFL	20,727,787,880,10000,			Ear
Ear pain	BIOM	3040; 95; 880; 1550; 802; 787; 776; 727; 4.9			Ear
Ears, general problems	BIOM	10000; 880; 787; 727; 776; 766; 688; 683; 652; 645; 542; 535; 440; 410; 340; 201; 158; 20; 9.19			Ear
Otolaryngologic Diseases	EDTFL	50,460,950,7500,32500,50000,67500,125910,546500,875470,			Ear
Otologic Diseases	EDTFL	70,350,700,45000,78250,114690,323000,637120,845870,973500			Ear
Ear Diseases Ear Infection	EDTFL	80,800,950,22300,57500,175000,419340,563160,813960,983170			Ear

Subject / Argument	Author	Frequencies	Notes	Origin	Target
Earaches	CAFL	727,787,880,5000			Ear
Ear Fungus	CAFL	854			Ear
Ear mycosis	BIOM	854; 858; 880; 787; 776; 766; 728; 727; 688; 683; 652; 645; 542; 535; 440; 410; 340; 250; 201; 158; 91.9			Ear
Otitis	EDTFL	30,240,700,1770,12330,27500,135520,550000,7 26290,875000	Ear infections.	Otitis	Ear
Otitis	BIOM	3.3; 3.6; 4.9; 5.8; 6; 9.19; 9.25; 9.8; 27; 29; 29.5; 52.75; 53; 53.5; 72.5; 98		Otitis	Ear
Inflammation in case of otitis basic	BIOM	2.5; 2.6; 3; 4; 4.9; 5.5; 9.4; 14.5; 20; 22; 25.5; 42; 49; 64; 63; 79.5; 85.5; 98; 91.5		Otitis	Ear
Otitis Interna	EDTFL	30,240,700,1770,12330,27500,135520,550000,7 25290,876000		Otitis	Ear
Otitis Externa	CAFL	727,787,880,174,482,5311,	Outer ear infection. See Ear, Ears, and Pseudomonas Aeruginosa sets.	Otitis	Ear
Otitis Externa	BIOM	27; 174; 464; 482; 728; 784; 880		Otitis	Ear
Otitis media	BIOM	683; 688; 776; 766; 316; 784; 786; 125; 802; 72; 522; 440; 880; 880; 720; 720; 1550; 1550		Otitis	Ear
Otitis Medinum	CAFL	683,688,776,766,316,784,786,125,802,72,522,4 40,880=600,720=600,1550=600,	Middle ear swelling and/or infection and fever. See Ear Cholesteatoma and Ears sets. Always use Streptococcus Pneumonia with this. If uncomfortable, lower Amplitude.	Otitis	Ear
Otitis Medinum	VEGA	316,	As mentioned above	Otitis	Ear
Mastoiditis	CAFL	287	Inflammation of bony structure of the skull behind ears below eye level.		Ear
Mastoiditis	EDTFL	230,620,750,5500,7500,33980,295300,327400,3 75430,522530	As mentioned above		Ear
Cholesteatoma	BIOM	453; 618; 793; 5057.5	Chronic otitis media form		Ear
Inner Ear Inflammation	XTRA	465,660,690,727.5,776,787,802,880,1550,			Ear
Eustachian Tube Inflammation	CAFL	1550,880,802,787,776,727,465,	Use General Antiseptic. See Ear(s), and Hearing sets.		Ear
Eustachian Tube Dysfunction	EDTFL	150,550,950,5250,25540,42500,162570,492570, 675510,828530			Ear
Eustachian Tube	XTRA	465,660,690,727.5,776,787,802,880,1550,	See Ear(s), and Hearing sets.		Ear
Clogged Auditory Tubes	XTRA	5092			Ear
Tympanic Membrane Perforation	EDTFL	90,310,440,58000,77900,126000,471680,48752 0,507120,622310,	Punctured eardrum. Causes include Otitis Media (see sets), trauma, ear surgery, extremely loud noises, or flying.		Ear
Eardrum Perforation	EDTFL	160,550,1850,8500,27300,57500,72500,207500, 412340,607000	As mentioned above		Ear
Labyrinth Diseases	EDTFL	70,490,600,800,32100,251500,382500,501690,6 18000,713540	Diseases of the inner ear.		Ear
Inner Ear Disease	EDTFL	80,800,950,22300,57500,175000,419340,56316 0,813960,983170,			Ear
Labyrinthitis	EDTFL	70,490,600,800,32100,47500,269710,450000,51 3540,686210	Inflammation of inner ear, leading to vertigo, hearing loss, or tinnitus (see sets for these).		Ear
Epidemic Neurolabyrinthitis [Labyrinthitis]	EDTFL	70,490,600,800,32100,47500,269710,450000,51 3539,686210,	Diseases of the inner ear. See Labyrinthitis, and Labyrinth Diseases.		Ear
Vestibular Neuronitis	EDTFL	30,250,870,2500,5870,85000,96500,175870,357 770,452590			Ear
Ears Discharges	CAFL	727,787,880,5000,10000,			Ear
Ear Discharge	XTRA	9.18,9.19,20.660,690,727.5,787,880,			Ear
Ear Wax	CAFL	311,320,750,984	See Cerumen set.		Ear
Cerumen Ear Wax	CAFL	311,320,750,984,720,	See Ear wax set.		Ear
Cerumen	VEGA	320,	Earwax.		Ear
Ear wax	BIOM	311; 320; 750; 984			Ear
Hearing	XTRA	10.7,		Hearing	Ear
Hearing Disorders	KHZ	10,500,930,2250,5290,30000,142500,350000,42 2060,775290,		Hearing	Ear
Hearing Disorders	EDTFL	140,290,900,8530,17500,72530,159030,322500, 408300,522280		Hearing	Ear
Auditory Hyperesthesia	EDTFL	40,240,570,17500,86530,132750,342510,72120 0,823100,919340,		Hearing	Ear
Hyperacusis	EDTFL	50,370,880,900,9400,115750,255830,485430,87 5580,943300	Increased sensitivity to everyday environmental sounds.	Hearing	Ear
Loudness Recruitment	EDTFL	140,210,6530,27300,61400,175310,347200,438 220,576380,683220		Hearing	Ear
Hearing Loss Sudden	EDTFL	30,290,620,970,17500,72530,159030,322500,40 8300,532280	It can be caused by Herpes Zoster.	Hearing	Ear
Deafness	CAFL	10000,1550,880,802,787,727,20,	Partial to complete. See Ears hard to hear set.	Hearing	Ear
Deafness 1	XTRA	9.18,9.19,65,660,690,727.5,760,787,802,880,15 50,10000,		Hearing	Ear

Subject / Argument	Author	Frequencies	Notes	Origin	Target
Deafness 2	XTRA	20,727,787,802,880,1550,5000,10000,		Hearing	Ear
Drum membrane, damage	BIOM	8; 29		Hearing	Ear
Ears Ringing	CAFL	20,727,787,880,5000,	See Tinnitus sets.	Tinnitus	Ear
Tinnitus	CAFL	20,2720,728,784,880,	Ringing or hissing/roaring in ears. See Circulatory Stasis, Dental, General Antiseptic, and Otitis sets.	Tinnitus	Ear
Tinnitus	EDTFL	50,240,15750,45000,93500,376290,512330,689 930,759830,925710	As mentioned above	Tinnitus	Ear
Tinnitus	XTRA	20,2720,728,784,880,	As mentioned above	Tinnitus	Ear
Pulsatile Tinnitus	EDTFL	50,240,15750,45000,93500,376290,512330,689 930,759830,925710		Tinnitus	Ear
Sonitus, dull	BIOM	27		Tinnitus	Ear
Sonitus, ringing	BIOM	29		Tinnitus	Ear
Cochlear nerve	BIOM	72.5		Hearing	Ear
Neuralgia, Geniculate	EDTFL	30,180,650,2500,8000,77500,270960,321800,50 5670,715280	Reactivation of Herpes Zoster virus (see sets) in ganglion of facial nerve, causing paralysis, pain, and taste loss. Also see Herpes Zoster Oticus.	Virus	Ear
Ramsay Hunt Auricular	EDTFL	70,180,1650,7930,102530,165500,320530,6935 00,875310,915930	As mentioned above	Virus	Ear
Otosclerosis	CAFL	9.19,	Abnormal growth of bone near middle ear which can lead to hearing loss.	Hearing	Ear
Deafness from Otosclerosis	XTRA	9.18,9.19,	Due to abnormal growth of bone near middle ear. See Otosclerosis.	Hearing	Ear
Otosclerosis	EDTFL	100,520,780,800,2250,5260,167500,352520,845 470,922530	As mentioned above	Hearing	Ear
Otosclerosis	BIOM	3.3; 5.8; 9.19	As mentioned above	Hearing	Ear
Otospongiosis	EDTFL	30,180,920,930,5500,10890,93400,210500,4243 70,978050	As mentioned above		Ear
Swimmers Ear	CAFL	728,784,880,464,174,482,5311,	See Pseudomonas Aeruginosa, and Otitis Externa sets.		Ear
Tympanitis	BIOM	10000; 5000; 1550; 880; 802; 787; 727; 465; 60.5; 20; 9.2			Ear
Dizziness	CAFL	4,5.8,60	See Vertigo, and Giddiness.	Dizziness	Ear
Dizziness	XTRA	5.8	See Vertigo, and Giddiness.	Dizziness	Ear
Dizziness	BIOM	5000; 1550; 880; 802; 787; 786; 784; 766; 727; 720; 688; 683; 652; 645; 522; 316; 92; 72; 60; 58; 40; 20; 5.8	See Vertigo, and Giddiness.	Dizziness	Ear
Dizziness 1	XTRA	40,58,60,72,92,316,522,645,652,683,688,720,72 7,766,784,786,787,802,880,1550,	See Vertigo, and Giddines.	Dizziness	Ear
Ears Dizziness	CAFL	20,727,787,880		Dizziness	Ear
Giddiness Dizziness	XTRA	20,10000		Dizziness	Ear
Giddiness	XTRA	20,727,787,880,5000,	Also see Vertigo, and Dizziness.	Dizziness	Ear
Vertigo	CAFL	60,5.8,4	Use Otitis medium, and Streptococcus pneumoniae sets. See General antiseptic set.	Dizziness	Ear
Vertigo	EDTFL	50,430,850,2750,5000,55180,269710,555300,70 7000,825500		Dizziness	Ear
Vertigo	BIOM	5000; 1550; 880; 802; 787; 786; 784; 766; 727; 720; 688; 683; 652; 645; 522; 316; 92; 72; 60; 58; 40; 20; 9.2; 5.8		Dizziness	Ear
Vertigo, Aural	EDTFL	50,430,850,2750,5000,55180,275090,410250,64 2060,978050		Dizziness	Ear
Lightheadedness [Nausea, Vertigo]	EDTFL	70,350,700,46000,78250,114690,323000,63708 0,845870,973500,	As mentioned above	Dizziness	Ear
Vertigo	XTRA	100	As mentioned above	Dizziness	Ear
Vestibular vertigo	BIOM	89.5; 95; 97.5			Ear
Meniere's 1	CAFL	8.8,8.9,9	Auditory vertigo associated with deafness and tinnitus. See Deafness, Otitis, and Tinnitus sets. Use General Antiseptic.	Dizziness	Ear
Meniere's Disease	CAFL	1550,802,880,787,727,465,428,33,329,5000=96 0,1130,782,9=1560,	As mentioned above	Dizziness	Ear
Meniere's Disease 1	CAFL	9,329,428,465,727,782=1560,787,802,808,1130 ,1550,5000=960,	As mentioned above	Dizziness	Ear
Meniere's Disease Meniere Disease Meniere's Syndrome	EDTFL	50,500,710,910,2560,33180,215470,402530,592 500,725370	As mentioned above	Dizziness	Ear
Meniere's syndrome	BIOM	5000; 1550; 802; 880; 832; 787; 727; 465; 428	As mentioned above	Dizziness	Ear

Subject / Argument	Author	Frequencies	Notes	Origin	Target

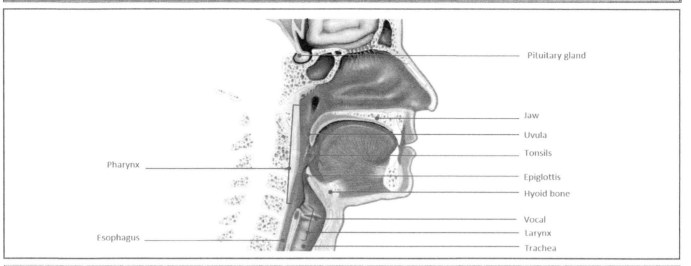

Pituitary gland — Jaw — Uvula — Tonsils — Epiglottis — Hyoid bone — Vocal — Larynx — Trachea

Pharynx — Esophagus

Subject / Argument	Author	Frequencies	Notes	Origin	Target
Throat	XTRA	12			Throat
Throat center	BIOM	20			Throat
Sore Throat	CAFL	2720,2489,1800,1600,1550,802,885,880,875,78 7,776,727,46.5,766,	See Pharyngitis, Streptococcus General, Streptococcus Pyogenes and Actinomyces Israelii sets.		Throat
Sore Throat	XTRA	1550	As mentioned above		Throat
Sore Throat [Group 10]	EDTFL	120,550,860,7500,12500,77500,120000,307250, 320000,615000,			Throat
Throat inflammation	BIOM	75.5; 82; 86; 89			Throat
Chronic throat diseases	BIOM	120; 666; 690; 727; 787; 800; 880; 1560; 1840; 1998; 776; 766			Throat
Epiglottitis	EDTFL	1210,4250,9790,28530,40310,157800,275830,3 36290,519320,613890			Throat
Supraglottitis	EDTFL	210,250,4520,42690,112250,321800,412500,64 3740,825520,971000	Inflammation of the epiglottis which can interfere with breathing.		Throat
Otolaryngologic Diseases	EDTFL	50,460,950,7500,32500,50000,67500,125910,31 9380,855820			Throat
Pharynx	BIOM	71.5			Throat
Pharyngeal Diseases	EDTFL	40,570,620,910,7500,295560,487500,605720,72 3820,935420	Disorders of that part of the throat situated immediately posterior to the nasal cavity, posterior to the mouth and superior to the esophagus and larynx.	Pharyngitis	Throat
Pharyngitis	CAFL	20,146,380,440,522,727,776,784,802,880,1550, 1600,	Inflammation of pharynx. Can cause chronic sore throat, halitosis and pharygeal ulcers. See Sore Throat and Halitosis sets.	Pharyngitis	Throat
Pharyngitis, acute	BIOM	75.5; 82; 86; 89		Pharyngitis	Throat
Pharyngitis, complex	BIOM	146; 2720; 2489; 1800; 1600; 1550; 880; 802; 787; 776; 727; 465; 440; 380; 1600; 20; 522; 146		Pharyngitis	Throat
Pharyngalgia	BIOM	2502; 2154; 2111; 1998; 1840; 1560; 1214; 1000; 885; 875; 625.5; 488; 452; 440; 432		Pharyngitis	Throat
Pharyngalgia, complex	BIOM	8450; 7880; 5004; 4192; 3552; 925; 875; 845; 380; 262; 222		Pharyngitis	Throat
Pharyngitis [Bacterial Infection]	EDTFL	120,550,860,7500,12500,77500,120000,307250, 320000,615000,		Pharyngitis	Throat
Glossopharyngeal Nerve	EDTFL	30,370,780,900,7500,20000,322060,377300,425 710,568430,	Severe pain localized in the distribution area of the 9th and 10th cranial nerve.	Nerve	Throat
Glossopharyngeal Neuralgia		30,370,780,900,7500,20000,322060,377300,425 710,568430,		Nerve	Throat
Cranial Nerve IX Diseases	EDTFL	40,200,700,880,5780,32500,181930,621690,705 530,815700,	Impaired functioning of one of the 12 cranial nerves.	Nerve	Throat
Retropharyngeal Abscess	EDTFL	40,570,620,910,7500,295560,487500,605720,72 3820,935420,	Abscess in throat tissues behind posterior pharyngeal wall. Also see Abscesses sets.		Throat
Esophagotracheal Fistula	EDTFL	180,240,10530,27500,35000,57500,96500,3251 10,475160,527000,			Throat
Tonsils	BIOM	1.7; 8.1; 9.6; 9.4; 20.5			Throat
Tonsillitis	CAFL	1.2,73,1550,802,1500,880,832,787,776,727,650, 625,600,465,144,452,582,	It can be caused by Adenovirus, Rhinovirus and Epstein Barr virus.	Tonsils	Throat
Tonsillitis	EDTFL	160,350,16030,43500,47500,269710,365250,45 7200,703260,889230,	As mentioned above	Tonsils	Throat
Tonsillitis	VEGA	452	As mentioned above	Tonsils	Throat
Tonsillitis	BIOM	35; 71.5; 87; 20.5; 75.5; 82; 86; 89		Tonsils	Throat

Subject / Argument	Author	Frequencies	Notes	Origin	Target
Tonsillitis 1	BIOM	2.2; 10; 12.5; 19.5; 26; 49; 55; 92.5		Tonsils	Throat
Tonsillitis 2	BIOM	1.6; 1.7; 9.44; 9.5; 20.5; 25.5; 35; 52; 52.75; 53; 53.5; 62; 62.5; 71.5; 75.5; 82; 85; 86; 87; 87.5; 89; 90; 91.5; 94.5; 98		Tonsils	Throat
Tonsillitis 3	BIOM	7.0; 9.4; 19.5; 40.5; 46.0; 50.0		Tonsils	Throat
Tonsillitis 4	BIOM	2.8; 3.3; 8.1; 9.19; 54.0; 54.25; 54.5		Tonsils	Throat
Tonsillitis 5	BIOM	0.7; 0.9; 2.5; 2.65; 3.3; 9.8; 56.0; 69.0		Tonsils	Throat
Tonsillitis 6	BIOM	2.5; 3.6; 3.9; 5.0; 6.3; 8.1; 34.0; 92.0		Tonsils	Throat
Tonsillitis, general	BIOM	1.2; 15; 73; 1550; 1500; 880; 832; 787; 776; 727; 650; 625; 600; 582; 542; 465; 452; 5000		Tonsils	Throat
Tonsillitis, chronic	BIOM	9.4; 20.5; 35; 52; 71.5; 75.5; 87		Tonsils	Throat
Hypertrophy of tonsils	BIOM	246; 151; 414		Tonsils	Throat
Tonsillar Pfropfe	CAFL	246,151,414	Also called tonsillar plugs. Actinomyces-like granules in tonsils.	Tonsils	Throat
Tonsillar Pfropfe	VEGA	246	As mentioned above	Tonsils	Throat
Adeno-associated Virus	XTRA	950.6,958.79,959.6,960.39,967.6,969.29,	Used in 'gene therapy.'		Throat
Adenoids	CAFL	1550,802,880,787,776,727,444,20,428,660,2720,2170,1.57,2,14,333,444,588,780,806.5,810,	Also called Naso/Pharyngeal Tonsil.		Throat
Adenoids	BIOM	1550; 802; 880; 787; 776; 727; 444; 20; 428; 660; 2720; 2170			Throat
Adenoiditis	BIOM	522; 572; 3343; 3833; 5311.5; 440; 441			Throat
Adenoids, adenoiditis	BIOM	428; 444; 523; 590; 660; 690; 768; 780; 786; 807; 810; 1550; 1570; 1865; 2000; 2170; 2720			Throat
Hoarseness	CAFL	880,760,727			Throat
Hoarseness	BIOM	13.5; 13.75; 21; 21.5; 100			Throat
Reinke's Edema	EDTFL	190,15000,33000,97500,157700,332410,426900,571000,836000,932000	As mentioned above	Voice	Throat
Vocal Cords	XTRA	12,		Voice	Throat
Vocal chords, irritation	BIOM	24; 94.5		Voice	Throat
Vocal chords, paresis	BIOM	94.5		Voice	Throat
Vocal Cord Disorders General Vocal Cord Paralysis Voice Disorders	EDTFL	50,730,2950,47500,222530,324530,452590,683000,712000,993410	Injury to laryngeal nerves, causing hoarseness, lack of vocal power, and severe shortness of breath.	Voice	Throat
Stammering	CAFL	10000,20,6000,7.83,		Voice	Throat
Stuttering	KHZ	70,530,37510,72560,315270,475270,527400,665760,732000,988100,		Voice	Throat
Angina Throat	CAFL	333,428,465,660,727,776,787,804,806.5,	Quinsy in throat. Also called Peritonsillar Abscess.		Throat

12f - Chest

Subject / Argument	Author	Frequencies	Notes	Origin	Target
Human Chest Cavity	XTRA	14648.1			Chest
Chest Infection Secondary	CAFL	72,333,452,683	Run Streptococcus pneumonia and General Antiseptic sets. See Chemtrail Detox set.		Chest
Chest Pain [Group 13]	EDTFL	70,410,700,970,2750,7500,15310,67500,115700,356720,			Chest
Funnel Chest [Pectus Excavatum]	EDTFL	70,280,650,2500,8000,77500,196500,315700,524940,660410,	Congenital deformity of wall of chest, causing 'caved-in' appearance.		Chest
Pectus Excavatum	EDTFL	70,280,650,2500,8000,77500,196500,315700,524940,660410,	As mentioned above		Chest
Costalgia	CAFL	10000,880,787,727,	Rib-cage pain.		Chest
Costalgia 1	XTRA	727,787,880,5000,10000,	Rib-cage pain.		Chest
Costalgia 2	XTRA	26,160,660,690,727.5,787,802,880,1500,1550,2720,3000,10000,	Rib-cage pain.		Chest
Hernia, Diaphragmatic	EDTFL	20,500,970,7500,22500,42500,125220,275560,322060,326160	Diaphragm defect that allows abdominal organs to move into chest cavity.	Hernia	Chest
Hernia, Esophageal	EDTFL	40,390,620,7500,22500,42500,125220,275560,635310,833200		Hernia	Chest
Hernia, Paraesophageal	EDTFL	150,220,730,7500,22500,42500,125220,275560,819340,915700	Also called Hiatal Hernia - see set. Protrusion of stomach into thorax through diaphragm defect. Also see Hiatal Hernia.	Hernia	Chest
Hernia, Hiatal	EDTFL	20,500,970,7500,118250,287560,367500,605220,800790,965000	Also called Esophageal Hernia. Protrusion of stomach into thorax through diaphragm defect. See Hernia Esophageal, and Hiatal Hernia.	Hernia	Chest
Hiatal Hernia 1	XTRA	128,134,333,411,423,424,436,453,478,542,550,555,563,576,634,639,643,644,647,674,678,686,718,727,728,738,745,784,786,787,824.39,876,878,880,882,884,934,943,958,960,985,999,1010,1050,1060,1089,1109,1902,2431,2600,7160,7270,8697,9646,20443.5,	Also called Esophageal Hernia. Protrusion of stomach into thorax through diaphragm defect. See Hernia Esophageal, and Hernia Hiatal.	Hernia	Chest

Subject / Argument	Author	Frequencies	Notes	Origin	Target
Hiatal Hernia 2	XTRA	727,784,787,800,802,848,875,876,877,878,879, 880=600,881,882,883,884,885,1266,2000,	As mentioned above	Hernia	Chest
Hiatal Hernia 3	XTRA	9.09,110,660,690,727.5,787,10000,	As mentioned above	Hernia	Chest
Costoclavicular Syndrome	EDTFL	130,550,850,7480,121200,315500,472500,7257 50,852000,975930			Chest
Neurovascular Syndrome, Thoracic Outlet	EDTFL	160,570,780,930,2750,7500,22500,40000,12500 0,433770,			Chest
Thoracic Outlet Syndrome	EDTFL	130,520,2610,110390,211110,351020,405850,6 22260,753080,832630	Due to compression of neurovascular bundle passing between two scalene muscles at upper chest/upper limb area. Also try Brachial Neuralgia, Brachial Plexus Neuritis, Hypochondrium, and Nerve Compression Syndromes.		Chest
Thoracic Outlet Nerve Compression Syndrome		30,370,780,900,7500,10720,40000,157500,3925 00,575560,			Chest
Scalenus Anticus Syndrome	EDTFL	40,240,730,7900,67220,127500,317500,665520, 831330,913500	As mentioned above		Chest
Thoracic Surgical Procedures	EDTFL	30,500,870,10470,37150,87500,135230,225680, 397500,597500			Chest

12g - Abdomen

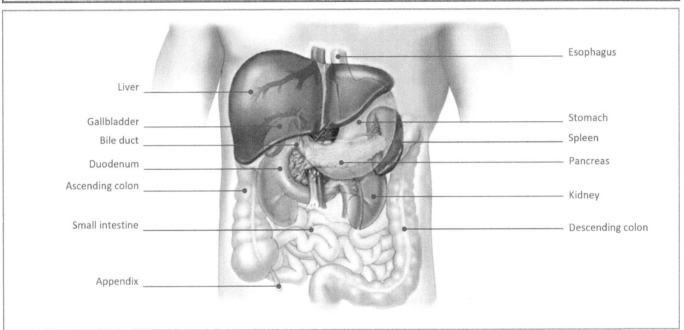

Subject / Argument	Author	Frequencies	Notes	Origin	Target
Solar plexus	BIOM	15			Abdomen
Hypochondrium Upper Abdomen 1	XTRA	20,727,787,880,10000,	Anatomical area of abdomen between bottom of breast and bottom of rib-cage.		Abdomen
Hypochondrium Upper Abdomen 2	XTRA	20,10000	Anatomical area of abdomen between bottom of breast and bottom of rib-cage.		Abdomen
Abdominal Inflammation	CAFL	2720,2489,2170,1865,1800,1600,1550,880,832, 802,787,776,727,660,465,450,444,440,428,380, 146,125,95,72,20,1.2,	Also see Gastroenteritis sets.		Abdomen
Pelvis organs disfunction	BIOM	2720; 2489; 2160; 2127; 2008; 1800; 1600; 1550; 802; 787; 776; 727; 690; 666; 650; 625; 600; 465; 444; 522; 95; 72; 450; 428; 1; 5000			Abdomen
Abdominal Pain	CAFL	10000,3000,95,3,3040,522,440,160,124,26,		Pain	Abdomen
Abdominal Pain	XTRA	5000,10000,	Commonly caused by Gastroenteritis, Irritable Bowel Syndrome, urinary tract problems and stomach inflammation.	Pain	Abdomen
Abdominal Cramps	XTRA	72,95,190,304,	Also see Gastroenteritis and Irritable Bowel Syndrome sets. Can also be caused by Appendicitis or Diverticulitis.	Pain	Abdomen
Cramping and Nausea	CAFL	72,95,190,880,832,787,727,20,4.9,		Pain	Abdomen
Colic			See Section 1 - Various Conditions	Colic	Abdomen
Colic Intestinal	XTRA	8,123,457,		Colic	Abdomen
Colic Stomach and Colon Pain	XTRA	20,727,787,800,880,		Colic	Abdomen
Distended Organs	XTRA	20,727,787,880,10000,	Abdominal bloating.		Abdomen

Subject / Argument	Author	Frequencies	Notes	Origin	Target
Peritoneal commissures		190; 660; 727; 787; 802; 880; 1550; 2170; 2720			Abdomen
Peritoneal cavity inflammation	BIOM	1.2; 20; 72; 95; 125; 146; 250; 380; 440; 450; 465; 727; 776; 787; 832; 880; 1550; 1600; 1800; 1865; 2000; 2170; 2489; 2720			Abdomen
Ascites	EDTFL KHZ	70,520,6230,37500,355080,475090,527000,667 000,789000,987230,	Fluid in peritoneal cavity.	Ascites	Abdomen
Ascites 1	XTRA	70,4160.24920,37500,31907,37605,31000,3916 7,18667,34577,	Fluid in peritoneal cavity.	Ascites	Abdomen
Ascites 2	XTRA	43379.96875,43380.03125,43380,41989.96875, 4190.03125,41990,19009.96875,19010.13125,1 9010,18949.96875,18950.03125,18950,	Fluid in peritoneal cavity. Converted from F165 format - may need Duty Cycle of 55%.	Ascites	Abdomen
Pseudomyxoma Peritonei 1	XTRA	80,4160,10400,35000,21060,35830,20590,3990 7,38400,36800,	Also called Gelatinous Ascites. Caused by cancerous cells (mucinous adenocarcinoma) that produce abundant mucin.		Abdomen
Ascites, Gelatinous	EDTFL	80,520,650,2500,355080,475090,527000,66700 0,789000,987230,			Abdomen
Pseudomyxoma Peritonei	EDTFL	160,170,870,2500,27500,82500,85520,165000,6 92500,825520	Also called Gelatinous Ascites.		Abdomen
Retroperitoneal Fibrosis	EDTFL	50,230,950,13390,121590,285430,325510,4725 00,612500,930000,	Proliferation of fibrous tissue in retroperitoneum, containing kidneys, aorta, renal tract and other structures. May cause lower back pain, kidney failure, hypertension and deep vein thrombosis.		Abdomen
Periaortitis, Chronic	EDTFL	40,520,83620,105950,179500,295540,487500,6 05720,723820,935420			Abdomen
Perianeurysmal Fibrosis, Inflammatory	EDTFL	70,370,950,7500,88000,193230,237500,487500, 706210,946500			Abdomen
Ormond Disease	EDTFL	50,400,920,2500,12710,13980,95470,233910,42 6300,571000			Abdomen
Hernia	EDTFL	180,560,950,7500,22500,42500,125220,275560, 533630,652430	Protrusion of organ through wall of its containing cavity.	Hernia	Abdomen
Hernia General	XTRA	9.09,110,660,690,727.5,787,2720,5000,10000,	Protrusion of organ through wall of its containing cavity.	Hernia	Abdomen
Umbilical Hernia	EDTFL	20,500,970,7500,22500,42500,125220,275560,8 22200,906070,	Congenital (normally resolves by age 3), or acquired (due to obesity, multiple pregnancies, heavy lifting, or a history of coughing).	Hernia	Abdomen
Groin hernia	BIOM	10000; 787; 727		Hernia	Abdomen
Enterocele	EDTFL	20,500,950,2250,12850,15220,90000,322060,32 3700,326160	Herniation of a loop of the small intestine	Hernia	Abdomen
Exomphalos	EDTFL	30,250,780,930,7500,95750,300000,454370,615 190,784810	Is a weakness of the baby's abdominal wall where the umbilical cord joins it.	Genetic Disease	Abdomen
Exomphalos-Beckwith	EDTFL	30,250,780,930,7500,95750,300000,454370,615 190,784810,		Genetic Disease	Abdomen
Omphalocele	EDTFL	170,350,830,7500,15910,47500,87500,392500,4 75520,575290		Genetic Disease	Abdomen
Peritonitis	CAFL	727,787,880,	Inflammation of peritoneum, the thin tissue that lines the inner wall of the abdomen and covers most of the organs.	Appendix	Abdomen
Encopresis	EDTFL	230,950,12870,25050,97500,110250,142540,33 1320,405030,522510	Voluntary or involuntary fecal soiling, usually in children.		Abdomen
Incontinence 1	CAFL	666,690,2050,2128,2250,			Abdomen
Incontinence 2	XTRA	465,660,690,727.5,787,802,880,1550,10000,			Abdomen
Urinary and fecal incontinence	BIOM	2250; 2050; 2128; 690; 666			Abdomen
Adhesions, Pelvic	EDTFL KHZ	20,2500,35160,67500,90000,355080,419340,56 7700,707260,930120,	Internal scar tissue following injury or surgery.		Abdomen
Adhesions	CAFL	2720,2170,1550,802,880,787,776,760,727,190	Internal scar tissue following injury or surgery.		Abdomen

13 - Digestive System

Subject / Argument	Author	Frequencies	Notes	Origin	Target
Eating Disorders	EDTFL	80,500,830,11700,58870,320650,330210,65302 0,822010,971320			Digestive System
Anorexia		*Can be caused by the protozoan Dientamoeba fragilis.*			
Anorexia nervosa		*Can be caused by Borrelia. In rare cases it may arise after infection with bacteria Streptococcus.*			
Bulimia nervosa		80,500,830,11700,58870,320650,330210,65302 0,822010,971320,			Bulimia
Anorexia Nervosa		80,500,830,11700,58870,320650,330210,65302 0,822010,971320,			Anorexia
Appetite Lack Of	CAFL	20,72,444,465,727,787,880,1865,10000,	Appetite stimulant.		Appetite
Appetite absence	BIOM	31			Appetite
Appetite regulation	BIOM	20; 35; 72; 94.5; 125; 444; 465; 727; 787; 880; 1865; 10000			Appetite
Obesity & eating disorders	EDTFL	180,320,800,5500,27900,45560,172500,392500, 553200,675290			Adiposity

Subject / Argument	Author	Frequencies	Notes	Origin	Target
Adiposity	BIOM	25.5; 26; 26.5; 34.5; 38; 38.5; 46; 60.5; 62; 63; 64.5; 67; 69; 75; 79; 79.5; 81; 85; 86.5; 95; 98			Adiposity
Adiposity basic	BIOM	0.7; 0.9; 1.2; 1.6; 1.7; 2.5; 2.6; 3.3; 4; 4.9; 6; 7; 8.1; 9.19; 9.4; 9.8; 11.5; 20; 23.5; 25.5; 26; 53; 98			Adiposity
Fat Obesity 1	XTRA	465,10000	Obesity is associated with Adenovirus 36.		Adiposity
Fat Obesity 2	XTRA	124,333,523,666,768,786,950,6,958.79,959,959.6,960.39,962,967.6,969.29,			Adiposity
Gastrointestinal tract	BIOM	25; 27.5; 30; 94			Digestive S.
Digestive tract	BIOM	0.9; 2.5; 2.6; 3.3; 6; 8.5; 9.8; 56; 56.25			Digestive S.
GIT regulation	BIOM	3.5; 3.8; 8.1; 8.6; 9.4; 10; 11.5			Digestive S.
Digestion center	BIOM	25			Digestive S.
Digestive tract regulation	BIOM	3.5; 3.8; 8.1; 9.4; 25; 59; 74; 95.5			Digestive S.
Digestive Disorders	BIOM	25.0			Digestive S.
Digestion	XTRA	727,787,880,5000			Digestive S.
Digestive System Diseases	EDTFL	260,550,850,2500,5500,27200,37500,123010,327230,533690	Stomach and intestines.		Digestive S.

13a - Mouth

Subject / Argument	Author	Frequencies	Notes	Origin	Target
Mouth	XTRA	8.22			Mouth
Eruptions Mouth	XTRA	5000			Mouth
Dental product intolerance	BIOM	522; 146; 10000; 125; 95; 72; 20; 4.9; 428; 1550; 802; 10000; 880; 787; 727; 465; 444; 20; 125; 95; 72			Mouth
Mouth Ulcer	XTRA	131		Stomatitis	Mouth
Oral Lesions	CAFL	2720,2489,2008,1800,1600,1550,802,880,787,727,465,444,522,146,	Chronic cases will always recur until metal dentalwork is replaced with uranium-free porcelain. See Herpes Simplex i, and use Stomatitis sets.	Stomatitis	Mouth
Stomatitis	CAFL	465,677,702,787,234,278,568,672,	Inflammation of mouth and lips. See Candida, Herpes Simplex i, Stomatitis Aphthous, Pyorrhea, and Gingivitis sets.	Stomatitis	Mouth
Stomatitis Aphthous - Canker	CAFL	478,487,498,788,955,982,	Also called Canker Sores - see sets. Repeated formation of benign and non-contagious mouth ulcers in otherwise healthy people. Also see Cancrum Oris sets.	Stomatitis	Mouth
Stomatitis	BIOM	10000; 5000; 880; 787; 727; 702; 677; 672; 568; 465; 278; 234; 20		Stomatitis	Mouth
Aphthous stomatitis, complex	BIOM	246; 322; 339; 343; 423; 424; 460; 465; 478; 480; 487; 498; 534; 556; 591; 685; 734; 742; 782; 788; 808; 831; 846; 848; 888; 944; 955; 982; 1043; 1901; 1902; 1903; 1904; 1905; 1906; 1907		Stomatitis	Mouth
Aphthae	EDTFL	50,410,920,5170,42500,119340,357100,527000,662710,789000,	As mentioned above	Stomatitis	Mouth
Aphtha	BIOM	880; 787; 727; 591; 465		Stomatitis	Mouth
Canker Sore	EDTFL	140,890,3220,15300,34190,72200,95000,150000,209600,434170	As mentioned above	Stomatitis	Mouth
Stomatitis, Aphthous [Mouth Ulcer]	EDTFL	150,240,650,830,2500,127500,265750,425710,745190,935700,	As mentioned above	Stomatitis	Mouth
Ulcer, Aphthous	EDTFL	150,240,650,830,2500,127500,265750,425710,745190,935700	As mentioned above	Stomatitis	Mouth
Periadenitis Mucosa Necrotica Recurrens	EDTF	190,570,1120,7900,27500,42600,96500,325430,415700,562910	As mentioned above	Stomatitis	Mouth
Stomatitis Aphthous 1	CAFL	1901,1902,1903,1904,1905,1906,1907,	As mentioned above	Stomatitis	Mouth
Stomatitis Aphthous V	CAFL	888,880,848,846,831,685,742,734,1043,944,782,591,480,423,343,339,322,832,556,808,534,460,424,246,	As mentioned above	Stomatitis	Mouth
Canker Sore 1	XTRA	246,322,339,342	Also see Stomatitis Aphthous. Painful recurrent benign mouth ulcers.	Stomatitis	Mouth
Canker Sore 2	XTRA	1901,1902,1903,1904,1905,1906,1907,	As mentioned above	Stomatitis	Mouth
Canker Sore 3	XTRA	234,278,465,568,672,677,702,787,	As mentioned above	Stomatitis	Mouth
Canker Sore 4	XTRA	478,487,498,788,955,982,1902,1904,1906,	As mentioned above	Stomatitis	Mouth
Burning Mouth Syndrome	EDTFL	260,650,5120,7000,42500,200000,458500,515150,683000,712420	Oral burning sensation with no medically identifiable cause.		Mouth
Glossitis, Benign Migratory	EDTFL	30,570,9000,12850,45000,92500,175750,450000,515160,689410	Inflammation of mucous membrane of tongue which moves over time.		Mouth
Glossitis Areata Exfoliativa	EDTFL	30,570,9000,12850,45000,92500,357530,651200,732590,973520	As mentioned above		Mouth
Oral mucosa, inflammation	BIOM	2720; 2489; 2008; 1800; 1600; 1550; 802; 880; 787; 727; 465; 444; 522; 146; 75.5			Mouth
Geographic Tongue	EDTFL	70,240,570,87500,175160,317350,322060,667000,742000,985670	As mentioned above	Tongue	Mouth

Subject / Argument	Author	Frequencies	Notes	Origin	Target
Tongue numbness	BIOM	87.5		Tongue	Mouth
Glossolysis	BIOM	91		Tongue	Mouth
Tongue ulcer	BIOM	2489; 2160; 2127; 1800; 1600; 880; 832; 802; 787; 727; 73		Tongue	Mouth
Alveolitis	BIOM	3000; 2720; 95; 47.5; 7.82			Mouth
Halitosis 1	CAFL	1550,802,880,787,727,20,	Bad breath. See Streptococcus Pneumonia, Streptococcus Aureus, Pharyngitis, Dental, Parasites General, and General Antiseptic sets.	Halitosis	Mouth
Halitosis (offensive breath)	BIOM	1550; 802; 880; 787; 727; 20		Halitosis	Mouth
Halitosis 2	XTRA	20,660,690,727.5,787,802,880,1550,	As mentioned above	Halitosis	Mouth
Halitosis	EDTFL	50,370,830,2500,3000,73300,95750,175000,269 710,336410	As mentioned above	Halitosis	Mouth
Halitosis	XTRA	1550	As mentioned above	Halitosis	Mouth
Bad Breath	CAFL	20,727,787,802,880,1550,	As mentioned above	Halitosis	Mouth
Mouth Eruptions White Patches	CAFL	465,666,690,727,2008,2127,	See Leukoplakia, Mucous Membrane general inflammation, EBV, BX virus, Papilloma, Cancer BX virus, and Carcinoma sets.	Virus	Mouth
Leukoplakia	CAFL	465,2127,2008,727,690,666,	White patches on mucous membranes. See EBV, Mouth Eruptions White Patches, Papilloma, and Cancer Carcinoma sets.		Mouth
Leukoplakia	BIOM	465; 2127; 2008; 727; 690; 666			Mouth
Macroglossia	EDTFL	130,350,870,7160,25000,35670,87500,93500,23 4510,519340	Enlargement of tongue, usually in children.		Mouth
Ranula	EDTFL	120,460,1560,5950,17500,127500,321750,4657 50,696500,819340	Swelling of connective tissue on floor of mouth composed of mucin (mucocele) from ruptured salivary gland.		Mouth
Stomatognathic Diseases	EDTFL	130,950,5780,12710,45000,125170,327550,479 930,743000,986220	Disorders of the mouth and jaws.		Mouth
Dental / Jaw Cavitations	EDTFL	60,200,650,5710,7000,42500,92500,478500,527 000,667000,	As mentioned above		Mouth
Upper Lip	XTRA	9.19		Lips	Mouth
Cheilitis	EDTFL	120,900,1220,17250,63210,119420,287200,403 030,435000,711170	Inflammation of lip - includes cracking, fissures, peeling, and chapping.	Lips	Mouth
Cheilitis Granulomatosa, Facial Neuropathy	EDTFL	120,900,1220,17250,125000,350000,425000,57 1000,828000,932000	Rare neurological disorder with recurring facial paralysis, swelling of face and lips, and folds and furrows in tongue.	Lips	Mouth
Granulomatous Cheilitis	EDTFL	20,120,950,13390,22500,370500,547500,65640 0,725370,825520		Lips	Mouth
Melkersson-Rosenthal [neurological]	EDTFL	90,320,950,3110,25000,45000,95000,100500,21 5790,414000,	Rare neurological disorder characterized by recurrent facial paralysis, swelling of the face and lips, and the development of folds and furrows in the tongue (fissured tongue).	Lips	Mouth
Mouth Eruptions Herpes Sores	CAFL	304,464,1488,1489,1550,1577,1900,2720,2950,	See Herpes General, and Herpes Simplex i sets.	Virus	Mouth
Cold Sores	CAFL	322,476,589,664,785,822,895,944,1043,1614,20 62,2950,	See Herpes simplex set (Section 17d - Virus).	Lips	Mouth
Cold Sores 2	XTRA	428,465,727,787,880,1500,1550,1800,1850,248 9,		Lips	Mouth
Cold Sores 3	XTRA	470,647,648,650,652,654,656,658,660,847,5641 ,8650,		Lips	Mouth
Cold Sores 5	XTRA	723.79,856.4,14537.81,17201.43,		Lips	Mouth
Cold Sore [Herpes Simplex]	EDTFL	40,300,620,51250,117250,245560,367500,6252 20,816720,905000,		Lips	Mouth
Herpes Labialis	EDTFL	40,300,620,51250,117250,245560,367500,6252 20,816720,905000		Lips	Mouth
Bulla	EDTFL	50,260,980,2500,12850,35330,57500,96500,322 060,475870	Fluid-filled blister.	Lips	Mouth
Vesication	EDTFL	190,350,17900,37100,210500,307050,476600,6 65340,789000,987230		Lips	Mouth
Fever Blister	EDTFL	70,220,620,2200,5500,42000,475030,527000,66 7000,742000		Lips	Mouth
Salivary gland	BIOM	8; 29.5		Saliva	Mouth
Salivary Gland Diseases Salivary Gland Virus Disease	EDTFL	80,240,570,6500,10720,36210,142500,321000,4 15700,775680		Saliva	Mouth
Salivary Gland Virus	BIO	126,597,1045,2145	Causes Infectious Mononucleosis (see sets), and retinitis. Also see Cytomegalovirus, CMV, Herpes Type 5, and HHV5 sets.	Saliva	Mouth
Sialorrhea [hypersalivation]	EDTFL	80,240,570,6500,10720,36210,142500,321000,4 15700,775680,	Excessive production of saliva. Can be caused by radiation, antipsychotics and other drugs, toxic metals, and pesticides.	Saliva	Mouth
Hypersalivation	EDTFL	80,240,570,6500,10720,36210,142500,321000,4 15700,775680,	As mentioned above	Saliva	Mouth
Hyposalivation	EDTFL	80,240,570,6500,10720,36210,142500,321000,4 15700,775680,	Dry mouth which may be due to changes in saliva composition or production. Commonly caused by drugs.	Saliva	Mouth
Mouth Dryness [Xerostomia]	EDTFL	190,520,5890,81200,127580,241520,471200,62 5300,853000,915090,	As mentioned above	Saliva	Mouth

Subject / Argument	Author	Frequencies	Notes	Origin	Target
Asialia	EDTFL	120,5810,25000,87500,228000,458500,522390, 683000,712230,992000,	As mentioned above	Saliva	Mouth
Xerostomia	EDTFL	190,520,5890,81200,127580,241520,471200,625300,853000,915090	As mentioned above	Saliva	Mouth
Taste	XTRA	10.3		Taste	Mouth
Taste Disorders	EDTFL	120,410,7900,17600,87500,95740,327050,476500,527000,662710	Dysgeusia/parageusia. Commonly caused by chemotherapy, administration of albuterol for asthma, and zinc deficiency.	Taste	Mouth
Taste Lack Of	CAFL	10000,20	Ageusia. Inability to detect sweetness, sourness, saltiness, bitterness, and savoriness. Causes, include radiation therapy, many different drugs, and vitamin B3 and zinc deficiency. See appropriate sets.	Taste	Mouth
Upper and lower jaw - Pilot frequencies	BIOM	20; 20.5; 83.5			Jaw
Jaw, inflammation	BIOM	1550; 880; 802; 787; 760; 20; 727; 10000; 465			Jaw
Jaw, festering	BIOM	36.5; 39; 74; 93.5			Jaw
Jaw Diseases	EDTFL	180,780,850,7500,13610,27500,95620,375670,523010,682020			Jaw
Prognathism	EDTFL	90,230,1950,8850,44160,72410,125210,433500,541500,621630	Protruding lower jaw, considered a disorder only if it affects chewing, speech, or social function.		Jaw
Lockjaw	CAFL	120,244,352,363,458,465,554,600,628,1142,	Due to wound infection with Clostridium Tetani - see set. Also see Tetanus sets.		Jaw
Lockjaw 2	XTRA	120,244,352,363,458,465,554,600,625,628,650, 660,690,727.5,787,880,1142,14625,	See Tetanus.		Jaw
Lockjaw Tetanus Secondary	XTRA	727,787,880,	See Tetanus.		Jaw
Lockjaw Tetanus	XTRA	20,120,234,244,352,363,400,458,465,554,600,628,700,880,1142,1200,15770,	See Tetanus.		Jaw
Ludwig's Angina	EDTFL	20,2500,60000,85000,220330,478500,526200,665300,741300,985630	Potentially life-threatening cellulitis of floor of mouth, almost always caused by untreated dental infection.		Jaw
Temporomandibular Joint Disorders	EDTFL	80,320,20000,85030,150000,219340,307250,453720,515150,683000	Pain and dysfunction of jaw muscles and joint, with restricted movement and noises.		Jaw
TMJ Disorders [Temporomandibular]	EDTFL	80,320,20000,85030,150000,219340,307250,453720,515150,683000,	As mentioned above		Jaw

13b - Gums

Subject / Argument	Author	Frequencies	Notes	Origin	Target
Gum Disease	CAFL	20,146,444,465,522,726,727,728,776,787,802,880,1550,1556,1600,1800,2008,2489,2720,	See Gingivitis, Pyorrhea, and Stomatitis sets.		Gums
Gum Disease 2	XTRA	20,465,726,728,776,787,802,880,1550,1556,			Gums
Gum Infection	XTRA	20,146,444,465,522,660,690,726,727.5,776,787, 802,880,1550,1556,1600,1800,1865,2008,2489, 2720,	Can be caused by MRSA, an antibiotic-resistant Staphylococcus infection.		Gums
Gingiva, inflammation	BIOM	95.5; 96			Gums
Gum Inflammation 1	XTRA	20,465,727,787,800,880,5000,			Gums
Gum Inflammation 2	XTRA	20,465,727,787,802,880,1550,			Gums
Gingivitis	CAFL	1550,880,802,787,728,726,465,20,1556,776,465,	Inflammation of gums caused by plaque leading to periodontitis. See Dental Infection, Dental Infection Roots and Gums, Pyorrhea, and Stomatitis.		Gums
Gingivitis [Group 5]	EDTFL	60,200,830,2750,3000,15000,85540,175000,225000,575830,	As mentioned above		Gums
Gingivitis 1	XTRA	20,146,444,465,522,660,690,726,727.5,776,787, 802,880,1550,1556,1600,1800,1865,2008,2489, 2720,	As mentioned above		Gums
Gingivitis - stomatitis	BIOM	222; 233; 254.2; 465; 685; 726; 728; 774; 1550; 1556			Gums
Trench Mouth	CAFL	20,465,726,728,776,787,802,880,1550,1556,	Ulcerative gingivitis Use Gingivitis set.		Gums
Pyorrhea	CAFL	2720,2489,2008,1800,1600,1550,802,880,787,776,727,465,444,522,146,	Infection of periodontium causing inflammation of gums and bone loss. Although it may be controlled or eliminated with treatment, infection always returns whenever subject experiences stress or poor diet until dental mercury is removed. Also see Gingivitis.	Pyorrhea	Gums
Pyorrhea	XTRA	444	As mentioned above	Pyorrhea	Gums
Pyorrhea Alveolaris [chronic periodontitis]	EDTFL	80,350,750,12930,50590,197500,482210,762200,891510,923790,		Pyorrhea	Gums
Pulpitis	BIOM	960; 660; 666; 690; 727; 784; 787; 800; 880; 1560; 1840; 1998; 2489			Gums

The most common bacteria concerning dental infections are:
Streptococcus mutans , the main organism causing dental caries
Streptococcus sanguinis , represents 50% of dental plaque streptococci
Streptococcus salivarius , represents 50% of streptocycchi contained in saliva
Streptococcus milleri , implicated in the formation of dental abscesses
Lactobacillus, secondary colonizer in caries, mainly affects dentin
Porphyrius monas gingivalis is associated with rapidly progressive periodontitis
Porphyromonas endodontalis appears to be specifically related to endodontic infections.
Infections can also be caused by: Actinobacillus actinomycetem-comitans, Porphyromonas gingivalis, Prevotella intermedia, Bacteroides forsythus,
Campylobacter rectus, Eubacterium species, Fusobacterium nucleatum, Eikenella corrodens and Pepto-streptococcus micros.

Subject / Argument	Author	Frequencies	Notes	Origin	Target
Teeth	BIOM	3.6; 4.9; 9.5			Teeth
Wisdom tooth	BIOM	93.5			Teeth
Dental	BIO	635,640,1036,1043,1094,			Teeth
Dental Diseases	EDTFL	60,200,830,2750,3000,15000,85540,175000,225000,575830,			Teeth
Dental 1	XTRA	48,60,465,635,640,685,1036,1043,1094,			Teeth
Dental 2	XTRA	47,48,60,95,146,190,333,465,470.5,518,521,522,523,547,555,600,			Teeth
Dental General	CAFL	728,784,635,640,1036,1043,1094,685,60,48,465,	Also see Toothache.		Teeth
Dental General	XTRA	1043			Teeth
Dental Comprehensive, Oral Health, includes Periodontal Disease	EDTFL	60,200,830,2750,3000,15000,85540,175000,225000,575830,			Teeth
Dental Abscess	XTRA	190,428,444,450,465,500,660,690,727.5,760,787,802,880,1550,1865,2170,2720,		Abscess	Teeth
Exposed Dental Nerve	XTRA	47.5,47-48			Teeth
Dental Foci	CAFL	5170,3000,2720,2489,1800,1600,1550,1500,880,832,802,787,776,727,666,650,646,600,465,190,95,47.5,	Neglecting this can prevent recovery from any illness if infection is a problem.		Teeth
Dental Foci 1	XTRA	47.5,95,190,465,600,646,650,666,727,776,787,802,832,880,1500,1550,1600,1800,2489,2720,3000,5170,	Addresses multiple dental issues. Use if infection recovery is slow.		Teeth
Dental Foci 2	XTRA	47.5,95,190,465,600,650,666,727,776,787,802,832,880,1500,1600,1800,2489,2720,3000,			Teeth
Caries	BIOM	10000; 3040; 2720; 1550; 880; 802; 787; 776; 727; 650; 600; 465; 100; 95; 87; 59; 57; 48; 20		Caries	Teeth
Root of tooth, inflammation	BIOM	30.5			Teeth
Incisive teeth, inflammation	BIOM	93			Teeth
Teeth, inflammatory tissues	BIOM	3040; 95; 190; 47.5; 2720; 2489; 1800; 1600; 1550; 802; 1500; 880; 10000; 2489; 787; 776; 727; 666; 650; 646; 600; 465			Teeth
Dental infections, complex	BIOM	64; 138; 148; 177; 183; 210; 534; 620; 626; 660; 723; 784; 799; 835; 960; 981; 1036; 1043; 1094; 1552; 1560; 1562; 1700; 1840; 1998; 3000; 3400; 5227; 7059; 7270		Infection	Teeth
Toothache, complex	BIOM	5170; 3040; 3000; 2720; 2489; 1800; 1600; 1550; 1500; 1093.9; 1043; 1036; 880; 832; 802; 787; 784; 776; 728; 727; 685; 666; 650; 646; 640; 635; 600; 465; 190; 95; 60; 47.5; 48; 8		Infection	Teeth
Dentofacial infections	BIOM	500		Infection	Teeth
Dental Infection	CAFL	960,660,666,690,727,784,787,800,880,1560,1840,1998,2489,	Roots and gums.	Infection	Teeth
Dental Infection	XTRA	190		Infection	Teeth
Dental Infection 1	CAFL	5170,3000,2720,2489,1800,1600,1550,1500,1094,1043,1036,880,832,802,787,776,727,685,666,650,646,640,635,600,465,190,95,60,48,47.5,		Infection	Teeth
Dental Infection 2	CAFL	20,254.2,464,620,664,727,728,774,776,784,787,799,800,880,1550,1552,1562,5000,10000,		Infection	Teeth
Dental Infection 3	XTRA	138,142,177,183,210,222,233,436,534,626,723,835,875,981,5227,7059,		Infection	Teeth
Dental Infection 4	XTRA	1560,1700,2489,3400,		Infection	Teeth
Dental and Jawbone Infections 1	XTRA	190,500,727,728,787,880,2170,2720,7270,		Infection	Teeth

Subject / Argument	Author	Frequencies	Notes	Origin	Target
Dental and Jawbone Infections 2	XTRA	15,326,465,727,787,880,		Infection	Teeth
Dental Infection and Earache	XTRA	518,521,547,622.29,635,640,646,646.29,650,66 6,680,685,727,750,760,768,775,776,787,800,80 2,832,880,900,930,960,		Infection	Teeth
Dental Infection and Earache 1	CAFL	518,521,547,622,635,640,646,646.3,650,666,68 0,685,727,750,760,768,775,776,787,800,802,90 0,930,960,		Infection	Teeth
Dental Infection Roots and Gums	XTRA	660,666,690,727,784,787,800,880,960,1560,184 0,1998,2489,		Infection	Teeth
Dental Infections Virus	CAFL	138,142,177,183,210,222,233,436,534,626,723, 835,875,981,5227,7057,		Infection	Teeth
Dental Bacteria	EDTFL	70,200,750,930,12850,22500,57500,672500,803 500,935310,		Infection	Teeth
Root Canal (Bacteria treatment)	EDTFL	70,520,7570,33800,282750,405750,523880,667 500,825280,915700		Infection	Teeth
Porphyromonas gingivalis	RL	867	From Dr. Richard Loyd. Common dental bacteria.	Infection	Teeth
Dental Ulcers	CAFL	727,776,787,880			Teeth
Dentigerous Cyst	EDTFL	130,200,730,830,18270,20000,85000,95310,122 530,150000,	Associated with the crown of an unerupted (or partially erupted) tooth.		Teeth
Fistula Dentalis	BIO	550,727,844,1122	Abnormal passage from the apical periodontal area of a tooth to the surface of the oral mucous membrane.		Teeth
Dental fistula	BIOM	1112; 880; 878; 844; 832; 787; 727; 550			Teeth
Fistula Dentalis	CAFL	550,844,786,727,878,1122,			Teeth
Fistula Dentalis 1	XTRA	550,660,690,727.5,844,878,1122,			Teeth
Tooth Extraction Follow Up	CAFL	7.82,47.5,95,2720,3000,	See General antiseptic set.		Teeth
Toothache	CAFL	3000,95,190,47.5,2720,2489,1800,1600,1550,80 2,1500,880,832,787,776,727,666,650,600,465,6 46,5170,	Neglecting this can prevent recovery from any illness. Should also be treated professionally, preferably a holistic dentist. Also see Gingivitis, and Pyorrhea sets.	Pain	Teeth
Toothache	XTRA	1550,		Pain	Teeth
Tooth ache	BIOM	7.8; 31; 47.5; 79.5; 95		Pain	Teeth
Toothache with ear ache	BIOM	518; 521; 547; 622.3; 635; 640; 646; 646.3; 768; 900; 930; 960; 7059		Pain	Teeth
Toothache - cold/hot	BIOM	31		Pain	Teeth
Toothache, pressing	BIOM	79.5		Pain	Teeth
Teeth, residual pain (in tissue)	BIOM	3040; 95; 47.5; 7.8		Pain	Teeth
Granuloma Dent	CAFL	441	Dental lesion which can occur in root canals - also try Granuloma.		Teeth
Granular periodontal tissue (dental granuloma)	BIOM	328; 441			Teeth
Paradontosis	BIO	424,1552	Also called periodontitis - see Bone Regeneration.		Teeth
Paradontosis	VEGA	1552	As mentioned above		Teeth
Paradontosis	BIOM	2720; 2489; 2008; 1800; 1600; 1550; 1552; 1461.7; 880; 802; 787; 776; 727; 522; 465; 444; 424; 146			Teeth
Parodontosis [Periodontosis/Periodontal]	EDTFL	80,350,750,12930,50590,197500,482210,76220 0,891510,923790,	As mentioned above		Teeth
Periodontitis	BIOM	2720; 2489; 2008; 1800; 1600; 1550; 802; 880; 787; 776; 727; 465; 444; 522; 146			Teeth
Periodontal Diseases	EDTFL	80,350,750,12930,50590,197500,482210,76220 0,891510,923790			Teeth
Periodontal Disease	CAFL	47.5,1800,1600,650,625,600,880,787,776,727,	See Paradontosis, Bone Regeneration, and Dental sets.		Teeth
Periodontal Disease	XTRA	1800	As mentioned above		Teeth
Pental periostitis	BIOM	2.65; 47.5; 1800; 1600; 650; 625; 600; 880; 787; 776; 727			Teeth
Endodontics	EDTFL	140,180,870,15830,23210,212530,247580,4653 50,695020,792510	Treatment of dental pulp, especially by root canals.		Teeth
Hutchinson's Teeth [Congenital syphilis]	EDTFL	320,600,6000,32500,67500,97500,325750,3743 00,586220,748600,	Malformation of the upper median incisors. Outcome in adult life of a congenital syphilis.		Teeth
Prosthodontics	EDTFL	130,570,830,2250,97500,325710,434140,52700 0,667000,742000	Dental prostheses.		Teeth
Bruxism	EDTFL	40,230,950,7500,10890,55150,376290,534250,6 55200,904100	Grinding of teeth.		Teeth
Teeth Grinding Disorder [Bruxism] (2023	EDTFL	40,230,950,7500,10890,55150,376290,534250,6 55200,904100,			Teeth

Subject / Argument	Author	Frequencies	Notes	Origin	Target

Subject / Argument	Author	Frequencies	Notes	Origin	Target
Esophagus	BIOM	57.5			Esophagus
Esophagus cartilages	BIOM	30.5			Esophagus
Esophageal Diseases	EDTFL	180,340,2330,17500,45750,375170,475000,527000,662710,723010			Esophagus
Dysphagia	EDTFL	510,800,980,37500,175300,275000,379930,450000,519610,883000	Conditions that interfere with swallowing.		Esophagus
Swallowing Disorders	EDTFL	510,800,980,37500,175300,275000,379930,450000,519610,883000	As mentioned above		Esophagus
Deglutition Disorders	EDTFL	510,800,980,37500,175300,275000,379930,450000,519610,883000	As mentioned above		Esophagus
Esophageal Achalasia	EDTFL	180,340,2330,17500,45750,375170,475000,527000,822060,925930	Muscle relaxation failure causing problems swallowing food.		Esophagus
Megaesophagus	EDTFL	30,500,930,10720,38100,47500,155650,297500,334250,757770	As mentioned above		Esophagus
Cardiospasm	EDTFL	120,7500,67500,92500,377910,453720,515160,688290,712000,993410			Esophagus
Esophageal Atresia	EDTFL	180,340,2330,17500,45750,375170,475000,527000,725470,925370	Birth defect where the esophagus fails to properly connect to the stomach.		Esophagus
Esophagitis Constriction	XTRA	660,690,727.5,787,880,	Inflammation of the esophagus, making swallowing food difficult.		Esophagus
Esophagitis	EDTFL	80,410,2830,15250,17300,356000,393000,425000,610500,826070	As mentioned above		Esophagus
Esophagitis	XTRA	727,787,880	As mentioned above		Esophagus
Hernia Esophageal	XTRA	40,300,620,51250,117250,245560,367500,625220,816720,905000,	Also called Hiatal Hernia - see set. Protrusion of stomach into thorax through diaphragm defect. Also see Hiatal Hernia.	Hernia	Esophagus
Hernia, Esophageal	EDTFL	40,390,620,7500,22500,42500,125220,275560,635310,833200	As mentioned above	Hernia	Esophagus
Hernia, Paraesophageal	EDTFL	150,220,730,7500,22500,42500,125220,275560,819340,915700	As mentioned above	Hernia	Esophagus
Esophageal Reflux	EDTFL	120,200,900,2250,17500,47500,135370,385940,591000,722530,		Reflux	Esophagus
Gastroesophageal Reflux	EDTFL	120,200,900,47500,2250,17500,135370,385940,591000,722530	Also called GERD. Esophageal damage caused by stomach acid.	Reflux	Esophagus
Regurgitation, Gastric	EDTFL	40,410,2620,4900,9230,23540,87530,442060,535350,634430		Reflux	Esophagus
Reflux; Barrett esophagus	BIOM	2127.5		Reflux	Esophagus
Barrett's Esophagus 1	XTRA	20,146,676,727,776,787,802,880,2127.5=360,10000,	Abnormal cell change of lower esophagus caused by chronic acid exposure.		Esophagus
Esophagus, Barrett [Acid Reflux]	EDTFL	120,200,900,2250,17500,47500,135370,385940,591000,722530,			Esophagus
Esophagotracheal Fistula	EDTFL	180,240,10530,27500,35000,57500,96500,325110,475160,527000,			Esophagus
Zenker Diverticulum	EDTFL	150,5500,12850,35160,93500,269710,426700,571000,822000,937410,			Esophagus
Pharyngoesophageal Diverticulum	EDTFL	150,5500,12850,35160,93500,269710,426700,571000,822000,937410,	Diverticulum (or pouch) in pharynx just above esophageal sphincter, causing swallowing difficulties, cough, and halitosis.		Esophagus

Subject / Argument	Author	Frequencies	Notes	Origin	Target
Gastroenteritis Calicivirus	XTRA	30,475,575,2750,5250,6250,9750=360,1500,362.5,	Also called Norwalk Virus or Winter Vomiting Virus.		Digestive S.
Gastroenteritis	EDTFL	120,200,900,47500,110250,322540,332410,684810,712230,992000	Inflammation of GI tract involving stomach and small intestine. Drink lots of fluids and replace salts.		Digestive S.
Gastroduodenitis	BIOM	20; 72; 95; 125; 150; 444; 465; 685; 727; 787; 802; 832; 880; 1500; 1600; 1800; 1865; 2127; 2160; 2720			Digestive S.
Gastrointestinal Disease	EDTFL	120,200,900,14280,17500,47500,237500,517500,696500,816500,			Digestive S.
Gastric Stomach and Colon	XTRA	20,727,787,880,5000,			Digestive S.
Gastrointestinal Hemorrhage	EDTFL	30,230,7500,12690,32500,67300,86230,93500,175000,526070,			Digestive S.
Hematochezia	EDTFL	150,240,700,870,2500,17500,432500,555910,625290,775520			Digestive S.
Melena [Gastrointestinal Bleeding]	EDTFL	120,200,900,43390,47500,105670,232400,342520,625350,975540,			Digestive S.
Gastroparesis	EDTFL	120,200,900,15670,47500,115900,434500,540000,670000,790000,	Delayed emptying of stomach into small intestine, usually due to vagus nerve damage.		Digestive S.
Gastroschisis	EDTFL	120,200,900,2500,5250,47500,142500,292500,326250,821060,	Congenital defect with opening in abdominal wall through which organs may protrude.		Digestive S.
Stomach	XTRA	5.14,10,			Stomach

Subject / Argument	Author	Frequencies	Notes	Origin	Target
Stomach, mid area	BIOM	55.5; 59; 59.75; 75			Stomach
Sphincter muscle of stomach	BIOM	74.5			Stomach
Stomach, pylorus	BIOM	58.25; 73			Stomach
Hiccups	CAFL	20,10000	Also spelled hiccoughs.		Stomach
Hiccups	BIOM	10.5; 10.55; 10000			Stomach
Enzyme defect	BIOM	10; 210; 250			Stomach
Stomach, enzymes	BIOM	80.5			Stomach
Stomach Disorders	CAFL	2127,2008,880,784,727,690,676,664,125,95,72, 20,3.9,450,802,1552,832,422,	Use appropriate E coli set, and Parasites general set if no lasting relief.		Stomach
Nausea	EDTFL	70,350,700,46000,78250,114690,323000,63708 0,845870,973500		Nausea	Stomach
Nausea	XTRA	396000		Nausea	Stomach
Nausea and Cramping	CAFL	72,95,190,880,832,787,727,20,4.9,	See Parasites Enterobiasis, Roundworm, Round Worms, and Roundworm General.	Nausea	Stomach
Motion Sickness	CAFL	10000,5000,648,624,600,465,440,648,444,1865, 522,190,146,125,95,72,20,	See Nausea and Cramping, Parasites Enterobiasis, Roundworm, Round Worms, and Parasites Roundworm General sets.	Sickness	Stomach
Motion sickness	BIOM	650; 625; 600; 465; 1865; 522; 146; 125; 95; 72; 20		Sickness	Stomach
Motion Sickness [Nausea]	EDTFL	70,350,700,46000,78250,114690,323000,63708 0,845870,973500,		Sickness	Stomach
Morning Sickness [Pregnancy Nausea]	EDTFL	70,350,700,46000,78250,114690,323000,63708 0,845870,973500,		Sickness	Stomach
Airsickness Altitude Sickness	EDTFL	90,10570,30420,88320,109500,257680,344200, 346260,572000,792330,	A sensation which is induced by air travel and altitudes.	Sickness	Stomach
Altitude Sickness	EDTFL	90,10570,30420,88310,109500,257680,344600, 346270,572000,792330,		Sickness	Stomach
Seasickness	EDTFL	30,1830,3230,11860,82360,95300,155260,3251 40,423200,760020		Sickness	Stomach
Mal de Debarquement [Seasickness]	EDTFL	30,1830,3230,11860,82360,95300,155260,3251 40,423200,760020,		Sickness	Stomach
Mal de Debarquement	XTRA	150,230,680,830,72520,137570,292610,537300, 822590,921050,	Also called Disembarkation Syndrome. Neurological condition with prolonged motion sickness and distress after travel.	Sickness	Stomach
Dyspepsia	EDTF	190,300,800,7200,27500,45580,96500,315700,4 19340,562960	See Indigestion, Acidosis, Heartburn, and Hernia. If chronic or with bloating, use appropriate Parasites General set(s).		Stomach
Dyspepsia	CAFL	10000,880,1550,832,800,787,727,465,444,20,12 5,95,72,4.9,	As mentioned above		Stomach
Dyspepsia	BIOM	1550; 880; 802; 800; 787; 727; 672; 444			Stomach
Dyspepsia 1	XTRA	727,787,802,880,1550,	As mentioned above		Stomach
Indigestion	CAFL	4.9,20,72,95,125,4444,465,727,787,880,10000	See Dyspepsia, Acidosis, Heartburn, and Hernia. If chronic or with bloating, use appropriate Parasites General set(s).		Stomach
Indigestion	BIOM	25			Stomach
Indigestion 1	XTRA	4.9,7.83,20,72,95,125,444,465,660,690,727.5,78 7,802,880,1550,1865,10000,	As mentioned above		Stomach
Indigestion 3	XTRA	4.9,20,72,95,125,444,465,727.5,787,800,832,88 0,1550,10000,	As mentioned above		Stomach
Emesis	EDTFL	220,340,930,2500,215610,355680,419340,6511 00,723030,868430			Stomach
Vomiting	EDTFL	150,260,5250,7000,37500,60000,119340,21050 0,458500,684810			Stomach
Vomiting center	BIOM	32.5			Stomach
Spasms and nausea	BIOM	880; 832; 787; 727; 20; 4.9			Stomach
Distended Stomach	XTRA	727,787,800,880,5000,	Abdominal bloating.		Stomach
Stomach, cardia	BIOM	49			Stomach
Gastrocardiac syndrome	BIOM	100			Stomach
Gastric Stasis	EDTFL	120,200,900,47500,96500,275030,534250,6912 40,775000,922530			Stomach
Gastritis	EDTFL	120,200,900,47500,96500,275030,534250,6912 40,753070,927100	Inflammation of stomach lining, commonly due to taking NSAIDS, or to Heliobacter Pylori.		Stomach
Gastritis	BIOM	3.8; 5.9; 7.7; 8.6; 9.4; 9.44; 10; 11.5; 21.5; 30.5; 55.5; 58.25; 59.75; 60.5; 61.5; 64.4; 67; 73; 74.5; 75.5; 79.5		Gastritis	Stomach
Gastritis 1-2	BIOM	880; 832; 802; 787; 727; 676; 422; 20		Gastritis	Stomach
Gastritis 2-2	BIOM	2127; 2008; 880; 787; 727; 659; 450; 400; 125; 95; 72; 20; 4		Gastritis	Stomach
Gastritis 3-2	BIOM	2127; 2008; 1552; 880; 832; 802; 784; 727; 690; 676; 664; 450; 422; 125; 95; 72; 20; 3.9		Gastritis	Stomach
Gastritis, acute	BIOM	2127; 2008; 880; 787; 727; 125; 95; 72; 20; 3.9; 450; 659; 400		Gastritis	Stomach
Gastritis, chronic	BIOM	3.9; 20; 72; 95; 125; 400; 450; 659; 727; 787; 880; 2008; 2127		Gastritis	Stomach

Subject / Argument	Author	Frequencies	Notes	Origin	Target
Menetrier Disease	EDTFL	30,120,930,7500,30300,147500,262500,315610, 505680,756500		Gastritis	Stomach
Gastritis and Flatus	CAFL	880,832,802,787,727,676,422,20,	As mentioned above	Gastritis	Stomach
Gastritis and Flatus 2	XTRA	**20,727,787,832**	As mentioned above	Gastritis	Stomach
Gastritis, Hypertrophic	EDTFL	120,200,900,47500,96500,275030,534250,6912 40,696500,796500	Premalignant condition with inflammation of gastric mucosa.	Gastritis	Stomach
Heartburn	BIOM	**444; 685; 788; 2170**			Stomach
Heartburn	BIOM	2720.0; 2170.0; 2127.0; 1865.0; 1800.0; 1600.0; 1550.0; 1500.0; 880.0; 832.0; 802.0; 787.0; 727.0; 685.0; 676.0; 465.0; 444.0; 125.0; 95.0; 72.0; 20.0			Stomach
Heartburn Chronic	CAFL	832,2720,2170,2127,1800,1600,1550,802,1500, 880,787,727,685,465,444,1865,125,95,72,20	Take a good calcium/magnesium supplement and use the Water Cure. See Acidosis, Hernia, Hyperacidity, **Staphylococcus**, and **Streptococcus** general, and **Heliobacter** sets.		Stomach
Gastric acidity regulation	BIOM	**59; 74; 95.5**		Acidity	Stomach
Hyperacidity	BIOM	**7.82; 230**		Acidity	Stomach
Peracidity	BIOM	10000; 2720; 2170; 1865; 1800; 1600; 1550; 1500; 880; 802; 787; 776; 727; 465; 444; 230; 125; 100; 95; 72; 20; 8	If chronic or with bloating, use appropriate Parasites general set(s). See Dyspepsia, Indigestion, Acidosis, Heartburn, and Hernia.	Acidity	Stomach
Hyperacidity Solar Plexus	XTRA	**230**	As mentioned above	Acidity	Stomach
Hyperacidity Stomach 1	XTRA	7.82,20,230,727,787,880,10000,	As mentioned above	Acidity	Stomach
Hyperacidity Stomach 2	CAFL	**7.82,20,230,**	See Acidosis, Heartburn, and Hernia sets.	Acidity	Stomach
Hypoacidity	BIOM	**20; 59; 74; 95.5**		Acidity	Stomach
Hypoacidity Stomach	XTRA	**20**	Low levels of digestive acid.	Acidity	Stomach
Hiatal Hernia	EDTFL	20,500,970,7500,118250,287560,367500,60522 0,800790,965000	Also called Esophageal Hernia. Protrusion of stomach into thorax through diaphragm defect. See Hernia Esophageal.	Hernia	Stomach
Hiatal Hernia 1	XTRA	128,134,333,411,423,424,436,453,478,542,550, 555,563,576,634,639,643,644,647,674,678,686, 718,727,728,738,745,784,786,787,824.39,876,8 78,880,882,884,934,943,958,960,985,999,1010, 1050,1060,1089,1109,1902,2431,2600,7160,727 0,8697,9646,20443.5,	As mentioned above	Hernia	Stomach
Hiatal Hernia 2	XTRA	727,784,787,800,802,848,875,876,877,878,879, 880=600,881,882,883,884,885,1266,2000,	As mentioned above	Hernia	Stomach
Hiatal Hernia 3	XTRA	9.09,110,660,690,727.5,787,10000,	As mentioned above	Hernia	Stomach
Ulcers General			See Section 1 - **Various Conditions**	Ulcers	Stomach
Ulcer Gastric	CAFL	**676**		Ulcer	Stomach
Ulcer, (Stomach)	EDTFL	150,240,650,830,2500,127500,255470,387500,6 96500,825910		Ulcer	Stomach
Antiulcer effect	BIOM	**8.6; 9.4; 10**		Ulcer	Stomach
Peptic Ulcer	EDTFL	150,240,650,830,2500,127500,255470,387500,6 96500,825910,	Break in lining of stomach, upper small intestine, or lower esophagus. Commonly caused by **Heliobacter Pylori** - see sets.	Ulcer	Stomach
Ulcer, gastric	BIOM	73; 83; 142; 566; 676; 232; 769; 760; 1000		Ulcer	Stomach
Gastric ulcer disease	BIOM	3.6; 3.8; 7; 8; 8.6; 9.4; 9.44; 10; 23.5; 46; 59; 61; 61.5; 63; 67; 73; 74; 79.5; 83; 95.5; 96		Ulcer	Stomach
Marginal Ulcer	EDTFL	150,240,650,830,2500,127500,255470,387500,6 96500,825910,	As mentioned above	Ulcer	Stomach
Gastric Gouty Ulcers	XTRA	**727,776,787,880**	Use for chancroid ulcers, dental ulcers, diabetic ulcers, and gastric gouty ulcers.	Ulcer	Stomach
Helicobacter Pylori			See section 17c - **Bacteria and Diseases**		
Gastrointestinal Post Surgery	EDTFL	120,200,900,7500,13930,47500,95470,329600,3 76290,422530,			Stomach

					13f - Intestines
Detox			See Section 2c - **Detox**	Detox	Intestines
Intestines	XTRA	**2.67,281**			Intestines
Intestines 1	XTRA	**800**			Intestines
Intestines 2	XTRA	**281**			Intestines
Duodenum	BIOM	**8.6; 67**			Intestines
Small Intestines	XTRA	**281.6**			Intestines
Small intestine	BIOM	2.6; 8; 9.4; 61.5; 62.5; 67			Intestines
Large Intestine Tonic	CAFL	**8,440,880**			Intestines
Large intestine	BIOM	23.5; 60; 60.5; 61; 62; 63; 64.5; 66; 68			Intestines
Colon	XTRA	**176**			Intestines
Colon Ascending	XTRA	**12207**	Right side of abdomen between cecum and transverse colon.		Intestines
Colon Descending	XTRA	**14160.15**	Left side of abdomen between the splenic flexure and the sigmoid colon.		Intestines

Subject / Argument	Author	Frequencies	Notes	Origin	Target
Anus	BIOM	68			Intestines
Hernia			See Section 12g - Abdomen	Hernia	Intestines
Intestinal tract, host defenses	BIOM	60.5; 64.5; 67			Intestines
Intestinal Problems General	CAFL	802	See Section 17e - Parasites		Intestines
Disbacteriosis	BIOM	6.3; 6.5; 23.5; 25; 60.5; 63; 64.5; 67	General alteration of human physiological bacterial flora		Intestines
Intestinal atony	BIOM	8.25; 23.5; 62; 63			Intestines
Bellyache	BIOM	3; 95; 3000; 5000; 10000			Intestines
Intestines Inflammation	CAFL	727,787,880,832,1550,105,791,	See Colitis sets.		Intestines
Inflammation of Intestine	BIOM	96			Intestines
Intestinal Inflammation	VEGA	105,791			Intestines
Intestines Inflammation 2	XTRA	105,727,787,791,832,880,1550,			Intestines
Inflammatory Bowel Diseases	EDTFL	80,250,700,850,7500,17500,185750,350000,425170,510500	Includes Crohn's Disease (see sets) and ulcerative colitis types (see Colitis Ulcerative).		Intestines
Intestinal Diseases	EDTFL	80,240,570,2500,7500,12050,191130,254080,343300,639180			Intestines
Inclusion Disease	EDTFL	80,420,770,7930,31210,122730,255610,371330,742600,955200	Serious congenital pathology characterized by malabsorption and diarrhea secondary to a lack of development of microvilli in the intestine.		Intestines
Leaky Gut Sweep	XTRA	6033=300,6027-6040=1300,	See also Candida sets.		Intestines
Leaky Gut Syndrome	EDTFL	180,570,1120,7600,27500,42500,96800,325430,415700,562910			Intestines
Leaky Gut	XTRA	6033			Intestines
Dysbiosis	BIOM	465.0; 880.0; 787.0; 727.0; 95.0; 125.0; 20.0			Intestines
SIBO (Small Intestinal Bacterial Overgrowth) or SBBOS(Small Bowel Bacterial Overgrowth Syndrome)	EDTFL	190,570,15160,52530,119340,357300,424370,561220,642910,930190		Small Int.	Intestines
Enteritis	BIOM	1.2; 73		Small Int.	Intestines
Enteritis, Granulomatous	EDTFL	70,460,3210,5170,17500,127500,351210,611000,706500,921200	Inflammation of the small intestine	Small Int.	Intestines
Enteritis, Pseudomembranous	EDTFL	70,460,3210,5170,392000,404370,515159,687620,689930,712810,		Small Int.	Intestines
Enteritis, Regional	EDTFL	70,460,3210,5170,392000,404370,515160,687620,712810,992000		Small Int.	Intestines
Ulcer, small intestine	BIOM	10; 440; 880		Small Int.	Intestines
Appendicitis	CAFL	1550,802,880,787,727,444,380,190,10,650,444,522,125,95,72,20,522,146,440,450,	If micro-perforation has occurred, infection must be eliminated before drinking any water. A few drops may be fatal.	Appendix	Intestines
Appendix	BIOM	9.4; 2.6; 1.7	As mentioned above	Appendix	Intestines
Appendicitis	EDTFL	140,460,7500,50000,93500,376290,524370,652430,752630,922530,	As mentioned above	Appendix	Intestines
Peritonitis	CAFL	727,787,880	Inflammation of peritoneum, the thin tissue that lines the inner wall of the abdomen and covers most of the organs.	Appendix	Intestines
Intestinal Gas	XTRA	20,422,465,660,676,690,727.5,760,787,802,832,880,1550,			Intestines
Intestines Spasms	XTRA	727,787,5000,			Intestines
Intestines to Release	XTRA	727,787,800,880,	Also see Autointoxication, Auto Intoxication, Constipation, Intestinal Obstruction, and Detox Autointoxication.		Intestines
Intestinal Obstruction	EDTFL	120,280,20050,125180,376910,414190,514210,685250,712000,993450	As mentioned above		Intestines
Irritable Bowel Syndrome IBS		Can be caused by the bacteria Escherichia coli and Mycobacterium avium subspecies paratuberculosis, the protozoan Giardia lamblia, and Blastocystis hominis. In those with HIV is associated with the protozoan Dientamoeba fragilis.			
Irritable Bowel Syndrome	CAFL	6766,5429,4334,2018,1550,880,832,829,812,802,787,727,465,422,407,334,20,	See Colitis and Parasites general sets.	IBS	Intestines
Irritable Bowel Syndrome	BIOM	407; 422; 829		IBS	Intestines
Irritable Bowel Syndrome IBS	EDTFL	80,250,700,850,7500,17500,185750,350000,425170,510500		IBS	Intestines
Irritable Bowel Syndrome 2	XTRA	20,422,465,727,787,802,832,880,1550,6766,		IBS	Intestines
Irritable Bowel Syndrome 3	XTRA	20,727,787,802,880,1550,		IBS	Intestines
Constipation	CAFL	1550,880,802,832,787,776,422,727,20,	Use Parasites General, and Roundworm sets if needed. See Auto Intoxication, Autointoxication, and Detox Autointoxication.	Constipation	Intestines
Constipation	BIOM	1550; 880; 802; 787; 776; 727; 20; 422; 440; 465; 800		Constipation	Intestines
Constipation	EDTFL	120,280,20050,125180,376910,414190,514210,685250,712000,993450		Constipation	Intestines
Constipation	XTRA	727,787,800,880		Constipation	Intestines
Constipation 2	XTRA	20,727,776,787,802,880,1550,		Constipation	Intestines

Subject / Argument	Author	Frequencies	Notes	Origin	Target
Constipation 3	XTRA	802,832,3176		Constipation	Intestines
Constipation due to Intestinal Paresis	BIOM	64.5		Constipation	Intestines
Laxative	BIOM	63.5		Constipation	Intestines
Laxative Mild 1	XTRA	20,727,787,800,802,880,		Constipation	Intestines
Laxative Mild 2	XTRA	802		Constipation	Intestines
Diarrhea	CAFL	1550,880,832,802,786,727,465,	See Clostridium Difficile, E. Coli and for chronic problems, Giardia, and IBS sets. Also see Parasites General if no relief after 2nd treatment.	Diarrhea	Intestines
Diarrhea	BIOM	1550; 880; 802; 787; 786; 727; 621; 465; 454; 443; 344; 152		Diarrhea	Intestines
Diarrhea Diarrhoeal Disease	EDTFL	120,200,900,47500,52500,110250,425140,570000,841000,932000,		Diarrhea	Intestines
Diarrhea, Gastroenteritis	EDTFL	120,200,900,47500,110250,322540,332410,684810,712230,992000,		Diarrhea	Intestines
Dysentery	CAFL	1552,802,832	Acute diarrhea with blood and mucus. Also see Entamoeba Histolytica, Shigella, and appropriate Salmonella and Campylobacter sets.	Diarrhea	Intestines
Dysentery [Diarrheal Diseases]	EDTFL	120,200,900,47500,52500,110250,425140,570000,841000,932000,	As mentioned above	Diarrhea	Intestines
Amoebic Dysentery	CAFL	148,166,308,393,631,778,	Also spelled Amebic.	Diarrhea	Intestines
Colitis	CAFL	440,802,832,880,1550,10000,	Inflammation of the colon.	Colitis	Colon
Colitis, General	EDTFL	150,550,850,5580,120000,315500,472500,527000,662710,752700,		Colitis	Colon
Colitis basic	BIOM	10000; 1550; 880; 832; 802; 800; 440; 96; 61.5; 20		Colitis	Colon
Colitis	BIOM	2.6; 3.5; 3.8; 4; 5.9; 7.7; 8.1; 9.4; 9.44; 23.5; 25; 75.5; 60.5; 61; 61.5; 62; 63; 64.5; 65; 66; 82.5; 96		Colitis	Colon
Colitis 2	XTRA	20,440,660,690,727.5,787,802,832,880,1550,10000,	Inflammation of the colon.	Colitis	Colon
Colitis and Diarrhea	CAFL	10000,5000,1550,880,832,802,787,727,621,465,454,440,433,344,152,	Inflammation of the colon.	Colitis	Colon
Colitis and Diarrhea	BIOM	10000; 5000; 1550; 880; 832; 802; 787; 727; 621; 465; 454; 440; 433; 344; 152; 96; 61.5		Colitis	Colon
Colitis and Diarrhea 2	XTRA	152,344,433,454,465,621,727,787,880,1550,5000,	Inflammation of the colon.	Colitis	Colon
Colitis Mucous Catarrh of Colon	XTRA	20,727,787,800,880,10000,	Inflammation of the colon with excessive production of mucus.	Colitis	Colon
Colitis, Granulomatous	EDTFL	240,700,970,72500,97500,336420,475120,527000,662710,752700		Colitis	Colon
Colitis, Mucous	EDTFL	110,550,900,5580,27400,291250,475120,527000,662710,752700,		Colitis	Colon
Colitis, Pseudomembranous	EDTFL	150,550,850,7460,120000,315500,472500,527000,662710,752700		Colitis	Colon
Ulcerative colitis	BIOM	61; 63; 65		Colitis	Colon
Colitis Ulcerative	EDTFL	150,550,850,7460,12500,40000,120000,313360,320000,615000	Inflammatory Bowel Disease with colonic inflammation and ulcers.	Colitis	Colon
Colitis, Rectal Ulcerative	EDTFL	150,240,650,830,2500,120000,127500,313360,320000,615000,		Colitis	Colon
Flatulence (tympany)	BIOM	1550; 880; 802; 787; 727; 465; 82.5; 74; 56; 50; 3.5			Intestines
Flatulence	CAFL	1550,880,832,802,787,727,465,			Intestines
Flatulence 1	XTRA	20,422,465,660,676,690,727.5,760,787,802,832,880,1550,			Intestines
Gastroduodenal Ulcer	EDTFL	40,9460,10330,22500,44300,45910,172500,292500,754030,825310,	Peptic ulcer in first part of small intestine.	Ulcer	Duodenum
Duodenal Ulcer	CAFL	676,727,750,880,10000,	As mentioned above	Ulcer	Duodenum
Ulcer, duodenal	BIOM	8.6; 9.4; 10; 67; 676; 750; 10000		Ulcer	Duodenum
Duodenal Ulcer	EDTFL	40,9460,10330,22500,44300,45910,172500,292500,754030,825310		Ulcer	Duodenum
Curling's Ulcer	EDTFL	150,240,650,830,2500,127500,255470,387500,696500,825910,	As mentioned above	Ulcer	Duodenum
Duodenal Ulcer 2	XTRA	1.1,1.19,73,250,660,664,676,690,727.5,750,776,784,787,802,832,880,1550,1600,1800,2127.5,2167,2170,2489,2950,10000,	As mentioned above	Ulcer	Duodenum
Duodenitis	CAFL	223,	Inflammation of the duodenum.		Duodenum
Duodenitis	BIOM	9.45; 10; 223			Duodenum
Intestinal Problems Colon	CAFL	10,440,880,787,727,	See Colitis, Parasites General, and General Antiseptic sets.		Colon
Colon Function Balance	XTRA	8,440,635,880,2500,			Colon

Subject / Argument	Author	Frequencies	Notes	Origin	Target
Colon Function Normalize Stimulate	XTRA	635			Colon
Colon Problems General	CAFL	20,440,880,1552,802,832,			Colon
Colonic Aganglionosis	EDTFL	150,520,720,5520,8220,47500,72510,126330,27 5560,475220,	It is a congenital malformation of the innervation of the lower intestine, which involves functional obstruction.		Colon
Hirschsprung Disease	EDTFL	110,550,930,5150,13980,137500,362500,69750 0,775000,922530	As mentioned above		Colon
Megacolon, Congenital	EDTFL	130,570,910,5250,37250,132700,237500,52253 0,675430,819340,	As mentioned above		Colon
Proctocolitis [Rectal]	EDTFL	150,240,650,830,2500,120000,127500,313360,3 20000,615000,	Inflammation of rectum and colon. Causes include Chlamydia Trachomatis, Lymphogranuloma Venereum, Neisseria Gonorrhoeae, HSV, and Campylobacter spp (see sets).	Bacteria	Colon
Proctosigmoiditis	EDTFL	30,330,1220,11090,62080,201510,372480,4175 20,625300,731210			Colon
Rectosigmoiditis [Rectal Colitis]	EDTFL	150,240,650,830,2500,120000,127500,313360,3 20000,615000,			Colon
Rectocolitis	EDTFL	150,550,850,7460,12500,40000,120000,313360, 320000,615000,			Colon
Rectocolitis, Hemorrhagic	EDTFL	150,550,850,7460,12500,40000,120000,313360, 320000,615000,			Colon
Rectocolitis, Ulcerative	EDTFL	150,240,650,830,2500,120000,127500,313360,3 20000,615000,			Colon
Crohn's Disease		Can be caused by an interaction between bacteria and fungi, and in particular between a Fungus, **Candida tropicalis**, and two bacteria: **Escherichia coli and Serratia marcescens**.			
Crohn's and Other Bowel Problems	CAFL	110,133,141,173,187,233,350,447,468,488,510, 543,604,664,672,782,866,972,979,1423,	Inflammatory bowel disease that can affect any part of GI tract.	Crohn	Intestines
Crohn's Disease	CAFL	10000,727,786,440,832,880,1550,20,	Inflammatory bowel disease that can affect any part of GI tract. See Colitis, Colon, and Parasites sets.	Crohn	Intestines
Crohn's Disease 1	XTRA	14,20,60,95,100,110,333,428,440,523,600,625,6 50,660,680,690,727,727.5,768,776,786,787,802, 810,832,880,1550,2000,3000,10000,	As mentioned above	Crohn	Intestines
Crohn's Disease	BIOM	1.2; 73; 133; 141; 173; 187; 233; 350; 407; 422; 447; 468; 510; 543; 604; 672; 782; 791; 866; 972; 979; 1423; 1552		Crohn	Intestines
Crohn's Disease	EDTFL	170,400,620,840,2500,25000,109320,362570,62 1680,775670		Crohn	Intestines
Crohn's Disease Protozoa	XTRA	200,206,249,298	As mentioned above	Crohn	Intestines
Crohn's Disease Viroid	XTRA	585,593,600	As mentioned above	Crohn	Intestines
Ileitis	BIOM	141; 133; 73; 1.2		Crohn	Intestines
Ileitis, Regional	EDTFL	80,380,650,880,9500,115710,354950,355350,36 8000,398400		Crohn	Intestines
Ileitis, Terminal	EDTFL	80,380,650,880,9500,115710,122500,282810,35 7770,426160		Crohn	Intestines
Ileocolitis [Crohns Disease]	EDTFL	170,180,620,840,2500,25000,109320,362570,62 1680,775670,		Crohn	Intestines
Ileocolitis Colon Inflammation	CAFL	802,832,440	Also called Crohn's Disease - see sets. Inflammatory bowel condition. Use Colitis, Parasites Roundworm, and Parasites General sets if necessary.	Crohn	Intestines
Ileocolitis Colon Inflammation 1	XTRA	20,727,787,800,802,880,		Crohn	Intestines
Ileocolitis Colon Inflammation 2	XTRA	440,802,832		Crohn	Intestines
Diverticulitis Acute	CAFL	120,500	Inflammation of diverticula in bowel wall caused by Diverticulosis. See Intestines Inflammation.	Diverticulum	Intestines
Diverticulitis	CAFL	154,934	As mentioned above	Diverticulum	Intestines
Diverticulitis	EDTFL	110,490,970,17300,29510,422500,602500,7153 10,803500,924310	Causes formation of pouches called diverticular in bowel wall. See Diverticulitis sets.	Diverticulum	Intestines
Diverticulosis	XTRA	154,400=1800,934,	As mentioned above	Diverticulum	Intestines
Diverticulosis	BIOM	154; 500; 934		Diverticulum	Intestines
Meckel Diverticulum	EDTFL	200,460,600,2250,12850,144900,323720,60253 0,720340,918280	Congenital bulge in small intestine causing severe pain, abdominal bloating, and rectal bleeding.	Diverticulum	Intestines
Peristalsis, motility	BIOM	23.5; 62; 63			Intestines
Intestinal Neuronal Dysplasia	EDTFL	80,240,570,2500,7500,12050,335690,587700,82 1000,975310	Inherited disorder inhibiting intestinal peristalsis, and thus digestion.		Intestines
Intestinal Polyps	EDTFL	40,440,620,2750,376910,414190,514210,52700 0,667000,685250		Polyps	Intestines
Rectal Diseases	EDTFL	110,250,5710,18500,41500,126510,431330,501 200,653800,825610			Intestines
Rectum inflammation	BIOM	2.6; 3.8; 4; 60.5			Intestines

Subject / Argument	Author	Frequencies	Notes	Origin	Target
Intestinal tract, rectum paresis	BIOM	63.5			Intestines
Rectal Prolapse	EDTFL	60,230,730,870,105720,237250,432500,526070,669710,819340			Intestines
Currarino Syndrome	EDTFL	70,200,850,2500,10890,25290,152500,324370,455720,879930,	Congenital malformation of sacrum, anus, or rectum.		Intestines
Sphincter muscle of intestinal tract	BIOM	68.5			Intestines
Fecal Incontinence	EDTFL	20,520,730,2250,5430,45440,269710,534250,682450,751870			Intestines
Encopresis	EDTFL	230,950,12870,25050,97500,110250,142540,331320,405030,522510	Voluntary or involuntary fecal soiling, usually in children.		Intestines
Anus Diseases	EDTFL	50,600,2250,7500,97500,317550,475000,667000,752700,986220,			Anus
Fissure in Ano	EDTFL	70,240,650,900,2500,27500,215700,347550,375540,522530			Anus
Anal Itching	CAFL	10000,880,787,760,727,465,125,120,95,72,444,1865,20,773,826,827,835,4152,	Pruritis. Use Parasites enterobiasis, and see Section 17e - Parasites		Anus
Perianal itch	BIOM	10000; 880; 787; 760; 727; 500; 465; 444; 125; 100; 95; 72; 20			Anus
Anus Prolapse	EDTFL KHZ	130,230,750,850,51310,327250,495000,681500,791950,953000,	Movement of rectal walls such that they protrude from anus, or result in internal intussusception.		Anus
Proctitis	CAFL	430,620,624,840,866,2213,	Inflammation of anus and lining of rectum, affecting only the last 6 inches. See Chlamydia Trachomatis set.	Bacteria	Anus
Fissures	CAFL	787,20,10000	Tears in skin or mucosa, usually in anus.	Fissures	Anus
Anal fissures	BIOM	10000; 787; 20			Anus
Fissures	XTRA	20,727,787,880,10000,	Tears in skin or mucosa, usually in anus.	Fissures	Anus
Hemorrhoids	EDTFL	50,520,710,930,2560,33180,215470,402530,592500,725370	Also called Piles. Also run circulation and circulatory sets alternatively on consecutive days for 10 days. Place electrodes on thighs.	Hemorrhoids	Anus
Hemorrhoids	CAFL	4474,6117,774,1550,447,880,802,727,	Circulation and circulatory sets should be run alternatively in conjunction with this set. For success, these sets are to be run on consecutive days for 10 days. Electrodes to be placed on upper legs.	Hemorrhoids	Anus
Hemorrhoids	BIO	447		Hemorrhoids	Anus
Hemorrhoids	BIOM	4474; 6117; 1550; 447; 880; 802; 727		Hemorrhoids	Anus
Hemorrhoidal boluses	BIOM	60.5; 66.5; 68.5; 99.5		Hemorrhoids	Anus
Hemorrhoids 1	XTRA	727,800,880,		Hemorrhoids	Anus
Hemorrhoids 2	XTRA	447,660,690,727.5,774,802,880,1550,4474,6117,		Hemorrhoids	Anus
Hemorrhoids 3	XTRA	727,802,880,1550,		Hemorrhoids	Anus
Hemorrhoids 4	XTRA	447,727,774,802,880,1550,4474,6117,		Hemorrhoids	Anus
Hemorrhoids Piles	XTRA	20,447,727,800,880,1550,		Hemorrhoids	Anus

13g - Liver

Subject / Argument	Author	Frequencies	Notes	Origin	Target
Liver	XTRA	10			Liver
Liver	BIOM	0.9; 2.5; 2.6; 3.3; 6; 8.5; 9.8; 56; 56.25			Liver
Liver 1	PROV	13427.72			Liver
Liver 2	PROV	317.82,33.13,1552,802,751,			Liver
Liver 4	XTRA	337,463,574,668,787,803,912,1862,3337,5546			Liver
Liver Support	CAFL	33.13,1552,802,751	Also try E coli, Parasites general, and Parasite flukes general.		Liver
Liver Support	BIOM	727.0; 33.13; 1552.0; 802.0; 751.0; 331.3			Liver
Liver, function regulation	BIOM	0.9; 2.5; 2.65; 3.3; 6; 8.5; 9.8; 56; 56.25; 69; 79			Liver
Liver Function Balance	XTRA	33.13,537,751,802,1550,1552,			Liver
Liver Function Stimulate & Normalize	XTRA	751			Liver
Liver Enlarged	XTRA	465,660,690,727.5,787,880,			Liver
Liver Enlargement	CAFL	727,787,880			Liver
Liver Diseases	EDTFL	200,220,680,2450,3000,7500,96500,326160,505510,632010			Liver
Caroli Disease	EDTFL	120,260,20000,125750,375170,464930,527000,662710,742000,985670	Dilation of the intrahepatic bile ducts.		Liver
Cholangitis	EDTFL	160,570,850,7500,52500,122530,375190,400000,564280,846960	Potentially life-threatening infection of bile duct.	Biliary Duct	Liver
Cholangitis	BIOM	0.2; 0.9; 2; 2.2; 2.7; 3.2; 2.5; 3.5			Liver
Choledochal Cyst, Choledochal Cyst, Type I	EDTFL	50,410,800,7500,125190,275000,424370,560000,642910,985900	Also called bile duct cysts.	Biliary Duct	Liver

Subject / Argument	Author	Frequencies	Notes	Origin	Target
Common Bile Duct Cyst	EDTFL	40,130,820,6030,21540,40350,90180,305430,410700,560940		Biliary Duct	Liver
Chronic Hepatitis [Group 4]	EDTFL	200,870,5290,27500,45560,95220,182500,414550,418800,421800,	Inflammation of liver. See other sets in Section 17d - Virus	Hepatitis	Liver
Cirrhosis Hepatitis	CAFL	291		Hepatitis	Liver
Hepatic cirrhosis	BIOM	56; 63.5; 74.5; 291; 331.3		Hepatitis	Liver
Hepatic Cirrhosis	EDTFL	140,250,950,7500,10530,87530,196500,551030,777300,866410		Hepatitis	Liver
Liver Fibrosis	EDTFL	50,230,950,10530,32509,62480,145440,372500,522500,792300,		Hepatitis	Liver
Liver Cirrhosis	EDTFL	190,520,650,1000,13960,110530,380000,447500,728980,825270,	Liver malfunction due to alcohol, hepatitis B or C, or non-alcoholic fatty liver disease.	Hepatitis	Liver
Cirrhosis of the Liver	XTRA	170,381,514,677,715,774,776,1250,2271,	Failure of liver function due to long-term damage.	Hepatitis	Liver
Fatty Liver	EDTFL	50,410,1000,5750,7250,15910,173300,435440,792500,915700	Abnormal accumulation of fat in the liver. Also see Liver sets.		Liver
Dysplasia, Arteriohepatic	EDTFL	170,520,620,850,20700,97500,155270,562500,753200,850000,	Genetic disorder affecting major organs.	Genetic disorder	Liver
Alagille Syndrome	EDTFL KHZ	80,800,950,22500,57500,176000,419340,563190,813960,983170,	As mentioned above	Genetic disorder	Liver
Budd-Chiari Syndrome	EDTFL	500,680,87400,95030,234510,347000,452590,684810,712230,997870,	Abdominal pain, ascites, and liver enlargement caused by hepatic vein blockage.		Liver
Chiari's Syndrome	EDTFL	850,2750,7500,12710,52500,97500,419340,566410,642910,930120			Liver
Hepatic venous outflow obstruction	EDTFL	140,250,950,7500,10530,20000,57500,325560,497610,660410	As mentioned above		Liver
Gilbert Disease	EDTFL	80,240,570,7500,12720,36210,142500,321000,415700,775680	Common genetic liver disorder with hyperbilirubinemia - see Hyperbilirubinemia Hereditary set.	Genetic disorder	Liver
Gilbert's disease	BIOM	0.9; 2.5; 3.3; 3.5; 9.8			Liver
Liver Necrosis 1	XTRA	33.13,329,331.3,377,471,626,628,634,635,714,724,751,774,802,847,867,1172.45,1552,2162,7867,9889,11774.63,	Liver cell death caused by external factors rather than by apoptosis.		Liver
Liver Necrosis 2	XTRA	33,33.13,802,1550,1552,			Liver
Enlarged Liver	EDTFL	30,250,730,7500,12850,35510,62580,125350,672910,924370	Enlarged liver. Also see Liver Enlarged, and Liver Enlargement.		Liver
Hepatomegaly	EDTFL	150,220,1950,17300,19530,95220,182500,233450,414550,421800	As mentioned above		Liver
Hepatomegaly	BIOM	2489; 880; 787; 727			Liver
Liver Trematode	BIOM	143; 238; 275; 676; 763; 1058.4; 6641; 6672			Liver
Liver Parasites	BIOM	143.0; 275.0; 676.0; 763.0; 238.0; 6640.5; 6671.5			Liver
Liver Parasites			See Section Section 17e - Parasites	Protozoa Parasites	Liver
Liver-Gall Bladder	BIOM	10000.0; 5000.0; 1550.0; 880.0; 832.0; 802.0; 787.0; 727.0; 465.0; 100.0; 20.0			Liver
Liver and Bile 1	BIOM	17; 38; 38.5; 56; 56.25; 63.5; 69; 79			Liver
Hepatobiliary system regulation	BIOM	0.7; 0.9; 2.5; 2.65; 3.3; 8.5; 9.8			Liver
Biliary ducts	BIOM	2; 2.2; 2.7; 3.2; 3.5; 8.5		Bile	Liver
Gall, production	BIOM	38; 38.5		Bile	Liver
Gall, regulation	BIOM	74.5		Bile	Liver
Liver Stores Bile Cholesterol	CAFL	21.34		Bile	Liver
Biliousness	CAFL	1550,802,10000,880,832,787,727,465,	Nausea and possible vomiting.	Bile	Liver
Biliousness 1	XTRA	21.33,465,660,690,727.5,787,802,832,880,1550,10000,	Nausea and possible vomiting.	Bile	Liver
Biliousness 2	XTRA	465,727,787,802,832,880,1550,5000,10000,	Nausea and possible vomiting.	Bile	Liver
Biliary Atresia	EDTFL	140,260,5620,42500,65110,90000,517500,688250,712230,997870	As mentioned above	Bile	Liver
Biliary Cirrhosis	BIO	381,514,677,2271	Inflammatory autoimmune disease in which bile flow through the liver is obstructed.	Bile	Liver
Biliary Cirrhosis	XTRA	170,381,514,677,715,774,776,1250,2271,	Inflammatory autoimmune disease in which bile flow through the liver is obstructed.	Bile	Liver
Biliary Headache	CAFL	8.5,3.5		Bile	Liver
Bile Duct Spasms and Pain	XTRA	2,2.2,2.5,2.7,3.2,3.5,	Can be caused by blockage due to cancer, gallstones, or injury.	Bile	Liver
Biliary Tract Diseases	EDTFL	140,260,5620,42500,65110,90000,517500,661710,742000,988900		Bile	Liver
Dyskinesia of bile passages - hypertonic type	BIOM	9.44		Bile	Liver
Dyskinesia of bile passages - hypotonic type	BIOM	3.5; 3.8; 8.1; 9.4		Bile	Liver

Subject / Argument	Author	Frequencies	Notes	Origin	Target
Biliary cirrhosis	BIOM	170; 381; 514; 677; 715; 774; 1250; 2271		Bile	Liver
Biliary obstruction	BIOM	23.3		Bile	Liver
Gallstone Attack	BIO	481,743,865,928		Bile	Liver
Gallstones 1	XTRA	2.64,20,30.5,444,660,690,727.5,787,800,880,15 52,1865,3000,6000.10000,		Bile	Liver
Gallstones	CAFL	2.65,3.5,3000,1552,800,880,787,727,20,6000,10 000,444,	See Gallstone attack and Cholecystitis acute.	Bile	Liver
Gallstone, dispersion	BIOM	17; 84; 85; 88.5; 94.5; 96		Bile	Liver
Cholelithiasis	BIOM	2.65; 3.5; 3.8; 5.9; 7.7; 9.19; 17; 27; 38; 63.5; 66.5; 74.5; 84; 85; 88.5; 90.5; 94.5; 96		Bile	Liver
Cholelithiasis	EDTFL	50,400,930,2500,12710,13980,95460,233910,42 6900,571000	Commonly called Gallstones- see sets.	Bile	Liver

13h - Gallbladder

Subject / Argument	Author	Frequencies	Notes	Origin	Target
Gallbladder	XTRA	10	It is a small hollow organ that has the function of storing the bile produced by the liver and then releasing it into the small intestine during digestion.		Gallbladder
Gall Bladder	BIOM	63.5			Gallbladder
Gallbladder 1	XTRA	20,727,787,880,5000,			Gallbladder
Gallbladder 2	XTRA	164.3			Gallbladder
Gallbladder, general problems	BIOM	1550; 802; 10000; 880; 832; 787; 727; 465			Gallbladder
Gallbladder Inflammation	CAFL	432,801,1551	See Cholecystitis chronic.		Gallbladder
Gallbladder Inflammation	BIO	432	Chronic.		Gallbladder
Gallbladder Pain	CAFL	800,1550		Pain	Gallbladder
Gallbladder Diseases	EDTFL	160,230,650,840,2500,127500,255470,387500,6 96500,825910			Gallbladder
Gallbladder distonia	BIOM	2.65; 20; 727; 787; 880; 3040			Gallbladder
Cholecystitis [Gall Bladder Inflamation]	EDTFL	80,200,750,17930,119000,255560,372580,5512 30,673290,713720,	Inflammation of the gallbladder.		Gallbladder
Chronic cholecystitis	BIOM	432; 481; 743; 801; 861; 865; 928; 1551			Gallbladder
Hepatocholecystitis	BIOM	10000.0; 5000.0; 1550.0; 880.0; 832.0; 802.0; 787.0; 727.0; 465.0; 100.0; 20.0			Gallbladder
Empyema, Gallbladder	EDTFL	160,230,650,840,2500,127500,255470,387500,6 96500,825910,			Gallbladder
Gallbladder Inflammation	EDTFL	190,300,720,840,2500,127500,255470,387500,6 96500,725540			Gallbladder
Cholecystitis	VEGA	481,743,865,928	Inflammation of the gallbladder. See Gallbladder sets.		Gallbladder
Cholecystitis Chronic	CAFL	432,801,1551	Long-term inflammation of the gallbladder. See Gallbladder sets.		Gallbladder
Gall Bladder Dystonia With Osteitis	CAFL	2.65,3000,880,787,727,20,			Gallbladder
Bilirubin	BIO	717,726,731,863	A bile pigment that may cause jaundice in high concentrations. Use Liver Support.	Bilirubin	Gallbladder
Bilirubin	BIOM	649; 717; 726; 734; 863		Bilirubin	Gallbladder
Bilirubin	CAFL	717,726,731,863,9305,649,734,	As mentioned above	Bilirubin	Gallbladder
Bilirubinemia	XTRA	1.19,10,20,72,95,125,146,250,444,600,625,649, 650,717,726,731,734,802,863,880,1500,1550,16 00,1865,9305,	Increased presence of bilirubin in blood.	Bilirubin	Gallbladder
Hyperbilirubinemia, Hereditary	EDTFL	150,180,800,5500,33200,172300,471200,55785 0,603440,921880,	Condition where bilirubin levels are elevated, for reasons that can be attributed to a metabolic disorder.	Bilirubin	Gallbladder
Rotor Syndrome [hyperbilirubinemia]	EDTFL	150,180,800,5500,33200,172300,471200,55785 0,603440,921880,	As mentioned above	Bilirubin	Gallbladder
Jaundice	CAFL	5000,1600,1550,1500,880,802,650,625,600,444, 1865,146,250,125,95,72,20,	See Liver Support, Gallbladder, Leptospirosis, Parasites General, and Flukes sets. Also see Icterus Haemolytic.	Jaundice	Gallbladder
Jaundice	BIOM	243; 5000; 250; 444; 600; 625; 650; 768; 1500; 10000		Jaundice	Gallbladder
Jaundice	EDTFL	160,490,620,850,7500,162500,281200,492520,6 75620,825230	See Liver Support, Gallbladder, Leptospirosis, Parasites General, and Flukes sets. Also see Icterus Haemolytic.	Jaundice	Gallbladder
Icterus [Juvenile Jaundice]	EDTFL	160,490,620,850,7500,162500,281200,492520,6 75620,825230,	As mentioned above	Jaundice	Gallbladder
Jaundice 1	XTRA	1.19,10,20,72,95,125,146,250,444,600,625,649, 650,717,726,731,734,802,863,880,1500,1550,16 00,1865,9305,	As mentioned above	Jaundice	Gallbladder
Jaundice, Chronic Idiopathic	EDTFL	160,490,620,850,7500,162500,281200,492520,6 91270,859830		Jaundice	Gallbladder
Dubin-Johnson Syndrome	EDTFL	410,570,600,102350,175140,475330,560060,60 0770,797680,891220		Jaundice	Gallbladder
Icterus Haemolytic	CAFL	243,768	A chronic form of jaundice involving anemia. See Jaundice set.	Jaundice	Gallbladder

Subject / Argument	Author	Frequencies	Notes	Origin	Target
Jaundice Hemolytic	EDTFL	160,490,620,850,7500,162500,281200,492520,859830,922530	As mentioned above	Jaundice	Gallbladder
Kernicterus	EDTFL	70,550,700,870,5250,7250,30000,55230,93500,325620	A pathological neonatal jaundice with deposit of free bilirubin in the brain tissue. Also see Bilirubinemia and Hyperbilirubinemia Hereditary.	Jaundice	Gallbladder
Bilirubin Encephalopathy	EDTFL	150,180,800,5500,33200,172300,471200,557850,603440,921880	Bilirubin-induced brain dysfunction. Also see Bilirubinemia and Hyperbilirubinemia Hereditary.	Jaundice	Gallbladder
Hyperbilirubinemic Encephalopathy	EDTFL	150,180,800,5500,33200,172300,471200,557850,603440,921880,	As mentioned above	Jaundice	Gallbladder

13i - Pancreas

Subject / Argument	Author	Frequencies	Notes	Origin	Target
Pancreas	CAFL	440,464,600,624,648,1552,727,787,880,			Pancreas
Pancreas	XTRA	10			Pancreas
Pancreas	BIOM	3.3; 4; 9.2; 9.7; 26; 52			Pancreas
Pancreas - Pilot frequencies	BIOM	25; 27.5; 30; 47.5; 50; 52.5; 94; 99.5			Pancreas
Pancreas 1	XTRA	14648.44			Pancreas
Pancreas 2	XTRA	440,464,600,624,648,727,787,880,1552,			Pancreas
Pancreas 3	XTRA	117.29			Pancreas
Pancreas Function Stimulate Normal	XTRA	654			Pancreas
Pancreas, regulation	BIOM	3.3; 4; 9.2; 9.7; 26; 52			Pancreas
Pancreas Balance 1	XTRA	1.19,250,654,660,690,727.5,2127.5,			Pancreas
Pancreas Balance 2	XTRA	10,15,20,26,440,444,464,465,537,600,624,625,648,650,776,787,802,832,880,1500,1550,1552,1600,1800,1865,2008,2170,2489,2720,			Pancreas
Pancreatic Diseases	EDTFL	70,570,23100,50000,72800,132200,220300,587300,722520,915200,			Pancreas
Pearson's Syndrome	EDTFL	190,230,3750,62500,162500,219110,321300,472530,888030,937390			Pancreas
Pancreas Disorder	XTRA	727,787,880,10000			Pancreas
Pancreas Fluke	XTRA	1850,2000,2003,2008,2013,2050,2080,6578,13135.94=1200,13156.25,20960.36,	See Section 17e - Parasites		Pancreas
Pancreatic Insufficiency	CAFL	20,250,650,625,600,465,444,26,2720,2489,2170,2127,2008,1800,1600,1550,802,1500,880,832,787,776,727,690,666,20,	Production of insulin has slowed. Run for Diabetes, but monitor blood sugar levels. If no improvement, test for insulin resistance.		Pancreas
Pancreatic Insufficiency	EDTFL	70,570,23100,2250,5290,30000,45370,57500,96500,233630			Pancreas
Pancreatic Insufficiency 2	XTRA	20,26,444,465,600,625,650,666,690,727,776,787,832,880,1500,1550,1600,1800,2008,2127,2170,2489,2720,	As mentioned above		Pancreas
Pancreatic Insufficiency 3	XTRA	10	As mentioned above		Pancreas
Exocrine Pancreatic Insufficiency [Digestion]	EDTFL	70,570,2250,5290,23100,30000,45370,57500,96500,233630,	Inability to digest food properly due to lack of pancreatic enzymes.		Pancreas
Pancreatic Degeneration 1	BIOM	26.5			Pancreas
Pancreatitis	EDTFL	70,570,23100,50000,85150,117170,453200,692230,824370,951000	Inflammation of pancreas, with upper abdominal pain, nausea, and vomiting.		Pancreas
Pancreatitis, chronic	BIOM	20; 26.5; 444; 465; 600; 625; 650; 666; 690; 727; 776; 787; 802; 832; 880; 1500; 1550; 1600; 2720			Pancreas
Phlegmon [Pancreatitis]	EDTFL	70,570,23100,50000,85150,117170,453200,692230,824370,951000,			Pancreas
Pancreas Parasites	BIOM	1850.0; 2000.0; 2003.0; 2008.0; 2013.0; 2050.0; 2080.0; 6577.5	See Section 17e - Parasites		Pancreas

Subject / Argument	Author	Frequencies	Notes	Origin	Target

14 - Urinary System

Subject / Argument	Author	Frequencies	Notes	Origin	Target
Urologic Diseases	EDTFL	140,320,950,5250,12710,45000,97500,150000,4 34080,985670,	Congenital or acquired dysfunction of the urinary system.		Urinary System
Urinary Tract Diseases	EDTFL	160,800,7500,30000,67500,125000,352930,563 180,642910,930120,			Urinary System
Urinary Tract Infections	CAFL	2050,880,1550,802,787,727,465,20,9.39,642,35 8,539,	UTI. See Bacterium Coli sets.	Infection	Urinary System
Urinary Tract Infection	XTRA	20	As mentioned above	Infection	Urinary System
Urinary Tract Infection	BIOM	2050; 880; 1550; 802; 787; 727; 465; 126; 20; 9.39; 642; 358; 539			Urinary System
Urinary Tract Infections	EDTFL	160,800,7500,30000,67500,125000,352930,563 180,642910,930120,	As mentioned above	Infection	Urinary System
Inflammation of the Genitourinary Tract	BIOM	5000.0; 2720.0; 2489.0; 1800.0; 1550.0; 802.0; 787.0; 776.0; 727.0; 625.0; 600.0; 522.0; 500.0; 465.0; 444.0; 428.0; 95.0			Urinary System

14a - Kidney

Subject / Argument	Author	Frequencies	Notes	Origin	Target
Kidney	PROV	319.87,8,20,727,787,800,880,5000,10000,9.2,10 ,40,440,1600,1550,1500,802,650,625,600,444,1 865,146,250,125,95,72,20,			Kidney
Kidneys	XTRA	4.11,10			Kidney
Kidneys	BIOM	2.8; 3.3; 3.5; 8.1; 9.2; 9.7			Kidney
Kidney 1	XTRA	8,20,727,787,800,880,5000,10000,			Kidney
Kidney 4	XTRA	248,463,522,622,658,917,932,1865,3374,5162			Kidney
Kidney Pattern	BIOM	2.8; 3.3; 8.1; 9.19; 54; 54.25; 54.5			Kidney
Renal duct	BIOM	86			Kidney
Kidney Tonic General	CAFL	440,248,8,880,20,10000,800,5000,3000,	Drink a minimum of 2.5 litres of water a day.		Kidney
Kidneys regulation and cleaning	BIOM	2.8; 3.3; 8.1; 9.19; 54; 54.25; 54.5; 63			Kidney
Juxtaglomerular apparatus regulation	BIOM	2.8	The Juxtaglomerular apparatus is a structure that is part of the kidney that controls the activity of individual nephrons.		Kidney
Juxtaglomerular Regulation	BIOM	2.8; 3.3; 8.1; 9.25			Kidney
Kidney Stimulation	XTRA	20,28,40,64,72,93,96,100,112,120,125,146,152, 240,250,334,440,442,465,524,582,600,625,644, 651,668,676,712,728,732,751,784,800,854,880, 1016,1134,1153,1500,1550,1600,1864,2112,222 2,2400,2720,4412,			Kidney
Kidneys, stimulation	BIOM	4412; 2720; 2400; 2112; 1864; 1600; 1550; 1500; 880; 854; 800; 784; 751; 732; 728; 712; 668; 651; 644; 625; 600; 524; 465; 442; 334; 250; 240; 152; 146; 28; 125; 120; 112; 100; 96; 93; 72; 64; 40; 20; 2222; 1153; 1134; 1016; 582; 676; 440			Kidney
Kidney Function Balance	XTRA	1.1,1.19,6.29,8,10,20,40,72,73,95,125,146,148,2 48,250,333,440,444,465,522,523,555,600,625,6 50,768,786,800,802,880,1500,1550,1600,1865,3 000,5000,10000,	As mentioned above		Kidney
Kidney Function Normalize Stimulate	XTRA	625	As mentioned above		Kidney
Kidneys, calcium/phosphorus balance	BIOM	4.6; 9.6; 15			Kidney
Body dehydration	BIOM	79			Kidney
Urinative effect	BIOM	8.1; 86			Kidney
Kidney Diseases	EDTFL	120,680,850,7500,12070,27500,97500,275620,5 23010,687450			Kidney
Colic			See Section 1 - Various Conditions		Kidney
Kidney Infection 1	XTRA	1.1,1.19,6.29,9.18,9.2,10,20,40,73,148,250,440, 444,465,594,660,690,727.5,776,787,802,880,15 00,1550,1600,1865,2008,10000,	Drink lots of pure water.	Infection	Kidney
Kidney Infection 2	XTRA	72,95,125,146,333,424,434,522,523,555,600,62 5,650,768,786,834,2045,	As mentioned above	Infection	Kidney
Kidney Insufficiency	CAFL	9.2,10,40,440,1600,1550,1500,880,802,650,625, 600,444,1865,146,250,125,95,72,20,	As mentioned above	Insufficiency	Kidney
Renal insufficiency	BIOM	10; 40; 440; 1600; 1550; 1500; 911; 880; 802; 650; 625; 600; 444; 1865; 146; 250; 125; 95; 72; 20; 9.7		Insufficiency	Kidney

Subject / Argument	Author	Frequencies	Notes	Origin	Target
Renal Excretory Insufficiency Diastolic Hypertensive	CAFL	9.2	Use for renal excretory insufficiency, diastolic hypertensive. See Kidney insufficiency.	Insufficiency	Kidney
Kidney Failure, Acute Kidney Failure, Chronic	EDTFL	160,410,770,8930,32280,43010,112520,421350, 422300,802590		Insufficiency	Kidney
Renal Failure, Chronic End-Stage	EDTFL	160,410,770,8930,32280,43010,112520,421350, 422300,802590,		Insufficiency	Kidney
End-Stage Renal Disease - ESRD	EDTFL	160,410,770,8930,32280,43010,112520,421350, 422300,802590,			Kidney
Kidney Papilloma	BIO	110,767,917	Small, supposedly benign growth on a kidney.		Kidney
Kidney Papilloma	PROV	110,148,264,634,767,848,917,760,762,1102,	As mentioned above		Kidney
Kidney Papilloma	VEGA	110,767	As mentioned above		Kidney
Urinary stone disease	BIOM	2.8; 3.8; 3.3; 3.5; 3.6; 5.9; 7; 7.7; 8.1; 9.19; 19.5; 43; 46; 53; 54; 54.25; 54.5; 63; 75.5; 79.5; 86; 90.5	Calculosis, of the urinary tract.	Kidney Stone	Kidney
Urinary stone disease basic	BIOM	2.5; 2.6; 3; 4; 4.9; 5.5; 9.4; 14.5; 20; 22; 25.5; 42; 49; 64; 63; 79.5; 85.5; 98; 91.5		Kidney Stone	Kidney
Urinary stone disease, general	BIOM	444; 727; 787; 800; 880; 10000; 6000; 5000; 3000; 1552; 20; 3.5; 2.65		Kidney Stone	Kidney
Sabulous urine	BIOM	3000; 880; 787; 727; 20; 2.65		Kidney Stone	Kidney
Renal Calculi	CAFL	3.5,444,727,787,880,1552,3000,30000,6000,100 00,	Drink at least 2.5 litres of water a day, and supplement with vitamins, minerals, and herbs.	Kidney Stone	Kidney
Kidney Stones	CAFL	444,727,787,880,10000,6000,3000,3.5,1552,	As mentioned above	Kidney Stone	Kidney
Kidney-stones, dispersion	BIOM	43; 53; 54; 54.25; 54.5; 62.5; 63; 65; 67.5; 86; 96		Kidney Stone	Kidney
Kidney Stones	EDTFL	40,180,700,850,5780,32500,60000,95670,12523 0,150000		Kidney Stone	Kidney
Kidney Stones 1	XTRA	30.5,444,660,690,727.5,787,880,1552,1865,300 0,6000,10000,	As mentioned above	Kidney Stone	Kidney
Kidney Stones 3	XTRA	727,787,880,10000	As mentioned above	Kidney Stone	Kidney
Gravel Deposits	XTRA	2.64,20,727,787,880,3000,5000,	Kidney stones passed in urination. See Gravel in Urine, Kidney Stones, and Kidney Calculi sets.	Kidney Stone	Kidney
Gravel In Urine 1	CAFL	2.65,20,727,787,880,3000,	As mentioned above	Kidney Stone	Kidney
Gravel In Urine 2	XTRA	2.64,20,727,787,880,3000,	As mentioned above	Kidney Stone	Kidney
Kidney Tubular Necrosis	EDTFL	70,180,570,7500,13610,122500,211000,305850, 452200,591430	Death of renal tubule cells due to drugs, low BP, or Renal Artery Obstruction (see set). Also called Stage 5 Chronic Kidney Disease (CKD).		Kidney
Lower Nephron Nephrosis	EDTFL	150,230,620,930,7500,12690,52500,72500,9350 0,96500			Kidney
Dialysis, Renal	EDTFL	80,570,900,5710,45200,152590,262500,695020, 715730,819340,		Dialysis	Kidney
Hemodialysis	EDTFL	190,550,940,7550,22200,42500,227150,275520, 515700,650000	Also see End Stage Renal Disease and appropriate kidney sets		Kidney
IgA Neuropathy	EDTFL	50,490,700,830,2400,32500,305050,431200,632 590,723010	Inflammation of glomeruli of kidney.		Kidney
Berger's Disease	EDTFL	180,17850,27500,47500,150000,225000,452590 ,684000,713000,993410	As mentioned above		Kidney
Bright Disease [Chronic Nephritis]	EDTFL	130,220,320,730,900,3870,19100,159320,35650 0,624370,	As mentioned above		Kidney
Glomerulonephritis	EDTFL	550,680,870,7500,13610,40000,90000,375950,5 75310,827000	As mentioned above		Kidney
Renal Osteodystrophy	EDTFL	60,500,890,12850,132600,347500,377650,5910 00,683560,825090	Changes in bone formation due to chronic kidney disease (CKD).		Kidney
Renal Rickets	EDTFL	190,1000,2580,17500,225000,323200,398400,6 82020,759830,932410,			Kidney
Hydronephrosis	EDTFL	80,250,750,800,2500,5780,95870,175560,52494 0,691270	Distension and dilation of the renal pelvis and calyces, usually caused by obstruction of the free flow of urine.		Kidney
Oxaluria {Hyperoxaluria]	EDTFL	80,110,810,7970,31220,42330,133630,352000,4 05720,623200,	Excessive urinary excretion of oxalate - may indicate presence of calcium oxalate Kidney Stones - see sets.		Kidney
Hyperoxaluria	EDTFL	80,110,810,7970,31220,42330,133630,352000,4 05720,623200	As mentioned above		Kidney
Medullary Sponge Kidney	EDTFL	70,240,600,7250,132280,427500,555950,69000 0,875000,936420	Congenital kidney disorder with cyst formation leading to increased risk of Kidney Stones (see sets) and Urinary Tract Infection (see sets).		Kidney
Bright's Syndrome	CAFL	10,20,274,423,465,636,688,727,880,1550,3000, 10000,	Can be caused by Streptococcus and Escherichia Coli.	Nephritis	Kidney
Bright's Syndrome 1	XTRA	727,787,880,1500	As mentioned above	Nephritis	Kidney
Nephritis	CAFL	1550,274,423,636,688,880,787,727,10,20,10000 ,40,73,465,3000,	Inflammation of the kidneys, commonly caused by urinary tract infections, toxins, and autoimmune disorders. Use Kidney Stones, and Kidney Tonic General.	Nephritis	Kidney
Nephritis	BIO	264,	As mentioned above	Nephritis	Kidney
Nephritis, acute	BIOM	1550; 274; 264; 423; 636; 688; 880; 787; 727; 10; 20; 10000; 40; 73; 465; 3000		Nephritis	Kidney

Subject / Argument	Author	Frequencies	Notes	Origin	Target
Nephritis 1	XTRA	1.1,10,20,40,73,264,274,423,465,636,660,688,6 90,727.5,787,1500,2045,3000,10000,	As mentioned above	Nephritis	Kidney
Nephritis 3	XTRA	20,727,787,800,880,10000,	As mentioned above	Nephritis	Kidney
Nephritis, chronic	BIOM	1.2; 7.3; 54; 73; 274; 423; 636; 638; 688; 1550; 3000; 10000		Nephritis	Kidney
Nephritis, Chronic	EDTFL	130,220,320,730,900,3870,19100,159320,35650 0,624370,		Nephritis	Kidney
Nephritis Hereditary	EDTFL	130,220,320,730,900,3870,19100,159320,72434 0,933910	As mentioned above	Nephritis	Kidney
Nephritis Nephrosis	XTRA	10,20,40,73,465,727,787,880,10000,	Degenerative disease of renal tubules which can be caused by nephritis, or other kidney diseases. Use Kidney Stones, and Kidney Tonic General.	Nephrosis	Kidney
Nephrosis	BIOM	20; 54; 240		Nephrosis	Kidney
Nephrosis Nephrotic Syndrome	EDTFL	60,490,730,1270,5870,12330,252500,317560,49 2500,675290	Kidney disorder with large Proteinuria (see set) leading to low protein blood levels, and Edema (use Ascites sets).	Nephrosis	Kidney
Minimal Change Disease	EDTFL	120,400,900,119340,175120,475030,527000,66 7000,753230,986220	Nephrotic syndrome.	Nephrosis	Kidney
Kidney Diseases Cystic	EDTFL	80,350,600,600,2750,5300,50000,62500,90000, 95670	Wide range of hereditary, developmental, and acquired kidney conditions involving cysts. Also see Polycystic Kidney Diseases and Medullary Sponge Kidney.		Kidney
Polycystic Kidney Diseases	EDTFL	80,350,600,600,2750,5300,50000,62500,90000, 95670,	Genetic disorder in which abnormal cysts develop and grow in the kidneys.	Genetic disorder	Kidney
Multicystic Dysplastic Kidney	EDTFL	40,240,950,2750,5810,178500,326500,571520,7 05850,827230	Genetic condition caused by malformed kidneys consisting of variously-sized cysts.	Genetic disorder	Kidney
Proteinuria	EDTFL	830,1870,5630,152300,328960,424210,482130, 502930,553700,591420	Excess serum proteins in urine, causing it to foam on micturition.		Kidney
Proteus Vulgaris	HC	408750-416450=3600,	Urinary tract pathogen.	Bacteria	Kidney
Pyelonephritis Pyelonephritis, Acute Necrotizing	EDTFL	50,500,1900,112870,312500,405400,652500,72 6070,802060,923200	Inflammation of kidney tissue, calyces, and renal pelvis. Also see Cysto Pyelo Nephritis.Can be caused by Escherichia coli and Proteus.		Kidney
Pyelitis (Proteus)	BIOM	434; 594; 776			Kidney
Pyelonephritis	BIOM	2.8; 3.8; 3.3; 3.6; 5.9; 7; 7.7; 8.1; 9.19; 19.5; 46; 75.5; 86; 90.5; 43; 54; 54.5; 54.25; 63; 86			Kidney
Cysto Pyelo Nephritis	VEGA	1385	Inflammation of bladder, pelvis of kidney, and kidney. Also see Pyelonephritis.		Kidney
Prune Belly Syndrome	EDTFL	100,520,870,3200,15890,32750,132000,437500, 525830,725310	Congenital disorder of urinary system, with abdominal wall muscle anomalies, cryptorchidism, and urinary tract abnormalities among others.		Kidney

14b - Bladder

Subject / Argument	Author	Frequencies	Notes	Origin	Target
Bladder	CAFL	727,787,800,880			Bladder
Bladder	XTRA	2.57			Bladder
Bladder	XTRA	352,727,787,800,880,			Bladder
Urinary bladder	BIOM	64.8; 68.5; 87			Bladder
Urinary bladder, urethra	BIOM	8.1; 9.39		Urethra	Bladder
Urethra	BIOM	88		Urethra	Bladder
Urinary bladder sphincter muscle weakness	BIOM	18.5			Bladder
Urinary Bladder Syndrome	BIOM	84			Bladder
Urinary Bladder Diseases	EDTFL	160,800,7500,30000,67500,125000,352930,563 180,642910,930120,			Bladder
Bladder Diseases	EDTFL	160,800,7500,30000,67500,125000,352930,563 180,642910,930120			Bladder
Bladder and Prostate Complaints	CAFL	9.39,20,465,727,787,802,880,1550,			Bladder
Bladder and Prostate Complaints	XTRA	9.39,20,465,727,787,802,880,1550,2050,			Bladder
Oliguria	EDTFL	190,1220,3720,17280,63210,119440,293240,40 3030,435000,711170	Low output of urine which may be due to dehydration, Kidney Failure, Urinary Tract Infections, or other serious problems - see appropriate sets.		Bladder
Urinary Retention	EDTFL	50,950,5250,12710,35750,96500,510250,65520 0,752630,926700			Bladder
Urinary Retention	BIOM	90.5			Bladder
Polyuria [Frequent Urination]	EDTFL	50,460,950,7500,32500,154310,325550,352570, 411120,634250,			Bladder
Nocturia [nocturnal polyuria]	EDTFL	50,460,950,7500,32500,154310,325550,352570, 411120,634250,	Having to wake from sleep to urinate. Also see Prostate sets.		Bladder
Nycturia [nocturnal polyuria]	EDTFL	50,460,950,7500,32500,154310,325550,352570, 411120,634250,	As mentioned above		Bladder

Subject / Argument	Author	Frequencies	Notes	Origin	Target
Enuresis	CAFL	10000,880,787,727	See Bed Wetting sets. Use Parasites General, Pinworms, and Ascaris sets.	Bed Wetting	Bladder
Enuresis	BIOM	45.5; 96		Bed Wetting	Bladder
Enuresis	BIOM	1550; 880; 802; 787; 727; 465; 120; 112; 96; 45.5; 7.83		Bed Wetting	Bladder
Enuresis-3	BIOM	10000.0; 5000.0; 1550.0; 880.0; 802.0; 787.0; 727.0; 465.0; 120.0; 112.0; 7.83		Bed Wetting	Bladder
Enuresis	EDTFL	170,230,620,930,7250,42500,231200,521400,739260,849420	As mentioned above	Bed Wetting	Bladder
Urination Disorders	EDTFL	50,950,5250,12710,35750,45000,97500,150000,229320,532410	As mentioned above	Bed Wetting	Bladder
Enuresis 2	XTRA	465,660,690,727.5,787,802,880,1550,2050,2128,2250,10000,	As mentioned above	Bed Wetting	Bladder
Bed Wetting	CAFL	7.83,20,112,120,465,727,787,802,880,1550,	As mentioned above	Bed Wetting	Bladder
Bed Wetting	XTRA	465,660,690,727.5,787,802,880,1550,2050,2128,2250,10000,	As mentioned above	Bed Wetting	Bladder
Incontinence 1	CAFL	666,690,2050,2128,2250,		Bed Wetting	Bladder
Incontinence 2	XTRA	465,660,690,727.5,787,802,880,1550,10000,		Bed Wetting	Bladder
Bladder Infection	XTRA	1.1,1.2,9.39,9.4,10,20,40,72,73,95,125,246,250,360,444,465,498,530,600,625,630,642,650,660,690,724,726,727.5,771,776,787,802,832,880,1500,1550,1600,1800,1865,2045,2127.5,2170,2250,2720,10000,	Proteus Vulgaris, P. Mirabilis, and P. Penneri includes pathogens responsible for many human urinary tract infections.	Infection	Bladder
Urinary Tract Infection - Cystitis	BIOM	246.0; 1550.0; 880.0; 802.0; 787.0; 727.0; 465.0; 20.0; 126.0; 597.0; 629.0; 682.0; 847.0; 867.0; 635.0; 329.0; 9888.5; 1045.0; 2145.0; 8847.5; 8855.5; 2050.0; 82.3; 165.0; 352.0		Infection	Bladder
Cystitis		*It can be caused by Escherichia coli, Streptococcus, Proteus, Klebsiella, Serratia, Enterobacter, Pseudomonas or other bacteria and can be exacerbated by Candida .*			
Cystitis	XTRA	9.39,9.4,20,465,498,530,630,660,690,727.5,787,802,880,1550,2045,	Urinary tract infection (UTI).	Cystitis	Bladder
Cystitis Bladder	XTRA	20,465,727,787,800,880,1550,5000,	Urinary tract infection (UTI).	Cystitis	Bladder
Cystitis	BIOM	2.8; 3.3; 3.8; 8.1; 9.4; 9.19; 52.75; 53; 53.5; 62; 62.5; 64.8; 68.5; 75.5; 84; 85; 86; 87.5; 90; 91.5; 97.5		Cystitis	Bladder
Cystitis, basic	BIOM	2020; 1550; 880; 802; 800; 787; 727; 465; 246; 20; 8.1; 9.4		Cystitis	Bladder
Cystitis 1	BIOM	2.2; 10.0; 12.5; 19.5; 26.0; 49.0; 55.0; 92.5		Cystitis	Bladder
Cystitis 2	BIOM	7.0; 9.4; 19.5; 40.5; 46.0; 50.0		Cystitis	Bladder
Cystitis 3	BIOM	2.8; 3.3; 8.1; 9.19; 54.0; 54.25; 54.5		Cystitis	Bladder
Cystitis 4	BIOM	2.8; 3.3; 3.8; 8.1; 9.4; 9.19; 52.75; 53.0; 53.5; 62.0; 62.5; 64.8; 68.5; 75.5; 84.0; 85.0; 86.0; 87.5; 90.0; 91.5; 97.5		Cystitis	Bladder
Cystitis 5	BIOM	0.7; 0.9; 2.5; 2.65; 3.3; 9.8; 56.0; 69.0		Cystitis	Bladder
Cystitis 6	BIOM	2.5; 3.6; 3.9; 5.0; 6.3; 8.1; 34.0; 92.0		Cystitis	Bladder
Cystitis, complex	BIOM	246; 1550; 880; 802; 787; 727; 465; 20; 126; 597; 629; 682; 847; 867; 635; 329; 9888.5; 1045; 2145; 8847.5; 8855.5; 2050; 82.3		Cystitis	Bladder
Chronic Cystitis	BIOM	246.0; 1550.0; 880.0; 802.0; 787.0; 727.0; 465.0; 20.0		Cystitis	Bladder
Cystitis Chronic	BIO	246	Long-term inflammation of the urinary bladder and ureters.	Cystitis	Bladder
Cystitis Chronic	CAFL	246,1550,880,802,787,727,465,20,	As mentioned above	Cystitis	Bladder
Cystitis, Interstitial	EDTFL	80,200,750,17930,119000,255560,372580,551230,673290,713720,		Cystitis	Bladder
Cystitis, Chronic Interstitial	EDTFL	80,200,750,17930,119000,255560,372580,551230,673290,713720,	Also called Bladder Pain Syndrome.	Cystitis	Bladder
Hematuria	EDTFL	30,700,830,890,2500,32500,305050,431200,632590,723020	Presence of blood in urine. May signal kidney stones or a tumor in the urinary tract.		Bladder
Bladder Exstrophy	EDTFL	160,800,7500,30000,67500,125000,352930,687620,712810,992000	Protrusion of bladder through abdominal wall.		Bladder
Cysto Pyelo Nephritis	VEGA	1385	Inflammation of bladder, pelvis of kidney, and kidney. Also see Pyelonephritis.		Bladder
Urinary bladder tuberculosis	BIOM	642; 771; 360; 726; 724			Bladder
Vesico-Ureteral Reflux	EDTFL	70,120,900,20000,40000,134250,357770,510250,752600,923700	Backflow of urine from bladder to kidneys, leading to UTIs (see UTI sets) and Pyelonephritis - see set. Also see Cysto Pyelo Nephritis.	Urethra	Bladder
Inflammation Urethra	XTRA	1.1,1.19,9.39,9.4,10,20,40,72,73,95,125,246,250,360,444,465,498,530,600,625,630,642,650,660,690,724,726,727.5,771,776,787,802,832,880,1500,1550,1600,1800,1865,2045,2127.5,2170,2250,2720,10000,		Urethra	Bladder

Subject / Argument	Author	Frequencies	Notes	Origin	Target
Urethral Stenosis	EDTFL	140,220,950,5250,12710,45000,97700,150000,7 22700,875800	Narrowing of urethra due to injury, medical procedures, infection, and some non-infectious types of Urethritis (see set).	Urethra	Bladder
Urethritis	CAFL	2720,2170,2127,1800,1600,1550,802,1500,880, 832,787,776,727,660,650,625,600,465,444,1865 ,125,95,72,1.2,	Inflammation of urethra. See Vaginosis, and Chlamydia Trachomatis sets.	Urethra	Bladder
Urethritis	BIOM	2720; 2160; 2127; 1800; 1600; 1550; 802; 1500; 880; 832; 787; 776; 727; 650; 625; 600; 465; 444; 1865			Bladder
Urethritis	EDTFL	140,320,950,5250,12710,45000,97700,150000,4 75090,985670	As mentioned above	Urethra	Bladder
Urethritis, desquamative	BIOM	9.4; 15.5; 19.5; 75.5; 88			Bladder
Urethrities, acute	BIOM	1.7; 3.6; 10; 15.5; 53.5; 75.5; 88			Bladder
Urogenital Urogenital Surgical Procedures	EDTFL	490,730,800,2500,7500,20000,50000,125710,37 7910,519340			Bladder

15 - Reproductive System and Genital apparatus

Subject / Argument	Author	Frequencies	Notes	Origin	Target
Reproductive System	XTRA	9,			Reproductive
Reproductive	CAFL	335,536,622,712			Reproductive
Reproductive	VEGA	622			Reproductive
Female Reproductive Disorders (General)	EDTFL	150,220,1210,5260,9570,21150,43290,193280,3 29080,488920			Reproductive System
Male Reproductive Disorders (General)	EDTFL	220,1820,3290,9030,34710,108330,288320,355 720,407330,629080			Reproductive System
Infertility of men	BIOM	5000; 10000; 2008; 2127; 880; 802; 787; 727; 690; 666; 650; 625; 600; 465; 40; 9.39			Reproductive System
Infertility	CAFL	2127,2008,465,880,802,787,727,690,666,650,62 5,600,9.39,	Can be caused by an infection of the endometrium with the A variant of human Herpesvirus 6 virus (HHV-6A).		Reproductive System
Infecundity	BIOM	2127; 2008; 465; 880; 802; 787; 727; 690; 666; 650; 625; 600; 98; 9.4			Reproductive System
Infertility	EDTFL	880,1840,5610,152300,328920,422210,482130, 532930,553700,595420	Inability to produce or fertilise a human egg. Also see Impotence (men), and Frigidity (women).		Reproductive System
Sterility	EDTFL	70,780,1300,21900,65190,322060,479930,5270 00,667000,742000,			Reproductive
Infertility 1	XTRA	9.39,9.4,335,465,536,600,622,625,650,660,690, 712,727.5,787,802,880,1550,2008,2127.5,	As mentioned above		Reproductive System

15a - Genitals

Subject / Argument	Author	Frequencies	Notes	Origin	Target
Sexuality	XTRA	9,221.23			Sex
Sexual center	BIOM	55			Sex
Libido	BIOM	97			Sex
Sexual Libido Boost	EDTFL	60,520,15170,42500,125710,376290,514350,68 2450,759830,918500			Sex
Women's libido	BIOM	2.5; 38			Sex
Women's lust	BIOM	19			Sex
Uteromania	BIOM	97.5			Sex
Men's libido	BIOM	4.5; 51; 51.5; 57			Sex
Men's lust	BIOM	57			Sex
Men's sexual regulation	BIOM	51; 57			Sex
Sexual excitement	BIOM	32			Sex
Sex Polarity Balance	CAFL	10000			Sex
Sexual Disorders (General Set)	EDTFL	70,780,1300,21900,65190,322060,479930,5270 00,667000,742000			Sex
Sexual Disorders [Frigidity]	EDTFL	220,970,7500,85190,95750,96500,175000,5243 70,655200,995200,			Sex
Sexual anesthesia	BIOM	20; 97; 625			Sex
Frigidity Female	CAFL	10000,20		Frigidity	Sex
Frigidity	XTRA	1.1,9.39,9.4,20,72,73,95,		Frigidity	Sex
Frigidity	EDTFL	30,140,930,7500,30000,147500,262500,315610, 505680,756500		Frigidity	Sex
Sexual Regulation - Female	BIOM	12.5; 38		Frigidity	Sex
Sexual Dysfunctions, Psychological	EDTFL	220,970,7500,85190,95750,96500,175000,5243 70,655200,995200			Sex
Sexual disfunction	BIOM	2127; 2008; 880; 802; 787; 727; 690; 666; 650; 625; 600; 465; 125; 95; 73; 72; 39; 20; 9			Sex
Paraphilias	EDTFL	80,330,1070,5200,27530,102380,145470,20305 0,486100,535910	Intense sexual arousal by atypical objects, situations, or individuals.		Sex

Subject / Argument	Author	Frequencies	Notes	Origin	Target
Sexual Weakness	CAFL	20,727,880,10000	Male-female.		Sex
Hereditary Sex Derangement	XTRA	5000			Sex
Sexual Diseases	CAFL	20,625,660,727,800,880,1500,1850,			Genitals
Pelvic Inflammatory Disease	BIOM	2950; 2976; 2720; 2489; 2170; 2127; 2008; 1800; 1600; 1550; 1488; 802; 787; 776; 727; 690; 666; 650; 625; 600; 465; 444; 522; 95; 72; 450; 428			Genitals
Inflammation of the Genitourinary Tract	BIOM	5000.0; 2720.0; 2489.0; 1800.0; 1550.0; 802.0; 787.0; 776.0; 727.0; 625.0; 600.0; 522.0; 500.0; 465.0; 444.0; 428.0; 95.0			Genitals
Gonadal Disorders	EDTFL	30,370,950,2500,7500,72500,96500,269740,375 370,377910	Diseases of ovaries or testes - also see Hydrocele, Orchitis, or appropriate organ sets.	Gonads	Genitals
Gonads	XTRA	9	Reproductive glands - ovaries in women, testes in men.	Gonads	Genitals
Genital Glands - Male	BIOM	51.0; 51.5; 57.0			Genitals
Genital Glands - Female	BIOM	98.0; 98.5; 98.75			Genitals
Gonads Inflammation 1	CAFL	9,20,72,95,125,600,625,650,666,690,727,776,78 7,802,832,880,1500,1550,	Inflammation of ovaries or testes - also see Hydrocele, Orchitis, or appropriate organ sets.	Gonads	Genitals
Gonads Inflammation 2	XTRA	727,787,880,10000	As mentioned above	Gonads	Genitals
Hypogonadism	EDTFL	30,500,850,7500,8000,127500,326600,525790,7 25000,825790	Diminished function of ovaries/testes with consequent lower levels of sex hormones.		Genitals
Phimosis	EDTFL	260,7500,22500,35050,95000,375330,424370,5 63190,714830,978050	Condition where penis foreskin cannot be fully retracted over the glans penis. May also refer to clitoral phimosis, whereby the clitoral hood cannot be retracted.		Genitals
Smegma	CAFL	153,180,638	Combination of shed skin cells, skin oils, and moisture occurring in female and male mammalian genitalia.		Genitals
Smegma	VEGA	180	As mentioned above		Genitals
Sexually Transmitted Diseases, Bacterial	EDTFL	40,410,730,900,65170,234250,300000,479500,5 27000,838900		Infections	Genitals
Venereal Diseases [Group 3]	EDTFL	950,23250,45560,47500,173210,182500,275030 ,367500,388900,456110,		Infections	Genitals
STD Comprehensive, Herpes, Gonorrhea, Syphilis, Chlamydia, HPV, HIV Symptoms	EDTFL	950,23250,45560,47500,173210,182500,275030 ,367500,388900,456110		Infections	Genitals
Chancre	XTRA	177,600,625,650,658,660,789,900,2776,6600,	Painless sore associated with syphilis or African Trypanosomiasis.		Genitals
Chancroid Ulcers	XTRA	727,776,787,880	STD (Sexually Transmitted Disease) with painful genital sores.		Genitals
Hard chancre	BIOM	177; 650; 625; 600; 658; 789; 900; 2776; 6600			Genitals
Chancroid	EDTFL	40,400,680,5090,7500,37000,180000,325650,79 2000,985670	STD with painful genital sores.		Genitals
Dyspareunia [Sexual Disorders]	EDTFL	220,970,7500,85190,95750,96500,175000,5243 70,655200,995200,	Painful sexual intercourse due to medical or psychological causes.		Genitals
Syphilis			Use Treponema Pallidum, and see Section 17c - Bacteria	Syphilis	Genitals
Luesinum and Syphilinum	CAFL	177,600,625,650,658,660,	Homeopathic. See Syphilis.	Syphilis	Genitals
Luesinum and Syphilinum 2	XTRA	177,600,625,650,658,660,789,900,2776,6600,	Homeopathic. See Syphilis.	Syphilis	Genitals
Luesinum and Syphilinum 3	XTRA	177	Homeopathic. See Syphilis.	Syphilis	Genitals
Vulvar Lichen Sclerosus	EDTFL	30,460,2500,7200,17500,96500,355080,517500, 687670,712420	Disorder with white patches of skin, mostly around genitals. Cause unknown. Also affects males. See Lichen Sclerosus et Atrophicus.		Genitals

Subject / Argument	Author	Frequencies	Notes	Origin	Target

Woman

Subject / Argument	Author	Frequencies	Notes	Origin	Target
Female Genitourinary System	BIOM	2.5; 4; 4.9; 5.5; 9.4; 9.5; 38; 97			

15b - Breast

Subject / Argument	Author	Frequencies	Notes	Origin	Target
Breast Inflammation	XTRA	654,698			Breast
Breast Diseases	EDTFL	150,490,620,800,5110,125000,426700,571000,838000,932000,			Breast
Breast Dysplasia	EDTFL	110,520,950,5250,21000,37500,62500,93500,150000,478500,			Breast
Mastalgia [Breast Pain]	EDTFL	190,490,820,9930,43390,103670,232500,342520,625350,975540,	Breast pain.		Breast
Breast Sore Nipples	XTRA	727,787,880,5000,			Breast
Mastitis	BIO	654	Also called Fibrocystic Breast Disease - see set. Inflammation of breast usually caused by bacteria. Try Staphylococcus Aureus, and other staph and strep sets.	Mastitis	Breast
Mastitis	BIOM	654.0; 698.0; 727.0; 787.0; 880.0; 5000.0		Mastitis	Breast
Mastitis 1	XTRA	654,698	As mentioned above	Mastitis	Breast
Breast Cysts	EDTFL	30,500,870,10470,37110,87500,135230,225680,397500,597500		Cysts	Breast
Breast Fibroid Cysts	CAFL	880,1550,802,787,776,727,690,666,267,1384,	Non-cancerous lump in breast.	Cysts	Breast
Breast Fibroid Cysts 2	XTRA	666,690,727,776,787,802,880,1550,	Non-cancerous lump in breast.	Cysts	Breast
Fibroid Cysts Breast	XTRA	267,660,690,727.5,776,787,802,880,1384,1550,	Non-cancerous breast lumps often related to menstrual cycle. Try Mastitis, and see Fascia sets.	Cysts	Breast
Fibrocyst	BIOM	1550; 1384; 880; 802; 787; 776; 727; 690; 666; 267; 523; 557; 478; 660; 778		Fibrocyst	Breast
Fibrocystic Breast Disease	EDTFL	90,370,910,128500,236500,302250,398400,682020,759830,932410	Non-cancerous breast lumps often related to menstrual cycle. Try Mastitis, and see Fascia sets.	Fibrocyst	Breast
Fibrocystic Mastopathy	EDTFL	90,370,910,128500,236500,302250,491610,651020,708570,879210	As mentioned above	Fibrocyst	Breast
Fibrocystic Mastopathy	BIOM	2128.0; 1550.0; 1384.0; 880.0; 802.0; 787.0; 776.0; 727.0; 690.0; 666.0; 267.0; 2189.0		Fibrocyst	Breast
Mastopathy basic	BIOM	2.5; 2.6; 3; 4; 4.9; 5.5; 9.4; 14.5; 20; 22; 25.5; 42; 49; 64; 63; 79.5; 85.5; 98; 91.5			Breast
Mammary Gland Fibroma	BIOM	5000.0; 1550.0; 880.0; 802.0; 787.0; 776.0; 727.0; 690.0			Breast
Lacteal gland fibromatosis	BIOM	2128; 1550; 1384; 880; 802; 787; 776; 727; 690; 666; 267; 2189			Breast
Breast Fibromatosis 1	XTRA	267,666,690,727,776,787,802,880,1384,1550,	Grouped non-cancerous breast lumps often related to menstrual cycle. Try Mastitis, and see Fascia sets.		Breast
Breast Fibromatosis 2	XTRA	267			Breast
Mammary Fibroid Cyst 1	XTRA	267,666,690,727,776,787,802,880,1384,1550,	Non-cancerous breast lumps often related to menstrual cycle. Try Mastitis, and see Fascia sets.		Breast
Mammary Fibroid Cyst 2	XTRA	666,690,727,776,787,802,880,1550,	As mentioned above		Breast
Breast Neoplasms	KHZ	20,800,5690,32500,85000,95750,150000,210500,759830,927100,			Breast
Fibroadenoma Breast	XTRA	1384	Non-cancerous nodules composed of fibrous and glandular tissue.		Breast
Fibroadenoma	BIOM	2950.0; 2189.0; 2128.0; 2127.0; 2008.0; 1744.0; 1552.0; 1550.0; 1488.0; 1384.0; 1234.0; 880.0; 802.0; 787.0; 776.0; 727.0; 690.0; 666.0; 465.0; 267.0	As mentioned above		Breast
Fibroadenoma Mamanae	CAFL	1384,2128,2189	As mentioned above		Breast
Insufficient Lactation	XTRA	5000			Breast
Galactorrhea	EDTFL	180,190,740,9000,11090,22500,107900,115700,377910,470120,			Breast
Lactation Disorders [Galactorrhea]	EDTFL	180,190,740,9000,11090,22500,107900,115700,377910,470120,			Breast
Hypogalactia	EDTFL	130,540,920,4540,17500,137500,262500,393500,775790,815700			Breast
Zuska's disease	EDTFL	930,2340,21670,55570,231200,293290,482680,653180,704840,855130	Subareolar abscess of the breast or galactophore fistula.		Breast

Subject / Argument	Author	Frequencies	Notes	Origin	Target
			15c - Uterus and Ovaries		
Cervical Inflammation	XTRA	20,60,72,95,125,660,690,727.5,740,787,790,880 ,5000,			Womb
Cervicitis	CAFL	20,727,787,880	Neck of womb inflammation		Womb
Crevicitis	BIOM	20.0; 727.0; 787.0; 880.0; 5000.0			Womb
Cerclage of Uterine / Cervix	EDTFL	20,220,25000,55780,125000,229320,450000,51 5160,712810,993410	Surgical procedure for cervical incompetence.		Womb
Cervix Incompetence	EDTFL	40,250,650,910,2500,7200,96500,450000,51555 9,686210,	Premature dilatation and thinning of cervix causing possible miscarriage or preterm birth.		Womb
Uterine Cervical Incompetence	EDTFL	40,250,650,910,2500,7200,96500,450000,51555 9,686210,	Abnormal changes in cells on surface of cervix.		Uterus
Cervix Dysplasia	EDTFL	40,250,650,910,2500,7200,96500,324940,47587 0,527000			Uterus
Uterus	BIOM	2.5; 3.5; 4; 4.9; 9.4; 9.5; 88; 99.5			Uterus
Urogenital Infections	BIOM	9.4			Uterus
Inflammation of the Uterus	BIOM	99.5			Uterus
Endometriosis 1	CAFL	142,246,275,284=300,438,524,651,676,763,800 ,830,846,854,945,1550=300,1850,2000,2003,20 08,2013,2082,2128,2150,6578,6641,6672,6766,	Growth of uterine tissue outside the uterus that may cause pain, infertility, and abnormal bleeding. Use Parasites General. See Dysmenorrhea and Menstrual Problems.	Endometriosis	Uterus
Endometriosis 2	XTRA	246,800,802,1550	As mentioned above	Endometriosis	Uterus
Endometriosis	EDTFL	130,570,780,12270,68290,355720,434150,5710 00,839000,932000	As mentioned above	Endometriosis	Uterus
Endometrioma	EDTFL	130,570,780,12270,68290,135250,272720,4255 30,733910,836420	Blood-filled cyst in ovary that begins as sloughed endometrial tissue. Also see Endometriosis.	Endometriosis	Uterus
Endometriosis, basic	BIOM	2008; 1850; 1550; 945; 854; 846; 830; 800; 763; 676; 651; 435; 275; 246; 800; 1550		Endometriosis	Uterus
Endometriosis, ecchondral	BIOM	922; 788; 765; 722; 625; 614; 613; 612; 611; 610; 609; 608; 607; 606; 605; 604; 603; 514; 461		Endometriosis	Uterus
Endometreosis	BIOM	6765.5; 6671.5; 6640.5; 6577.5; 2150; 2128; 2082.0; 2013; 2008; 2003; 2000; 1850; 1550; 945; 854; 846; 830; 800; 763; 676; 651; 524; 435; 275; 246; 142		Endometriosis	Uterus
Endometriosis Chronic	CAFL	246,800,1550	Use with Parasites Flukes and General. See Dysmenorrhea and Menstrual Problems sets.	Endometriosis	Uterus
Endometriosis Chronic	BIO	246	As mentioned above	Endometriosis	Uterus
Endometritis Tuberculosa	CAFL	461,514,620,625,722,765,722,765,788,922,	Inflammation of womb lining. See Echo Virus, Dysmenorrhea, and Menstrual Problems sets.	Endometriosis	Uterus
Endometritis Tuberculosa	XTRA	461,514,603,604,605,606,607,608,609,610,611, 612,613,614,620,625,722,765,788,922,	As mentioned above	Endometriosis	Uterus
Pelvic Inflammatory Disease	CAFL	2720,2489,2170,2127,2008,1800,1600,1550,802 ,787,776,727,690,666,650,625,600,465,444,522, 95,72,450,428,	Infection of uterus, fallopian tubes, ovaries, and inside of pelvis, usually by Neisseria Gonorrheae, or Chlamydia Trachomatis (see sets). See Fallopian Tube Infection, Salpingitis, Gonorrhea, and General Antiseptic sets.	Bacteria	Uterus
Pelvic Inflammatory Disease	EDTFL	80,400,830,5470,105000,215470,325510,63100 0,801910,931220	As mentioned above		Uterus
Uterine Cervical Dysplasia	EDTFL	150,550,810,7950,32500,35540,337570,376290, 515500,689930,	Abnormal changes in cells on surface of cervix.		Uterus
Uterine Inversion	EDTFL	40,520,680,830,2500,27500,67500,95750,32265 0,375160	Dangerous but rare childbirth complication where placenta fails to detach on expulsion, turning the uterus inside out.		Uterus
Uterine Prolapse	EDTFL	70,490,600,930,2250,5810,95090,324520,37500 0,525710	Vertical slippage of uterus due to weakening of support ligaments.		Uterus
Amniotic Band Syndrome	EDTFL KHZ	70,180,5620,37500,100000,275160,525710,655 200,750000,926700,	Congenital - due to trapping of fetal limbs by fibrous bands while in utero		Uterus
Amputation, Intrauterine	EDTFL	80,580,620,900,2500,32500,305050,431200,632 590,723010	As mentioned above		Uterus
Ring Constrictions, Intrauterine	EDTFL	130,180,830,5250,127500,212500,335280,5600 00,695950,997500	As mentioned above		Uterus
Streeter Syndrome	EDTFL	130,570,38500,87500,90000,367400,452590,68 4810,712230,997860	As mentioned above		Uterus
Uterine Polyp	CAFL	689	Mass in inner lining of uterus. Can cause menstruation problems.	Polyp	Uterus
Uterine Polyps	EDTFL	1220,3270,4230,6870,9030,74050,103830,2743 50,388320,482230		Polyp	Uterus
Cervical Polyp	CAFL	277,288,867,687,744,	Benign, often asymptomatic growth in cervical canal.	Polyp	Uterus
Ovary	BIOM	2.5; 2.6; 4.0; 4.9; 9.4; 64.0; 98.0			Ovary
Ovaries - Pilot frequencies	BIOM	2.5; 2.6; 4; 4.9; 9.4; 64; 98			Ovary
Ovary	BIOM	4.0; 4.9			Ovary

Subject / Argument	Author	Frequencies	Notes	Origin	Target
Ovaries - dysfunction	BIOM	650; 625; 600; 465; 444; 26; 2720; 2489; 2160; 2127; 2008; 1800; 1600; 1550; 802; 1500; 880; 832; 776; 727; 690; 666; 20			Ovary
Ovarian dysfunction	BIOM	2720; 2489; 2170; 2127; 2008; 1800; 1600; 1550; 1500; 982; 880; 832; 802; 787; 776; 727; 711; 690; 666; 650; 625; 600; 567; 465; 444; 26; 20			Ovary
Ovarian Disorders General	CAFL	650,625,600,465,444,26,2720,2489,2170,2127,2 008,1800,1600,1550,802,1500,880,832,787,776, 727,690,666,20,			Ovary
Ovarian Elimination Stimulation	CAFL	20,800,1550			Ovary
Ovum	BIO	752			Ovary
Adnexitis	CAFL	440,441,522,572,3343,3833,5312,	Swelling of the ovaries or fallopian tubes.	Adnexitis	Ovary
Adnexitis	VEGA	522,572,3343,3833,5312,440,441,	As mentioned above	Adnexitis	Ovary
Adnexitis	EDTFL	40,460,33010,72500,117590,231900,509020,64 5440,798720,915000,	As mentioned above	Adnexitis	Ovary
Adnexitis	BIOM	10000; 2720; 2489; 2160; 1800; 1600; 1550; 802; 880; 787; 727; 650; 600; 440; 600		Adnexitis	Ovary
Adnexitis	BIOM	5311.5; 3833.0; 3343.0; 2489.0; 2127.0; 1600.0; 1500.0; 880.0; 832.0; 802.0; 800.0; 787.0; 776.0; 727.0; 650.0; 625.0; 572.0; 522.0; 465.0; 441.0; 440.0; 20.0; 1.0		Adnexitis	Ovary
Polycystic Ovary Syndrome	EDTFL	170,520,680,830,2500,387500,452500,621810,8 70530,921050,	Symptoms due to high male hormone level in women, including irregular, heavy, or no periods, excess body and facial hair, acne, pelvic pain, trouble conceiving, and patches of thick, darker, velvety skin.		Ovary
Stein-Leventhal Syndrome	EDTFL	180,640,750,19500,28100,52900,201160,27400 0,391000,801210	As mentioned above		Ovary
Puerperal Infection	EDTFL	100,260,680,7500,11020,45000,325430,515700, 653430,750000	Bacterial infection of female reproductive tract following childbirth or miscarriage, commonly by Streptococcus Pyogenes and anaerobic Streptococcus spp, Staphylococcus spp, E Coli, and Clostridium spp.		F. Genitals
Fallopian tubes, inflammation	BIOM	8.5; 13; 29; 89			F. Genitals
Fallopian Tube Infection	XTRA	440,441,522,552,572,3343,3833,5312,			F. Genitals
Salpingitis	EDTFL	180,570,1850,17200,309520,329220,353220,38 7270,575280,724370,	Also see Fallopian Tube Infection, and Pelvic Inflammatory Disease.		F. Genitals

15d - Female pathologies

Subject / Argument	Author	Frequencies	Notes	Origin	Target
Female Disorder	XTRA	727,787,880			F. Genitals
Genital Diseases, Female	EDTFL	50,240,940,950,2500,7500,32500,125370,31934 0,519299,			F. Genitals
Gynecologic Diseases	EDTFL	30,120,930,7500,132340,247520,362530,59652 0,695610,819340			F. Genitals
Menstrual cycle, disturbance	BIOM	20; 22; 42; 49; 63			F. Genitals
Menstrual Problems	CAFL	880,1550,802,787,727,465,20,	Douche with plain water first. See Dysmenorrhea, and Endometriosis sets.		F. Genitals
Menstruation Disorders Menstruation Disturbances	EDTFL	120,230,970,2530,30000,155680,262100,31564 0,527500,725370			F. Genitals
Adenomyosis	EDTFL	30,250,730,3720,7500,35510,62580,125350,672 910,924370,	Presence of glandular tissue in muscle, causing painful and/or profuse menses.		F. Genitals
Amenorrhea	CAFL	10000,880,1550,802,787,760,727,465,20,	Absence of menstruation.	Amenorrhea	F. Genitals
Amenorrhea	BIOM	10000; 1550; 880; 802; 787; 760; 727; 465; 100; 20		Amenorrhea	F. Genitals
Amenorrhoea	BIOM	10000.0; 1550.0; 880.0; 802.0; 787.0; 760.0; 727.0; 465.0; 100.0; 20.0		Amenorrhea	F. Genitals
Algodismenorrhea	BIOM	26.0; 4.9; 1550.0; 880.0; 802.0; 787.0; 727.0; 465.0			F. Genitals
Algodismenorrhea (Pain in emmenia)	BIOM	26; 3.5; 4.9; 1550; 880; 802; 787; 727; 465			F. Genitals
Dysmenorrhea	CAFL	26,4.9,1550,880,802,787,727,465,	Painful menstruation. Use pure water douche during treatment. If no relief after 3rd treatment, use appropriate Endometriosis set(s). See Menstrual Problems.	Dysmenorrhea	F. Genitals
Dysmenorrhea	BIOM	2.5; 3.5; 3.8; 4; 4.9; 5.5; 6.3; 8; 8.5; 9.4; 9.5; 13; 20; 22; 42; 49; 55; 63; 89		Dysmenorrhea	F. Genitals
Dymenorrhoea	BIOM	10000.0; 1550.0; 880.0; 802.0; 787.0; 760.0; 727.0; 465.0; 100.0; 26.0; 20.0; 4.9		Dysmenorrhea	F. Genitals
Dysmenorrhea (of infectious aetiology)	BIOM	10000; 1550; 880; 802; 787; 760; 727; 465; 100; 26; 20; 4.9			F. Genitals
Menstrual Cramps	XTRA	26	Also see Dysmenorrhea, and Endometriosis sets.		F. Genitals
Menstruation, Retrograde	EDTFL	50,910,930,2520,30000,155680,262600,315640, 865830,937410			F. Genitals

Subject / Argument	Author	Frequencies	Notes	Origin	Target
Hypermenorrhea	BIOM	2.5; 3; 9.44			F. Genitals
Hypomenorrhea [menstrual disorder]	EDTFL	120,230,970,2530,30000,155680,262100,315640,527500,725370,			F. Genitals
Polymenorrhea [Menstrual]	EDTFL	120,230,970,2530,30000,155680,262100,315640,527500,725370,	As mentioned above		F. Genitals
Menopause 1	BIOM	2.2; 10.0; 12.5; 19.5; 26.0; 49.0; 55.0; 92.5		Menopause	F. Genitals
Menopause 2	BIOM	7.0; 9.4; 19.5; 40.5; 46.0; 50.0		Menopause	F. Genitals
Menopause 3	BIOM	1.2; 2.5; 3.6; 3.8; 4.0; 4.59; 4.9; 5.5; 6.3; 8.0; 9.4; 9.44; 9.5; 9.6; 15.0; 42.0; 72.0; 88.0; 92.5		Menopause	F. Genitals
Menopause 4	BIOM	2.8; 3.3; 8.1; 9.19; 54.0; 54.25; 54.5		Menopause	F. Genitals
Menopause 5	BIOM	0.7; 0.9; 2.5; 2.65; 3.3; 9.8; 56.0; 69.0		Menopause	F. Genitals
Menopause 6	BIOM	2.5; 3.6; 3.9; 5.0; 6.3; 8.1; 34.0; 92.0		Menopause	F. Genitals
Climax, basic	BIOM	10000; 880; 832; 802; 787; 727; 660; 650; 600; 465; 444; 125; 95; 92.5; 72; 20		Menopause	F. Genitals
Climax basic	BIOM	1.2; 2.5; 3.6; 3.8; 4; 4.59; 4.9; 5.5; 6.3; 8; 9.4; 9.44; 9.5; 9.6; 15; 42; 72; 88; 92.5		Menopause	F. Genitals
Climax, dysmenorrhea	BIOM	1.2; 2.5; 3.6; 3.8; 4; 4.59; 4.9; 5.5; 6.3; 8; 9.4; 9.44; 9.5; 9.6; 15; 42; 72; 88; 92.5		Menopause	F. Genitals
Climax, sweating	BIOM	98.5		Menopause	F. Genitals
Hot Flashes	CAFL	10000,880,787,727	Also called Hot Flushes. Form of flushing due to reduced levels of estradiol, usually seen in menopause..		F. Genitals
Hot Flashes (Hot Flushes)	EDTFL	80,130,350,7500,85000,193930,237500,487500,706210,946500	As mentioned above		F. Genitals
Hot Flashes 2	XTRA	537,660,690,727.5,787,880,10000,	As mentioned above		F. Genitals
Leucorrhoea	BIOM	880; 787; 727			F. Genitals
Cystocele Bladder Prolapse	EDTFL	160,230,7500,30000,67500,125000,352930,563180,642910,930120,	Bladder prolapse, or cystocele, is characterized by protrusion of the bladder through the anterior wall of the vagina.		F. Genitals
Vagina	BIOM	2.5; 9.4; 83			F. Genitals
Vaginosis, vaginitis	BIOM	414; 542; 642; 652; 800; 832; 845; 866; 942; 728; 784; 880; 464			F. Genitals
Vaginosis	CAFL	414,542,642,652,800,832,845,866,942,728,784,880,464,	A non-specific infection. See Gardnerella, Candida, and Trichomonas sets.	Vagina	F. Genitals
Vaginal Disease	EDTFL	400,680,830,5250,7500,35090,96500,175000,519340,689930,		Vagina	F. Genitals
Vagina and uterus prolapse	BIOM	2.5; 9.4; 45.5		Vagina	F. Genitals
Vaginal Prolapse	EDTFL	70,490,600,930,2250,5810,324520,519340,689930,931000		Vagina	F. Genitals
Mycotic vaginosis	BIOM	331; 336; 555; 587; 632; 688; 757; 882; 884; 887		Vagina	F. Genitals
Vaginitis, Monilial	EDTFL	70,2500,5500,25160,45000,125090,269710,479930,527000,667000		Vagina	F. Genitals
Vulvar Diseases	EDTFL	400,680,830,5250,7500,35090,96500,175000,519340,689930,		Vagina	F. Genitals
Pruritus Vulvae	EDTFL	170,720,1650,16850,55250,127500,455870,565000,752000,975310,	Genital itch (vulval).	Vagina	F. Genitals
Candidiasis Vulvovaginal	EDTFL	30,460,17500,27500,40000,85160,95000,150000,210500,434170	Also called Vaginal Thrush.	Yeast	F. Genitals
Moniliasis Moniliasis, Vulvovaginal	EDTFL	20,220,900,7500,22700,85370,155470,285000,416500,605410	Candidiasis	Yeast	F. Genitals
Episiotomy	EDTFL	70,190,870,900,5710,7250,22500,97500,375350,500000	Surgical incision of perineum during childbirth.		F. Genitals
Hydatidiform Mole	EDTFL	70,350,700,5590,17250,22500,150000,413020,550000,719340	Also called Molar Pregnancy. Abnormality in which a non-viable fertilized egg implants in the uterus and will fail to come to term.		F. Genitals
Hyperemesis Gravidarum	EDTFL	70,350,500,600,2720,5500,50000,62500,90000,95670	Intractable nausea, vomiting, and dehydration in pregnant women which can last till the birth.		F. Genitals
Rhesus Gravidatum	CAFL	312,322,536,684	Rhesus disease is a condition where antibodies in a pregnant woman's blood destroy her baby's blood cells.		F. Genitals
Hydramnios	EDTFL	60,370,870,7500,8000,62500,95550,325870,473000,742060	Excess of amniotic fluid in the amniotic sac, seen in about 1% of pregnancies.		F. Genitals
Polyhydramnios	EDTFL	60,370,870,7500,8000,62500,95550,325870,473000,742060,	As mentioned above		F. Genitals
Embryopathies	EDTFL	150,190,780,7500,68000,115440,327700,545430,612370,779930,	Developmental disorders or diseases in embryos.		F. Genitals
Fetal diseases (General)	EDTFL	20,500,890,172500,207500,315230,425620,691220,735540,962070	As mentioned above		F. Genitals
Polyhydramnios	EDTFL	170,180,870,2750,22010,41580,187520,265290,692500,742060			F. Genitals

Man

Subject / Argument	Author	Frequencies	Notes	Origin	Target
Male Genitourinary System	BIOM	2.6; 4; 4.5; 4.9; 9.4; 19.5; 55; 97			
Regulation of men's urogenital system	BIOM	2.6; 4; 4.9; 5.5; 9.4; 19.5; 57			
Hormone Balance - Male	BIOM	3.5			
Prostate gland and urinary bladder regulation	BIOM	4; 4.9; 9.4; 20; 60; 72; 73; 95			
Regulation of testicle and prostate gland function	BIOM	2.6; 4; 9.4			

15e - Prostate

Subject / Argument	Author	Frequencies	Notes	Origin	Target
Prostate	CAFL	727,787,880,5000			Prostate
Prostate Gland	CAFL	5000	Stimulate.		Prostate
Prostate Gland	BIOM	2.6; 4; 4.9; 9.4; 19.5			Prostate
Prostatitis and urinary bladder	BIOM	880; 1550; 802; 787; 727; 465; 72; 20; 9.39			Prostate
Prostate Complaints	CAFL	9.39,20,72=360,73,95,125,465,666,690,727=360,880,2008,2127,	See Prostatitis and other prostate sets. Use Streptococcus General, and Propionibacterium Acnes, and practise metals avoidance.		Prostate
Prostate Problems	XTRA	9.4	As mentioned above		Prostate
Prostate Problems General	PROV	2720,2128,2008,880,802,787,728,727,690,666,465,408,125,95,72,20,9,	See Streptococcus sets, and practise metals avoidance.		Prostate
Prostate Enlarged	PROV	2250,2128,2050,920,690,666,	See Prostatitis and other prostate sets. Use Streptococcus General, and Propionibacterium Acnes, and practise metals avoidance.		Prostate
Prostate – Enlarged	EDTFL	180,220,3520,13810,7500,88500,151790,285000,335790,819340	As mentioned above		Prostate
Prostate – Infection / Pain	EDTFL	180,220,3520,13810,7500,88500,151790,285000,335790,839340	As mentioned above		Prostate
Benign Prostatic Hyperplasia	BIOM	2720.0; 2489.0; 2127.0; 2008.0; 1550.0; 802.0; 787.0; 776.0; 727.0; 465.0; 444.0; 410.0; 125.0; 100.0; 95.0; 72.0			Prostate
Prostate Hyperplasia	PROV	920,	Non-cancerous enlargement of prostate.		Prostate
Prostate gland, sclerosis	BIOM	9.4; 17; 28; 85; 85.5			Prostate
Prostate Tumor	CAFL	666,690,727,2008,2127,	Malignant. See Cancer prostate sets.		Prostate
Prostatic Diseases	EDTFL	180,220,3520,7500,13810,40000,275650,475680,527000,667000,	Disorders include Prostate Cancer, Prostatitis, and Prostate Hyperplasia (see sets).		Prostate
Prostate Adenominum	PROV	442,688,1875,748,766,920,	Homeopathic remedy for prostate tumor.		Prostate
Prostatitis	CAFL	100,410,522,146,2720,2050,2489,2170,2127,2008,1550,802,787,776,727,690,666,465,125,95,72,20,444,522,9.1,	Inflammation of prostate. Can be caused by Mycoplasma Hominis, Neisseria gonorrhoeae, Chlamydia trachomatis, Escherichia coli, Enterobacter aerogenes, Serratia marcescens, Pseudomonas aeruginosa, Proteus mirabilis.	Prostatitis	Prostate
Prostatitis 1	CAFL	2050,2250	Inflammation of prostate.	Prostatitis	Prostate
Prostatitis basic	BIOM	1.7; 2.5; 2.6; 3.3; 3.6; 4; 4.9; 7; 9.4; 19; 19.5; 20; 46; 51; 57; 60; 72; 73; 79.5; 88.5; 93.5; 95; 97		Prostatitis	Prostate
Prostatitis	BIOM	9.39; 2127; 2008; 727; 690; 666; 465; 880; 787; 727; 125; 95; 73; 72; 20		Prostatitis	Prostate
Prostatitis	BIOM	100; 410; 522; 146; 2720; 2489; 210; 2127; 2008; 1550; 802; 787; 776; 727; 690; 666; 465; 444; 522; 125; 95; 72; 20; 9.1		Prostatitis	Prostate
Prostatitis 1		2.2; 10.0; 12.5; 19.5; 26.0; 49.0; 55.0; 92.5		Prostatitis	Prostate
Prostatitis 2		2.5; 2.6; 4.0; 4.9; 9.4; 51.0; 57.0; 97.0		Prostatitis	Prostate
Prostatitis 3		2.8; 3.3; 8.1; 9.19; 54.0; 54.25; 54.5		Prostatitis	Prostate
Prostatitis 4		1.7; 3.3; 3.6; 4.0; 4.9; 7.0; 9.4; 19.0; 19.5; 20.0; 46.0; 60.0; 72.0; 73.0; 79.5; 88.5; 93.5; 95.0		Prostatitis	Prostate
Prostatitis 5		0.9; 2.5; 2.6; 3.3; 6.0; 8.5; 9.8; 56.0		Prostatitis	Prostate
Prostatitis 6		2.5; 3.6; 3.9; 5.0; 6.3; 8.1; 34.0; 92.0		Prostatitis	Prostate
Prostatitis with complications	BIOM	2050; 2250; 666; 690; 465; 298; 249; 200		Prostatitis	Prostate
Congestion prostatitis, hyperplasia	BIOM	727; 690; 666; 920		Prostatitis	Prostate
Congestion Prostatitis	BIOM	2250; 2128; 2050; 920; 690; 666		Prostatitis	Prostate
Prostatitis, dishormonal	BIOM	1.7; 3.3; 3.6; 4; 4.9; 7; 9.4; 19; 19.5; 20; 46; 60; 72; 73; 79.5; 88.5; 93.5; 95		Prostatitis	Prostate

Subject / Argument	Author	Frequencies	Notes	Origin	Target
Androgen Insensitivity Syndrome	EDTFL	60,7500,67500,95000,357250,376290,475050,6 65340,761850,987230,	Impairs male sexual development		M. Genitals
Testicular Feminization	EDTFL	120,900,5250,27500,57500,83580,222530,4251 10,571000,937410			M. Genitals
Femininity Inner (Male)	XTRA	420.82			M. Genitals
Sexual Dysfunction Men	CAFL	9.39,20,72,73.95,124,465,600,625,650,666,690, 727,787,802,880,2008,2112,2127,	See Erectile Dysfunction, Impotence, Nitric Oxide Generate, and Sacral, Zinc Etc. Also see Circulation, and Circulatory sets, and Orchitis.	Erectile Dysf.	M. Genitals
Erectile Dysfunction	EDTFL	60,520,15170,42300,125710,376260,514350,68 2450,759830,918500,	Also see Impotence and Circulatory Stasis sets.	Erectile Dysf.	M. Genitals
Sexual (Male) erectile dysfunction	EDTFL	60,520,15170,42300,125710,376260,514350,68 2450,759830,918500	As mentioned above	Erectile Dysf.	M. Genitals
Psychopotency	BIOM	5.5; 6.3; 19; 27.5; 92.5; 93.5; 95; 98.5		Erectile Dysf.	M. Genitals
Impotence	CAFL	9.39,2127,2008,465,10000,880,802,787,727,690 ,666,125,95,73,72,20,650,625,600,	Not sterility but failure to achieve or maintain erection. Use Circulatory Stasis.	Erectile Dysf.	M. Genitals
Potency, weakening	BIOM	14; 15.5; 55; 55.5; 57; 19.5		Erectile Dysf.	M. Genitals
Impotency	BIOM	9.4; 2127; 2008; 465; 880; 802; 787; 727; 690; 666; 125; 95; 73; 72; 20; 650; 625; 600		Erectile Dysf.	M. Genitals
Strengthening of potency	BIOM	9.4; 20; 50; 55; 72; 73; 95; 97		Erectile Dysf.	M. Genitals
Impotence 2	XTRA	1.1,9.39,9.4,20,72,73,95,124,125,335,465,536,6 00,622,625,650,660,690,712,727.5,787,802,880, 1550,2008,2127.5,10000,	As mentioned above	Erectile Dysf.	M. Genitals
Nitric Oxide Generate	XTRA	32,64,128	For Erectile dysfunction.	Erectile Dysf.	M. Genitals
Sacral, Zinc, etc.	ALT	32,64,128,147,210.42,256,272,303,324,337,384, 400,440,448,480,537,586,635,999,1444=1200,1 351,1413,1534,1550,	Impotence support (males).	Erectile Dysf.	M. Genitals
Penis	BIOM	15.5			M. Genitals
Foreskin	BIOM	75			M. Genitals
Idiopathic Scrotal Calcinosis	EDTFL	120,260,700,2490,31000,72750,122500,282810, 357770,426160,	It is a skin condition characterized by calcification of the skin resulting from the deposition of calcium and phosphorus that occur on the scrotum.		M. Genitals
Penile Induration	EDTFL	30,120,920,2750,12710,50000,321150,325440,4 33630,560000	Also called Peyronie's Disease (see set) and Fibrous Cavernitis (see Cavernitis Fibrous). Abnormal curvature of penis.		M. Genitals
Cavernitis, Fibrous [Peyronies]	EDTFL	100,350,950,13610,27500,47520,60000,110250, 425050,932000,	Also called Peyronie's Disease and Penile Induration. Abnormal curvature of penis.		M. Genitals
Peyronie's Disease	EDTFL	100,350,950,13610,27500,47520,60000,110250, 425050,932000	As mentioned above		M. Genitals
Genital Diseases, Male	EDTFL	50,240,940,950,2500,7500,32500,125370,67223 0,775870,			M. Genitals
Male Urogenital Diseases	EDTFL	130,310,820,7190,29330,35640,83200,93200,20 4340,534320			M. Genitals
Penile Diseases	EDTFL	170,180,830,2500,27500,73980,135410,367020, 497500,625830	As mentioned above		M. Genitals
Seminal Vesiculitis	XTRA	393,433,2712	Inflammation of seminal vesicles, glands which contribute to semen manufacture. Usually bacterial. Can be caused by Gonococco, Streptococco, Enterococco, Trichonomas.		M. Genitals
Balanitis	EDTFL	30,250,930,7500,13610,95000,310250,451170,5 19679,688290,	Inflammation of the glans penis, with many possible causes.		M. Genitals
Hypospadias	EDTFL	130,260,800,5500,20000,32500,45680,57700,92 500,93500	Birth defect in males where the urethra is not located on top of the glans penis.		M. Genitals
Testicles	BIOM	2.6; 4; 4.5; 4.9; 9.4; 14; 51			M. Genitals
Testicles, inflammation	BIOM	2720; 2489; 210; 2127; 2008; 1800; 1600; 1550; 802; 1500; 880; 832; 787; 776; 727; 690; 666; 650; 625; 600; 125.5; 72; 20			M. Genitals
Spermatic Cord Torsion	EDTFL	310,600,6000,32500,67500,97500,325750,5193 40,691230,754190	Twisting of spermatic cord, cutting off testicle's blood supply.		M. Genitals
Hydrocele	CAFL	880,787,727	Fluid in body cavity. Most common is Hydrocele testis, affecting the testicles. Also see Gonads Inflammation and Orchitis sets.	Hydrocele	M. Genitals
Hydrocele	BIOM	2.5; 2.6; 4; 4.9; 9.4		Hydrocele	M. Genitals
Hydrocele 1	XTRA	727,787,880,10000	As mentioned above	Hydrocele	M. Genitals
Hydrocele 2	XTRA	660,690,727.5,787,80,	As mentioned above	Hydrocele	M. Genitals
Hydrocele 3	XTRA	727,787,880	As mentioned above	Hydrocele	M. Genitals
Varicocele	EDTFL	180,930,3730,42500,71500,96500,323500,4340 00,642910,983170	Abnormal enlargement of testicular veins which can cause Infertility - see sets.		M. Genitals
Orchitis	CAFL	2720,2489,2170,2127,2008,1800,1600,1550,802 ,1500,880,832,787,776,727,690,666,650,625,60 0,125,95,72,20,9,	Inflammation of testes due to TB, Mumps, Gonorrhea, Cancer, bacteria, etc. See causative condition if known. See Gonads inflammation, Testicle Fluid, Testicular Diseases, and Hydrocele sets.	Orchitis	M. Genitals

Subject / Argument	Author	Frequencies	Notes	Origin	Target
Orchitis Secondary	CAFL	**727,787,880,10000**	As mentioned above	Orchitis	M. Genitals
Testicular Diseases	EDTFL	120,900,5250,27500,57500,222530,425110,571500,838000,937410			M. Genitals
Testicular Torsion	EDTFL	120,900,5250,27500,57500,222530,425110,571000,838000,937420			M. Genitals
Testicle Fluid	CAFL	**727,787,880**	See Hydrocele, Orchitis, Gonads, Gonadal Disorders, and Testicular Diseases sets.		M. Genitals
Cryptorchidism	EDTFL	40,170,780,1210,52780,122850,328850,487500,725790,915700,	Absence of one or both testicles from scrotum - usually undescended.		M. Genitals
Epididymitis	CAFL	2250,1500,880,787,727,20,	Inflammation of testicle area, ducts. Also see Orchitis set. Can be caused by **Chlamydia trachomatis, Gonorrea** e **Candida albicans**.		M. Genitals
Epididymitis	EDTFL	30,180,930,970,5500,10890,93000,210500,424370,978050	As mentioned above		M. Genitals
Epididymitis 2	XTRA	20,660,690,727.5,787,880,1500,	As mentioned above		M. Genitals
Hematospermia	EDTFL	20,410,940,2750,5860,15560,73300,192500,533630,734250	Presence of blood in semen. Most often benign, but thought to be a slight predictor of prostate cancer.		M. Genitals
Gonorrhea			See Section **17c - Bacteria and Diseases**		M. Genitals
Testosterone and hormones			See Section **7 - Endocrine System**		M. Genitals

Subject / Argument	Author	Frequencies	Notes	Origin	Target

16 - Neoformation

Polyp :is a pathological excrescence that is formed on a mucosa, a synovial or serous within the connective, projecting into a body cavity or into a channel.

Cysts: is a cavity or bag, normal or pathological, closed by a membrane distinct, containing a liquid material or semi-solid.

Tumor or neoplasia: is an abnormal cell proliferation and may be limited to the site of origin, or it can give rise to metastases.

Adenoma : is a benign epithelial tumor whose cells take on the appearance of a gland, or deriving glandular epithelium of an organ.

Neuroma : (more properly called traumatic neuroma) is a non-neoplastic proliferation, but hyperplastic, of Schwann cells and nerve fibers, which follows to a trauma to a peripheral nerve which has led to its complete interruption and that is the outcome of a attempt ineffective regeneration of the nerve itself.

Cancer: only indicates a malignant tumor can produce metastases.

Carcinoma: malignant tumor of epithelial origin, or malignancy that is derived from any epithelial tissue, be it fabric lining (mucous membranes, skin) or glandular.

Sarcoma: cancer of the connective tissue, namely of the supporting tissue of the organism.

Lymphoma: a group of lymphoid tissue tumors (T and B lymphocytes and their precursors).

Melanoma: malignant tumor that originates in melanocytes, the skin cells that is responsible for the synthesis of melanin.

16a - Polyps

Subject / Argument	Author	Frequencies	Notes	Origin	Target
Polyp General	CAFL	522,146,2720,2489,2170,2127,2008,1800,1600, 727,690,666,650,625,600,465,444,20,	Abnormal growth of tissue from mucous membrane.		Polyps
Polyps (General)	EDTFL	1220,3270,4230,6870,9030,74050,103830,2743 50,388320,482230			Polyps
Polyopsia [Cerebal Polyopia]	EDTFL	70,410,730,5860,72500,135000,367500,550300, 725340,920320,		Brain	Polyps
Polyp Nasal	CAFL	542,1436		Nose	Polyps
Larynx Polyp	XTRA	202,675		Larynx	Polyps
Intestinal Polyps	EDTFL	40,440,620,2750,376910,414190,514210,52700 0,667000,685250		Intestines	Polyps
Gardner Syndrome	EDTFL	200,280,650,2500,3000,7500,96500,336160,534 250,652430,			Polyps
Uterine Polyp	CAFL	689	Mass in inner lining of uterus. Can cause menstruation problems.	Uterus	Polyps
Uterine Polyps	EDTFL	1220,3270,4230,6870,9030,74050,103830,2743 50,388320,482230		Uterus	Polyps
Cervical polypus	BIOM	277; 288; 522; 687; 744		Uterus	Polyps
Cervical Polyp	CAFL	277,288,867,687,744,	Benign, often asymptomatic growth in cervical canal.	Uterus	Polyps
Endometrial Polyps	EDTFL	1220,3270,4230,6870,9030,74050,103830,2743 50,388320,482230		Uterus	Polyps
Cervical Polyp	CAFL	277,288,867,687,744,	Benign, often asymptomatic growth in cervical canal.	Uterus	Polyps
Polyposis Coli, Familial [Colon Cancer]	EDTFL	20,30,40,5030,119340,350000,434330,691270,7 59830,927100,			Polyps
Polyposis Syndrome, Familial	EDTFL	20,750,2420,5350,8520,125690,323650,561500, 795340,953000			Polyps

16b - Cysts

Subject / Argument	Author	Frequencies	Notes	Origin	Target
Cysts	EDTFL	130,200,730,830,18270,20000,85000,95310,122 530,150000,	Closed sac with abnormal walls containing air, fluids, or semi-solids.		Cysts
Cyst Other	XTRA	75,76,543			Cysts
Arachnoid Cysts	EDTFL	160,190,600,2450,4000,56000,221500,225330,3 44500,490000	Cysts in brain meninges or spinal cord.	Brain	Cysts
Leptomeningeal Cysts [Scull Fracture]	EDTFL	80,250,570,7500,10530,12500,40000,173300,32 9370,675000,	As mentioned above	Brain	Cysts
Arachnoid Diverticula	EDTFL	160,190,600,2350,3000,55000,201500,225330,3 44500,490000	As mentioned above	Brain	Cysts
Tarlov Cysts	EDTFL	110,190,410,2250,8300,12050,347950,523000,5 42500,622730	Meningeal cysts in spinal canal containing nerve fibres.		Cysts
Perineurial Cysts	EDTFL	80,320,730,3870,19120,159300,285000,654030, 724340,933910			Cysts
Neurenteric Cyst	EDTFL	150,520,730,13610,125270,255560,372580,551 230,673290,713720			Cysts
Dentigerous Cyst	EDTFL	130,200,730,830,18270,20000,85000,95310,122 530,150000,	Associated with the crown of an unerupted (or partially erupted) tooth.	Teeth	Cysts
Breast Cysts	EDTFL	30,500,870,10470,37110,87500,135230,225680, 397500,597500	Fluid-filled sac in breast. Generally benign.	Breast	Cysts
Breast Fibroid Cysts	CAFL	880,1550,802,787,776,727,690,666,267,1384,	Non-cancerous lump in breast.	Breast	Cysts
Breast Fibroid Cysts 2	XTRA	666,690,727,776,787,802,880,1550,	Non-cancerous lump in breast.	Breast	Cysts
Mammary Fibroid Cyst 1	XTRA	267,666,690,727,776,787,802,880,1384,1550,	Non-cancerous breast lumps often related to menstrual cycle. Try Mastitis, and see Fascia sets.	Breast	Cysts
Mammary Fibroid Cyst 2	XTRA	666,690,727,776,787,802,880,1550,	As mentioned above	Breast	Cysts
Cyst Ovarian	BIO	982	Fluid-filled sac in ovary, sometime causing pain or bloating.	Ovary	Cysts
Ovarian Cyst	CAFL	567,982,711	See Cyst ovarian set.	Ovary	Cysts

Subject / Argument	Author	Frequencies	Notes	Origin	Target
Ovarian Cyst	BIOM	567.0; 982.0; 711.0; 75.0; 76.0; 543.0		Ovary	Cysts
Dermoid Cyst	BIOM	694.0; 719.0; 784.0; 228.0; 231.0; 237.0; 887.0; 2890.0; 222.0; 262.0; 2154.0; 465.0; 488.0; 567.0; 7879.5; 10000.0; 787.0; 747.0; 727.0; 20.0		Ovary	Cysts
Ovarian Cysts	EDTFL	170,520,680,830,2500,387500,452500,621810,870530,921050		Ovary	Cysts
Corpus Luteum Cyst	EDTFL	70,250,2980,38170,132790,199270,332300,659250,670150,781950,		Ovary	Cysts
Cyst Sebaceous 1	XTRA	20,222,228,231,237,262,465,488,567,694,719,727,747,784,787,887,2154,2890,7880,10000,	Due to blocked sebaceous glands, swollen hair follicles, high testosterone, and some steroids.	Skin	Cysts
Cyst Sebaceous 2	XTRA	75,76,543	As mentioned above	Skin	Cysts
Sebaceous Cyst	EDTFL	170,2230,4300,7210,72740,165280,362500,414700,734840,840150		Skin	Cysts
Dermoid Dermoid Cyst	EDTFL	20,200,900,5950,8500,125690,262500,592500,758520,823440,	Tumor, usually benign, that contains tissue types inconsistent with its location.	Skin	Cysts
Epidermal Cyst Epidermoid Cyst	EDTFL	70,180,6750,40870,172690,201250,421500,597500,835350,923070	Benign cyst usually found on skin.	Skin	Cysts
Mediastinal Cyst	EDTFL	60,260,750,2250,7500,52500,329450,371050,373010,687620			Cysts
Pericardial Cyst	EDTFL	170,490,920,9920,42390,105670,232500,342520,625350,975540			Cysts
Thoracic Cyst	EDTFL	50,290,650,6210,7870,45000,135210,302160,329550,409220			Cysts
Thymic Cyst	EDTFL	170,490,770,890,2250,9000,327780,334260,421000,802210		Thyme	Cysts
Tracheal Cyst	EDTFL	160,230,12850,55750,125000,210400,479930,593200,761850,987230	Tumors found in the cavity containing heart, trachea, and esophagus - include neurogenic, thymoma, lymphoma, pheochromocytoma, and germ cell tumors including teratoma, thyroid tissue, and parathyroid lesions.	Trachea	Cysts
Papillomavirus Cyst	XTRA	6.29,110,148,264,634,760,762,767,848,874,907,917,1102,	Also called verrucous cyst, or cystic papilloma. Use Human Papilloma Virus HPV sets.		Cysts
Pilonidal Cyst	EDTFL	180,490,720,950,95500,175330,327150,527000,634000,762400	Painful cyst or abscess near or on the natal cleft of the buttocks that often contains hair and skin debris.		Cysts
Pilonidal Sinus	EDTFL	180,490,720,950,95500,300000,327850,655300,755000,805120			Cysts
Popliteal Cyst [Bakers Cyst]	EDTFL	170,380,8850,57500,117500,237520,357500,691020,810500,915700,	Benign swelling of the semimembranosus or other synovial bursa behind the knee joint. Found in Lyme Disease.	Knee	Cysts
Baker's Cyst	EDTFL	170,380,8850,57500,117500,237520,357500,691020,810500,915700,	As mentioned above	Knee	Cysts
Cyst on artificial limb	BIOM	81.5			Cysts
Solitary Cyst	BIO	75,543	Most commonly manifests as Breast Cyst - see set.		Cysts
Solitary Cyst	VEGA	75	As mentioned above		Cysts
Syringomyelia	EDTFL	70,270,850,35230,63020,125050,235680,396500,575680,751710	Disorder where a cyst or cavity forms within spinal cord, resulting in pain, paralysis, weakness, and stiffness.		Cysts
Hydrosyringomyelia [Syringomyelia]	EDTFL	70,270,850,35230,63020,125050,235680,396500,575680,751710,	As mentioned above		Cysts
Choledochal Cyst, Choledochal Cyst, Type I	EDTFL	50,410,800,7500,125190,275000,424370,560000,642910,985900	Also called bile duct cysts.	Liver	Cysts
Common Bile Duct Cyst	EDTFL	40,130,820,6030,21540,40350,90180,305430,410700,560940		Liver	Cysts

16c - Tumor

Subject / Argument	Author	Frequencies	Notes	Origin	Target
Papillomatosis	EDTFL	50,400,650,7530,12850,17500,72500,233910,426200,571000	Presence of numerous papillomas, benign tumors derived from the exuberant proliferation of the epithelium lining the skin or a mucosa.		Tumor
Tumor Any Kind	XTRA	2127	See Cancer sets.		Tumor
Tumor, General Non Malignant	EDTFL	80,400,730,900,5110,47500,222700,323150,527000,663710			Tumor
Benign Tumor	RL	688	From Dr. Richard Loyd.		Tumore
Tumor Benign	XTRA	1,10,10.19,10.4,10.59,10.8,11,	Also see Cancer sets.		Tumor
Cancer Adenoma	CAFL	433	Benign form of adenocarcinomas. Use Blood Cleanser.	Adenoma	Tumor
Adenoma, basic	BIOM	3.5; 0.4; 4.9; 9.4; 20; 60; 72; 73; 95		Adenoma	Tumor
Adenoma	EDTFL	40,5810,22500,52500,224370,434000,527000,667000,721000,987230,	Benign epithelial tumor with glandular associations.	Adenoma	Tumor
Adenoma, Basal Cell [Salivary Gland Tumor]	EDTFL	120,270,9330,34210,205690,317250,434500,692500,776950,838250,		Adenoma	Tumor
Adenoma, beta-Cell	EDTFL	40,5810,22500,52500,92500,434000,529000,668000,721000,987230,		Adenoma	Tumor

Subject / Argument	Author	Frequencies	Notes	Origin	Target
Adenoma, Papillary [Renal Tumor]	EDTFL	100,520,7500,30000,225030,434150,527000,662710,749000,986220,		Adenoma	Tumor
beta-Cell Tumor	EDTFL	80,570,15750,52500,62500,95000,250000,434370,682020,753070,		Adenoma	Tumor
Adenoma, Follicular [Thyroid Tumor]	EDTFL	180,490,750,950,2500,7500,112360,325950,434290,534250,		Adenoma	Tumor
Adenoma, Microcystic [Pancreatic Tumor]	EDTFL	70,570,23100,50000,375180,434500,527000,667000,753230,986220,	Also called Pancreatic Serous Cystadenoma - benign pancreatic tumour.	Adenoma	Tumor
Adenoma, Monomorphic [Salivary Gland Tumor]	EDTFL	120,270,9330,34210,205690,317250,434500,692500,776950,838250,	Also called Warthin's Tumor - benign cystic tumor of salivary glands.	Salivary glands	Tumor
Angioma	EDTFL	170,240,700,830,2500,17500,432500,555910,625290,775520,	Blood vessel malformation resembling tumor in children, usually benign and self-correcting.	b.vessels	Tumor
Chorioangioma	EDTFL	60,490,570,12000,72500,225000,475190,527000,667000,752700	Vascular tumor (angioma) of the placenta.	b.vessels	Tumor
Hemangioma	EDTFL	60,430,900,7500,8000,77500,187500,358810,721000,986220	Benign tumor of endothelial cells, which normally line blood vessels.	b.vessels	Tumor
Hemangioma, Cavernous	EDTFL	60,430,900,7500,8000,77500,512330,655200,750000,927100	Form of angioma (benign vascular lesion) located in the brain.	b.vessels	Tumor
Hemangioma, Histiocytoid	EDTFL	60,430,900,7500,8000,77500,225300,438950,633100,823410		b.vessels	Tumor
Hemangioma, Intramuscular	EDTFL	60,430,900,7500,8000,77500,325400,450000,695830,895870	Localized intramuscular vascular malformation	b.vessels	Tumor
Hemangioma, Sclerosing	EDTFL	60,430,900,7500,8000,77500,252500,307550,492500,675290	Rare benign neoplasm affecting the skin, found mostly in the legs and less frequently in the hands and feet	b.vessels	Tumor
Port Wine Stain [nevus flammeus]	EDTFL	20,400,900,20000,55000,93500,222700,391500,421220,515700,		b.vessels	Tumor
Angiomyxoma	EDTFL	50,310,1590,5030,7290,125440,321560,625910,732500,815030,	Frequently recurring benign tumor of vulva or pelvis.		Tumor
Breast Fibromatosis 1	XTRA	267,666,690,727,776,787,802,880,1384,1550,	Benign tumor clusters with aggressive growth.	Breast	Tumor
Breast Fibromatosis 2	XTRA	267	Benign tumor clusters with aggressive growth.	Breast	Tumor
Breast Tumors	XTRA	727,787,880,2008,2127,5000,		Breast	Tumor
Tumor, Breast, Non Malignant	EDTFL	80,400,730,900,5110,47500,222700,320250,527000,663710		Breast	Tumor
Breast Tumors Benign	XTRA	174,178,191,405,482,633,731,739.79,785,1132,1234,2959.4,3672,3702,3965,5311,6646,7344,7760,10357,10380,10406.25,		Breast	Tumor
Cementoma	EDTFL	40,570,620,940,7500,295550,487500,605720,723820,935420	Tumor on root of tooth, usually mandibular molar.		Tumor
Cholesteatoma, [Middle Ear Osteoma]	EDTFL	80,800,950,22300,57500,175000,419340,563160,813960,983170,	Benign tumor usually found in middle ear and mastoid region.		Tumor
Middle Ear Cholesteatoma	EDTFL	80,410,800,5250,42500,117500,326520,395680,725000,956500		Ear	Tumor
Cholesteatoma	CAFL	453,618,793,5058	As mentioned above	Ear	Tumor
Cholesteatoma	VEGA	453,618,793	As mentioned above	Ear	Tumor
Chondroma	EDTFL	20,520,700,900,2500,5250,142500,292500,325900,821060	Benign tumor in cartilage.	Cartilage	Tumor
Ollier's Disease Enchondromatosis	EDTFL	170,490,570,5250,13320,20000,35520,60000,93500,315700		Cartilage	Tumor
Enchondrosis, Multiple	EDTFL	420,960,7530,15630,25570,33820,125000,300000,328500,527810			Tumor
Enchondroma Enchondroma, Multiple	EDTFL	460,950,7500,15690,25540,40000,125000,300000,326400,527810	Bone tumor of a benign nature that originates in a cartilage cell of the bone marrow.	Bones	Tumor
Chordoma	EDTFL	180,620,930,9600,17510,162810,292100,317300,433950,805190	Skull and spinal tumours.	Bones	Tumor
Craniopharyngioma	EDTFL	70,200,7500,25160,27250,42500,95950,427500,605000,862020,	Rare brain tumor derived from embryonic pituitary tissue.	Brain	Tumor
Craniopharyngioma [Adamantinous]	EDTFL	80,200,600,2270,27250,42500,95950,427500,605000,862020,	As mentioned above	Brain	Tumor
Craniopharyngioma, Papillary	EDTFL	60,260,950,5130,27250,42500,95950,427500,605000,862020	As mentioned above	Brain	Tumor
Rathke Pouch Tumor	EDTFL	160,450,900,5910,137500,372900,416600,418000,420200,824370	As mentioned above	Brain	Tumor
Ependymoma	EDTFL	20,120,950,12300,13580,41200,245540,262020,692330,892500	Central nervous system tumor, usually intracranial in children and spinal in adults.		Tumor
Ependymoma, Papillary Ependymoma, Myxopapillary	EDTFL	20,120,950,12300,13580,41200,275.83, 419.35, 611.78, 858.52	As mentioned above		Tumor
Fibroids General	CAFL	267,465,666,690,727,776,787,802,880,1384,1488,1550,1744,2008,2127,2128,2189,2950,	Benign smooth muscle tumors. See Parasites General Flukes and Fascia sets.	Fibroma	Tumor

Subject / Argument	Author	Frequencies	Notes	Origin	Target
Fibroid	EDTFL	160,550,900,5580,27500,291240,292000,293050,345500,824370	As mentioned above	Fibroma	Tumor
Fibroid Tumor	EDTFL	160,550,900,5580,27500,291240,584230,684810,712420,995380	As mentioned above	Fibroma	Tumor
Fibroma	CAFL	2127,2008,727,690,666,1550,802,465,	Benign tumor composed of fibrous or connective tissue.	Fibroma	Tumor
Fibroma	BIOM	2127.0; 2008.0; 727.0; 690.0; 666.0; 1550.0; 802.0; 465.0		Fibroma	Tumor
Fibroma 1	XTRA	272,273,465,660,690,727.5,802,1550,2008,2127.5,	As mentioned above	Fibroma	Tumor
Fibroma 2	XTRA	465,660,690,727.5,802,1550,2008,2127.5,	As mentioned above	Fibroma	Tumor
Fibroma 3	XTRA	465,666,690,727,802,1550,2008,2127,	As mentioned above	Fibroma	Tumor
Fibroma Secondary	XTRA	465,802,1550	As mentioned above	Fibroma	Tumor
Fibromatosis, Aggressive Fibromatosis, Juvenile Hyaline	EDTFL	850,900,980,17530,213230,321290,423690,597500,862500,915540	Very rare disease with pearly or tan nodules or papules on face, scalp, and back. Often mistaken for Neurofibromatosis.		Tumor
Desmoid [Fibromatosis]	EDTFL	850,900,980,17530,213230,321290,423690,597500,862500,915540,			Tumor
Fibropendulum	CAFL	661,7465,211,233,766,	Pendulous fibrous tumor of the skin.		Tumor
Gastrointestinal Stromal Tumors	EDTFL	120,200,900,5260,47500,127250,335910,487500,692490,752010,	GI tract connective tissue tumors. Also see Sarcoma, and Cancer Sarcoma sets.		Tumor
GIST [Gastrointestinal Stromal Tumor]	EDTFL	120,200,900,5260,47500,127250,335910,487500,692490,752010,			Tumor
Bannayan-Riley-Ruvalcaba Syndrome	EDTFL	60,260,900,9000,10890,45910,125290,526160,652480,750000,	Multiple non-malignant tumors composed of normal tissue growing in a disorganized mass.		Tumor
Hamartoma	EDTFL	70,200,700,5580,17200,22500,150000,413020,550000,719340,	As mentioned above		Tumor
Hamartoma Syndrome, Multiple	EDTFL	70,200,700,5580,17200,22500,150000,413020,550000,719340,	As mentioned above		Tumor
PTEN Hamartoma Tumor Syndrome	EDTFL	70,200,700,5580,17200,22500,150000,413020,550000,719340,	As mentioned above		Tumor
Cowden Disease [multiple hamartoma]	EDTFL	70,200,700,5580,17200,22500,150000,413020,550000,719340,	As mentioned above		Tumor
Lhermitte-Duclos Disease	EDTFL	50,900,1520,55150,375060,479930,527000,662710,789000,987230	As mentioned above		Tumor
Zollinger-Ellison Syndrome	EDTFL	150,5500,12850,32160,93500,269710,426900,507220,782800,881290	Gastrin-secreting tumor of pancreas (or other abdominal locations) that stimulates acid-secreting cells of stomach with consequent GI ulceration.	Pancreas	Tumor
Insulinoma Insuloma	EDTFL	20,450,650,2210,6150,10230,15910,30250,77500,327110	It is an endocrine tumor of the pancreas that affects beta cells located in the islets of Langerhans, mostly benign.	Pancreas	Tumor
Darier-White Disease	EDTFL	160,550,5860,81500,127550,241520,471500,625300,853000,915090	As mentioned above		Tumor
Seborrheic Keratosis	EDTFL	150,350,620,930,7500,37500,131980,285000,624110,881190,	Flat rounded benign skin tumor originating from keratinocytes that can appear with basal cell carcinoma (see appropriate sets).	Skin	Tumor
Keratosis Seborrheic	EDTFL	150,350,620,930,7500,37500,131980,285000,624110,881190	As mentioned above		Tumor
Fibroid Uterus Fibroids, Uterine	EDTFL	160,550,900,5580,27500,257510,291240,302580,592490,875430,		Uterus	Tumor
Fibroma, Uterine [Fibroid]	EDTFL	160,550,900,5580,27500,257510,291240,302580,592490,875430,		Uterus	Tumor
Leiomyoma [Uterine Fibroids]	EDTFL	160,550,900,5580,27500,257510,291240,302580,592490,875430,	Smooth muscle benign tumor most commonly found in uterus, esophagus, and small bowel.	Uterus	Tumor
Leiomyoma	XTRA	465,666,690,727,802,1550,2008,2127,	As mentioned above	Uterus	Tumor
Fibromyoma	EDTFL	850,900,980,17530,213230,321290,423690,597500,862500,915540	As mentioned above		Tumor
Leiomyosarcoma	EDTFL	110,570,960,5230,23250,37510,262500,523690,691000,797500	Smooth muscle malignant tumor most commonly found in uterus, intestines, blood vessels and skin.		Tumor
Leiomyosarcoma, Epithelioid	EDTFL	150,900,5580,30000,47500,96500,125000,375750,434330,563190,	As mentioned above		Tumor
Leiomyosarcoma, Myxoid	EDTFL	150,900,5580,30000,47500,96500,434220,562500,725690,975230,	As mentioned above		Tumor
Lipoma	BIO	47	Benign, soft tumor of fatty tissue. Use Liver support set.	Lipoma	Tumor
Lipoma	CAFL	47,606,709	As mentioned above	Lipoma	Tumor
Lipoma	EDTFL	130,400,620,3830,35250,132205,282500,327500,522600,748000	As mentioned above	Lipoma	Tumor
Lipomatosis [Multiple Lipoma]	EDTFL	130,400,620,3830,35250,132250,282500,327500,522600,748000,	Also see Adiposis Dolorosa, also known as Dercum's Disease.	Lipoma	Tumor
Lipoma, Pleomorphic	EDTFL	130,400,620,3830,35250,132205,355080,517600,687620,712420	Also see Adiposis Dolorosa, also known as Dercum's Disease.	Lipoma	Tumor

Subject / Argument	Author	Frequencies	Notes	Origin	Target
Adiposis Dolorosa Dercum's Disease	EDTFL	160,970,27500,110250,325000,476500,527000, 665340,749000,985660,	Multiple painful lipomas. See Lipomatosis and Lipoma sets.	Lipoma	Tumor
Hibernoma	EDTFL	160,17850,27500,47500,150000,227000,452520 ,683000,714000,993410		Lipoma	Tumor
Fatty Tumor	EDTFL	260,380,890,6310,11590,48900,181280,327150, 433830,509210		Lipoma	Tumor
Mammary Fibromatosis 1	XTRA	267,666,690,727,776,787,802,880,1384,1550,	Grouped non-cancerous breast lumps often related to menstrual cycle. Try Mastitis, and see Fascia sets.		Tumor
Mammary Fibromatosis 2	XTRA	267	As mentioned above		Tumor
Mammary Tumor Benign	XTRA	174,178,191,405,482,633,731,739.79,785,1132, 1234,2959.4,3672,3702,3965,5311,6646,7344,7 760,10357,10380,10406.25=1800,			Tumor
Mammary Tumor	XTRA	727,787,880,2008,2127,5000,			Tumor
Meningioma	CAFL	446,535,537	Benign, slow-growing tumor of meningeal membranes enveloping brain and spinal cord.	Meningioma	Tumor
Meningioma	VEGA	535	As mentioned above	Meningioma	Tumor
Meningioma	EDTFL	150,230,730,850,5260,127250,335910,487800,6 92470,752010	As mentioned above	Meningioma	Tumor
Benign Meningioma	EDTFL	150,230,730,850,5260,127250,335910,487800,6 92470,752010,	As mentioned above	Meningioma	Tumor
Malignant Meningioma	EDTFL	350,930,7500,17500,52500,70000,215700,3254 00,434000,523010,	As mentioned above	Meningioma	Tumor
Meningiomas, Multiple Meningiomatosis	EDTFL	150,230,730,850,5260,127250,335910,592500,6 25230,723010	As mentioned above	Meningioma	Tumor
Myoma	CAFL	253,420,453,832	Benign tumor of the uterus. Also see Leiomyoma.	Myoma	Tumor
Myoma	VEGA	453,832	As mentioned above	Myoma	Tumor
Myxoma	EDTFL	70,350,700,45000,77220,114690,323000,63708 0,805870,973500	It is a mixoid tumor of primitive connective tissue. It is most commonly formed in the heart.	Myoma	Tumor
Myoma	BIOM	1.7; 2.5; 3.5; 4; 4.9; 8.5; 9.4; 9.5; 12.5; 45.5; 57; 42; 57.5; 79.5; 97.5		Myoma	Tumor
Myoma	BIOM	253; 420; 453; 832		Myoma	Tumor
Myoma, of infectious aetiology	BIOM	253; 420; 453; 832		Myoma	Tumor
Neurilemmoma [Schwannoma]	EDTFL	60,500,980,9000,12850,132500,337500,524370, 758570,955720,	Benign nerve sheath tumor composed of Schwann cells, which normally produce insulating myelin sheath covering peripheral nerves.		Tumor
Neurilemmosarcoma {Nerve Sarcoma]	EDTFL	150,2120,20000,45150,47500,96500,125000,37 5750,434330,563190,	As mentioned above		Tumor
Neurinoma	EDTFL	190,470,500,970,14630,42500,196500,320100,4 52930,777500	As mentioned above		Tumor
Schwannoma	EDTFL	60,500,980,9000,12850,132500,337500,524370, 758570,955720	As mentioned above		Tumor
Schwannomatosis, Plexiform	EDTFL	60,500,980,9000,12850,132500,345750,587500, 695270,875980	As mentioned above		Tumor
Schwannoma, Vestibular	EDTFL	60,500,980,9000,12850,132500,337500,524370, 757570,975340			Tumor
Schwannoma, Acoustic	EDTFL	60,500,980,9000,12850,132500,337500,519340, 524370,653690			Tumor
Neuroma, Acoustic	EDTFL	340,970,2750,15030,71500,196500,275870,419 240,612740,858570	Also called Vestibular schwannoma. Benign intracranial tumor which arises from Schwann cells which create myelin sheaths.		Tumor
Odontogenic Tumors [Epithelial]	EDTFL	80,400,730,900,5110,47500,222700,323150,527 000,663710,	Neoplasms arising out odontogenic (tooth-forming) tissues or cells - also see Cancer sets.	Tooth	Tumor
Papilloma Kidney	CAFL	110,148,264,634,767,848,917,760,762,1102,	Small, usually benign growth on a kidney.	Kidney	Tumor
Rectal Tumors	EDTFL	180,250,5710,18500,41500,126510,434400,526 070,669710,819340			Tumor
Teratoma	EDTFL	300,12710,49000,150000,347500,358570,47950 0,662710,749000,986220	Usually benign tumor that may contain hair, teeth, bone, of other disparate tissues originating from different germ cell layers.		Tumor
Teratoma, Cystic	EDTFL	300,12710,49000,150000,357600,358570,47950 0,662710,749000,986220	As mentioned above		Tumor
Teratoma, Mature	EDTFL	300,12710,49000,150000,357600,358570,47950 0,527000,667000,987230	As mentioned above		Tumor
Teratoid Tumor [Rhabdoid]	EDTFL	160,570,780,950,8500,95640,217520,491000,52 4370,892410,	As mentioned above		Tumor
Dysembryoma	EDTFL	140,350,870,7150,25000,35680,87600,93500,23 4510,519340	As mentioned above		Tumor
Tumor Benign Papilloma Virus	XTRA	6.29,110,148,264,634,760,762,767,848,874,907, 917,1102,	See Cancer, HPV, and Papilloma sets.	Virus	Tumor
Warthin's Tumor [papillary cystadenoma]	EDTFL	30,12710,35330,72500,97500,122530,222700,5 63190,640000,978050,	As mentioned above	Salivary glands	Tumor
Tumor, Malignant [General]	EDTFL	2750,5030,15610,17500,37000,95500,200000,4 34390,739100,905310,	See Heading under Cancer for exact identification		Tumor

Subject / Argument	Author	Frequencies	Notes	Origin	Target
Cancer Prevention	BIOM	3.5; 5; 12.5; 45.5; 53.5; 57; 90; 95			Cancer
Carcinogen	BIOM	10000.0; 2130.0; 2128.0; 2127.0; 2120.0; 2008.0; 880.0; 787.0; 727.0; 690.0; 465.0			Cancer
Neoplasms (All individual listings for Neoplasms are listed under CANCER)	EDTFL	70,550,900,22500,47500,434030,527000,667000,752700,988900	Abnormal growth of a tissue caused by the rapid division of cells that have undergone a certain form of the mutation.		Neoplasms
Dr. Rife's specialized MOR		1860,7270,7660,7870,8020,8450,17220,20060,21270,28160	Uses Dr Rifes 3.30 Mhz MOR Sideband. Cancer and Virus Specific Includes BX Virus Carcinoma, BY Sarcoma, Ecoli, Meningitis, Strep & Staph		Cancer
Dr. Rife RED BEAM RAY		17220,20080,21270,28160,93500,221500,350000,434000,739100,753070			Cancer
Cancer Always	XTRA	11162.11,11503.9	Always include in your targeted Program.		Cancer
Cancer	CAFL	6.8,20,55.56,440,663,778,1050,1550,2180,3672,	Experimental additional frequencies. Use Blood Cleanser.		Cancer
Cancer: Comprehensive RDPV3 GROUP 6	EDTFL	2750,5030,15610,17500,37000,95500,200000,434390,739100,905310,	Focus on Leukemia, Lymphoma, Brain, Sarcomas, Blood, Bone Cancer		Cancer
Cancer	XTRA	10022-10028=2400,5890000,	Basic comprehensive set.		Cancer
Cancer All Tumors	XTRA	727,727.5,728,2008,2128,			Cancer
Cancer 1 Healing	XTRA	568,1538,1829,2726,3445,6149,	See Cancer sets.		Cancer
Cancer Frequencies	XTRA	2127,2008,880,787,727,690,666,			Cancer
Cancer Additional Frequencies 1	CAFL	618,20,55.56,440,663,778,1050,1550,2180,3672,	See Cancer sets. Use Blood Cleanser.		Cancer
Cancer Additional Frequencies 2	CAFL	2180,2182,2184	See Cancer sets. Use Blood Cleanser.		Cancer
Cancer Experimental Additional Frequencies	CAFL	55.56,6.8,440,778,1050,1550,2180,663,3672,	Use Blood Cleanser.		Cancer
Cancer Experimental Additional	XTRA	6.79,55.56,66.5,440,663,778,1050,1550,2180,3672,	Use Blood Cleanser.		Cancer
Cancer Cells	XTRA	0.16-1.35=6250,6.8,440,	0.16-1.34 Hz=inhibit murine malignant tumor growth, induce cancer cell apoptosis, and arrest angiogenesis.		Cancer
Cancer Cell Repair Octal	XTRA	5877968.080734,2938984.040367,1469492.020183,734746.010092,367373.005046,183686.502523,91843.251261,45921.625631,22960.812815,11480.406408,5740.203204,2870.101602,1435.050801,717.5254,358.7627,179.38135	Use sine. Octal sub-harmonics of 380nm light per Dr. Fritz-Albert Popp's biophoton research.		Cancer
Cancer Cell Repair Scalar	XTRA	598209.060162,29783.075377,1482.81201,73.824863	Experimental. Use sine. Scalar sub-harmonics of 380nm light per Dr. Fritz-Albert Popp's biophoton research.		Cancer
Cancer General	RL	93046-93194,128438-128522,136118-136202,2857425-2857575,2944925-2945075	From Dr. Richard Loyd. Includes BX, BY, and tumor reduction frequencies.		Cancer
Cancer: General <SWEEP> Set	EDTFL	60,230,730,32500,90000,175000,321730,653690,753070,922530	Main cancer higher sub-harmonics. Use Blood Cleanser.		Cancer
Cancer General 1	CAFL	10000,5000,3176,2720,2489,2189,2184,2128,2084,2050,2008,880,854,800,784,728,666,524,464,333,304,120,	Use Blood Cleanser.		Cancer
Cancer General 2	CAFL	10000,3176,3176,3040,2720,2489,2182,2127,2048,2008,1862,1552,880,802,786,727,665,664,465,304,125,96,72,64,20,	Use Blood Cleanser.		Cancer
Cancer General 3	CAFL	10000,3176,2720,2489,2180,2128,2049,2008,1865,943,886,866,776,732,728,690,676,650,523,442,414,304,240,128,	Use Blood Cleanser.		Cancer
Cancer General Set 1	CAFL	120,304,464,524,666,728,800,854,880,2008,2050,2084,2128,2184,2489,2720,3176,5000,10000,	Use Blood Cleanser.		Cancer
Cancer General Set 2	CAFL	20,72,96,304,465,664,665,727,786,802,880,1552,1862,2008,2048,2127,2182,2489,2720,3040,3176,10000,	Use Blood Cleanser.		Cancer
Cancer General Set 3	CAFL	128,240,304,414,442,523,650,676,690,728,732,776,866,943,1865,2008,2049,2128,2180,2489,2720,3176,10000,	Use Blood Cleanser.		Cancer
Cancer Basic 1	CAFL	588.2,666,690,727,1250,2008,2127,2128,	Use Blood Cleanser.		Cancer

Subject / Argument	Author	Frequencies	Notes	Origin	Target
Cancer Basic 1	XTRA	20,50,64,72,95=600,96,120,125,128,130,222,227,240,282,304,333,523,768,786,383,413,414,421,430,442,444,1865,464=300,465,484,489,524,555,676,600,625,650,620,644,660,690,727.5=600,712,732,776,779,784,787,800,802,1550,854,875,792,880,886,901,943,957,965,1027,1032,1122,1127,1217=120,1227=120,1320=120,1352=120,1489,1551,1552=120,1722=120,1862=150,1988=90,2006,2008,2013,2048,2049,2050,2084,2098,2123,2126,2127.5,2132,2133,2180,2182,2184,2450,2452,2454,2489,2720,3040,3176=300,3524,5000,6000,6064,9999,10000	Use Blood Cleanser.		Cancer
Cancer Basic 2	CAFL	120,464,524,666,728,800,854,880,**2008**,2048,2084,**2128**,2184,2452,2720,3040,3176,5000,6064,10000,	Use Blood Cleanser.		Cancer
Cancer Basic 2	XTRA	6.79,55.56,95,440,644,660,663,690,727.5,778,901,1050,1352,2008,2098,2127.5,2180,2182,2184,2720,3000,3672,10000,10022,10025,10026,10027,11162,11503.9=900,19611.45,	Use Blood Cleanser.		Cancer
Cancer Basic 3	XTRA	588.2,666,690,727,1250,**2008**,2127,**2128**,11162.11=900,588.2,666,690,727,1250,2008,2127,2128,11162.11=900,11503.9=900,	Use Blood Cleanser.		Cancer
Cancer Basic 4	XTRA	120,464,524,666,728,784,800,854,880,**2008**,2048,2084,**2128**,2148,2452,2720,3040,3176,5000,6064,10000,11162.11=900,11503.9=900,	Use Blood Cleanser.		Cancer
Cancer Basic 5	XTRA	120,464,524,666,728,784,800,854,880,**2008**,2048,2084,**2128**,2184,2452,2720,3040,3176,5000,6064,10000,1162.11=900,11503.9=900,	Use Blood Cleanser.		Cancer
Cancer Basic 6	XTRA	657.03,776.03,1935.99,8008.06,8485.01,9149.05,10646.03,10975.01,11162.11=900,11250,11289.05,11503.9,11659.62,11710.03,11812.52,11875,12031.25,12531.25,13031.25,16634.43,16910.68,21238.97,21726.04,	Use Blood Cleanser.		Cancer
Cancer Basic 7	XTRA	20,120,333,464,524,666,676,683,690,728,766,776,784,800,854,880,1489,1552,1604,**2008**,2048,2084,2127,**2128**,2182,2189,2452,2720,2790,2876,2950,3040,3176,3713,5000,6064,6766,10000,10025,11162.11=900,11430,11503.9=900,11780,17034,21275,	Use Blood Cleanser.		Cancer
Cancer Basic 8	XTRA	6.79,55.56,440,663,778,1050,1550,2180,3672,11162.11=900,11503.9=900,	Use Blood Cleanser.		Cancer
Cancer Basic 9	XTRA	663,727,778,787,880,1050,1550,2008,2050,2127,11162.11=900,11503.9=900,20507.81,	Use Blood Cleanser.		Cancer
Cancer Basic A	XTRA	663,727,778,787,802,880,1050,1550,2008,2050,2127,3022,5122,11162.11=900,11503.9=900	Use Blood Cleanser.		Cancer
Cancer Basic Set	CAFL	120,464,524,66,728,784,800,854,880,2008,2084,2184,2452,2720,3040,3176,5000,6064,10000,	Use Blood Cleanser.		Cancer
Cancer Tumor Reduction	XTRA	1604368,1604850.01	Use Blood Cleanser.		Cancer
Cancer Not Killed by Freqs 2008 and 2128	CAFL	2180,2182,2184	Use Blood Cleanser.		Cancer
Cancer Maintenance	CAFL	120,250,428,465,600,626,650,661,664,667,690,728,776,784,800,802,832,880,1489,1500,1600,1865,2000,2012,2100,2170,2490,2730,	Use Blood Cleanser.		Cancer
Cancer: Comprehensive (Alternative Set), Focus on Leukemia, Lymphoma, Brain, Sarcomas, Blood, Bone Cancer	EDTFL	120,250,700,5030,15610,17500,31200,95500,425580,434720			Cancer
Residual Cancer Residual Tumor	EDTFL	20,30,40,5030,119340,350000,434330,691270,759830,927100,	Residual Cancer Burden (RCB) after neoadjuvant treatment.		Cancer
Cancer Pain	CAFL	3000,95,2127,2008,727,690,666,	Use Blood Cleanser.		Cancer
Cancer Pain	XTRA	95,660,690,727.5,2008,2127.5,2720,3000,10000	Use Blood Cleanser.		Cancer
BXBY Sweep	RL	11429800-11430200, 11779700-11780300	From Dr. Richard Loyd. Cancer BX and BY sweep.	Virus	Cancer
Cancer BXBY	XTRA	782937.42	Hits BX and BY viruses simultaneously. This is a fundamental frequency, so don't apply multipliers, modulation, or harmonics addition.	Virus	Cancer

Subject / Argument	Author	Frequencies	Notes	Origin	Target
Bacillus X Cancer Carcinoma	CUST	12832000	Determined by the British Rife Research Group	Virus	Cancer
Bacillus X Filter Cancer Carcinoma	*Rife*	1604000	Crane=2128, Rife (1936)=21275. (3rd octave lower than the previous one)	Virus	Cancer
Bacillus X BX Cancer Carcinoma	XTRA	12531.25	Cancer virus that causes Carcinoma (7th octave lower than the previous one).	Virus	Cancer
Bacillus X Cancer Carcinoma	RL	12833 *or* 1604125 *or* 3133	From Dr. Richard Loyd. The best frequency for cancer.	Virus	Cancer
BX Virus	CUST	2128	Crane - Dr. Robert P. Stafford, used to modulate a carrier signal of frequency 3.1MHz.	Virus	Cancer
BX Virus	CAFL	2128,3713	As mentioned above	Virus	Cancer
Cancer Carcinoma Original Crane	CAFL	2127.5,21275	John Crane, associate of Dr. Rife.	Virus	Cancer
BX Virus Carcinoma	XTRA	3214900	Hoyland MOR	Virus	Cancer
Cancer BX	XTRA	1607450	(lower octave than the previous one)	Virus	Cancer
Bacillus X Cancer Carcinoma	XTRA	17.6,**2128**,11503.9,12531.25,16634.43,21275,	As mentioned above	Virus	Cancer
Bacillus X	XTRA	12375,12531.25,21275,	As mentioned above	Virus	Cancer
BX Virus 1	XTRA	1604,2008,**2128**,2790,2876,3713,10025,11503.89,11503.9,12534.12,16634.43,17034,21275,	As mentioned above	Virus	Cancer
BX Virus 2	XTRA	263.11,334,1566.4,1675,2008,2127,2127,2127.5,**2128**,2385,2521,2655,2663,2787.5,3324,5013,5013.5,5020,5278.3,5318.8,5388.5,5575,6687.3,7037.5,7356,8020,8368.2,8610,8836.89,10025,10026,10027,	As mentioned above	Virus	Cancer
Cancer BX Virus	CAFL	1603.9-1604.1=600, 1604.1-1603.9=600, **2008,2128,** 2789.9-2790.1=600, 2790.1-2789.9=600, 2875.9-2876.1=600, 2876.1-2875.9=600, 3713,11503,	Virus causing carcinomas. Also use Blood Cleanser.	Virus	Cancer
Cancer BX Carcinoma Virus 1	XTRA	10025,10026,10027,55,127,462,590,660,690,7275,787,852,856,880,1582,1755,2008,2120,2127.5,2008,	Virus causing carcinomas. Also use Blood Cleanser.	Virus	Cancer
Cancer BX Carcinoma Virus 2	XTRA	2008,2005	Virus causing carcinomas. Also use Blood Cleanser.	Virus	Cancer
Cancer BX Carcinoma Virus 3	XTRA	2127,2008,880,787,727,690,666,		Virus	Cancer
Cancer BX Carcinoma Virus 4	XTRA	2127,2127.5,**2128**,2876,3713,10025,10026,10027,11503.9,12534.12,	Virus causing carcinomas. Also use Blood Cleanser.	Virus	Cancer
Cancer Carcinoma	CAFL	727,787,880,2008,2120,2127,7130,	Use Blood Cleanser. See EBV, Leukoplakia, Mouth Eruptions White Patches, Papilloma, BX Virus, and Cancer BX Virus sets.		Carcinoma
Cancer Carcinoma General	CAFL	340,690,728,**2008**,2104,2112,2120,**2128**,2136,2144,2152,2160,2168,2176,2184,2192,2200,2217,5000,9999,	Use Blood Cleanser. See BX Virus, and Cancer BX Virus sets.		Carcinoma
Cancer Carcinoma Scan	CAFL	728,690,**2008**,2104,2112,2120,**2128**,2136,2144,2152,2160,2168,2176,2184,2192,2200,2217,500 0,9999,304,	Main low sub-harmonics of carcinoma. Use Blood Cleanser. See BX Virus, and Cancer BX Virus sets.		Carcinoma
Carcinoma	EDTFL	50,520,600,940,12690,125000,269780,434030,571000,839000			Carcinoma
Carcinoma, Anaplastic	EDTFL	50,160,520,940,12690,125000,328900,434030,571000,839000			Carcinoma
Carcinoma, Basal Cell	EDTFL	50,520,600,940,12690,125000,269710,434030,571000,839000			Carcinoma
Carcinoma, Spindle-Cell	EDTFL	50,520,600,940,12690,125000,269710,434030,571000,839000			Carcinoma
Squamous Cell Carcinoma	EDTFL	50,520,600,940,12690,125000,269710,434030,571000,839000			Carcinoma
Carcinoma, Undifferentiated	EDTFL	60,180,970,5830,22000,47280,87220,97500,355720,434000			Carcinoma
Carcinomatosis	EDTFL	50,520,600,940,12690,125000,326650,434030,571000,839000			Carcinoma
Carcinoma 1	XTRA	462,852,1582,**2128**,	Also see Cancer Carcinoma.		Carcinoma
Carcinoma 2	XTRA	55,127,304,462,590,644,660,690,727.5,787,852,856,880,901,1352,1582,1820,2008,2098,2104,2112,2120,2127.5,**2128**,2136,2144,2152,2160,2168,2176,2184,2192,2200,2217,5000,9999,10025,10026,10027,	Also see Cancer Carcinoma.		Carcinoma
Carcinoma 3	XTRA	666,690,727,787,880,2008,2127,**2128**,	Also see Cancer Carcinoma.		Carcinoma
Cancer Carcinoma 1	XTRA	**1570,1820,2008,2128**	Epithelial cell cancer - begins in tissue lining inner or outer surfaces of the body.		Carcinoma

Subject / Argument	Author	Frequencies	Notes	Origin	Target
Cancer Carcinoma 3	XTRA	303,690,728,**2008**,2104,2112,2120,**2128**,2136,2144,2152,2160,2168,2176,2184,2192,2200,2217,5000,9999,	Epithelial cell cancer - begins in tissue lining inner or outer surfaces of the body.		Carcinoma
Carcinoid Carcinoid Tumor	EDTFL	80,120,850,20000,40000,352930,434720,517500,684810,712420	Also see Cancer Carcinoid Tumor Gastrointestinal, and Argentaffinoma.		Carcinoma
Cancer Carcinoma Scan 2	XTRA	304,690,728,**2008**,2104,2112,2120,**2128**,2136,2144,2152,2160,2168,2176,2184,2192,2200,2217,5000,9999,	Main low sub-harmonics of carcinoma. Use Blood Cleanser. See BX Virus, and Cancer BX Virus sets.		Carcinoma
Carcinoma Small Cell	KHZ	30,460,750,850,2500,7500,17500,96500,350000,450000,	Also see Cancer Carcinoma.		Carcinoma
Carcinomatosis	XTRA	43-193,	Also called Carcinosis. Disseminated or metastasized cancer.		Carcinoma
BY Virus	CUST	2008	Crane - Dr. Robert P. Stafford, used to modulate a carrier signal of frequency 3.1MHz.	Virus	Sarcoma
BY Virus	CAFL	2008,3524,	Cancer virus that causes Sarcoma.	Virus	Sarcoma
Bacillus Y Cancer Sarcoma	XTRA	**2008**,11162.11,20080,	As mentioned above	Virus	Sarcoma
BY Virus 3	XTRA	**2008**,**2128**,3524,11162,11430,11780,17034,20080,	As mentioned above	Virus	Sarcoma
Bacillus Y BY Cancer Sarcoma	XTRA	11162.11	As mentioned above	Virus	Sarcoma
BY Sarcoma	XTRA	3059040	Hoyland MOR. Cancer virus causing Sarcoma.	Virus	Sarcoma
Cancer BY Virus	XTRA	1529520	(lower octave than the previous one)	Virus	Sarcoma
Cancer BY Sarcoma Virus 1	XTRA	1503.9,16634.43,12534.43,12534.12,21275,17934,11503.89,11503.89,11503.89,10025,3713,2876,2790,**2128**,**2008**,1604,	Virus causing Sarcomas. Also use Blood Cleanser.	Virus	Sarcoma
Cancer BY Sarcoma Virus 2	XTRA	263.11,334,1566.4,1675,**2008**,2127,2127.5,**2128**,2385,2521,2655,2663,2787.5,3324,5013,5013.5,5020,5278.3,5318.8,5388.5,5575,6687.3,7037.5,7356,8020,8368.2,8610,8836.89,10025,10026,10027,	Virus causing Sarcomas. Also use Blood Cleanser.	Virus	Sarcoma
Cancer BY Sarcoma Virus 3	XTRA	1604,2008	Virus causing Sarcomas. Also use Blood Cleanser.	Virus	Sarcoma
BY Human to Human Contact	XTRA	334	As mentioned above	Virus	Sarcoma
Cancer Sarcoma General	CAFL	1755,2008,3524	Malignant tumors not originating from epithelial cells. See BY Virus, and Cancer BY Virus. Use Blood Cleanser.	Connective	Sarcoma
Cancer Sarcoma	CAFL	727,787,880,2000,**2008**,2127,	As mentioned above	Connective	Sarcoma
Sarcoma	EDTFL	150,2120,20000,45150,47500,96500,125000,375750,434330,563190		Connective	Sarcoma
Sarcoma 2	XTRA	2008,2005	See Cancer Sarcoma, and BY Virus sets.	Connective	Sarcoma
Cancer Sarcoma 2	XTRA	728,785,802,880,1755,2005,2007.5,2015.9,2083.8,3524,	As mentioned above	Connective	Sarcoma
Cancer: Sarcoma General – Resonant Light Alternate Set1	EDTFL	130,570,750,12270,68290,135250,272720,434530,733910,836420	As mentioned above	Connective	Sarcoma
Cancer: Sarcoma General – Resonant Light Alternate Set2	EDTFL	100,550,730,870,67200,172850,230000,434200,535230,608210		Connective	Sarcoma
Sarcoma, General Sarcoma, Osteogenic Sarcoma, Soft Tissue	EDTFL	140,220,720,2580,47500,96500,125000,375750,434330,563190		Connective	Sarcoma
Sarcoma, Epithelioid	EDTFL	150,900,5580,30000,47500,96500,125000,375750,434330,563190		Connective	Sarcoma
Sarcoma, Germinoblastic [see Cancer: LYMPHOMA]	EDTFL	80,350,37500,47500,96500,115700,125000,375750,434330,563190,		Connective	Sarcoma
Sarcoma, Nerve	EDTFL	150,2120,20000,45150,47500,96500,125000,375750,434330,563190,		Connective	Sarcoma
Sarcoma, Spindle Cell	EDTFL	50,520,600,940,12690,125000,269710,434030,571000,839000,		Connective	Sarcoma
FibroSarcoma	BIO	1744	Malignant tumor containing connective tissue and developing rapidly from fibrous tissues of bone. See Cancer sets.	Connective	Sarcoma
FibroSarcoma	XTRA	744	As mentioned above	Connective	Sarcoma
Histiocytoma, Fibrous	EDTFL	140,520,750,5520,12530,145830,262500,397500,633910,825170		Connective	Sarcoma
Histiocytoma, Benign Fibrous	EDTFL	150,520,9730,11640,12530,145830,262500,434500,633910,825170		Connective	Sarcoma
Histiocytoma, Malignant Fibrous	EDTFL	150,520,9730,11640,12530,145830,262500,434500,633910,825170,	Also called Pleomorphic undifferentiated Sarcoma. See Cancer Sarcoma, Sarcoma, and Cancer BY sets.	Connective	Sarcoma
Histiocytoma, Cutaneous	EDTFL	130,520,800,8500,12530,145830,262500,397500,633910,825170		Connective	Sarcoma
Sarcoma, Ewing's	EDTFL	70,500,37500,75560,47500,96500,125000,375750,434330,563190	Rare bone/soft tissue tumor, most commonly occurring in pelvis, femur, humerus, ribs, or clavicle. Also see OsteoSarcoma, Cancer Sarcoma, and BY Virus sets.	Connective	Sarcoma

Subject / Argument	Author	Frequencies	Notes	Origin	Target
Ewing's Tumor [Bone Cancer]	EDTFL	20,30,40,5030,119340,350000,434330,691270,7 59830,927100,		Connective	Sarcoma
Cancer: Ewing's (PNET=Primitive Neuroectodermal Tumor)	EDTFL	80,120,850,85030,119340,326150,350000,6912 70,759830,927100	One of Ewing family of tumors not generally associated with bones.	Connective	Sarcoma
Cancer: Soft Tissue Sarcoma	EDTFL	150,2120,20000,45150,73300,96500,125000,37 5750,434330,563190,		Connective	Sarcoma
Kaposi's Sarcoma		*Can be caused by **Kaposi's Sarcoma herpesvirus and HIV**.*			
Kaposi's Sarcoma	BIO	**249,418**	Systemic disease caused by human herpesvirus 8 (HHV8) with cutaneous tumors.	Connective	Sarcoma
Kaposi's Sarcoma	XTRA	**249,418,647**	Usually cutaneous tumor caused by **Human Herpesvirus 8 (HHV-8)**. Found in AIDS and immunosuppressed conditions.	Connective	Sarcoma
Cancer: RhabdomyoSarcoma	EDTFL	40,550,780,50000,97500,229320,329570,51968 0,684810,712000	Aggressive highly malignant cancer that develops from skeletal (striated) muscle cells that have failed to fully differentiate, usually in the young. Also see appropriate Cancer sets.	Connective	Sarcoma
RhabdomyoSarcoma	EDTFL	120,250,620,2500,3000,315750,425280,697500, 869710,925280	As mentioned above	Connective	Sarcoma
Cancer RhabdomyoSarcoma Embryonal Vega 1	CAFL	**2586,4445,5476**	Rare connective tissue cancer with cells resembling embryonic skeletal muscle. Use Blood Cleanser.	Connective	Sarcoma
Cancer RhabdomyoSarcoma Embryonal	CAFL	6384,6024,2586,2217,2184,**2128**,2127,2100,209 3,2084,2060,2048,2040,2032,2016,2008,2005,2 000,880,784,728,464,	Rare connective tissue cancer with cells resembling embryonic skeletal muscle. Use Blood Cleanser.	Connective	Sarcoma
Cancer RhabdomyoSarcoma	CAFL	464,728,784,880,2000,2005,2008,2016,2048,20 84,2093,2100,2127,**2128**,2184,2217,6024,6384,	Also called RMS. Connective tissue cancer. May arise from progenitor cells. Use Blood Cleanser.	Connective	Sarcoma
Epithelioma	EDTFL	80,350,5190,55000,72500,73300,92500,98500,1 25230,527810	Abnormal growth of the epithelium, the layer of tissue that covers the surfaces of organs and other structures in the body.	Connective	Sarcoma
Epithelioma, Basal Cell	EDTFL	80,350,5190,55000,72500,73300,92500,475270, 827000,967000,		Connective	Sarcoma
Epithelial Neoplasms, Malignant	EDTFL	40,250,650,930,2500,7500,96500,334250,43440 0,792200,		Connective	Sarcoma
Granuloma, Malignant	EDTFL	70,500,970,9000,12850,39500,132810,434210,5 06530,925370		Connective	Sarcoma
Leukemia		*Can be caused by **human T-cell leukemia virus-1**.*			
Leukemia	CAFL	666,690,727,787,880,2008,2127,	Cancer involving the blood-forming tissues in bone marrow. See Cancer Leukemia sets.	Blood	Cancer
Leukemia	EDTFL	110,1490,32570,102250,212500,434500,672500 ,735340,893500,930100,	As mentioned above	Blood	Cancer
Leukemia	BIO	424,830,901,918,	As mentioned above	Blood	Cancer
Leukemia	XTRA	**690,666**	As mentioned above	Blood	Cancer
Myeloid Leukemia	BIO	**422,822**	Characterized by rapid growth of incompletely-formed white blood cells. AML - see Cancer and Leukemia.	Blood	Cancer
Cancer Leukemia	BIO	**424,830,901,918**	Begins in bone marrow, causing white blood cell abnormalities. Use Blood Cleanser.	Blood	Cancer
Cancer Leukemia	CAFL	2127,2008,880,787,727,690,666,2217,	See Leucosis. Use Blood Cleanser.	Blood	Cancer
Cancer: Leukemia	EDTFL	110,1490,32570,102250,212500,434500,672500 ,735340,893500,930100,	Begins in bone marrow, causing white blood cell abnormalities. Use Blood Cleanser.	Blood	Cancer
Cancer: Leukemia, Acute Myeloid	EDTFL	130,570,770,12270,68290,135250,272720,4345 30,733910,836420	As mentioned above	Blood	Cancer
Cancer: Leukemia, Chronic Lymph	EDTFL	130,570,780,12270,68290,135250,272720,4345 30,733910,836420	As mentioned above	Blood	Cancer
Cancer: Leukemia, Hairy Cell	EDTFL	70,120,600,800,2500,22500,72500,434390,7391 00,905310	As mentioned above	Blood	Cancer
Cancer: Leukemia, Lymphoblastic	EDTFL	50,520,600,930,12690,125440,269710,434030,5 71000,839000	As mentioned above	Blood	Cancer
Cancer: Leukemia, Myelogenous	EDTFL	30,870,2500,17300,35150,97500,434610,56200 0,840960,985900	As mentioned above	Blood	Cancer
Chronic Lymphocytic Leukemia	EDTFL	130,570,780,12270,68290,135250,272720,4345 30,733910,836420,		Blood	Cancer
Cancer Leukemia 2	XTRA	6.79,14,15,422,428,440,450,465,590,666,690,72 7,787,822,880,1850,2008,2030,2127,10000,	As mentioned above	Blood	Cancer
Cancer Leukemia Hairy Cell	CAFL	122,622,932,5122,488,781,	Characterized by abnormal blood cells & shortage of others. See Cancer Leukemia sets.	Blood	Cancer
Leukemia Hairy Cell	BIO	**122,622,932,5122**	Typified by abnormal blood cells and shortage of others. Use Blood Cleanser.	Blood	Cancer
Cancer Hairy Cell	BIO	122,622,932,5122,1522,	As mentioned above	Blood	Cancer
Leukemia T Cell	XTRA	222,262,822,3042,3734,	Cancer of white blood cells. See Cancer Leukemia, and Leukemia sets.	Blood	Cancer

Subject / Argument	Author	Frequencies	Notes	Origin	Target
Cancer Blood Multiple Melanoma	XTRA	728	Multiple melanomas/moles.	Blood	Cancer
Cancer: Plasma Cell Neoplasm	EDTFL	570,900,15750,62500,95000,250000,434000,52 4370,682020,753070,	Plasma cell tumor, closely related to Multiple Myeloma, Plasmacytomas, or Primary Amyloidosis.	Blood	Cancer
Plasmacytoma	CAFL	275	Tumor with plasma cells that occurs in bone marrow, as in Multiple Myeloma, or outside bone marrow, as in tumors of inner organs and lining of nose, mouth, and throat. See Cancer Plasmacytoma.	Blood	Cancer
Cancer Plasmacytoma	BIO	475	Malignant plasma-cell tumor in soft tissue or axial skeleton.	Blood	Cancer
Cancer Multiple Myeloma	CAFL	249,263,418,422,475,526,647,781,822,1488,200 8,2107,**2128**,2145,2950,4213,4750,5122,11780, 21275,	Plasma cell blood cancer arising in bone marrow. Use Blood Cleanser.	Blood	Cancer
Multiple Myeloma	EDTFL	100,500,680,830,190890,312600,452500,68750 0,795690,892500	Cancer of plasma cells in bone marrow. Also see Cancer Multiple Myeloma, Cancer Plasma Cell Neoplasm, and Plasmacytoma sets.	Blood	Cancer
Multiple Myeloma	RL	967	From Dr. Richard Loyd.	Blood	Cancer
Myeloma, Plasma-Cell	EDTFL	100,500,680,830,190890,312600,452500,68750 0,795690,892500,	As mentioned above	Blood	Cancer
Cancer Myeloid	BIO	422,822	Characterized by rapid growth of incompletely-formed white blood cells. Acute Myeloid Leukemia (AML).	Blood	Cancer
Cancer: Myelodysplastic Syndrome	EDTFL	130,460,830,12690,93500,221500,434710,5123 30,667000,753070	Bone marrow stem cell disorder causing blood production problems.	Blood	Cancer
Cancer: Myeloproliferative Disorders	EDTFL	100,520,7500,30000,225030,434150,527000,66 2710,749000,986220	Bone marrow diseases in which excess cells are produced.	Blood	Cancer
Macroglobulinemia	EDTFL	150,640,25080,87950,194380,229430,409950,5 37390,605480,787270		Blood	Cancer
Waldenstrom Macroglobulinemia [B Cell Cancer]	EDTFL	350,930,7500,17500,52500,70000,215700,3243 00,434000,523010,	As mentioned above	Blood	Cancer
Lymphoma [See Cancer, Lymphoma all variables]	EDTFL	80,570,15750,52500,62500,95000,250000,4343 70,682020,753070,	See multiple and specific selections	Lymph	Lymphoma
Cancer: Lymphoma	EDTFL	70,120,600,800,2500,22500,72500,434390,7391 00,905310	As mentioned above	Lymph	Lymphoma
Cancer: Lymphoma, Malignant	EDTFL	110,520,81300,135710,221500,434500,570510, 691510,775480,971550		Lymph	Lymphoma
Leukemia Lymphatic	BIO	478,833	See Cancer leukemia sets.	Lymph	Lymphoma
Lymphatic Leukemia 1	XTRA	833	As mentioned above	Lymph	Lymphoma
Lymphatic Leukemia 2	XTRA	478	As mentioned above	Lymph	Lymphoma
Burkitt Lymphoma Burkitt Cell Leukemia	EDTFL	110,1490,32570,102250,212500,434500,672500 ,735340,893500,930100,	B lymphocyte neoplasm	Lymph	Lymphoma
African Lymphoma	EDTFL	80,570,15750,52500,62500,95000,250000,4343 70,682020,753070,	Also called Burkitt's Lymphoma.	Lymph	Lymphoma
Cancer Lymphoma	KHZ	120,350,930,7500,17500,52500,70000,93500,21 5700,523010,	White blood cell tumors developing from lymphatic cells.	Lymph	Lymphoma
Cancer Lymphoma 1	XTRA	2116,2180,2182,	As mentioned above	Lymph	Lymphoma
B-Cell Lymphoma	EDTFL	80,570,15750,52500,62500,95000,250000,4343 70,682020,753070,	Blood cancers in lymph glands. Includes Hodgkin's and Non-Hodgkin's Lymphomas.	Lymph	Lymphoma
Cancer: Lymphoma, B-Cell	EDTFL	80,570,15750,52500,62500,95000,250000,4343 70,682020,753070	White blood cell tumors developing from lymphatic B-Cells.	Lymph	Lymphoma
Germinoblastoma Lymphoma	EDTFL	80,570,15750,52500,62500,95000,250000,4343 70,682020,753070,	As mentioned above	Lymph	Lymphoma
Schuman B Cell	CAFL	322,425,561,600,620,623,780,781,950,952,1023 ,1524,1097,1100,	As mentioned above	Lymph	Lymphoma
Schuman B Cell	BIO	322,425,428,561,600,620,623,780,781,950,952, 1023,1524,	As mentioned above	Lymph	Lymphoma
Cancer: Lymphoplasmacytic	EDTFL	350,930,7500,17500,52500,70000,215700,3243 00,434000,523010	Tupe of lymphoma affecting B cells. See Lymphoproliferative Disorders, B-Cell Lymphoma, Lymphoma Non Hodgkins, and non-Hodgkin's sets.	Lymph	Lymphoma
Cancer LymphoSarcoma	CAFL	482	Type of Lymphoma. Use Blood Cleanser.	Lymph	Lymphoma
Reticulolymphosarcoma [See Cancer, Lymphoma]	EDTFL	50,410,620,15750,87500,324650,434000,65520 0,750000,927100,		Lymph	Lymphoma
Lymphoma Non Hodgkins		*Can be caused by HIV and Simian Virus 40 .*			
Non-Hodgkin Lymphoma	EDTFL	50,410,620,15750,87500,324650,434000,65520 0,750000,927100,	90% of all Lymphomas are non-Hodgkin's.	Lymph	Lymphoma
Lymphoma Non Hodgkins	XTRA	574,588,666,778,1078,1120,1340,1440,1744,20 04,2008,2012,2016,2128,3524,3672,3713,7760,	See B-Cell Lymphoma, and Cancer Lymphoma Non-Hodgkin's.	Lymph	Lymphoma
Cancer Non Hodgkins 1	PROV	574,588,666,778,1078,1120,1340,1744,3524,37 13,	Use Cancer Melanoma, and Blood Cleanser. Also helps with blood cell production problems in Morgellons.	Lymph	Lymphoma
Cancer Non Hodgkins 2	PROV	2008,2004,2012,2116,2128,3672,7760,	As mentioned above	Lymph	Lymphoma

Subject / Argument	Author	Frequencies	Notes	Origin	Target
Hodgkin's Lymphoma		Can be caused by **Epstein-Barr virus, Hepatitis C virus**, and **HIV**.			
Hodgkin Lymphoma	EDTFL	80,570,15750,52500,62500,95000,250000,4343 70,682020,753070,	Malignant tumor of the lymphatic system.	Lymph	Lymphoma
Hodgkin Disease [Lymphoma]	EDTFL	80,570,15750,52500,62500,95000,250000,4343 70,682020,753070,	As mentioned above	Lymph	Lymphoma
Granuloma, Hodgkin	EDTFL	70,500,970,9000,12850,267000,320850,602210, 733630,925000	As mentioned above	Lymph	Lymphoma
Hodgkin Disease 3	XTRA	10,440,552,880,1522,	As mentioned above	Lymph	Lymphoma
Cancer Hodgkin's Disease	BIO	552,1522	Also called Hodgkin's lymphoma. Cancer of the lymphatic system that is both chronic and progressive.	Lymph	Lymphoma
Cancer Hodgkin's Disease 2	XTRA	263.11,334,552,1552,1566.4,1675,2008,2127,32 85,2521,2655,2663,2787,3324,5013,5013.5,500 0,5278.3,5388.5,5575,6687.3,7037.5,7356,8020, 8368.2,8610,8836.89,10025,10026,10027,	Also called Hodgkin's lymphoma. Cancer of the lymphatic system that is both chronic and progressive.	Lymph	Lymphoma
Cancer Lymphogranuloma Lymphoma 2	XTRA	304,360,361,362,363,364,365,366,367,368,369, 373,464,465,528,532,540,556,665,685,716,717, 718,731,732,733,776,802,808,832,846,848,880, 888,1402,1488=1800,1489=1800,1550,1577,19 00,2950=900,8778,	As mentioned above	Lymph	Lymphoma
Cancer Lymphogranuloma Venereum	CAFL	430,620,624,840,866,2213,	As mentioned above	Lymph	Lymphoma
Cancer Lymphogranuloma Venereum Secondary	XTRA	430,555.7,620,624,840,866,1111.4,2213,2222.8,	As mentioned above	Lymph	Lymphoma
Carcinoid tumors		Can be caused by **Enterovirus infections**.			
Endocrine Cancer	KHZ	140,460,750,2090,32500,47500,117500,396500, 655720,825540,	Pineal, pituitary, thyroid, thymus, adrenal, pancreas, and ovary/testis gland cancers. Also see appropriate Cancer sets.	Endocrine S.	Cancer
Cancer: Endocrine Gland Endocrine Cancer Neuroendocrine Tumors	EDTFL	570,830,2850,32500,97500,322530,434420,566 410,835960,978850	Tumors arising from cells of endocrine and nervous systems, some benign, some malignant, most commonly in intestines.	Endocrine S.	Cancer
Carcinoid, Goblet Cell	EDTFL	60,230,20000,60500,125750,150000,357300,53 2410,653650,759830		Endocrine S.	Cancer
Adrenocortical Cancer	EDTFL	60,490,570,2500,7500,30000,225750,329530,41 9340,561930		Endocrine S.	Cancer
Cancer Thyroid		Can be caused by **EBV** and **Simian virus 40**.			
Cancer: Thyroid	EDTFL	180,490,750,950,2500,7500,112360,325950,434 290,534250	Use Blood Cleanser.	Thyroid	Cancer
Cancer: Parathyroid	EDTFL	70,550,900,22500,47500,434030,527000,66700 0,752700,988900	Rare progression of parathyroid adenoma to Carcinoma.	Thyroid	Cancer
Carcinoma, Thymic	EDTFL	50,520,600,930,12690,125000,269740,434030,5 71000,839000	Uncommon tumor of thymus, most associated with Myasthenia Gravis (see set).	Thymus	Tumor
Cancer: Thymoma	EDTFL	50,520,600,930,12630,125000,269710,434030,5 71000,839000	As mentioned above	Thymus	Cancer
Thymoma	EDTFL	70,500,1000,7600,17100,127500,335290,56575 0,725950,919340		Thymus	Cancer
Cancer Neuroblastoma	CAFL	878,1757,2635,3513,4392,5270,6148,	Mainly a childhood neuroendocrine cancer. Use Blood Cleanser.		Cancer
Neuroblastoma	EDTFL	60,350,620,970,12500,27500,142500,434870,62 3010,815580,	Neuroendocrine Tumors (see set) - most common form of childhood cancer.		Cancer
Neuroblastoma, Retinal	EDTFL	20,970,5690,32500,175030,434170,517500,683 000,712420,995380,			Cancer
Adrenal tumor		Can be caused by **BK virus** and **Simian virus 40**.			
Pheochromocytoma Pheochromocytoma, Extra-Adrenal	EDTFL	140,220,730,5250,7250,52010,157510,290200,6 75350,821370	Neuroendocrine tumor of the medulla of the adrenal glands. See Neuroendocrine Tumors, and Adrenal sets.		Tumor
Cancer: Pheochromocytoma	EDTFL	70,550,900,22500,47500,434030,527000,66700 0,752700,988900	Neuroendocrine tumor of medulla of adrenal glands.		Tumor
Paraganglioma	KHZ	10,300,650,900,2500,57220,113930,293500,358 570,479500,	Rare neuroendocrine neoplasm found at various body sites. See Neuroendocrine Tumors and other appropriate Cancer sets.		Tumor
Paraganglioma Paraganglioma, Gangliocytic	EDTFL	70,350,25400,52000,60000,150000,475110,527 000,667000,987230	As mentioned above		Tumor
Cancer: Nervous System Neoplasms	EDTFL	170,220,930,2750,27500,132500,255580,43485 0,724940,825870	Includes brain and nerve sheath tumors, arachnoid cysts, and optic nerve gliomas.	Nerve	Cancer
Neurofibromatosis Neurofibromatoses	EDTFL	850,900,980,17530,213230,321290,423690,597 500,862500,915540,	Collection of genetically inherited conditions which are clinically and genetically different and present a high chance of tumor formation.	Nerve	Cancer
von Recklinghausen Disease	EDTFL	80,120,15330,83000,90000,357300,527000,657 110,830200,987230		Nerve	Cancer
Tumor Brain	BIO	543,641,857	See Cancer Astrocytoma, Gliomas, Glioblastoma, and Astrocytoma sets.	Brain	Tumor

Subject / Argument	Author	Frequencies	Notes	Origin	Target
Tumor Brain	CAFL	7.69,8.25,9.19,20,543,641,664,666,690,720,728, 800,832,855,857,880,2008,2127,**2128**,2170,218 0,2182,	As mentioned above	Brain	Tumor
Brain Tumor 1	XTRA	7.69,7.7,8.25,9.18,9.19,20,463,466,543,590,641, 660,664,690,720,727.5,800,832,853,855,857,88 0,2008,2127.5,2127,2170,2180,2182,	Also see Cancer sets.	Brain	Tumor
Brain Tumor 2	XTRA	7.69,8.25,9.18,543,641,666,690,853,857,880,21 27,2170,	Also see Cancer sets.	Brain	Tumor
Tumor Brain 2	XTRA	7.69,7.7,8.25,9.18,9.19,20,463,466,543,590,641, 660,664,690,720,727.5,800,832,853,855,857,88 0,2008,2127.5,2170,2180,2182,	As mentioned above	Brain	Tumor
Tumor Brain 3	XTRA	7.69,8.25,9.18,463,466,470,543,641,666,690,85 7,880,2127,2170,	As mentioned above	Brain	Tumor
Tumor Brain 4	XTRA	7.69,8.25,9.18,543,641,666,690,853,857,880,21 27,2170,	As mentioned above	Brain	Tumor
Tumor Brain 5	XTRA	543,641,857=720,	As mentioned above	Brain	Tumor
Cancer Brain Tumor	KHZ	10,20,30,5030,119340,350000,512330,691270,7 59830,927100,	See Astrocytoma and Cancer Astrocytoma. Use Blood Cleanser.	Brain	Cancer
Cancer: Brain Tumor [Medulloblastoma]	EDTFL	160,350,930,35780,112500,212710,396500,434 790,597500,751170,		Brain	Cancer
Medulloblastoma, Desmoplastic Medullomyoblastoma	EDTFL	160,350,930,35780,112500,212710,396500,434 790,597500,751170,	As mentioned above	Brain	Cancer
Cancer: Brain Tumor, Ependymoma	EDTFL	80,5750,7250,50000,97500,210500,434370,655 200,750000,927100,		Brain	Cancer
Cancer: Brain Tumor, Brain Stem Glioma	EDTFL	40,970,5690,32500,175030,434170,517600,683 000,712420,995380,		Brain	Cancer
Cancer: Brain Tumor, S.P.N.& Pineal Tumors	EDTFL	20,30,40,5030,119340,350000,434330,691270,7 59830,927100,		Brain	Cancer
Cancer: Brain Tumor, Visual Pathway and Hypothalamic Glioma	EDTFL	20,30,40,5030,119340,350000,434330,691270,7 59830,927100,		Brain	Cancer
Cancer Astrocytoma	CAFL	857,9.19,8.25,7.69,2170,543,641,2127,880,690, 666,	Common tumor of brain and central nervous system. Use Blood Cleanser.	Brain	Cancer
Astrocytoma Astrocytoma, Giant Cell Astrocytoma, Grade IV	EDTFL	2750,5030,15610,17500,37000,95500,350000,4 34390,739100,905310,		Brain	Cancer
Cancer: Brain Tumor, Cerebellar Astrocytoma	EDTFL	2750,5030,15610,17500,37000,95500,350000,4 34390,739100,905310,		Brain	Cancer
Brain Tumor, Cerebral Astrocytoma	EDTFL	60,180,980,6050,22000,47280,87220,97500,355 720,434500		Brain	Cancer
Oligoastrocytoma, Mixed	EDTFL	2750,5030,15610,17500,37000,95500,350000,4 34390,739100,905310,		Brain	Cancer
Astrocytoma	PROV	7.69,8.25,9.19,20,543,641,666,690,857,2127,21 70,	As mentioned above	Brain	Cancer
Astrocytoma	VEGA	857	As mentioned above	Brain	Cancer
Arachnoidal Cerebel Sarcoma	EDTFL	140,220,720,2580,193110,247590,385210,5216 80,651300,729340,	Most common malignant primary brain tumor in children, commonly metastasizing via spinal canal. Also see appropriate Cancer sets.	Brain	Sarcoma
Sarcoma, Cerebellar, Circumscribed Arachnoidal	EDTFL	70,520,6820,7570,47500,96500,125000,375750, 434330,563190	As mentioned above	Brain	Sarcoma
Glioblastoma		*Can be caused by **Cytomegalovirus, BK virus, JC virus**, and **Simian virus 40**.*			
Cancer Glioblastoma	CUST	200000	TTFields - Cell line name: U-118 and U-87	Brain	Cancer
Cancer Glioblastoma	CAFL	720,2008,**2128**,2180,2182,728,832,800,664,20,8 55,543,641,857,	Tyoe of brain/brain stem tumor. Use Blood Cleanser.	Brain	Cancer
Glioblastoma	EDTFL	80,350,600,800,212030,305210,434240,565610, 690000,826320		Brain	Cancer
Giant Cell Glioblastoma	EDTFL	80,350,600,800,212030,305210,434240,565610, 690000,826320,		Brain	Cancer
Glioblastoma Multiforme	EDTFL	80,350,600,800,212030,305210,434240,475160, 527000,541220		Brain	Cancer
Glioblastoma, Retinal	EDTFL	80,350,600,800,7250,32500,137500,326070,490 000,515700		Brain	Cancer
Cancer Glioblastoma Tremor	CAFL	463,466,470	Tremor due to brain/brain-stem tumor. Use Blood Cleanser.	Brain	Cancer
Cancer Gliomas	CAFL	543,641,857	Largest group of brain cancers. Use Blood Cleanser.	Brain	Cancer
Glioma	EDTFL	180,230,720,890,5360,147250,327350,487900,6 95810,875360		Brain	Cancer
Glioma, Astrocytic	EDTFL	180,230,720,890,5360,147250,337550,651200,7 32590,973520		Brain	Cancer

Subject / Argument	Author	Frequencies	Notes	Origin	Target
Glioma, Retinal	EDTFL	180,230,720,890,77220,111620,337550,651200, 732590,973520		Brain	Cancer
Brain Tumor, Brain Stem Glioma	EDTFL	40,970,5690,32500,175030,434170,517500,683 000,712420,995380		Brain	Cancer
Glial Cell Tumors [Astrocytoma]	EDTFL	2750,5030,15610,17500,37000,95500,350000,4 34390,739100,905310,	Brain or spinal tumor that arises from glial cells. See Cancer Gliomas, and Tumor Brain sets.	Brain	Cancer
Glioma	VEGA	543,641	As mentioned above	Brain	Cancer
Cancer Droglioma	CAFL	853	As mentioned above	Brain	Cancer
Cancer: Pituitary	EDTFL	60,500,47500,150000,210500,219340,321250,4 34500,515160,688290	May be invasive or benign adenoma, or malignant carcinoma.	Brain	Cancer
Cancer: Extracranial Germ Cell Tumor	EDTFL	140,460,750,840,96500,355720,434150,571000, 839000,932000	Germ cell. As mentioned above.	Brain	Cancer
Cancer: Head and Neck	EDTFL	900,920,32750,293700,329050,415840,423460, 472120,512140,629900,			Cancer
Head Cancer Head and Neck Cancer Neck Cancer Upper Aerodigestive Tract Neoplasms	EDTFL	900,920,32750,293700,329050,415840,423460, 472120,512140,629900		Neck	Cancer
Cancer Head and Neck	XTRA KHZ	100,520,7500,30000,225030,475150,527000,66 2710,749000,986220,		Neck	Cancer
Neck Neoplasms	EDTFL	900,920,32750,187500,293700,329050,415840, 455300,672230,775870,		Neck	Cancer
Cancer: Eye Eye Cancer Retinoblastoma	EDTFL	70,2120,5690,20000,93500,175750,434500,527 000,667000,873290	Use Retyne™ Light mat combined with Rife Healing Mat	Eyes	Cancer
Eye Cancer Intraocular Melanoma	KHZ	60,230,730,32500,90000,175000,344510,65369 0,753070,922530,	Also called Uveal Melanoma. Arises from eye colour pigments.	Eyes	Cancer
Auricular Cancer	EDTFL	80,120,850,85030,119340,325250,434220,6912 70,759830,927100,	Cancer of the ear, head, and neck.	Ear	Cancer
Cancer: Ear	EDTFL	20,460,5120,27900,85000,95750,150000,43471 0,682450,753070,	As mentioned above.	Ear	Cancer
Cancer: Salivary Gland	EDTFL	120,270,9330,34210,205690,317250,434500,69 2500,776950,838250	Can be caused by cell phone use.	Face	Cancer
Adenoma Basal Cell	XTRA	40,5810,22500,52500,92500,434000,527000,66 7000,721000,987230,	Low-grade malignant salivary gland neoplasm. See Cancer sets.	Face	Cancer
Cancer: Lip and Oral Cavity	EDTFL	150,230,680,860,72570,137570,434250,537500, 822590,921050,		Face	Cancer
Cancer Lip and Oral Cavity	XTRA KHZ	80,570,15750,52500,62500,95000,250000,5243 70,682020,753070,		Face	Cancer
Cancer: Mouth	EDTFL	150,230,680,860,72570,137570,434250,537500, 822590,921050		Mouth	Cancer
Cancer: Oral Cancer Oral Cancer Oral Neoplasms	EDTFL	150,230,680,860,72570,137570,434250,537500, 822590,921050,		Mouth	Cancer
Mouth Cancer	EDTFL	150,230,680,860,72570,137570,434250,537500, 822590,921050,		Mouth	Cancer
Cancer Mouth	XTRA KHZ	80,570,15750,52500,62500,95000,250000,5243 70,682020,753070,	Use Blood Cleanser.	Mouth	Cancer
Cancrum Oris	CAFL	20,727,787,802,880,	Rapidly growing oral or nasal ulcer. Use Blood Cleanser.	Face	Cancer
Cancrum Oris 2	XTRA	20,660,690,727.5,787,802,880,1550,	As mentioned above	Face	Cancer
Cancer: Paranasal Sinus and Nasal Cavity	EDTFL	70,550,900,22500,47500,434030,527000,66700 0,752700,988900		Nose	Cancer
Cancer: Otorhinolaryngologic	EDTFL	70,320,620,850,5000,22500,60000,352930,4345 30,563190	Ear, nose, and throat cancers.		Cancer
Cancer: Tonsil	EDTFL	160,350,47500,269710,434760,515150,684810, 723000,841200,997870	Use Blood Cleanser.	Tonsil	Cancer
Cancer Tonsil	XTRA KHZ	80,120,40000,85000,136420,357300,425750,57 1000,840000,937410,	Use Blood Cleanser.	Tonsil	Cancer
Cancer Throat BX Sweep 1	XTRA	1605450-1609450,	Alternare quotidianamente con Cancro alla gola BX Sweep 2.	Throat	Cancer
Cancer Throat BX Sweep 2	XTRA	1527520-1531520,	Alternare quotidianamente con Cancro alla gola BX Sweep 1.	Throat	Cancer
Cancer Throat Tumor 1	XTRA	128,29000,38300,39007	Experimental. Dowsed by Nancy Sliwa for David Bourke.	Throat	Cancer
Cancer Throat Tumor 2	XTRA	46015.6,23007.8,11503.9,10025,3713,2876,204 80,1604,	As mentioned above	Throat	Cancer
Cancer Oropharyngeal		*Can be caused by Human Papilloma Virus (HPV).*			
Cancer: Oropharyngeal	EDTFL	50,410,600,950,5780,30000,57500,97500,43487 0,675960	Middle throat - base of tongue, tonsils, soft palate, and pharynx.	Throat	Cancer

Subject / Argument	Author	Frequencies	Notes	Origin	Target
Cancer Oropharyngeal	XTRA KHZ	100,830,10890,2500,52500,87500,95190,20435 0,512590,709680,	As mentioned above	Throat	Cancer
Nasopharyngeal carcinoma		*Can be caused by Epstein-Barr virus.*			
Cancer Nasopharyngeal	CAFL	105,172,253,274,660,663,667,669,738,825,1013 ,1920,6618,8768,	Cancer of upper throat, nasal and auditory passages. See Epstein Barr Virus. Use Blood Cleanser.	Throat	Cancer
Cancer: Nasopharyngeal	EDTFL	570,900,15750,62500,95000,250000,52 4370,682020,753070	As mentioned above	Throat	Cancer
Cancer Nasopharyngeal 2	XTRA	105,172,253,274,465,660,663,667,669,727,738, 744,776,778,787,825,880,929,52,941.92,1013,1 032,1920,6618,8768,18670.15,18919.09,	As mentioned above	Throat	Cancer
Cancer: Hypopharyngeal	EDTFL	30,460,17500,27500,40000,85160,95000,15000 0,210600,434170	Cancer of tissue area where larynx and esophagus meet.	Throat	Cancer
Cancer: Respiratory Tract	EDTFL	70,120,600,800,2500,22500,72500,434390,7391 00,905310	Includes Laryngeal and Lung Cancers.	Throat	Cancer
Larynx Neoplasms [Squamous-cell carcinoma]	EDTFL	50,520,620,940,12690,125000,307700,434030,5 71000,839000,		Larynx	Cancer
Cancer: Larynx	EDTFL	110,320,970,2600,11090,20000,57500,225000,4 34010,565360,		Larynx	Cancer
Cancer Carcinoma Larynx	CAFL	327,524,731,1133	Use Blood Cleanser. See BX Virus,and Cancer BX Virus sets.	Voice Box	Carcinoma
Cancer Metasatic Squamous Neck	KHZ	100,520,7500,30000,225030,475150,527000,66 2710,749000,986220,	Head, neck, and parts of throat, metastasizing to lymphatic system. See Epstein Barr Virus, and use Blood Cleanser.		Cancer
Cancer Carcinoma Bronchial	CAFL	462,776,852,1582,2104,2144,2184,3672,	Use Blood Cleanser. See Cancer Bronchial, BX Virus, and Cancer BX Virus sets.	Lung	Carcinoma
Carcinoma Bronchial	VEGA	462,852,1582	Also see Cancer Carcinoma.		Carcinoma
Cancer Lung		*Can be caused by the bacterium Chlamydia Pneumoniae, with Human Papillomaviruses, and with Merkel cell Polyomavirus. Also from a bacterium called Pseudomonas Solanacearum.*			
Pulmonary Neoplasms [see Cancer: Lung] [2 types listed]	EDTFL	70,120,600,800,2500,22500,72500,434390,7391 00,905310,		Lung	Cancer
Pulmonary Cancer [Lung Cancer]	EDTFL	70,120,600,800,2500,22500,72500,434390,7391 00,905310,	Lung cancer/carcinoma. See appropriate Cancer sets.	Lung	Cancer
Cancer Lung	XTRA	462,776,852,1582,2104,2144,2184,3672,		Lung	Cancer
Cancer: Lung, Non-Small Cell Cancer: Lung, Small Cell	EDTFL	70,120,600,800,2500,22500,72500,434390,7391 00,905310		Lung	Cancer
Carcinoma, Small Cell Carcinoma, Oat Cell	EDTFL	50,520,600,940,12690,125000,269710,434030,5 71000,839000	Also see Cancer Lung Small Cell.	Lung	Carcinoma
Cancer Lung Non-Small Cell	CUST	150000	TTFields - Cell line name: NCI-H1299	Lung	Cancer
Carcinoma, Non-Small Cell Lung	EDTFL	70,120,600,800,2500,22500,72500,434390,7391 00,905310,	See also Cancer Lung Non-Small Cell, and Non-Small Cell Lung Carcinoma.	Lung	Carcinoma
Mesothelioma		*Can be caused by Simian Virus 40, especially in conjunction with asbestos exposure.*			
Mesothelioma	CUST	150000	TTFields - Cell line name: NCI-H2052	Lung	Cancer
Mesothelioma	EDTFL	430,930,2760,17500,35670,87500,236420,3242 00,434000,519340,	Rare cancer of lining of organs, most commonly lungs, usually due to asbestos exposure. Also see Cancer Malignant Mesothelioma, and Simian Virus 40.	Lung	Cancer
Cancer: Malignant Mesothelioma	EDTFL	430,930,2760,17500,35670,87500,236420,3242 00,434000,519340	Affects lungs and organ linings. Asbestos-related.	Lung	Cancer
Cancer: Thoracic	EDTFL	150,2120,20000,45150,73300,96500,125000,37 5750,434330,563190,	Cancers located in the thorax. Use Blood Cleanser.	Thorax	Cancer
Cancer Adenocarcinoma Esophageal	CAFL	47,2182,2219,832,2084,2127,2160,2452,2876,	Malignant growths of glandular origins or with glandular traits (such as secretion). Use Blood Cleanser.	Throat	Carcinoma
Cancer: Esophageal	EDTFL	50,520,600,930,12690,125000,265710,434030,5 71000,839000	May be caused by Porphyromonas gingivalis.	Throat	Cancer
Cancer Gastric	XTRA	676	Use Blood Cleanser.	Stomach	Cancer
Cancer Stomach		*Can be caused by Helicobacter pylori.*			
Cancer Stomach	CAFL	676,728,880,2167,2950,	See Heliobacter Pylori. Use Blood Cleanser.	Stomach	Cancer
Cancer: Stomach	EDTFL	150,2120,20000,45150,73300,96500,125000,37 57500,434330,563190	As mentioned above	Stomach	Cancer
Cancer Stomach	XTRA KHZ	30,180,2500,15030,96500,125150,377910,6470 00,789000,985670,	As mentioned above	Stomach	Cancer
Cancer Stomach 2	XTRA	660,676,690,727.5,880,2167,2950,	As mentioned above	Stomach	Cancer
Cancer Stomach 3	XTRA	347,352,676,695,705,728,880,2167,2779,2819,2 950,	As mentioned above	Stomach	Cancer
Cancer Stomach 4	XTRA	0.2,0.4,0.59,0.8,695,705,728,880,2167,2779,281 9,2950,	As mentioned above	Stomach	Cancer
Cancer Carcinoid Tumor Gastrointestinal	KHZ	50,520,600,930,12690,125000,269710,425030,5 71000,839000,	Slow-growing and potentially malignant.		Carcinoma

Subject / Argument	Author	Frequencies	Notes	Origin	Target
Cancer: Digestive System	EDTFL	20,30,40,5030,119340,350000,434330,691270,7 59830,927100	As mentioned above		Cancer
Cancer: Gastric (Stomach) Cancer: Gastrointestinal	EDTFL	150,230,730,850,5260,127250,335910,487500,6 92490,752010	As mentioned above		Cancer
Gastrointestinal Cancer	EDTFL	150,230,730,850,5260,127250,335910,487500,6 92490,752010,			Cancer
Cancer: Intestinal [Gastrointestinal]	EDTFL	150,230,730,850,5260,127250,335910,487500,6 92490,752010,	As mentioned above		Cancer
Cancer Intestinal	KHZ	50,520,600,930,12690,125000,269710,425030,5 71000,839000,	As mentioned above	Intestines	Cancer
Cancer Intestinal	XTRA	15,55,1070.81,1075.77,2000,21508,21607.59,	As mentioned above	Intestines	Cancer
Intestinal Cancer	EDTFL	150,230,730,850,5260,127250,335910,487500,6 92490,752010,		Intestines	Cancer
Cancer: Small Intestine	EDTFL	300,2120,2330,17500,45750,375170,434000,52 7000,662710,723010,		Intestines	Cancer
Cancer: Colon	EDTFL	20,30,40,5030,119340,350000,434330,691270,7 59830,927100		Intestines	Cancer
Cancer Carcinoma Colon	CAFL BIO	656	Use Blood Cleanser. See BX Virus, and Cancer BX Virus sets.	Colon	Carcinoma
Colorectal cancer		Can be caused by Escherichia Coli, Helicobacter pylori, Streptococcus bovis and Fusobacterium nucleatum, with Human Papillomaviruses, and with the helminth Schistosoma japonicum. JC virus may be a risk factor for colorectal cancer.			
Cancer: Rectal (Rectum) Rectal Cancer	EDTFL	180,250,5710,18500,41500,126510,434400,472 000,538100,614010	Also called Colorectal, Colon, or Bowel Cancer.	Rectum	Cancer
Anal Cancer		Can be caused by Human Papilloma virus (HPV)			
Cancer Liver		Can be caused by Hepatitis B virus, Hepatitis C virus, and by the helminth Schistosoma japonicum.			
Cancer Liver	XTRA	214,393,479,520,734,3130,		Liver	Cancer
Cancer: Liver Cancer	EDTFL	70,120,600,800,2500,22500,72500,434390,7391 00,905310,		Liver	Cancer
Cancer Liver Cancer	XTRA KHZ	110,520,81300,135710,221500,434500,570510, 691510,775480,971550,	Use Blood Cleanser. See BX Virus, and Cancer BX Virus sets.	Liver	Cancer
Cancer Carcinoma Liver 1	CAFL	393,479,520,734,3130,	As mentioned above	Liver	Carcinoma
Cancer Carcinoma Liver 2	XTRA	143,238,275,334,433,477,574,676,752,763,767, 779,869,876,1023.72,6641,6672,20562.06,	As mentioned above	Liver	Carcinoma
Cancer Liver Carcinoma 1	XTRA	393,479,520,734,3130,	As mentioned above	Liver	Carcinoma
Cancer Liver Carcinoma 2	XTRA	143,238,275,334,433,477,574,676,752,763,767, 779,869,876,1023.72,6641,6672,20562,	As mentioned above	Liver	Carcinoma
Cancer Carcinoma Liver Fermentative	CAFL	214	Use Blood Cleanser. See BX Virus, and Cancer BX Virus sets.	Liver	Carcinoma
Cancer Extrahepatic Bile Duct	KHZ	10,370,830,2500,70000,95030,175000,269710,3 55720,755000,	Type of liver cancer.	Liver	Cancer
Cancer: Extrahepatic Bile Duct	EDTFL	30,930,2120,2500,15690,115900,434500,54000 0,670000,790000	Type of liver cancer.	Liver	Cancer
Cancer Gallbladder		Can be caused by the bacterium Salmonella typhi.			
Cancer: Gallbladder	EDTFL	50,520,600,930,12690,125000,260710,301000,4 34030,812200	Use Blood Cleanser.	Gallbladder	Cancer
Cancer Pancreatic		Can be caused by Hepatitis B virus and the bacterium Helicobacter pylori.			
Cancer Pancreatic	CUST	150000	TTFields - Cell line name: AsPC-1	Pancreas	Cancer
Pancreatic Cancer	EDTFL	70,570,23100,50000,375180,434500,527000,66 7000,753230,986220		Pancreas	Cancer
Cancer Pancreatic 1	XTRA	47,832,2084,2127,2160,2182,2219,2452,2876,	See also Cancer Islet Cells Carcinoma and Cancer Pancreatic Exocrine and Islet Cell.	Pancreas	Cancro
Cancer Pancreatic 2	XTRA	545,547,556,600,625,650,660,690,727.5,784,78 7,1560,2000,2008,2127.5,2184,2455,2489,2492	As mentioned above	Pancreas	Cancer
Cancer Pancreatic Exocrine and Islet Cell	KHZ	60,500,47500,150000,219340,225150,210500,4 54500,515160,688290,	Also see Cancer Islet Cells Carcinoma and Cancer Pancreatic.	Pancreas	Cancer
Cancer: Pancreatic, Exocrine & Islet Cell	EDTFL	70,570,23100,50000,375180,434500,527000,66 7000,753230,986220	Also see Cancer Islet Cells Carcinoma and Cancer Pancreatic.	Pancreas	Cancer
Cancer: Islet Cell Carcinoma	EDTFL	160,550,850,7500,20000,47500,95310,210500,4 34950,527000	Pancreatic Neuroendocrine Tumor. Most are benign.	Pancreas	Carcinoma
Cancer: Kidney [Renal]	EDTFL	100,520,7500,30000,225030,434150,527000,66 2710,749000,986220,		Kidney	Cancer
Cancer: Renal Cell (kidney)	EDTFL	100,520,7500,30000,225030,434150,527000,66 2710,749000,986220		Kidney	Cancer
Wilms Tumor [nephroblastoma]	EDTFL	30,460,750,850,2500,7500,96500,328850,43493 0,451170,	Also called Nephroblastoma. Kidney cancer occurring mostly in children.	Kidney	Cancer

Subject / Argument	Author	Frequencies	Notes	Origin	Target
Rhabdoid Tumor	EDTFL	160,570,780,950,8500,95640,217520,491000,52 4370,892410	Very aggressive form of tumour originally described as a variant of Wilms' tumour, mainly a kidney tumour occurring mostly in children. Also see Cancer Wilms' Tumor, Wilms Tumor, and Nephroblastoma.	Kidney	Tumor
Cancer Bladder		*Can be caused by* **Schistosoma helminths, Bilharzia, Human Papilloma virus (HPV).**			
Cancer Bladder	CAFL	**329,635,847,9889**	Also see Bladder TBC, Cancer Bladder TBC, Cancer Urethral, Parasites, and Schistosoma. Use Blood Cleanser.	Bladder	Cancer
Cancer: Bladder Cancer	EDTFL	130,350,47500,159300,352930,475150,527000, 662710,742000,988900,		Bladder	Cancer
Cancer Bladder	XTRA KHZ	80,5750,7250,50000,97500,210500,524370,655 200,750000,927100,	As mentioned above	Bladder	Cancer
Cancer Bladder 2	XTRA	1015.99,1076.82,1093.47,1236.71,1272.83,1286 .84,1378.98,1248.53,1577.75,1759.04,1778.38,1 863.21,11031.25,13671.87,	As mentioned above	Bladder	Cancer
Cancer Bladder 3	XTRA	329,1035.49,1087.17,1089.25,1238.74,1257.39, 1261.5,1272.83,1350.21,1431.24,1564.68,1734. 8,1799.56,1910.33,9889,11031.25,13671.87,	As mentioned above	Bladder	Cancer
Cancer Bladder 4	XTRA	1013.25,1076.82,1228.66,1277.15,1288.03,1331 .18,1373.96,1423.15,1564.68,1622.97,1742.8,17 82.57,11031.25,13671.87,	As mentioned above	Bladder	Cancer
Cancer Bladder TBC	XTRA	360,642,724,726,771,	As mentioned above	Bladder	Cancer
Bladder TBC	CAFL	642,771,360,726,724,	Transitional Bladder Cancer. Can also cause kidney cancer. Also see Cancer Bladder and Cancer Urethral.	Bladder	Cancer
Bladder TBC	VEGA	**771**	As mentioned above	Bladder	Cancer
Cancer Urologic Neoplasms	XTRA KHZ	30,460,750,850,2500,7500,17500,96500,352930 ,451170,	Includes all bladder cancers, renal cell cancer, and prostate cancer.		Cancer
Urologic Cancer	EDTFL	130,350,47500,159300,352930,475150,527000, 662710,742000,988900,			Cancer
Cancer: Urethral (Urinary) Cancer: Urinary Bladder Cancer: Urologic Neoplasms Urinary Tract Cancer	EDTFL	140,320,950,5250,12710,45000,97500,150000,4 34080,985670	Also see Bladder TBC, Cancer Bladder, Cancer Bladder TBC, Parasites, and Schistosoma. Use Blood Cleanser.	Urethra	Cancer
Cancer Prostate		*Can be caused by* **Xenotropic murine leukemia virus, BK virus, Propionibacterium Acnes, Trichomonas vaginalis (protozoan)** . *In addition by* **Human Papilloma virus (HPV)** *along with the* **Epstein Barr virus (EBV)** .			
Prostate Tumor	CAFL	666,690,727,2008,2127,	Malignant. See Cancer prostate sets.	Prostate	Tumor
Cancer: Prostate	EDTFL	180,220,3520,13810,57630,291140,434800,608 110,771420,795020	As mentioned above	Prostate	Cancer
Cancer Prostate	KHZ	666,2125,**2128**,2131,2140,2145,3672,	Also see Prostate Adenomium, and Prostate Hyperplasia. Use Blood Cleanser.	Prostate	Cancer
Cancer Prostate	PROV	20,72,304,442,666,690,727,766,787,790,800,92 0,1875,1998,**2008**,2050,2120,2127,**2128**,2130,2 217,2250,2720,5000,	As mentioned above	Prostate	Cancer
Cancer Prostate 1	CAFL	666,2125,**2128**,2131,2140,2145,3672,	As mentioned above	Prostate	Cancer
Cancer Prostate 2	XTRA	20,60,72,95,125,304,408,442,660,688,690,727.5 ,748,766,787,790,800,854,920,1840,1875,1998, 2008,2050,2120,2125,2127,2130,2131,2140,214 5,2217,2250,2288,2720,3672,5000,10025,	As mentioned above	Prostate	Cancer
Cancer Prostate 3	XTRA	20,60,72,95,125,304,442,666,690,727,766,787,7 90,800,920,1875,1998,**2008**,2050,2120,2127,**21 28**,2130,2217,2250,2720,5000,	As mentioned above	Prostate	Cancer
Cancer Prostate 4	XTRA	**854,1840,2145,2288**	As mentioned above	Prostate	Cancer
Cancer: Penile (Penis)	EDTFL	70,550,900,22500,47500,434030,527000,66700 0,752700,988900		Genital	Cancer
Cancer Genital Neoplasms Male	KHZ	10,550,780,50000,97500,229320,454370,51968 0,684810,712000,	Abnormal growths or tumors. Use Blood Cleanser.	Genital	Cancer
Cancer: Testicular (Testis)	EDTFL	110,400,12710,42500,95000,210480,434750,57 1000,837000,932000	Use Blood Cleanser.	Genital	Cancer
Cancer: Genital, Female	EDTFL	80,850,2500,43000,97230,175000,434000,7910 00,853000,972100	Use Blood Cleanser.	Genital	Cancer
Cancer Genital Neoplasms Female	KHZ	30,460,27500,17500,40000,85160,95000,15000 0,210500,451170,	Abnormal growths or tumors. Use Blood Cleanser.	Genital	Cancer
Gynecologic Neoplasms [Cancer Genital Female]	EDTFL	80,850,2500,43000,97230,175000,434000,7910 00,853000,972100,		Genital	Cancer
Cancer Uterine	XTRA	127,443,2288,2944=1800,	Cervical cancer associated with Human Papilloma Virus (HPV).	Uterus	Cancer
Cancer: Uterine , Sarcoma	EDTFL	80,120,40000,85900,136420,328050,357300,57 1000,840000,937410	As mentioned above	Uterus	Sarcoma
Cancer: Uterine Cervical	EDTFL	130,7500,35130,67500,96500,275160,434160,5 27000,663710,752700,		Uterus	Cancer

Subject / Argument	Author	Frequencies	Notes	Origin	Target
Cancer Carcinoma Uterine Fermentative	CAFL BIO	127	Use Blood Cleanser. See EBV, Leukoplakia, Mouth eruptions white patches, Papilloma, BX Virus, and Cancer BX Virus sets.	Uterus	Carcinoma
Endometrial Cancer	EDTFL	400,780,5290,7500,37000,95500,185000,43400 0,792000,985670	Cancer arising from womb's lining, most commonly after menopause, and associated with obesity, hypertension, diabetes, and excess estrogen.	Womb	Cancer
Adenoma Cervical	CAFL	433	Epithelial tumor of the cervix that can be benign or malignant. See Cancer Adenoma and Cervical sets.	Uterus	Cancer
Cervical Cancer		*Can be caused by Human Papilloma virus (HPV)*			
Cervix Adenocarcinoma	CUST	150000	TTFields - Cell line name: HeLa	Utero	Carcinoma
Cervical Cancer	XTRA	2288,2944=2400	See Cancer Cervical and Cancer Carcinoma Uterine Fermentative sets.	Womb	Cancer
Cancer Cervical	CAFL	466,907	Use Blood Cleanser.	Uterus	Cancer
Cancer: Womb	EDTFL	50,520,620,940,2500,127600,235370,434500,79 2200,875470,			Cancer
Cancer: Cervical [/Uterus]	EDTFL	130,7500,35130,67500,96500,275160,434160,5 27000,663710,752700,	As mentioned above	Uterus	Cancer
Cancer Cervical 1	XTRA	466,907,2288,2944=2880,	As mentioned above	Uterus	Cancer
Cancer Cervical 2	XTRA	16816.25,16813.5,16970,9609,9258,5657,1051, 1011,907,874,767,489,466,404,265,110,45,1000 0,5000,3176,2489,186,372,427,446,465,484,503 ,522,541,560,579,598,617,636,655,674,693,712, 731,750,769,788,807,826,845,864,883,902,921, 940,959,978,997,1016,1035,1054,1073,1488,15 50,1568,1644,1865,1909,2976,5310,5952,	As mentioned above	Uterus	Cancer
Cancer Uterine Cervical Neoplasms	KHZ	10,400,780,5290,7500,37000,95500,185000,792 000,985670,	Cervical cancer associated with Human Papilloma Virus (HPV).	Uterus	Cancer
Cancer Ovarian		*Can be associated with Mumps virus.*			
Cancer Ovarian	CUST	200000,	TTFields - Cell line name: A2780	Ovary	Cancer
Cancer: Ovarian Epithelial	EDTFL	40,250,650,930,2500,7500,96500,334250,43440 0,792200		Ovary	Cancer
Cancer: Ovarian Germ Cell	EDTFL	80,570,15750,52500,62500,95000,434400,5243 70,682020,792200		Ovary	Cancer
Cancer: Ovarian Low Malignant Potential Tumor	EDTFL	170,520,680,830,2500,127600,204350,235370,4 34590,792200		Ovary	Cancer
Cancer: Germ Cell	EDTFL	50,520,600,930,12690,125000,263710,434030,5 71000,839000,	Starts in an ovary, producing abnormal invasive cells which spread.	Ovary	Cancer
Ovarian Cancer	EDTFL	170,520,680,830,2500,127600,235370,434500,7 92200,875470	As mentioned above	Ovary	Cancer
Cancer Ovarian	XTRA	20,26,444,465,600,625,650,660,690,727.5,776,7 87,802,832,880,1500,1550,1600,1800,1865,200 8,2127.5,2170,2489,2720,	As mentioned above	Ovary	Cancer
Krukenberg Tumor [Ovary Tumor]	EDTFL	170,520,680,830,2500,127600,204350,235370,4 34590,792200,	Metastasized malignancy in ovary, usually from GI tract primary cancer. See appropriate Cancer sets.	Ovary	Cancer
Cancer: Vaginal	EDTFL	30,2750,7500,17500,96500,358570,434820,518 920,683000,712230			Cancer
Cancer: Vulvar Vulvar Cancer	EDTFL	170,930,5120,17600,35750,73300,434250,4922 20,830000,939000	Malignant invasive growth in vulva. May be melanotic, squamous or basal cell carcinoma.		Cancer
Cancer: Gestational Tumor	EDTFL	50,520,620,940,2500,127600,235370,434500,79 2200,875470,			Cancer
Trophoblastic Cancer [Gestational] Trophoblastic Tumor	EDTFL	50,520,620,940,2500,127600,235370,434500,79 2200,875470,			Cancer
Cancer Gestational Trophoblastic Tumor	XTRA KHZ	250,780,930,10890,7500,95900,322530,415700, 562910,742060,	Pregnancy-related tumor.		Cancer
Cancer Trophoblastic Neoplasms	KHZ	130,7500,35160,67500,96500,275160,475160,5 27000,663710,752700,	As mentioned above		Cancer
Cancer: Trophoblastic	EDTFL	20,370,22500,52500,90000,275000,275160,310 250,425110,838000	As mentioned above		Cancer
Breast Cancer		*Can be caused by Bacteroides fragilis, Mouse mammary tumor virus (MMTV), Epstein-Barr virus, Human Papilloma virus (HPV), Bovine leukemia virus (BLV).*			
Breast Adenocarcinoma	CUST	120000,	TTFields - Cell line name: MCF-7 and MDA-MB-231	Breast	Cancer
Breast Cancer	EDTFL	20,460,5120,27500,85000,95750,150000,43471 0,682450,753070,	Also see Cancer sets.Use Blood Cleanser.	Breast	Cancer
Cancer Breast 1	CAFL	120,166,666,676,732,802,866,1550,2008,2100,2 104,2112,2116,2120,2127,**2128**,2152,2182,2184 ,2187,2189,2191,2876,2950,3072,	Use Blood Cleanser.	Breast	Cancer
Cancer Breast 2	CAFL	28,96,317,422,477,690,728,808,942,1234,1552, 1830,1862,2084,2112,2136,2145,2160,2720,304 0,3176,4412,	Use Blood Cleanser.	Breast	Cancer

Subject / Argument	Author	Frequencies	Notes	Origin	Target
Cancer Breast 3	CAFL	48,72,444,1865,**2008**,2063,2103,**2128**=3360,21 33,2146,2162,2173,2180,2189,2208,2263,2289, 2333,2672,	Use Blood Cleanser.	Breast	Cancer
Cancer Breast 4	CAFL	127,304,478,656,982,1582,2120,2134,9000,999 9,	Use Blood Cleanser.	Breast	Cancer
Cancer Breast 4	XTRA	28,96,317,422,477,690,728,808,942,1234,1552, 1830,1862,2048,2112,2136,2145,2160,2720,304 0,3176,4412,	Use Blood Cleanser.	Breast	Cancer
Cancer Breast 5	CAFL	33,1131,**2128**=3360,	Use Blood Cleanser.	Breast	Cancer
Cancer Breast 5	XTRA	64,95,96,240,317,422,524,664,808,854,942,943, 1234,1552,1830,1862,2048,2050,2125,2136,214 5,2160,2189,2450,2452,2876,3040,3176,4412,5 000,	Use Blood Cleanser.	Breast	Cancer
Cancer Breast 6	XTRA	127,304,478,656,982,1582,2120,2134,9000,999 9,	Use Blood Cleanser.	Breast	Cancer
Paget's Disease of Breast Paget's Disease, Mammary	EDTFL	230,320,620,950,5000,22500,419340,651100,72 3030,868430	Type of malignant breast cancer with appearance of eczema, usually affecting nipple and areola. Also see appropriate Cancer sets.	Breast	Cancer

Subject / Argument	Author	Frequencies	Notes	Origin	Target
Skin neoplasm		*Can be caused by Human Papilloma virus (HPV).*			
Cancer: Skin Cancer: Skin, Kaposi's Sarcoma	EDTFL	110,400,830,5500,25000,125170,225750,47519 0,527000,662710	See Cancer Basal Cell Skin Carcinoma, Cancer Squamous Cell Carcinoma, and Cancer Melanoma. Use Blood Cleanser.	Skin	Cancer
Cancer: Skin, Melanoma	EDTFL	350,930,7500,17500,52500,70000,215700,3254 00,434000,523010,		Skin	Cancer
Cancer Skin	XTRA	666,760=1800,**2008**,2116=1800,2125,**2128**,213 1,2140,2145,2280=480,3672,6130,6601,6672	As mentioned above	Skin	Cancer
Lentigo, Malignant	EDTFL	60,120,850,7510,32520,43060,151180,225530,4 34620,659020	Form of skin cancer (melanoma), which occurs mainly in the face of elderly people.	Skin	Melanoma
Cancer: Melanoma	EDTFL	350,930,7500,17500,52500,70000,215700,3254 00,434000,523010	Most dangerous form of skin cancer, sometimes occurring in mouth, intestines, or eyes. See appropriate Cancer sets.	Skin	Melanoma
Melanoma Melanoma Amelanotic	EDTFL	350,930,7500,17500,52500,70000,215700,3254 00,434000,523010,	Type of skin cancer where cells do not make melanin, making them more difficult to recognise.	Skin	Melanoma
Cancer Melanoma 1	CAFL	100,1000,10000,666,728,1050,2050,**2128**,2008, 2217,60,80,95,880,450,495,45,465,787,125,20,1 0,7.5,	As mentioned above	Skin	Melanoma
Cancer Melanoma 2	XTRA	7.5,10,20,45,60,80,95,100,110,125,450,465,466, 495,666,728,787,802,880,907,979,1000,1050,11 02,1552,**2008**,2050,**2128**,2217,	As mentioned above	Skin	Melanoma
Cancer Melanoma Metastasis	CAFL	979	Mostly affects skin, but can appear in mouth, intestines, or eyes. Use Blood Cleanser.	Skin	Melanoma
Cancer HPV (Moles and Tumors)	XTRA	1603750	From JW. Use sine wave. See Human Papilloma Virus, and Papilloma HPV.	Skin	Cancer
Cancer Basal Cell Skin Carcinoma	XTRA	760=300,2116=1800,2280=300	Malignant but rarely fatal. Affects skin of face, head, neck, and sometimes trunk. See Cancer Carcinoma Basal Cell Skin, EBV, Leukoplakia, Mouth Eruptions White Patches, **Papilloma**, BX Virus, and Cancer BX Virus.	Skin	Cancer
Cancer Carcinoma Basal Cell Skin 1	XTRA	11276.06,11276.10,11276.11,11276.12,11276.2 3,11276.27,	As mentioned above	Skin	Carcinoma
Cancer Carcinoma Basal Cell Skin	CAFL	2116=1800,760,2280,**2128**,2876,	As mentioned above	Skin	Carcinoma
Carcinoma Skin Basal Cell	XTRA	760,2116=1800,2280,	As mentioned above	Skin	Carcinoma
Carcinoma Basal Cell	XTRA KHZ	80,120,850,5160,20000,40000,85000,97500,355 720,454500,515000,	As mentioned above	Skin	Carcinoma
Basal Cell Carcinoma	XTRA	760=1800,2116=1800,2280=480,666,**2008**,2125 ,**2128**,2131,2140,2145,2280=480,3672,6130,66 01,6672,	Common skin cancer, mostly found on head or neck. Rarely fatal or metastatic.	Skin	Carcinoma
Basal Cell Nevus Syndrome	EDTFL	100,570,800,7500,15200,52800,95110,655200,7 50000,923700,	Genetic predisposition to Basal Cell Carcinoma development.	Skin	Cancer
Nevoid Basal Cell Carcinoma	EDTFL	50,160,520,940,12690,125000,328800,434030,5 71000,839000	As mentioned above	Skin	Cancer
Rodent Ulcer	EDTFL	150,240,650,830,2500,127500,255470,387500,6 96500,825910,	Is an old term for what is now called nodular basal cell carcinoma.	Skin	Cancer
Gorlin Syndrome	EDTFL	370,950,2500,7500,67500,96500,375520,47591 0,525910,801290,		Skin	Cancer
Cancer: Skin, T-Cell Lymph	EDTFL	110,400,830,5500,25000,125000,125170,37575 0,434330,563190,		Skin	Cancer
Cancer: Lymphoma, T-Cell	EDTFL	50,410,620,15750,87500,324650,434000,65520 0,750000,927100		Skin	Cancer
T-Cell Lymphoma, Cutaneous	EDTFL	50,410,620,15750,87500,325750,434000,65520 0,750000,927100,		Skin	Cancer
Granulomatous Slack Skin	EDTFL	140,1000,5500,12310,45000,370500,547500,65 6400,725370,825520	It is a form of cutaneous T-cell lymphoma and a variant of mycosis fungoides.	Skin	Lymphoma

Subject / Argument	Author	Frequencies	Notes	Origin	Target
Sezary Syndrome [T Cell Lymphoma]	EDTFL	50,410,620,15750,87500,325750,434000,65520 0,750000,927100,	Cutaneous T Cell Lymphomas. Sometimes considered to be late Mycosis Fungoides with Lymphadenopathy.	Skin	Lymphoma
Carcinoma, Merkel Cell	EDTFL	350,930,12330,25240,35680,87500,93500,2336 30,434000,519340,	Rare aggressive skin cancer due to Merkel cell **Polyomavirus (MCV)**.	Skin	Cancer
Squamous cell carcinoma		*Can be caused by **Human Papilloma virus (HPV)**.*			
Cancer: Squamous Cell Carcinoma	EDTFL	50,520,620,940,12690,125000,307700,434030,5 71000,839000		Skin	Carcinoma
Squamous Cell Carcinoma	XTRA	666,760,2008,2116=1800,2125,**2128**,2131,2140 ,2145,2280=480,3672,6130,6601,6672,	Also see Cancer Squamous Cell Carcinoma, Bowen's Disease, and Cancer Lung Non-Small Cell sets.	Skin	Carcinoma
Bowen's Disease	EDTFL	40,350,2500,35160,93500,458500,517500,6894 10,712000,993410	Also called Squamous Cell Carcinoma in Situ. Can manifest on skin and sex organs.	Skin	Cancer
Cancer: Mycosis Fungoides	EDTFL	80,120,850,5170,22400,43300,87220,97500,355 720,434500	Skin cancer resembling eczema. Use Blood Cleanser.	Skin	Cancer
Cancer Mycosis Fungoides	BIO	852	Skin cancer resembling eczema. Use Blood Cleanser.	Skin	Cancer
Mycosis Fungoides	BIO	532,662,678,852,1444,	Form of cutaneous cancer resembling Eczema. Cutaneous T Cell lymphoma, sub-type of non Hodgkin's - see sets for these.	Skin	Cancer
Cancer: Bone	EDTFL	20,30,40,5030,119340,350000,434330,691270,7 59830,927100,	Can be benign or malignant.	Bone	Cancer
Cancer Bone	XTRA	**2008**,2125,**2128**,2131,2140,2145,3524,3672,371 3,6130,6601,6672,	As mentioned above	Bone	Cancer
OsteoSarcoma	EDTF KHZ	10,240,730,7900,67220,127500,317500,665520, 831330,913500,	Cancerous tumor of bone. See appropriate Cancer and Sarcoma sets.	Bone	Sarcoma
Cancer OsteoSarcoma	KHZ	140,300,830,7500,128000,202430,340000,4500 00,575370,719340,	Aggressive malignant bone tumor in children and young adults.	Bone	Sarcoma
ChondroSarcoma	EDTFL	50,290,15750,45000,93500,376290,512330,689 930,759830,925710	Skeletal system cancer. See Cancer BY Virus, Cancer BXBY, and Cancer Sarcoma sets.	Bone	Sarcoma
Cancer FibroSarcoma	PROV	1744	Originates in fibrous tissues of bone.	Bone	Sarcoma
Cancer Fibrous Tumor Secondary	CAFL	1340	Originates in fibrous tissues of bone.	Bone	Cancer
Argentaffinoma	EDTLF	50,520,600,930,12640,125000,269710,434030,5 71000,839000,	Also called Carcinoid Syndrome - refers to symptoms secondary to carcinoid tumor - malignant tumor composed of Argentaffini cells, that is, those that are stained with silver salts.		Tumor
Cancer Cells Conidium Head	CAFL	728	Caused by fungal spores. Use Blood Cleanser.		Cancer
Cancer Germ Cell Tumor Extragonadal	KHZ	160,550,850,7500,20000,47500,95310,210500,4 75950,527000,	Class of tumors originating from gonadal germ cells. Sites: cranium, mouth, neck, mediastinum, pelvis, ovary, testis.		Cancer
Cancer Tertiary	CAFL	20,421,965,50,383,	Use Blood Cleanser.		Cancer
Tumor Staphylococcus Aureus	XTRA	424,478,555,644,647,727,728,738,745,784,787, 824,943,999,1050,7270,8697,	Also see **Staphylococcus aureus** sets.		Tumor
Tumor Virus Infections	EDTFL	20,320,620,970,12630,112500,265750,425710,7 45190,935700	Oncoviruses that can cause cancer. See appropriate Cancer sets.		Tumor
Metastasis (Cancer)(Organ)	EDTFL	130,460,830,12690,93500,221500,434710,5123 30,667000,753070		Metastasis	Cancer
Cancer: Metastasis Squamous	EDTFL	50,520,620,940,12690,125000,307700,434030,5 71000,839000,		Metastasis	Cancer
Cancer: Metastasis (Organ)	EDTFL	130,460,830,12690,93500,221500,434710,5123 30,667000,753070		Metastasis	Cancer
Cancer: Metastasis (Alternative Set) Comprehensive Breast, lung, prostate, bowel/colon/rectal, Liver, Endometrial	EDTFL	350,930,12330,25230,35690,87500,93500,2336 30,434000,519340		Metastasis	Cancer

Notes on TTFields:	*Tumor Treating Fields or TTFields represent an innovative method of destroying cancer cells. The method consists in applying a high frequency electric field, capable of stopping the proliferation of cancer cells. The electric field, produced by frequency generators in the 100-300 kHz range, is applied by means of electrodes positioned on the skin, so as to invest the cancerous mass. To be effective, this therapy requires a very high number of hours of application. For further information, consult the book "**Therapeutic Waves**", by the same Author.*

Subject / Argument	Author	Frequencies	Notes	Origin	Target
Paraneoplastic Autonomic Dysfunction	EDTFL	20,220,900,7500,22700,85370,155470,262500,3 92500,591000	Set of signs or symptoms due to cancer but not caused by local cancer cells.		
Paraneoplastic Encephalomyelitis	EDTFL	50,960,5830,7500,12330,113230,425000,57100 0,865830,937410,	As mentioned above		
Paraneoplastic Syndromes	EDTFL	20,220,900,7500,22700,85370,155470,355350,3 68000,398400	As mentioned above		
Lambert-Eaton Myasthenic Syndrome	EDTFL	200,460,600,2750,122000,275690,327500,6495 40,735000,833690	Rare autoimmune disorder with weakness of limb muscles, often accompanying cancer, typically small cell lung cancer (see sets).		

Subject / Argument	Author	Frequencies	Notes	Origin	Target
Eaton-Lambert Syndrome	EDTFL	30,520,620,930,7500,12710,96500,225540,3000 00,323530	As mentioned above		

17 - Pathogens and Parasites

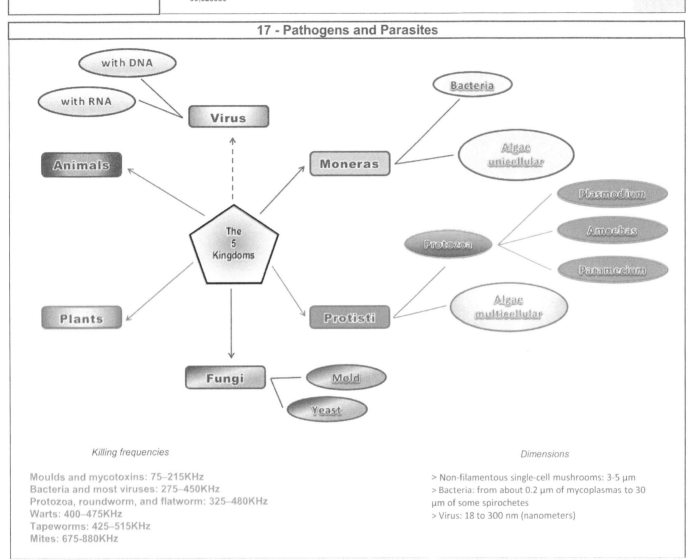

Killing frequencies

Moulds and mycotoxins: 75–215KHz
Bacteria and most viruses: 275–450KHz
Protozoa, roundworm, and flatworm: 325–480KHz
Warts: 400–475KHz
Tapeworms: 425–515KHz
Mites: 675-880KHz

Dimensions

> Non-filamentous single-cell mushrooms: 3-5 μm
> Bacteria: from about 0.2 μm of mycoplasmas to 30 μm of some spirochetes
> Virus: 18 to 300 nm (nanometers)

Note: *diseases caused by pathogens are indicated in blue*

17a - Infections

Herxheimer reaction	EDTFL	120,500,850,5910,137500,372500,416600,4180 00,420200,824370		Infections
Infection Any	XTRA	**880,787,727,465**		Infections
Infections General	CAFL	1550,880,802,786,728,465,444,125,95,72,48,20, 304,1.2,5500,676,422,766,	See General antiseptic.	Infections
Basic Infection	BIOM	1550; 880; 802; 786; 728; 465; 444; 125; 95; 72; 48; 20; 304; 1.2; 5499.5; 676; 422; 766		Infections
Infection of Various Classes	BIOM	1600; 1550; 1500; 880; 832; 787; 776; 760; 727; 700; 690; 666; 650; 625; 600; 465; 444; 125; 95; 72; 20; 1865; 500; 450; 440; 428; 660		Infections
Infections (various types)	BIOM	5500; 1865; 1600; 1550; 1500; 880; 832; 802; 787; 776; 760; 727; 690; 666; 650; 625; 600; 465; 444; 125; 95; 72; 20; 1865; 500; 450; 440; 428; 660		Infections
Infections	BIOM	1550; 1500; 1000; 880; 832; 802; 787; 776; 760; 727; 700; 690; 685; 666; 650; 625; 600; 465; 444; 440; 428; 125; 20		Infections
Infections 1	XTRA	1.19,20,48,72,95,125,250,304,333,422,444,465, 523,660,676,690,727.5,766,768,786,802,880,15 50,1865,5500	See General antiseptic.	Infections
Infections 2	XTRA	428,440,600,625,650,700,760,776,787,832,1500 ,1600,2112,2170,5000,	See General antiseptic.	Infections

Subject / Argument	Author	Frequencies	Notes	Origin	Target
Infections General Secondary	CAFL	428,440,450,500,600,625,650,660,666,690,700, 760,776,832,1500,1600,1865,2112,5000,	See General antiseptic.		Infections
Infections General Tertiary	CAFL	610,732,751,832,1800,1850,2008,2489,2720,30 40,40000,	See General antiseptic.		Infections
Infection: basic, secondary, and tertiary	BIOM	5000; 3040; 2112; 832; 751; 732; 610			Infections
Infections General Tertiary	XTRA	610,732,751,832,1800,1850,2008,2489,2720,30 40,20000,	See General antiseptic.		Infections
Infection Bone	XTRA	47,600,625,650,660,690,727.5,776,787,880,160 0,1800,10000,	Also see Osteomyelitis sets.		Infections
Infection Diabetic	XTRA	20,80,190,660,690,727.5,800,2020,			Infections
Infection Allergies	XTRA	10000,	Use for infection OR allergies.	Allergy	Infections
Sepsis	EDTFL	80,240,650,900,2500,27700,55910,119340,3937 00,536420	Or septicemia. Condition where immune response to infection harms tissues or organs. Usually bacterial, but can be fungal, viral, or parasitical.		Infections
Sepsis Syndrome	EDTFL	80,240,650,900,2500,27700,55910,688290,7120 00,995380			Infections
Septic Shock	EDTFL	80,240,650,900,12330,27600,135520,551000,72 5290,875000,	Serious condition that occurs when Sepsis leads to dangerously low blood pressure and cell metabolism abnormalities.		Infections
Shock, Toxic	EDTFL	170,450,900,5910,137500,372500,416600,4180 00,742000,985660	As mentioned above		Infections
Toxic Shock Syndrome	EDTFL	170,450,900,5910,137500,372500,416600,4180 00,742000,985660,	As mentioned above		Infections
Shock, Endotoxic	EDTFL	170,450,900,5910,137500,372500,416600,4180 00,742000,985660,	As mentioned above		Infections
Surgery Pre-op Post-op Prevent Infections	CAFL	146,428,444,465,522,727,776,787,802,832,880, 1500,1550,1600,1800,2170,	Use General Antiseptic, Staphylococci, and Streptococcus Infection sets.		Infections
Cross Infection	EDTFL	190,310,680,9080,112830,217500,335000,5475 00,725280,925000,	The transfer of infection, especially to a hospital patient with a different infection or between different species of animal or plant.		Infections
Nosocomial Infections	EDTFL	40,180,780,2500,7500,55290,95520,225290,326 250,519340			Infections
Iatrogenic Infections	XTRA	146,333,424,428,434,444,465,522,523,590,594, 660,690,727.5,768,776,786,787,802,832,834,88 0,1500,1550,1600,1800,1865,2170,	Infections contracted in a hospital/medical facility, or caused by a medical professional.		Infections
Infections Fungi, Bacteria and Viruses			See the following paragraphs dedicated to these Pathogens.		Infections
General Antiseptic	CAFL	10000,5000,2145,1550,1488,880,802,786,776,7 66,760,728,688,683,676,666,660,464,450,444,4 28,120,20,			Infections
Antiseptic General	CAFL	428,444,450,465,660,727,760,787,802,880,1550 ,5000,10000=300,	Common pathogens.		Infections
Antiseptic, General	BIOM	10000; 1550; 880; 800; 787; 727; 522; 146; 100; 20	Common pathogens.		Infections
Antiseptic	BIOM	727; 880; 787; 465; 802; 1550; 555; 428; 660; 760; 450; 1.7			Infections
General Antiseptic 1	XTRA	428,444,450,465,660,727,760,787,802,880,1550 ,5000,10000,			Infections
General Antiseptic 3	XTRA	14,333,428,450,465,523,555,590,660,690,728,7 60,768,786,787,802,804,880,1360,1550,1770,18 65,2000,2720,3176,5000,10000,			Infections
General Antiseptic and Circulation Stimulation	XTRA	1.19,20,786,832,1050,5000,			Infections
Antiseptic effect	BIOM	666; 690; 728; 802; 880; 1550; 1865			
Clark 2.5KHz Zapper Contact	XTRA	2500=420,0=1260,2500=420,0=1260,2500=420,	On 7 mins, off 21 (7-21-7-21-7), Amplitude=9.5, Offset=100%.	Sweep	Infections
Clark 30KHz Zapper Contact	XTRA	30000=420,0=1260,30000=420,0=1260,30000= 420,	30KHz 7 mins, pause 21 (7-21-7-21-7-21 mins), 9.5V, 100% Pos Offset. Contact Mode.	Sweep	Infections
Hulda C Zap 2500	XTRA	2500	Flukes.	Sweep	Infections
Hulda C Zap 3000	XTRA	15000	Flukes.	Sweep	Infections

PRION			PRoteinaceus Infective ONly particle		
Prions 3	RL	656,956,957,958,959,960	From Dr. Richard Loyd. Misfolded proteinaceous material that can pass its defective structure on to other correctly formed proteins.		Prions
Prion Diseases [CJD GSS]	EDTFL	40,200,860,2500,5870,85000,96500,175870,357 770,452590,	As mentioned above		Prions
Prions	ODD	0.07,0.12,0.75,0.93,15.09,24.4,417.5,505,791.5, 995.15,	As mentioned above		Prions
Spongiform Encephalopathy, Subacute	EDTFL	130,250,620,5750,17250,37300,129560,345430, 415700,682020,	Neurodegenerative disease due to Prions.		Prions

Subject / Argument	Author	Frequencies	Notes	Origin	Target
Creutzfeldt-Jakob Syndrome	EDTFL	40,250,860,2500,5870,85000,96500,175870,357770,452590			Prions
Creutzfeldt-Jakob, New Variant	EDTFL	40,200,860,2500,5870,85000,234510,347050,482500,717520,	Neurodegenerative disease due to Prions (PRoteinaceus Infective ONly particl).		Prions
CJD Variant: (V-CJD)	EDTFL	120,350,900,22500,130000,251230,493500,555080,754370,815680	(Creutzfeldt-Jakob Disease Variant)		Prions
Kuru Encephalopathy	EDTFL	130,280,520,1730,7250,27500,37500,123040,327230,533690	Transmissible spongiform encephalopathy caused by a prion. See Creutzfeldt-Jakob and Prions sets.	Brain	Prions
Gerstmann-Straussler Syndrome	EDTFL	80,350,600,870,2250,5000,172500,317950,397500,796500	Very rare inherited prion disease, usually familial.		Prions

Subject / Argument	Author	Frequencies	Notes	Origin	Target
Biofilms 01	XTRA	641.18,543.75,28500,280000,400,80,28.48	Includes chronic Rhinitis (see set) with nasal polyposis, E Coli (see sets), and Staphylococcus Epidermis biofilms (see Staphylococcus Pyogenes Albus).		Biofilms
Bisphenol A	XTRA	1055.525	Plastic pollutant which forms biofilms when Staphylococcus Epidermis (see sets) is present.		Biofilms
Biofilm	RL	477	From Dr. Richard Loyd.		Biofilms

17b - Fungi, Molds, Algae and Diseases

Subject / Argument	Author	Frequencies	Notes	Origin	Target
Fungus General	CAFL	2222,1552,1550,1153,1134,1016,880,802,787,784,727,582,465,422,254,72,20,	See Candida and Yeast sets as well as other specific types.		Fungus
Fungi - Basic Programme	BIOM	2222; 1552; 1550; 1152.9; 1134; 1015.9; 880; 802; 787; 784; 727; 582; 465; 422; 254; 72; 20			Fungus
Fungal and Yeast Infection	XTRA	465			Fungus
Fungal Infections	BIOM	37; 53.5; 100			
Fungal Infection	XTRA	20,465,727,802,880,1550,			Fungus
Fungus Adams	XTRA	943,2644			Fungus
Fungus Black Nail	XTRA	612,644,766,1000,190,465,	Toenail and fingernail Fungus. Also try Onychomycosis.	Nail	Fungus
Fungus EW Range	CAFL	823,824,825,826,827,828,829,			Fungus
Fungus Flora 1	CAFL	331,336,555,587,632,688,757,882,884,887,			Fungus
Fungus Flora	VEGA	632			Fungus
Fungus Foot and General 1	CAFL	1550			Fungus
Foot Fungus	BIOM	200; 727; 787; 880; 5000; 644; 766; 464; 802; 1552; 9998.5; 3176; 304; 379			Fungus
Yeast-like fungi in uterine neck	BIOM	706; 771			Fungus
Fungus Suttons Bar	XTRA	854			Fungus
Fungus and Mold	CAFL	4442,2411,1833,1823,1333,1155,1130,1016,942,933,886,880,866,784,774,766,745,743,728,623,623,594,592,565,555,524,512,464,414,374,344,337,321,254,242,222,158,132,	General set. See Candida and Yeast sets as well as other specific types.		Fungus and Mold
Mold and Fungus General	CAFL	132,245,321,337,344,374,414,464,524,555,728,743,766,784,866,880,886,942,1823,2411,	Also see specific types. See Mold sets.		Fungus and Mold
Fungi and mold	BIOM	4442; 2411; 1833; 1823; 1333; 1155; 1130; 1016; 942; 933; 886; 866; 784; 774; 766; 745; 743; 728; 660; 659; 623; 594; 592; 565; 555; 524; 512; 464; 414; 374; 344; 337; 327; 321; 254; 242; 222; 158; 132			Fungus and Mold
Fungus and Mold 2	XTRA	132,254,321,337,344,374,414,464,524,555,728,743,766,784,866,880,886,942,1823,2411,	General set. See Candida and Yeast sets as well as other specific types.		Fungus and Mold
Mold Spectrum Sweep	XTRA	185385.792-186614.208		Sweep	Mold
Molds General Alternative Set	EDTFL	40,240,62230,135000,235510,329560,340040,592520,654320,779500			Mold
Mold	CAFL	222,242,523,565,592,623,745,933,1130,1833,4442,	General. Also see specific types.		Mold
Mold	BIO	222,242,523,565,592,623,745,933,1130,1155,1333,1833,4442,			Mold
Mold	VEGA	222,242,523,592,745,933,1155,1333,1833,4442			Mold
Molds (Moulds) Human Fungal	EDTFL	77000,126000,133000,177000,181000,188000,232000,242000,277000,288000			Mold
Slime Molds 1	XTRA	81000,126000,21000	From Dr. Hulda Clark. Targets Arcyria, Lycogala, and Stemonitis. Common in Morgellons.		Mold
Slime Molds Sweep	XTRA	145286.417-146713.583	Common in Morgellons. Arcyria, Lycogala, and Stemonitis.		Mold
Mould Infections	BIOM	1550.0; 880.0; 802.0; 727.0; 465.0; 20.0			Mold
Mold A and C	VEGA	331,732,923,982			Mold
Mold Mix A	BIO	594			Mold
Mold Mix B	BIO	158,512,623,774,1016,1463,			Mold

Subject / Argument	Author	Frequencies	Notes	Origin	Target
Mold Mix C	VEGA	1627			Mold
Mold Vac II	VEGA	257			Mold
Yeast General	CAFL	72,254,375,522,876,987,414,422,465,582,787,1016,2222,	See Candida, and Candidiasis sets. Use Parasites General, Roundworm, and Ascaris sets if no lasting relief achieved.		Yeast
Yeast-like fungi, general	BIOM	582; 778; 861; 863; 864; 865; 871; 873; 876; 906; 908; 974; 982; 984; 986; 987; 1016; 1134			Yeast
Yeast General V	CAFL	72,422,582,787,1016,2222,1134,254,987,986,984,982,980,974,908,906,878,876,873,871,866,865,864,863,861,778,	As mentioned above		Yeast
Yeast Infections	XTRA	465	As mentioned above		Yeast
Yeast Ultimate	VEGA	72,422,582,787,1016,2222,	As mentioned above		Yeast
Yeast Baker's	CAFL	843	Leavening agent in breads. Also found in and on human body.		Yeast
Yeast Cervical	CAFL	788,706,771	Use Candida, and Candidiasis sets. Also see Parasites General, Roundworm, and Ascaris sets		Yeast
Aflatoxin	CAFL	344,510,943,474,476,568,	Liver-damaging mold toxin produced by Aspergillus spp.- carcinogenic toxin.	Liver	Mold
Aflatoxin	VEGA	344	As mentioned above	Liver	Mold
Aflatoxin 1	HC	177000	As mentioned above	Liver	Mold
Aflatoxins	BIOM	334; 438.7; 466; 474; 476; 510; 568; 943; 8812.3; 9360		Liver	Mold
Aflatoxin 1	XTRA	344,438.74,474,476,510,568,943,8812.30,9359.96,11079.69,	As mentioned above	Liver	Mold
Aflatoxin 2	XTRA	438.74,466,8812.30,9359.96,	As mentioned above	Liver	Mold
Agyfla	HC	71000,	Mold toxin.		Mold
Agyfla	XTRA	175.99,3534.88	Mold toxin.		Mold
Alternaria Tenuis	VEGA	853	Fungus causing upper respiratory problems and asthma.	Lung	Fungus
Alternaria Tenuis	XTRA	304,853	As mentioned above	Lung	Fungus
Alternaria blight	BIOM	304; 853			Fungus
Aspergillus, complex	BIOM	247; 339; 374; 524; 697; 743; 758; 1823; 1972			Fungus
Aspergillus Flavus	CAFL	1823,247,1972	Mold found on corn, peanuts, and grain that produces Aflatoxin.	Lung	Mold
Aspergillus Flavus	VEGA	1823	As mentioned above	Lung	Mold
Aspergillus Flavus	RL	364	From Dr. Richard Loyd.	Lung	Mold
Aspergillus flavus	BIOM	247; 1823; 1972			Mold
Aspergillus Glaucus	CAFL	524,758	Blue mold occurring in some human infectious processes.	Brain	Mold
Aspergillus Glaucus	BIO	524	As mentioned above	Brain	Mold
Aspergillus glaucus	BIOM	524; 758			Mold
Aspergillus Fumigatus	RL	248	From Dr. Richard Loyd. Species involved in about 90 per cent of aspergillus infections.		Mold
Aspergillus Niger	BIO	374	Common mold that may produce severe and persistent infection.		Mold
Aspergillus niger	BIOM	374; 697; 758			Mold
Aspergillus Terreus	CAFL	743,339	Mold occasionally associated with infection of the bronchi and lungs.	Lung	Mold
Aspergillus Terreus	VEGA	743	As mentioned above	Lung	Mold
Aspergillus terreus	BIOM	339; 743		Lung	Mold
Aspergillus versicolor	RL	488	From Dr. Richard Loyd. Aspergillus versicolor is a slow-growing filamentous Fungus. Is a major producer of the hepatotoxic and carcinogenic mycotoxin sterigmatocystin.	Lung	Mold
Aspergillosis	EDTFL	120,830,5000,7250,37500,357300,434250,563190,709830,978050,	Infection by Aspergillus fungi, mainly pulmonary. Also see Aspergillus and Aflatoxin.	Lung	Mold
Sterigmatocystin_1	HC	88000	Mycotoxin produced by molds of the genus Aspergillus.		Mold
Sterigmatocystin_2	HC	96000	As mentioned above		Mold
Sterigmatocystin_3	HC	126000	As mentioned above		Mold
Sterigmatocystin_4	HC	133000	As mentioned above		Mold
Basidiomycetes	CAFL	751	Also called Basidiomycota. Filamentous fungi.	Skin	Mold
Basidiomycetes	BIOM	224; 289; 302; 375; 377; 546; 643; 751; 1447; 1642			Mold
Beth Sutton's Bar Fungus	VEGA	854	.		Mold
Blastomyces Dermatitidis	RL	1233	From Dr. Richard Loyd. Blastomyces dermatitidis is the causal agent of blastomycosis, an invasive and often serious fungal infection found occasionally in humans and other animals in regions where the Fungus is endemic.		Mold
Botrytis cinerea	BIOM	114; 212; 1545			Mold
Candida 1	CAFL	3176,2644,1403,1151,943,886,877,866,762,742,661,465,464,450,414,386,381,254.2,120,95,64,20,	Yeast. Includes Candida Carcinomas and C. Tropicalis.		Yeast

Subject / Argument	Author	Frequencies	Notes	Origin	Target
Candida 2	CAFL	10000,5000,3176,2489,1395,1276,1160,1044,928,877,812,728,696,580,464,381,348,232,116,58,20,	As mentioned above		Yeast
Candida 3	CAFL	20,60,95,125,225,427,464,727,	As mentioned above		Yeast
Candida 4	XTRA	20,60,95,125,225,427,464,465,675,709,727,1403,2128,2167,2128,	As mentioned above		Yeast
Candida	BIOM	10000; 3175; 2182; 2167; 1403; 1395; 1276; 1160; 1044; 928; 877; 465; 427; 381; 348; 232; 225; 125; 116; 60; 58			Yeast
Candida	EDTFL	40,400,780,5290,7500,37000,320050,434000,792000,985670			Yeast
Candida	XTRA	4640	Experimental. As mentioned above		Yeast
Candida Sweep	XTRA	12006.25	Yeast species. See Parasites General, Roundworm, and Ascaris if these do not work long-term.		Yeast
Monilia	BIO	866,886	Former name for Candida.		Yeast
Candida Albicans 1	CAFL	464,464.5,465,465.5,841,	As mentioned above		Yeast
Candida Albicans 2	CAFL	72,412,422,543,582,727,787,802,1016,1134,1153,1550,2222,	As mentioned above		Yeast
Candida Albicans 3	CAFL	20,152,225,240,427,442,650,688,751,880,1146,8146,	Addresses some causal factors.		Yeast
Candida Albicans 4	CAFL	188,250,376.9,464,465,753.9,841,1507,3015,	As mentioned above		Yeast
Candida Secondary	CAFL	72,422,582,727,787,802,1016,1134,1153,1550,2222,412,543,2128,	As mentioned above		Yeast
Candida Tertiary	CAFL	880,95,125,20,60,225,427,240,650,688,152,442,8146,751,1146,	Addresses some causal factors.		Yeast
Candida Albicans	BIOM	110; 342; 414; 420; 423; 587; 688; 757; 956.8			Yeast
Candida Albicans	BIOM	20; 60; 95; 125; 225; 414; 427; 465; 727; 787; 880			Yeast
Candida Albicans 1	XTRA	414,952.34,956,79,962.75,12006.25,12062.5,12137.5,	As mentioned above		Yeast
Candida Albicans 2	XTRA	412,414,464,8146,11092.5,11310,11742,11742.5,11745,	As mentioned above		Yeast
Candida Albicans 3	XTRA	464,464.5,465,465.5,841,	Yeast species. See Parasites General, Roundworm, and Ascaris if these do not work long-term.		Yeast
Candida Albicans 7	XTRA	956.79,19217.81	As mentioned above		Yeast
Candida Albicans	VEGA	414	Yeast species. See Parasites General, Roundworm, and Ascaris if these do not work long-term.		Yeast
Candida Albicans	RL	574	From Dr. Richard Loyd.		Yeast
Candida Auris	RL	888,563	From Dr. Richard Loyd. Is a species of Fungus which grows as yeast. It is one of the few species of the genus Candida which cause candidiasis in humans.		Yeast
Candida and Organ Support 1	XTRA	956.79,11126.5,1145.75,11162.25,11387.25,11434.5≈1200,11979,12006.25≈1200,	Combination treatment and support.		Yeast
Candida and Organ Support 2	XTRA	20,60,72,95,100,125,152,225,240,254.19,344,381,386,422,427,442,450,465,510,543,582,600,625,650,660,661,688,690,727.5,742,751,762,784,787,802,866,877,880,886,943,1016,1134,1146,1151,1153,1403,1550,2127.5,2222,2644,8146,	Combination treatment and support.		Yeast
Candida HiPower	XTRA	23485,51155,51156,53940,58914,58916,88740,23484,57420,99180,8146,22620,29580,	From Pulsed Technologies. Alternate daily with Candida LoPower, and run with Candida Organ Support set.		Yeast
Candida LoPower	XTRA	31724,31725,33060,46980,50460,54404,54405,55250,55251,60900,64380,67860,412,	From Pulsed Technologies. Alternate daily with Candida HiPower, and run with Candida Organ Support set.		Yeast
Candida Organ Support	XTRA	23958,24354,28251,29766,32121,32670,36735,38281,44506,44583,45549,45738,54531,56133,56376,57519,58806,63336,67977,71874,84942,86394,87000,89298,	Run with Candida HiPower and Candida LoPower sets. From Pulsed Technologies.		Yeast
Candida Overgrowth	XTRA	13427.72	As mentioned above		Yeast
Candida Krusei	RL	698	From Dr. Richard Loyd.		Yeast
Candida Parapsilosis	XTRA	634	From Dr. Richard Loyd. Causes Sepsis (see set), and wound and tissue infections in the immunocompromised. Also infects nails. See Onchomycosis.	Skin Nail	Yeast
Candida Robusta	RL	468	From Dr. Richard Loyd. Candida robusta is rarely identified in humans, but has been reported as a cause of VVC in pregnant women.		Yeast
Candida Rugosa	RL	588	From Dr. Richard Loyd. Candida rugosa has been described as an 'emerging' human fungal pathogen.		Yeast
Candida Tropicalis	BIO	1403	As mentioned above		Yeast
Candida Tropicalis	BIOM	675; 709			Yeast
Candida Tropicalis 1	XTRA	233,344,438,510,776,943,	As mentioned above		Yeast
Candida Tropicalis 2	XTRA	675,709,1403,	As mentioned above		Yeast

Subject / Argument	Author	Frequencies	Notes	Origin	Target
Candida Lusitania	XTRA	878777.778	Weaponized biofilm. From Newport. Wave=square, Duty=82.4%. Causes Arrythmia, Peritonitis, Sinusitis (see sets for these three), dacrocystitis, and neurological problems.		Biofilm
Candida Carcinomas	CAFL	2167,2128,2182,465			Yeast
Candida Carcinomas	XTRA	465,2128,2167,2128			Yeast
Candida and Helminth	BIOM	3176; 2644; 1403; 1150.9; 943; 886; 877; 866; 762; 742; 661; 465; 464; 450; 414; 412; 386; 381; 254.2; 120; 95; 64; 20			Yeast
Candida and Parasites	BIOM	414; 464; 386; 877; 866; 886; 254.2; 381; 661; 762; 742; 1150.9; 450; 943; 1403; 2644			Yeast
Candidiasis	EDTFL	40,400,780,5290,7500,37000,321510,434000,792000,985670	Candida infection, commonly called Thrush.		Yeast
Candidiasis - Basic v	BIOM	72; 422; 582; 787; 1015.9; 2222; 1134; 254; 987; 986; 984; 982; 980; 974; 908; 906; 878; 876; 873; 871; 866; 865; 864; 863; 861; 778			Yeast
Candidiasis, secondary	BIOM	8146; 1146; 751; 688; 650; 442; 427; 240; 225; 152; 125; 95; 60			Yeast
Moniliasis Moniliasis, Vulvovaginal	EDTFL	20,220,900,7500,22700,85370,155470,285000,416500,605410	Candidiasis		Yeast
Candidiasis, Vulvovaginal	EDTFL	40,400,780,5290,7500,37000,321510,434000,792000,985670,	Also called Vaginal Thrush.		Yeast
Thrush	CAFL	414,465	Candidiasis, usually oral, with white or light brown tongue coating, or vaginal (see sets). Also see Stomatitis sets.		Yeast
Thrush	EDTFL	130,400,7250,42800,92500,322530,479500,527000,667000,987230	Oral moniliasis		Yeast
Candida Glabrata	XTRA	558777.777	Biofilm. From Newport. Wave=square, Duty=82.4%. Common biofilm-forming yeast causing disease for those in weakened condition, with suppressed immune function, or Lyme/Morgellons Disease.		Biofilm
Candida Glabrata	RL	595	From Dr. Richard Loyd.		Yeast
Torulopsis	BIO	354,522,872,2121	Now called Candida Glabrata. A common yeast causing disease for those in weakened condition or with suppressed immune function.		Yeast
Torulopsis	VEGA	522,2121	As mentioned above		Yeast
Central Spores (Bacillus Smear)	HC	372450-378650=3600,			Fungus
Central Spores (Bacillus Smear)	XTRA	923.21,932,938.58,11639.05,11750,11832.8,			Fungus
Parasites: Sub terminal spores bacillus Smear	EDTFL	680,900,2500,5500,13930,93500,404250,407000,412000,415250			Fungus
Cephalosporium	BIO	481,3966	Fungi that are the source of some broad-spectrum antibiotics.		Fungus
Cephalosporium	BIOM	481; 3966; 544			Fungus
Cephalothecium Trichothecium Roseum	CAFL	371,574,6933	Plant pathogen.		Fungus
Chaetomium Globosum	CAFL	221,102,862	Mold causing mycosis and neurological infections. Can be found indoors.	Allergies	Fungus
Chaetomium Globosum	BIO	221,867	As mentioned above		Fungus
Cladosporium Fulvum Passalora Fulva	CAFL	438,233,776,510	Pathogenic Fungus.	Skin	Fungus
Cladosporium Fulvum	VEGA	438	As mentioned above	Skin	Fungus
Cladosporium Fulvum	BIOM	233; 438; 510; 775; 776			Fungus
Cladosporium Fulvum 1	XTRA	233,438,510,776	As mentioned above	Skin	Fungus
Cladosporium Fulvum 2	XTRA	233,344,438,510,776,943,	As mentioned above	Skin	Fungus
Hormodendrum Cladosporium cladosporioides	CAFL	663,678,695,532,627,	Fungal plant pathogen that can affect man.		Fungus
Hormodendrum	XTRA	695	As mentioned above		Fungus
Coccidiodes Immitis	XTRA	336,337,20000	Causes Coccidioidomycosis, or Valley Fever - see these sets.		Fungus
Coccidioidomycosis	EDTFL	170,520,620,880,20300,97500,155270,562500,753200,850000	Fungal infection by Coccidiodes Immitis. Usually respiratory, and can involve fever, muscle/joint pain, rash/lesions, and headache.		Fungus
Valley Fever 4 Coccidioidomycosis	XTRA	80000=2400,336,337,	As mentioned above		Fungus
Colletotrichum	CAFL	1482	Pathogenic plant Fungus.		Fungus
Cryptococcus Gattii	RL	578	From Dr. Richard Loyd. Is an encapsulated yeast found primarily in tropical and subtropical climates. Appearing several months after exposure to the Fungus, the infection causes a bad cough and shortness of breath, among other symptoms.		Yeast
Cryptococcus neoformans	RL	636	From Dr. Richard Loyd.		Yeast

Subject / Argument	Author	Frequencies	Notes	Origin	Target
Cryptococcosis [Fungal Diseases]	EDTFL	60,260,820,9800,67500,215500,332500,441120, 625290,810500,	Yeast infection that starts in lungs and can cause meningitis and other problems. Also see Torulopsis sets.		Yeast
Cryptococcosis	BIOM	367; 428; 444; 476; 478; 522; 579; 594; 597; 613; 624; 785; 792; 872; 2121; 5880; 5884			Yeast
Chromomycosis	BIOM	532; 627; 695	It is a chronic infection of the skin and underlying tissues caused by fungi.		Fungus
Torulosis [Cryptococcosis]	EDTFL	60,260,820,9800,67500,215500,332500,441120, 625290,810500,			Fungus
Cryptococcus Neoformans	CAFL	367,428,444,476,478,522,579,594,785,792,872, 2121,5880,5884,597,613,624,	Yeast causing respiratory infection that can turn into meningitis.	Lung	Fungus
Cunninghamella	CAFL	311,323	Fungus which can infect humans.		Fungus
Cytochalasin	XTRA	190.86,225.56,3833.59,4530.61,	Cell-permeable mycotoxin. Used in cloning.		Mold
Cytochalasin B_1	HC	77000	As mentioned above		Mold
Cytochalasin B_2	HC	91000	As mentioned above		Mold
Mold Cytochalasin 1	XTRA	19250,190.86	As mentioned above		Mold
Mold Cytochalasin 2	XTRA	11375,225.56	As mentioned above		Mold
Dan's Mold	VEGA	222,333,421,822,1233,1351,1711,1832,	.		Muffe
Dematium Nigrum	CAFL	243,738	Soil Fungus found in human lesions.		Fungus
Dematium Nigrum	BIO	243	As mentioned above		Fungus
Dermatomycosis	BIOM	5000; 800; 732; 442; 440; 422; 128; 92; 76; 60			Fungus
Epicoccum	CAFL	734,778	Mold producing allergic reaction on inhalation.	Allergies	Fungus
Epicoccum	VEGA	734	As mentioned above		Fungus
Epidermophytia	BIOM	345; 465; 644; 766; 784			Fungus
Epidermophyton Floccosum	CAFL	465,784,644,766	Fungus that attacks skin and nails, including some athlete's foot and jock itch ringworms. Use correct Microsporum and Fungus General sets. See Tinea Cruris and Parasites sets.	Skin Nail	Fungus
Epidermophyton floccosum	RL	856	From Dr. Richard Loyd.	Skin Nail	Fungus
Epidermophyton Floccosum 2	CAFL	20,345,465,634,644,660,690,727.5,766,784,802, 880,1550,	As mentioned above	Skin Nail	Fungus
Trichophyton	BIO	132,812,2422,9493	Fungus causing Athlete's Foot, Ringworm, Jock Itch (see sets), and similar infections of nail, beard, skin and scalp.	Skin Nail	Fungus
Trichophyton General	CAFL	132,725,808,812,2422,9493,	As mentioned above	Skin Nail	Fungus
Trichophyton Mentagrophytes	CAFL	311,414	As mentioned above	Skin Nail	Fungus
Trichophyton Nagel	CAFL	381,585,593,812	Fungus that mostly infects nails.	Skin Nail	Fungus
Trichophyton Nagel, main	BIOM	132; 133; 142; 373; 376; 378; 385; 387; 420; 425; 428; 576; 578; 580; 581; 583; 584; 585; 587; 588; 592; 593; 597; 724; 725; 726; 732; 733; 738; 748; 750; 765; 766; 771; 777; 778; 779.5; 794; 794; 797; 801; 805; 808; 809; 817; 886; 1256; 2422; 6887; 7688; 7697; 7885			Fungus
Trichophyton Nagel Secondary	CAFL	133,142,373,376,378,385,387,420,425,428,576, 578,580,581,583,584,587,588,592,595,597,724, 725,726,750,794,797,801,805,808,809,817,886, 2422,6887,7688,7697,7885,584,587,592,732,73 3,738,748,765,766,771,777,778,779,1256,	As mentioned above	Skin Nail	Fungus
Nagel Trichophyton	BIO	133,381,812,2422	As mentioned above	Skin Nail	Fungus
Trichophyton Rubrum	BIO	752,923	As mentioned above	Skin Nail	Fungus
Trichophyton Tonsurans	CAFL BIOM	454,765	As mentioned above	Skin Nail	Fungus
Ringworm	CAFL	422,442,732,5000,60,76,92,120,128,440,800,	Fungal skin infection in man and animals. See Microsporum Audouini, and Canis, Trichophyton, and/or Epidermophyton.	Skin	Fungus
Ringworm	EDTFL	40,120,950,14030,118520,251290,365280,5900 00,722700,977500		Skin	Fungus
Athlete's foot Onychomycosis Tinea			See Section 11a - Skin and 11c - Nails	Skin	Fungus
Claviceps Purpurea	XTRA	660,690,727.5,731.23,14687.19,18437.5,	Ergot Fungus.		Fungus
Ergot	HC	295000	Also called Ergotism (see set). Rye and cereal mold which causes convulsive and gangrenous symptoms when ingested long-term.		Mold
Ergot	XTRA	660,690,727.5,731.23,14687.19,18437.5,	As mentioned above		Mold
Ergot	XTRA	660,690,727.5,18437.5,731.23,14687.19,	As mentioned above		Mold

Subject / Argument	Author	Frequencies	Notes	Origin	Target
Mold Ergot	XTRA	18437.5,731.23,	As mentioned above		Mold
Ergot Poisoning Ergotism	EDTFL	80,120,850,5160,20000,40000,85000,97500,355 720,434500	Ergot Poisoning		Mold
Saint Anthonys Fire [Ergotism]	EDTFL	80,120,850,5160,20000,40000,85000,97500,355 720,434500,			Mold
St. Anthonys Fire	EDTFL	80,120,850,5160,20000,40000,85000,97500,355 720,434500,			Mold
Fusarium General	CAFL	768,625,746	Pathogenic plant and soil Fungus which can cause corneal infections as well as more serious illnesses and birth defects in humans. Weaponized, and common in Morgellons.		Fungus
Fusarium General 2	XTRA	600,625,650,746,768,	As mentioned above		Fungus
Fusariose, complex	BIOM	790; 780; 768; 746; 705; 102			
Fusarium Oxysporum	CAFL	102,332,705,795,780,	As mentioned above		Fungus
Fusarium Oxysporum	BIO	102,705	As mentioned above		Fungus
Fusarium Oxysporum	VEGA	102	As mentioned above		Fungus
Eye Fusarium General	XTRA	600,625,650,746,768,	Eye infection due to pathogenic plant Fungus. Bioweapon.	Eyes	Fungus
Geotrichum Candidum	CAFL	350,355,384,386,403,404,407,409,410,412,415, 418,543,544,687,987,988,737,700,	Candida-like plant Fungus used in some dairy products that can infect man - found in skin, sputum, and feces.		Fungus
Geotrichum Candidum	VEGA	412	As mentioned above		Fungus
Geotrichum candidum	BIOM	350; 355; 386; 403; 404; 407; 409; 410; 412; 415; 418; 543; 544; 687; 700; 737; 987; 988			Fungus
Geotrichum Candidum 2	XTRA	412,543	As mentioned above		Fungus
Gliocladium 1	XTRA	469,633,855	Filamentous Fungus which can cause disease in humans and animals.		Fungus
Gliocladium 2	XTRA	855	As mentioned above		Fungus
Griseofulvin	HC	288000	Oral antifungal drug derived from Penicillium mold which can cause nasty side effects.		Mold
Griseofulvin	XTRA	713.87,14338.68			Mold
Mold Griseofulvin	XTRA	18000,713.87	As mentioned above		Mold
Parasites Helminthosporium	CAFL	793,969,164,5243	Pathogenic plant fungi, some of which can infect man.		Fungus
Parasites: helminthosporium (worm eggs)	EDTFL	680,900,2500,5500,13930,93500,386400,38680 0,393000,395600	As mentioned above		Fungus
Helminthosporium	BIO	793,969	As mentioned above		Fungus
Histoplasma	CAFL	424,616,749	Fungus found in bat and bird droppings that causes lung disease Histoplasmosis - see sets.	Lung	Fungus
Histoplasma Capsulatum 1	XTRA	727.01,748.58,754.4,18331.25,18875,19021.88,	As mentioned above	Lung	Fungus
Histoplasma Capsulatum 2	XTRA	748.58,15035.69	As mentioned above	Lung	Fungus
Histoplasmosis	BIOM	424; 6164; 749			Fungus
Histoplasmosis	EDTFL	120,140,810,7500,12690,39220,48820,224940,4 26160,503140	Serious lung disease.	Lung	Fungus
Histoplasmosis	XTRA	424,616,749,15035.69,18348.5=1200,18875,	As mentioned above	Lung	Fungus
Jim Adams Fungus	VEGA	943,2644			Fungus
Katy Luce Foot Fungus	VEGA	634			Fungus
Katy Luce Finger Wart	VEGA	495	Fungus	Skin	Fungus
Lycogala	HC	126000,	Slime mold.		Mold
Lycogala	XTRA	312.31,6273.17	Slime mold.		Mold
Mold Lycogala	XTRA	15750,312.31	Slime mold. Implicated in Morgellons.		Mold
Madura Foot	EDTFL	70,230,830,2750,30000,30000,50000,134250,32 5650,425680	Caused by Madurella Fungus. Implicated in Morgellons Disease. Also use Staphylococcus Aureus, S. Coagulae Positive, S. Haemolyticus, and S. General.	Foot	Fungus
Maduromycosis	EDTFL	150,620,25050,87500,124330,222530,479930,5 27000,667000,987230		Foot	Fungus
Malassezia Furfur	CAFL	222,225,491,616,700,	Yeast causing Tinea Versicolor. See Fungus General, and Tinea Versicolor sets. May also be implicated in Morgellons.	Skin	Yeast
Malassezia	BIOM	222; 225; 491; 616; 700			Fungus
Mycogone	BIOM	1123			Fungus
Microsporum Audouini	CAFL	422,831,1222,285	Fungus commonly causing Ringworm of the scalp and other areas.	Skin	Fungus
Microsporum Audouini	BIOM	285; 831; 1222			Fungus
Microsporum Canis	VEGA	1644	As mentioned above	Skin	Fungus
Microsporum Canis	BIOM	347; 402; 970; 1644			Fungus
Mucor Mucedo	BIO	612,1000	Fungus that causes rot in fruit and baked goods, sometimes found on feet and skin.		Fungus
Mucor Mucedo	CAFL	612,1000,488,766,9788,735,	As mentioned above		Fungus
Mucor Mucedo	HC	288000	As mentioned above		Fungus
Mucor Mucedo	BIOM	488; 612; 735; 766; 1000; 6788			Fungus

Subject / Argument	Author	Frequencies	Notes	Origin	Target
Mucor Plumbeus	BIO	361	Soil and grain Fungus also found in buildings and causing an immune response.		Fungus
Mucor Plumbeus	BIOM	361; 578; 785; 877			Fungus
Mucor Racemosus	CAFL	310,474,875	Fungus that grows on decaying vegetation and bread, and can cause ear infection.		Fungus
Mucor Racemosus Secondary	CAFL	473,686,713,729,731,751,760,778,871,873,876, 878,887,1200,7768,7976,8788,	As mentioned above		Fungus
Mucor Racemosus, complex	BIOM	309.9; 473; 474; 686; 713; 729; 731; 751; 760; 778; 871; 873; 876; 878; 887; 1200; 7768; 7976; 8788			Fungus
Mucor Racemosus Sinus	BIO	310,474	As mentioned above		Fungus
Mucormycosis	CAFL	623,733,942	Fungal infection. Also see Zygomycosis set.	Mouth	Fungus
Mycetoma	KHZ	20,120,850,7500,32500,40000,60000,115700,92 500,423010,563190,640000,985900,	Chronic fungal or bacterial infections. Also see Streptothrix, Actinomyces spp, Actinomycosis.		Fungus
Mycogone Fungoides	CAFL	488,532,662,764,852,1444,	Type of mold that infects mushrooms - has also been found in skin.		Mold
Mycogone Fungoides Secondary	CAFL	328,367,490,491,495,496,628,678,709,714,729, 746,757,761,766,768,1055,1074,9979,	As mentioned above		Mold
Mycoses	KHZ	170,220,930,2750,27500,132500,255580,47585 0,724940,825870,	Fungal infection affecting the skin, hair, nails and mucous membranes.	Skin	Fungus
Fungus Diseases	EDTFL	60,260,650,5150,7300,42500,92500,475950,527 000,661710		Skin	Fungus
Mycosis Fungoides	BIO	532,662,678,852,1444,	As mentioned above	Skin	Fungus
Mycosis Fungoides	VEGA	852	As mentioned above	Skin	Fungus
Feet and nails mycosis	BIOM	2222; 1552; 1550; 1153; 1134; 1016; 880; 802; 787; 784; 727; 582; 254; 465; 422; 72; 200; 1550; 1552; 454; 455		Skin	Fungus
Head mycosis	BIOM	76; 92; 120; 128; 132; 378; 578; 725; 732; 766; 800; 808; 812; 2422; 6887; 7688; 7697; 7885; 9493		Skin	Fungus
Mycosis fungoides	BIOM	367; 491; 495; 496; 628; 678; 709; 714; 29; 757; 761; 768; 1055; 1074; 9979		Skin	Fungus
Mycosis spp.	BIOM	446; 748; 1123		Skin	Fungus
Nagel Mycosis	BIO	462,654,	Disaccharide from which glucose can be hydrolized.	Skin	Fungus
Neurospora sitophila	BIOM	705; 878			Fungus
Nigrospora spp.	BIOM	350; 764			Fungus
Oat Smut	CAFL	806	Fungal grain disease where parts of the fruited ears change to black powder.		Fungus
Oospora	CAFL	9599,5346	Spores of fertilized oospheres in some algae, fungi, and oomycetes. May be implicated in Morgellons Disease.		Mold
Penicillium Chrysogenum	BIO	344,868,1070,2411	Formerly called Penicillium Notatum - see sets. Fungus mostly found in damp or water-damaged buildings.		Fungus
Penicillium Chrysogenum	CAFL	129,249,344,967	As mentioned above		Fungus
Penicillium Chrysogenum	VEGA	344,2411	As mentioned above		Fungus
Penicillium Chrysogenum	BIOM	129; 249; 344; 345; 688; 728; 764; 765; 868; 967; 1070; 2411			Fungus
Penicillium Chrysogenum Secondary	CAFL	345,688,728,764,765,868,1070,2411,	As mentioned above		Fungus
Penicillium Notatum	BIO	321,555,629,825,942,	Now called Penicillium Chrysogenum.		Fungus
Penicillium Notatum	BIOM	321; 334; 412; 550; 555; 556; 560; 562; 566; 572; 629; 644; 715; 835; 922; 942; 4870; 7780			Fungus
Penicillium Notatum	VEGA	321,555,942	As mentioned above		Fungus
Penicillium Rubrum	CAFL	332,457,460,462,766,1015,1018,	Fungus similar to Penicillium Chrysogenum and found in corn and soybeans.		Fungus
Penicillium Rubrum	BIOM	332; 457; 460; 462; 766; 1015; 1018			Fungus
Penicillium Rubrum	VEGA	332,766	As mentioned above		Fungus
Rhizopus Nigricans	BIO	132	Commonly called bread mold, but also found in spoiled food, soil, and playground sandboxes. Its spores contain 31 allergens.		Fungus
Rhizopus Nigricans	CAFL	132,327,775,659,660,	As mentioned above		Fungus
Rhodo Torula	CAFL	833,598,778	Common type of unicellular pigmented yeast, usually afflicting immunosuppressed persons and/or those with central lines installed. Also see Basidiomycetes sets.		Yeast
Rhodotorula Mucilaginosa	RL	674	From Dr. Richard Loyd.		Yeast
Rhodotorula glutinis Rhodotorula minuta Raoultella ornithinolytica	RL	385	From Dr. Richard Loyd.		Yeast
Sporobolomyces	BIO	753	Type of yeast.		Yeast
Sporotrichum Pruinosum	CAFL	584,598,687,755,715,	Type of yeast which can infect lungs. Also use Basidiomycetes set.		Yeast
Sporotrichum Pruinosum	VEGA	755	As mentioned above		Yeast

Subject / Argument	Author	Frequencies	Notes	Origin	Target
Sporotrichum Pruinosum	BIOM	584; 598; 687; 755; 715			Yeast
Stachybotrys Chartarum	XTRA	540.1,577.9,604.39,747.39,764.5,765,844,922.2, 952.39,969.6,	Very toxic black mold most common in damp or water-damaged buildings.		Mold
Stemonitis	HC	21100	Slime mold.		Mold
Stemphylium	CAFL	461,340,114	Plant pathogen.		Fungus
Sterigmatocystine	BIOM	6621.68; 6273.17; 4779.56; 4381.26; 329.67; 312.32; 237.96; 218.13			Fungus
Talaromyces Marneffei	RL	689	From Dr. Richard Loyd. Formerly called Penicillium Marneffei, is now regarded as one of the world's ten most feared fungi. It is a particularly important cause of disease due to weakened immunity in people living in southeast Asia whose immune systems have been weakened by HIV infection.		Fungus
Trichoderma	BIO	711	Common soil Fungus that also infects homes. Very toxic. Also use Fungus General sets.		Fungus
Trichosporon beigelii/cutaneum/ovoides	RL	556	From Dr. Richard Loyd. As well as being a member of the normal flora of mouth, skin and nails, it is the causative agent of superficial and deep infections in humans.		Yeast
Wallemia Sebi	RL	657	From Dr. Richard Loyd. Wallemia sebi is a xerophilic Fungus of the phylum Basidiomycota. It is commonly found on highly sugared or salted materials. It is also found in indoor air, house dust, and soil.		Fungus
Wheat Smut Wheat Bunt	CAFL	10163,156,375	Type of pathogenic Fungus infecting wheat. Also see Bisidiomycetes set.		Fungus
Wheat Stem Rust 1	CAFL	643	As mentioned above		Fungus
Zearalenone	HC	100000	Potent myctotoxin produced by some Fusarium (see sets) and Gibberella fungi.		Fungus
Zearalenone	BIOM	247.9			Fungus
Zygomycosis	CAFL	942,623,733	Also known as Mucormycosis. Serious fungal infection usually associated with uncontrolled Diabetes Mellitus or immunosuppressive drugs.		Fungus
Zygomycosis	BIOM	623; 733			Fungus
Zygomycosis	EDTFL	240,7600,22500,35050,95000,375330,424370,5 63190,714820,978050	As mentioned above		Fungus
Entomophthoramycosis	EDTFL	230,320,840,2300,35000,43300,114300,306300, 553730,624520			Fungus
Blue-green Algae	HC	256000	Former name for Cyanobacteria.		
Stigeoclonium_1	HC	404250-415250=3600,	A genus of green algae		
Stigeoclonium_2	HC	407000	A genus of green algae		
Stigeoclonium_3	HC	405000	Toxic green algae.		
Parasites: Stigeoclonium	EDTFL	680,900,2500,5500,13930,93500,353000,38640 0,387000,388000	A genus of green algae in the family Chaetophoraceae.		
Bryozoa Cristatalla	HC	396000	Microscopic aquatic/moss invertebrate.		
Bryozoa Cristatalla	XTRA	981.59,12375	As mentioned above		
Rotifer	CAFL	4500	Phylum of microscopic aquatic animals.		
Rotifer	HC	1151000	As mentioned above		

17c - Bacteria and Diseases

Note: *diseases caused by pathogens are indicated in blue*

Subject / Argument	Author	Frequencies	Notes	Origin	Target
Bacteria General	XTRA	20,465,660,664,690,727.5,784,787,800,802,832, 866,880,1550,			Bacteria
Gram Positive Bacterial Infections	EDTFL	120,550,860,7500,12500,275290,307250,43537 0,587500,795520		Infections	Bacteria
Gram (+) Bacterial Infections	EDTFL	120,550,860,7500,12500,275290,307250,43537 0,587500,795520		Infections	Bacteria
Gram (-) Bacterial Infections	EDTFL	120,550,860,7500,12500,307250,435370,58750 0,795570,901030	Many species of bacteria with outer membranes which can cause toxic shock, and defeat antibiotics.	Infections	Bacteria
Bacterial Gram (+) and (-) Bacterial infections Specific to cold & flu inc. Pneumonia	EDTFL	120,550,860,7500,12500,77500,120000,307250, 320000,615000,		Infections	Bacteria
Bacterial Infections	CAFL	20,465,866,664,690,727,787,832,800,880,1550, 784,	If infection is chronic, type is accurately diagnosed, and frequencies or antibiotics are ineffective long-term, use Parasites General, and Roundworm sets.	Infections	Bacteria
Basic Bacterial Infection	BIOM	1550.0; 880.0; 866.0; 832.0; 800.0; 787.0; 784.0; 727.0; 690.0; 664.0; 465.0; 200.0; 20.0		Infections	Bacteria
Bacterial infections, basic	BIOM	1550; 866; 832; 800; 784; 690; 664; 465		Infections	Bacteria
Puerperal Infection	EDTFL	100,260,680,7500,11020,45000,325430,515700, 653430,750000	Bacterial infection of female reproductive tract following childbirth or miscarriage, commonly by Streptococcus Pyogenes and anaerobic Streptococcus spp, Staphylococcus spp, E Coli, and Clostridium spp.	Infections	Bacteria

Subject / Argument	Author	Frequencies	Notes	Origin	Target
Bacteremia	EDTFL KHZ	350,870,2500,11090,40000,90000,275160,4257 10,564280,640000,	The presence of bacteria in the blood	Infections	Bacteria
Bacteriosis-1	BIOM	60.5; 64.5; 67.0		Infections	Bacteria
Bacillus Infections	CAFL	787,880,802,727,1552,800,	B Coli, B Coli Rod.	Infections	Bacteria
Bacillus Infections	EDTFL	50,370,830,2500,3000,73300,355080,359000,36 3000,393000,	B Coli, B Coli Rod.	Infections	Bacteria
Bacterial Infections and Mycoses	EDTFL	50,370,900,2500,3000,73300,95750,175000,269 710,355080,	Microbial and fungal infections.	Infections	Bacteria
Wide Spectrum Antibiotic	XTRA	727,787,802,880,465,	The five most important frequencies for pathogens.	Infections	Bacteria
Nisin	XTRA	1279784.646	Natural broad-spectrum antibiotic. May also be useful for tumors, periodontal problems, biofilms, yeasts, and molds (MW).	Infections	Bacteria
Wide-Spectrum ABX	XTRA	12,666,690,727,1840	Hits Staphylococcus Aureus, E Coli, Pseudomonas, and others.	Infections	Bacteria
Bacterial Capsules (Capsular)	HC	416050-418750=3600,	Outer envelope of bacterial cell wall		Bacteria
Bacterial Capsules	HC	362400-357600=3600,	Outer envelope of bacterial cell wall.		Bacteria
Bacterial Capsules 1	XTRA	886.39,886.39,892.35,898.29,11175,11250,1132 5,	Outer envelope of bacterial cell wall.		Bacteria
Bacterial Capsules 2	XTRA	892.35,1034.88,17923.34,20786.09,	Outer envelope of bacterial cell wall.		Bacteria
Actinobacillus	CAFL	488,565,672,674,678,766,768,777,885,887,7877 ,9687,42664,42666,46668,46787,773,776,778,8 22,	Pathogenic bacteria found in oral/respiratory tract. May help cause Endocarditis.	Respiratory	Bacteria
Actinobacillus	VEGA	773,	As mentioned above	Respiratory	Bacteria
Actinobacillosis	BIOM	488; 565; 672; 674; 678; 773; 766; 768; 776; 777; 778; 822; 885; 887; 7877; 9687		Respiratory	Bacteria
Actinomyces Bovis	XTRA	1.10,20,73,160,220,465,660,690,727.5,787,1000 0,	Bacteria causing Actinomycosis in animals, infections, swelling.		Bacteria
Actinomyces Israelii	BIO	222,262,2154,	Bacterium normally found in colon, throat, or vagina causing deep, pus-filled holes in tissue. Also see Streptothrix.		Bacteria
Actinomyces Israelii	VEGA	262,2154,	As mentioned above		Bacteria
Actinomyces Israelii	BIOM	160; 222; 262; 488; 567; 690; 727; 747; 2154; 7880			Bacteria
Actinomyces Israelii 1	XTRA	46.5,727,766,776,787,802,880,1550,1600,1800, 2489,2720,	As mentioned above		Bacteria
Actinomyces Israelii 2	XTRA	20,23,222,262,465,488,567,727,747,787,2154,7 880,10000,	As mentioned above		Bacteria
Actinomycosis	CAFL	20,465,727,787,880,10000,	Painful oral, lung, or GI tract abscesses. See Actinomyces and Streptothrix.	Mouth	Bacteria
Actinomycosis 1	XTRA	1.1,20,23,73,160,220,222,262,465,488,567,660, 690,727.5,787,2154,7880,10000,12000,	As mentioned above	Mouth	Bacteria
Actinomycosis 2	XTRA	20,157,192,222,228,231,237,262,465,488,567,6 78,727,747,784,787,887,2154,2890,7870,7880,1 0000,12000,	As mentioned above	Mouth	Bacteria
Actinomycosis (Streptothrix)	Rife	192000,	Rife (1936)=7870,687000,186554. See Actinomyces spp and Streptothrix.		Bacteria
Streptothrix	CUST	784	Crane - Dr. Robert P. Stafford, used to modulate a carrier signal of frequency 3.1MHz.		Bacteria
Actinomycosis Streptothrix MOR	XTRA	784,1607,7870,11659.62,12000,21093.75,21187 .5,	As mentioned above		Bacteria
Actinomycosis (streptotrichosis)	BIOM	10000; 7880; 7870; 2890; 2154; 887; 787; 784; 747; 727; 678; 567; 488; 465; 262; 237; 231; 228; 222; 192; 157; 20			Bacteria
Streptothrix	CAFL	784,228,231,237,887,2890,222,262,2154,465,48 8,567,7880,10000,787,747,727,20,	Includes Actinomycosis, Nocardia, and Actinomyces Israelii - see sets.		Bacteria
Streptothrix	XTRA	3260650	Hoyland MOR. Includes Actinomycosis, Nocardia, and Actinomyces Israelii - see sets.		Bacteria
Aggregatibacter actinomycetemcomitans	RL	358	From Dr. Richard Loyd. Previously Actinobacillus actinomycetemcomitans is a Gram-negative, facultative anaerobe, non-motile bacterium that is often found in association with localized aggressive periodontitis, a severe infection of the periodontium.		Bacteria
Anaplasma Marginale 2nd	HC	415300-424000=3600,	As mentioned above		Bacteria
Anaplasma Marginale	HC	386400-388000=3600,	As mentioned above		Bacteria
Parasites: Anaplasma marginale	EDTFL	20,220,910,7500,22500,85390,155470,285000,4 16500,605410	Tick- and fly-borne Rickettsia-like bacteria which live in blood cells. Found in some Lyme Disease cases.		Bacteria
Parasites: Anaplasma marginale (2nd range)	EDTFL	20,220,910,7500,22500,72500,135470,296600,5 56720,879930	As mentioned above		Bacteria
Anaplasma Marginale 1	XTRA	957.78,959.27,961.75,12075,12093.75,12125,	As mentioned above		Bacteria
Anaplasma Marginale 2	XTRA	959.27,1046.02,19267.59,21010.13,	As mentioned above		Bacteria
Anaplasma Marginale 3	XTRA	1029.43,1046.02,1050.99,12978.12,13187.5,132 50,	As mentioned above		Bacteria
Anaplasma Lyme	XTRA	387	As mentioned above		Bacteria

Subject / Argument	Author	Frequencies	Notes	Origin	Target
Anaplasmosis	EDTFL KHZ	100,240,800,15200,32500,97500,322060,37791 0,492500,723000,	Condition caused by anaplasma (Rickettsia bacteria).		Bacteria
Bacillus Anthracis	HC	393500-398000=3600,	Weaponised bacteria that causes Anthrax.		Bacteria
Bacillus Anthracis 2nd	HC	363200-365300=3600,	As mentioned above		Bacteria
Bacillus Anthracis 3rd	HC	359400-370500=3600,	As mentioned above		Bacteria
Bacillus Anthracis Spores	HC	391450-386950=3600,	As mentioned above		Bacteria
Bacillus Anthracis	XTRA	975.38,979.11,986.53,12296.87,12343.75,12437 .5,	As mentioned above		Bacteria
Bacillus Anthracis 1	XTRA	622,623,624,627,628,629,632,633,634,637,638, 639,642,643,644,	As mentioned above		Bacteria
Bacillus Anthracis 2	XTRA	129,224,273,400,414,420,500,633,768,900,930, 1365,1370,4000,16655,	As mentioned above		Bacteria
Bacillus Anthracis 2nd range	XTRA	11350	As mentioned above		Bacteria
Bacillus Anthracis 3	XTRA	900.27,902.26,905.49,11350,11375,11415.62,	As mentioned above		Bacteria
Bacillus Anthracis 4	XTRA	890.86,912.17,918.37,11231.25,11500,11578.12 ,	As mentioned above		Bacteria
Bacillus Anthracis 5	XTRA	902.26,912.17,961.75,979.11,18122.49,18321.6 3,19317.38,19665.88,	As mentioned above		Bacteria
Bacillus Anthracis Spores	XTRA	959.14,961.75,970.30,12092.19,12125,12232.8,	As mentioned above		Bacteria
Anthrax	Rife	139200	Serious disease of lungs, intestines, and skin. Weaponised.	Skin Lung Intestines	Bacteria
Anthrax	CAFL	500,633,1365,768,414,900,	As mentioned above	Skin Lung Intestines	Bacteria
Anthrax	EDTFL	70,680,930,5500,11090,119340,150000,175330, 545000,705000,	As mentioned above	Skin Lung Intestines	Bacteria
Bacillus Cereus	HC	373650-375850=3600,	Can cause food poisoning.		Bacteria
Bacillus Cereus 1	XTRA	928.28,18645.25	As mentioned above		Bacteria
Bacillus Cereus 2	XTRA	926.19,928.28,931.6,11676.55,11703.12,11745. 3,	As mentioned above		Bacteria
Bacillus Licheniformis	XTRA	2655,21554	Also spelled Lichenoformis. Degrades feathers. Used in nanotech. Mutagenic immunomodulator present in cancer and Morgellons/Lyme.		Bacteria
Bacillus lichenoformis	BIOM	2655			Bacteria
Bacillus Subtilis	CAFL	432,722,822,1246	Can cause conjunctivitis and disease in the immunocompromised, but also functions as a probiotic - as in natto.		Bacteria
Bacillus Subtilis Niger_1	HC	371850-387100=3600,	As mentioned above		Bacteria
Bacillus Subtilis Niger_2	HC	380000,	As mentioned above		Bacteria
Bacillus Subtilis Niger_3	HC	375000,	As mentioned above		Bacteria
Bacillus Subtilis Niger 1	XTRA	921.72,954.32,959.51,11620.3,12031.25,12096. 87,	Metabolically-changed form of B Subtilis due to presence of Aspergillus Niger mold.		Bacteria
Bacillus Subtilis Niger 2	XTRA	921.72,941.92,959.51,11620.3,11875,12096.87,	As mentioned above		Bacteria
Bacillus Subtilis Niger 3	XTRA	921.72,929.52,959.51,11620.3,11718.75,12096. 87,	As mentioned above		Bacteria
Bacillus Subtilis Niger 4	XTRA	929.52,941.92,954.32,18670.15,18919.09,19168 .02,	As mentioned above		Bacteria
Bacillus Thuringiensis	CAFL	520,2551,902,1405	Also known as BT. Pesticidal, with genes spliced into GMO plant foods.		Bacteria
Bacteroides Fragilis	CAFL	556776.6677	Biofilm. From Newport. Pleomorphic bacteria in the gut. Implicated in colon cancers. Use with Parasites Ascaris set..		Biofilms
Bacteroides Fragilis	CAFL	633,634,635,636,637,	Pleomorphic bacteria in the gut. Implicated in colon cancers. Use with Parasites Ascaris set.		Bacteria
Bacteroides Fragilis	HC	324300-325000=3600,	As mentioned above		Bacteria
Bacteroides Fragilis	RL	565	From Dr. Richard Loyd. Bacteroides fragilis is an obligately anaerobic, Gram-negative, rod-shaped bacterium.		Bacteria
Bacteroides Fragilis	BIOM	633; 634; 635; 636; 637			Bacteria
Bacteroides Fragilis 1	XTRA	803.86,805.59,20268.75,20312.5,	As mentioned above		Bacteria
Bacteroides Fragilis 2	XTRA	633	As mentioned above		Bacteria
Bacteroides Fragilis 3	XTRA	805.59,808.07,16180.79,16230.57,	As mentioned above		Bacteria
Bacteroides Fragilis 4	XTRA	807.33,808.07,20356.25,20375,	As mentioned above		Bacteria
Balantidium Coli Cysts	HC	458800-462900=3600,	Caused by Balantidiasis.		Bacteria
Parasites: Balantidium coli cysts	EDTFL	680,900,2500,5500,13930,93500,383000,40000 0,415300,424000	As mentioned above		Bacteria
Balantidium Coli Cysts 1	XTRA	1137.25,1140.23,1147.41,14337.5,14375,14465. 62,	As mentioned above		Bacteria
Balantidium Coli Cysts 2	XTRA	1140.23,11451.02	As mentioned above		Bacteria

Subject / Argument	Author	Frequencies	Notes	Origin	Target
Bartonella		*May cause : **Major depressive disorder • Panic disorder • Depression • ALS • Cat Scratch Fever***			
Bartonella Alsatica	XTRA	236.32	Associated with Lymphadenitis and Endocarditis (see sets).		Bacteria
Bartonella Bacilliformis	XTRA	745.4	Invades red blood cells, and is transmitted by sandflies.		Bacteria
Bartonella Birtlesii	XTRA	857.5			Bacteria
Bartonella Bovis	XTRA	344.6	First found in European cattle.		Bacteria
Bartonella Weisii	XTRA	877.4	Now called Bartonella Bovis - see set.		Bacteria
Bartonella Clarridgeiae	XTRA	716.8	Zoonotic pathogen causing Cat Scratch Fever (see sets).		Bacteria
Bartonella Doshiae	XTRA	856.4			Bacteria
Bartonella Elizabethae	XTRA	867.4			Bacteria
Bartonella Grahamii	XTRA	545.6			Bacteria
Bartonella Henslae	CAFL	364,379,645,654,786,840,842,844,846,848,850, 857,967,6878,634,696,716,1518,	Causes Bacteremia, Endocarditis, Angiomatosis, Peliosis hepatis, and Cat Scratch Fever (see sets).		Bacteria
Bartonella Henselae	RL	878	From Dr. Richard Loyd .		Bacteria
Bartonella Henselae	XTRA	354.15	As mentioned above		Bacteria
Bartonella Henselae Comp	XTRA	576656.5577, 7776665.6666	Includes toxin removal. Also use Herpes Simplex 1 sets. Dowsed by Newport.		Bacteria
Bartonella Koehlerae	XTRA	763.25	First found in cats and birds.		Bacteria
Bartonella Lyme	XTRA	832,39936	As mentioned above		Bacteria
Bartonella Melophagi	XTRA	643.6	Known to cause infection in humans.		Bacteria
Bartonella Quintana	XTRA	356,357,547	As mentioned above		Bacteria
Bartonella Quintana 2	XTRA	476.3	Transmitted by body lice and other arthropods, causing trench fever.		Bacteria
Bartonella Rochalimae	XTRA	588.1	Closely related to B. Quintana, B. Henselae, and B. Clarridgeiae.		Bacteria
Bartonella Rochalimae	XTRA	66697.6755	Dowsed by Newport. See Bartonella and Cat Scratch Fever sets.		Bacteria
Bartonella Schoenbuchensis	XTRA	665.3	First found in deer fly, whose bite causes human Dermatitis - see set.		Bacteria
Bartonella Tamiae	XTRA	878,4	First found in human blood in Thailand.		Bacteria
Bartonella Taylorii	XTRA	573.41			Bacteria
Bartonella Tribocorum	XTRA	456.6	First found in wild rats.		Bacteria
Bartonella Vinsonii subsp Arupensis	XTRA	432.44	Found in humans in Thailand.		Bacteria
Bartonella Vinsonii subsp Berkhoffii	XTRA	466.7	Subspecies found in Bartonella Vinsonii - see set. First found in dog with endocarditis.		Bacteria
Bartonella Vinsonii subsp Vinsonii	XTRA	654.1	As mentioned above		Bacteria
Bartonella Vinsonii	XTRA	654.6	As mentioned above		Bacteria
Bartonella Washoensis	XTRA	968.84	Causes Meningitis - see sets. Also found in dogs and rodents.		Bacteria
Bartonella Species Self-Test	XTRA	236.32,745.4,857.5,344.6,716.8,856.4,867.4, 545.6,354.15,763.25,643.6,476.3,588.1,665.3,87 8.4,573.41,456.6,654.6,654.1,466.7,432.44,968. 84,877.4	All species 60 secs each. Run in Contact or Plasma Modes. Note running frequency when 'hits' are felt, then use Reverse Lookup.		Bacteria
Bartonella Toxin	XTRA	7776665.6666	Toxin removal. Apply: Frequencies Directly. Dowsed by Newport. See Bartonella and Cat Scratch Fever sets.		Bacteria
Bartonella Infections	EDTFL	70,120,900,20000,40000,134270,357770,51025 0,752630,923700,	Bacterium which causes Cat Scratch Fever. Common in Lyme and Morgellons.		Bacteria
Bartonellosis	EDTFL	70,120,900,20000,40000,134270,357730,51025 0,752630,923700,	As mentioned above		Bacteria
Rochalimaea Infections {Rickettsiaceae]	EDTFL	150,190,900,55750,322060,477500,527000,662 710,742000,988900,	As mentioned above		Bacteria
Carrion's Disease [Oroya Fever]	EDTFL	680,900,2500,13930,205530,331000,337600,40 8000,409700,435850,	As mentioned above		Bacteria
Oroya Fever	EDTFL	680,900,2500,13930,205530,331000,337600,40 8000,409700,435850	As mentioned above		Bacteria
Verruga Peruana	EDTFL	120,650,13980,87500,96500,222530,325000,47 5160,749000,986220	As mentioned above		Bacteria
Cat Scratch Fever	XTRA	364,379,634,645,654,696,716,786,840,842,844, 846,848,850,857,967,1518,6878,	Regional lymphadenopathy caused by Bartonella spp. after cat bite or scratch. Also use Bartonella.		Bacteria
Cat's scratch disease	BIOM	10000; 6878; 1518; 967; 857; 850; 848; 846; 844; 842; 840; 786; 716; 696; 654; 645; 634; 379; 364			Bacteria
Inoculation Lymphoreticulosis	EDTFL	20,250,450,650,2210,6150,10230,15910,30280, 77500	Cat Scratch Fever		Bacteria
Bordetella Pertussis	HC	329850-332250=3600,	Bacteria causing Pertussis (whooping cough).		Bacteria
Bordetella Pertussis 1	XTRA	20615.63	Bacteria causing Pertussis (whooping cough).		Bacteria
Bordetella Pertussis 2	XTRA	817.62,820.47,823.57,20615.63,20687.5,20765. 63,	Bacteria causing Pertussis (whooping cough).		Bacteria

Subject / Argument	Author	Frequencies	Notes	Origin	Target
Bordetella Pertussis 3	XTRA	46,284,526,660,690,697,727.5,765,906,9101,12 775.30,12819.84,12868.28,16479.52,20615.63,2 0687.5,20765.63,	Bacteria causing Pertussis (whooping cough).		Bacteria
Bordetella Pertussis 4	XTRA	776,787,802,832,880,1234,1550,7344,12775.3,1 2819.84,12868.28,16479.52,20615.63,20687.5,2 0765.63,	Bacteria causing Pertussis (whooping cough).		Bacteria
Bordetella Parapertussis 1	XTRA	46,484,526,660,690,697,727.5,765,906,9101,12 775.3,12819.84,12868.28,16479.52,20615..63,2 0687.5,20765.63,	Bacteria causing generally milder form of Pertussis (whooping cough).		Bacteria
Bordetella Parapertussis 2	XTRA	776,787,802,832,880,1234,1550,7344,12775.3,1 2819.84,12868.28,16479.52,20615.63,20687.5,2 0765.63,	Bacteria causing generally milder form of Pertussis (whooping cough).		Bacteria
Bordetella Bronchiseptica	RL	655	From Dr. Richard Loyd. Kennel cough in dogs. Rarely infects humans.		Bacteria
Whooping Cough	CAFL	46,284,526,697,765,906,9101,	See Pertussis, and Pertussis secondary sets.	Whooping Cough	Bacteria
Whooping Cough [Pertussis]	EDTFL	110,900,1220,17250,63220,119420,287210,403 020,435000,711170,	Infectious bacterial disease highly contagious	Whooping Cough	Bacteria
Whooping Cough	BIOM	9101; 7344; 1234; 906; 832; 802; 765; 697; 526; 284; 46; 28.5		Whooping Cough	Bacteria
Whooping Cough	KHZ	100,350,950,13610,27500,47500,60000,110250, 425050,932000,	Infectious bacterial disease highly contagious	Whooping Cough	Bacteria
Pertussis	BIO	526,765	Whooping cough.		Bacteria
Pertussis Secondary	CAFL	880,832,802,787,776,727,1234,7344,	Whooping Cough - see sets.		Bacteria
Branhamella Catarrhalis	XTRA	579	Also called Moraxella and Neisseria Catarrhalis. Causes respiratory, ear, eye, CNS, and joint infections.		Bacteria
Branhamella Catarrhalis 2	XTRA	2013	As mentioned above		Bacteria
Branchamella catarrhalis	BIOM	2013; 579; 581; 687; 770; 772; 775; 778; 2013			Bacteria
Branhamella Moraxella Catarrhalis	CAFL	2013,579,581,687,770,772,775,778,2013,	As mentioned above	Respiratory	Bacteria
Branhamella Neisseria Catarrhalis 1	XTRA	978.86,981.59,983.32,12340.62,12375,12396.87 ,	As mentioned above	Respiratory	Bacteria
Branhamella Neisseria Catarrhalis 2	XTRA	981.59,19715.68	As mentioned above	Respiratory	Bacteria
Moraxella catarrhalis	RL	678	From Dr. Richard Loyd.		Bacteria
Borrelia		*May cause : Lyme disease • Anorexia nervosa • ADHD • Bipolar disorder • Dementia • Depression • Obsessive–compulsive disorder • Rheumatoid arthritis • Schizophrenia*			
Borrelia	VEGA	254,644	As mentioned above		Bacteria
Borrelia Afzelii	RL	796	From Dr. Richard Loyd.		Bacteria
Borrelia Lyme 1	XTRA	485,490,495,500,505,610,615,620,625,630,690, 785,790,795,864,	As mentioned above		Bacteria
Borrelia Lyme 2	XTRA	3,230,254,306,338,344,345,432,484,485,490,49 5,500,505,510,525,533,534,597,605,610,615,62 0,625,630,644,660,664,673,688,690,699,727,73 2,758,785,790,795,797,800,864,880,884,885,92 0,943,1455,1520,2016,2050,272,	As mentioned above		Bacteria
Borrelia Lyme 3	XTRA	3422.86,13542.86,17187.52,21576.29,	As mentioned above		Bacteria
Borrelia Lyme 4	XTRA	615,625,1520,2016,2050,	As mentioned above		Bacteria
Borrelia Lyme 5	XTRA	920	As mentioned above		Bacteria
Borrelia Afzelli Lyme 6	XTRA	12109.37	As mentioned above		Bacteria
Borrelia Lyme A	XTRA	776,786,802,828,863,880,885,1433,1455,1519,1 550,1600,1800,2016,2720,2899,4879,6675,	As mentioned above		Bacteria
Borrelia Lyme B	XTRA	62,144,250,345,432,451,464,581,600,604,672,7 26,749,758,765,	As mentioned above		Bacteria
Borrelia Lyme JB	XTRA	13542.86	As mentioned above		Bacteria
Borrelia Lyme Secondary	XTRA	254,525,597,644,699,885,	As mentioned above		Bacteria
Borrelia Lyme Tertiary	XTRA	306,432,484,610,625,690,790,864,2016,	As mentioned above		Bacteria
Borrelia Burgdorferi Lyme Disease	HC	378950-382000=3600,	As mentioned above		Bacteria
Borrelia Burgdorferi Lyme Disease	PROV	939.32,941.92,946.87,11842.19,11875,	As mentioned above		Bacteria
Borrelia Burgdorferi 1	XTRA	941.92,18919.09	As mentioned above		Bacteria
Borrelia Burgdorferi 2	XTRA	11875	As mentioned above		Bacteria
Borrelia Burgdorferi Lyme	XTRA	432,864,345,612,2016,38304,	As mentioned above		Bacteria
Borrelia Garinii Lyme	XTRA	11937.5	As mentioned above		Bacteria
Borrelia Spirochete A	XTRA	444	Chain before Borrelia Spirochete B in a Program.		Bacteria

Subject / Argument	Author	Frequencies	Notes	Origin	Target
Borrelia Spirochete B	XTRA	20,70,324,644,736,544,444,333,367,243,331,13 3,332,73,445,43,776,24,566,	Chain after Borrelia Spirochete A in a Program.		Bacteria
Borrelia Spirochete Inhabited Microbes	XTRA	13888.87=3000,19599.93,20148,17013.88,2085 4.18,15208.19,16666.5,18361.25,21888,12283,	Targets Borrelia-infected organisms.		Bacteria
Borrelia Hatchlings and Eggs	XTRA	203,214,414,589,640,667,840,1000,1072,1087,1 105,8554,	Spirochete involved in Lyme disease.		Bacteria
Borrelia Spp. Cysts	XTRA	840.6	Experimental. Encysted bacterial agent of Lyme disease.		Bacteria
Borreliosis	CAFL	338,344,345,432,533,534,605,673,732,758,797, 800,884,1455,4200,6863,6870,	Also called Lyme Disease.	Joints	Bacteria
Borreliosis	BIO	254,345,525,605,644,673,797,884,1455,	As mentioned above		Bacteria
Borreliosis A (Lyme's disease)	BIOM	6675; 4879; 2899; 2720; 2016; 1800; 1519; 1455; 1433; 885; 863; 828; 786; 699; 644; 597; 525; 254			Bacteria
Borreliosis B (Lyme's disease)	BIOM	2016; 864; 790; 765; 758; 749; 726; 672; 610; 604; 581; 484; 464; 451; 432; 345; 306; 250; 144; 62			Bacteria
Borreliosis(Lyme's disease)	BIOM	6870; 6863; 4200; 2720; 2050; 2016; 1520; 1455; 920; 864; 800; 797; 785; 758; 732; 699; 688; 673; 664; 673; 644; 630; 615; 610; 605; 597; 534; 533; 525; 510; 505; 500; 495; 490; 485; 484; 432; 345; 344; 338; 306; 254; 230; 3			Bacteria
Borreliosis (Lyme's disease) tertiary	BIOM	640; 8554; 203; 412; 414; 589; 667; 1072; 1087; 1105			Bacteria
Rocky's borreliosis	BIOM	7989; 1590; 239; 846; 422; 417; 1455; 797; 758; 693; 673; 577; 4870; 4880; 579			Bacteria
Borreliosis 1	XTRA	3,42,125,230,254,306,338,432,484,525,533,597, 600,610,625,644,650,652,660,664,673,690,727. 5,785,797,800,884,885,1064,1455,2016,2050,27 20,4200,6863,6870,10000,	As mentioned above		Bacteria
Borreliosis 2	XTRA	344,345,432,485,495,510,534,605,615,620,644, 688,699,732,758,810,864,920,943,1520,	As mentioned above		Bacteria
Borreliosis 3	XTRA	939.32,941.92,946.87,1500,2127,2416,2624,342 2.86,9664,11842.19,11875,11937.5,12382,1354 2.86,17187.52,18368,18919.09,20393.88,21576. 29,	As mentioned above		Bacteria
Lyme 1	CAFL	864,495,485,490,495,500,505,620,610,615,620, 625,630,690,790,785,790,795,	Also called Borreliosis. Relapsing fever in humans and animals caused by parasitic spirochetes from ticks. Use Borreliosis, Babesia, and Parasites blood flukes sets.	Lyme	Bacteria
Lyme 2	CAFL	2050,1520,615,2016=600,625=600,	As mentioned above	Lyme	Bacteria
Lyme 3	CAFL	920	As mentioned above	Lyme	Bacteria
Lyme Secondary	CAFL	525,597,644,885,699,	As mentioned above	Lyme	Bacteria
Lyme Tertiary	CAFL	306,432,484,610,625,690,864,2016,790,	As mentioned above	Lyme	Bacteria
Lyme Disease	CAFL	46866,46851,34170,34112,6870,6863,4200,205 0,2016,1520,1455,920,884,800,797,758,673,625 ,615,605,432,345,344,338,254,	As mentioned above	Lyme	Bacteria
Lyme	RL	587	From Dr. Richard Loyd.	Lyme	Bacteria
Chronic Lyme Borreliosis (inc Myamotoi)	EDTFL	110,490,730,2250,7500,30000,270280,333910,7 91030,905070		Lyme	Bacteria
Lyme Borreliosis Lyme Disease	EDTFL	110,490,730,2250,7500,30000,270280,333910,7 91030,905070		Lyme	Bacteria
Lyme Disease	KHZ	650,2500,7500,25230,70000,42500,95670,1750 00,523010,682020,	Also called Borreliosis.	Lyme	Bacteria
Lyme	VEGA	605,673,1455,797	Also known as Borreliosis.	Lyme	Bacteria
Lyme 1	XTRA	485,490,495,500,505,610,615,620,625,630,690, 785,790,795,864,	As mentioned above	Lyme	Bacteria
Lyme 2	XTRA	6425,6575,6625,6727,6777,6929,6957,7033,707 9,7181,7329=180,8215,8515,8935,9255,	As mentioned above	Lyme	Bacteria
Lyme 3	XTRA	485,490,495,500,505,610,615,620,625,630,690, 785,790,795,864,	As mentioned above	Lyme	Bacteria
Lyme 5	XTRA	615,625=600,1520,2016=600,2050,	As mentioned above	Lyme	Bacteria
Lyme 7	XTRA	3422.86,13542.86,17187.52,21576.29,	As mentioned above	Lyme	Bacteria
Lyme 9	XTRA	920	As mentioned above	Lyme	Bacteria
Lyme General	XTRA	2016,2016.44,612,432,432.89,686868.7777,	Also known as Borreliosis.	Lyme	Bacteria
Lyme Disease	BIO	254,345,525,605,644,673,797,884,1455,	Also called Borreliosis.	Lyme	Bacteria
Lyme Disease 3	XTRA	27,735,768,939.32,941.92,946.87,1500,2127,24 16,2624,3422.86,9664,11842.19,11875,11937.5, 12382,17187.52,18368,18919.09,20393.88,2157 6.29,	Also called Borreliosis.	Lyme	Bacteria
Lyme Disease 5	XTRA	605,673,797,1455,2016,		Lyme	Bacteria

Subject / Argument	Author	Frequencies	Notes	Origin	Target
Lyme Disease 6	XTRA	432,450,465,484,610,652,690,790,864,1103,1500,4200,		Lyme	Bacteria
Lyme Disease 8	XTRA	254,345,525,605,644,673,797,884,1455,		Lyme	Bacteria
Lyme Disease 9	XTRA	450,465,652,1103,1500,4200,		Lyme	Bacteria
Lyme Disease A	XTRA	2016		Lyme	Bacteria
Lyme Disease B	XTRA	776,786,802,828,863,880,885,1433,1455,1519,1550,1600,1800,2016,2720,2899,4879,6675,		Lyme	Bacteria
Lyme Disease C	XTRA	605,673,797,1455		Lyme	Bacteria
Lyme Disease D	XTRA	12109.37		Lyme	Bacteria
Lyme Disease E	XTRA	62,144,250,345,432,451,464,581,600,604,672,726,749,758,765,		Lyme	Bacteria
Lyme Disease F	XTRA	11875		Lyme	Bacteria
Lyme Disease G	XTRA	11937.5		Lyme	Bacteria
Lyme Disease W1	XTRA	337,463,467,576,688,728,786,803,856,882,912,1554,1862,2128,3337,5762,6667,		Lyme	Bacteria
Lyme Disease W2	XTRA	611,615,625,650,673,690,724,736,783,786,787,789,793,796,787,		Lyme	Bacteria
Lyme Disease W3	XTRA	799,803,840,847,1087,1455,2016,2050,4320,6870,		Lyme	Bacteria
Lyme Cramp	XTRA	748=1500	Muscle cramp.	Lyme	Bacteria
Lyme Doug's	XTRA	20,27,305,306,432,610,611,612,625,727,787,802,880,920,4200,4320,10000,	Also called Borreliosis.	Lyme	Bacteria
Lyme Envita	XTRA	1550,803,8300,800,8020,880,8450,784,7870,728,7270,444,20,31930.4,38934.1,	Also called Borreliosis.	Lyme	Bacteria
Lyme Hatchlings Eggs	CAFL	640,8554,203,412,414,589,667,840,1000,1072,1087,1105,	Also called Borreliosis.	Lyme	Bacteria
Lyme and Rocky Mountain Spotted Fever V	CAFL	128,239,417,422,577,578,579,673,693,758,797,846,1455,1590,4870,4880,7989,39975,40439,	See Rocky Mountain set.	Lyme	Bacteria
Lyme jb	XTRA	13542.86	.	Lyme	Bacteria
Lyme Main Co-infections	XTRA	2016,364,570,5776	Main frequencies for Lyme co-infections.	Lyme	Bacteria
Lyme Pain and GI Tract	XTRA	438.8,386.4,650=1200,376,	Abdomen, indigestion, anal, urethral.	Lyme	Bacteria
Lyme Pain and Repair Liver	XTRA	397=600,311.12=1200,478.5=3600,	Liver repair and regeneration.	Lyme	Bacteria
Lyme Pain and Repair Organs 1	XTRA	243.2=1200,450,655=360,625,440.15,	Kidney, lung, ovary, pancreas.	Lyme	Bacteria
Lyme Pain and Skeletal	XTRA	428=1800,655=360,444=1200,625=1200,	Bones, joints, spine, skull.	Lyme	Bacteria
Lyme Pain and Tissue	XTRA	397,727,257.51,592.49,418.05,363.35,519.34,760,748,	Nerve, breast, muscle.	Lyme	Bacteria
Lyme Parasites	XTRA	560.2,423,519.34,451.04=240,524,645.25,478.5,	Flukes: lung, pancreatic, liver.	Lyme	Bacteria
Lyme Spirochete Inhabited Microbes	XTRA	12283,13888.87,15208.19,17013.88,18361.25,19599.93,20148,20854.18,21888,		Lyme	Bacteria
Lyme Herxheimer Helper 1	XTRA	10000,880,787,727,522,3,300,330,146,555,33,12595,72,444,1865,20,		Lyme	Bacteria
Lyme Herxheimer Helper 2	XTRA	444,148,555,333,10000,880,787,727,125,95,72,522,146,20,		Lyme	Bacteria
Botulinum	CAFL	518,533,639,172,1372,691,683,	Bacillus that causes Botulism, an often fatal form of food poisoning.		Bacteria
Botulinum	VEGA	518	As mentioned above		Bacteria
Botulinum	XTRA	172,253,435,518,533,639,660,668,683,690,691,727,775,802,831,1372,1550,1552,2688,10000,	As mentioned above		Bacteria
Bacillus Botulinus 6	XTRA	172,518,533,639,660,683,690,691,727.5,802,831,1372,1550,1552,10000,	As mentioned above		Bacteria
Botulism Botulism, Infantile	EDTFL	120,250,700,2540,2740,10540,32500,92500,356720,425580	Often fatal form of food poisoning, caused by Botulinum - see set.		Bacteria
Botulism	XTRA	172,518,533,639,660,683,690,691,727.5,802,831,1372,1550,1552,10000,	As mentioned above		Bacteria
Botulism	BIOM	253; 897.31			Bacteria
Brucella Abort Bang	XTRA	1423	Also called Brucella Abortus, Bang's Disease, and Brucellosis. Causes fever, GI tract and other serious problems.		Bacteria
Brucella Melitensis	CAFL	748,643,695	Form of Brucella found in goats and sheep. May cause reproductive problems in humans.		Bacteria
Brucella Melitensis	VEGA	748	As mentioned above		Bacteria
Brucellosis	EDTFL	50,400,830,2500,3000,73300,95030,175000,275750,358570	Also called Bang's Disease. Causes fever, GI tract and other serious problems.		Bacteria
Brucellosis, complex	BIOM	1423; 748; 643; 695			Bacteria
Malta Fever	EDTFL	80,410,1000,5780,7250,15870,92500,215700,324590,519340	As mentioned above		Bacteria

Subject / Argument	Author	Frequencies	Notes	Origin	Target
Undulant Fever	EDTFL	330,900,2770,37210,98130,123400,205300,418150,633100,823410	As mentioned above		Bacteria
Campylobacter	CAFL	733,1834,2222,378,705.86,2823.5,	Bacteria causing food poisoning, usually found in poultry.		Bacteria
Campylobacter 1	XTRA	333,378,523,705.86,732,733,768,786,1633,1834,2222,2823.5,	As mentioned above		Bacteria
Campylobacter 2	XTRA	333,378,523,732,768,786,872.51,879.96,885.4,1633,1834,2222,11093.75,22000,	As mentioned above		Bacteria
Campylobacter Fetus Smear	HC	365300-370600=3600,	As mentioned above		Bacteria
Campylobacter Fetus Smear 1	XTRA	912.17,18321.63	As mentioned above		Bacteria
Campylobacter Fetus Smear 2	XTRA	905.49,912.17,918.62,11415.62,11500,11581.25,	As mentioned above		Bacteria
Campylobacter jejuni	BIOM	732; 733; 1633; 1834; 2222; 786; 768; 523; 378; 705.86; 2823.5; 912.18; 879.96			Bacteria
Campylobacter pylori	BIOM	2950; 2819; 2799; 2167; 880; 728; 705; 695; 676; 352			Bacteria
Campylobacter Infections	EDTFL	60,230,20000,62500,125750,150000,357300,532460,653690,759830	As mentioned above		Bacteria
Campylobacter Pyloridis			See Helicobacter (or Heliobacter) Pylori.		Bacteria
Chlamydia	BIO	430,620,624,840,2213,	Usually a sexually-transmitted bacterial infection causing trachoma, inclusion conjunctivitis, lymphogranuloma venereum, urethritis, and proctitis. See Trachoma.		Bacteria.
Chlamydia General	CAFL	3773,3768,2223,2218,2213,942,866,840,622,555,470,430,			Bacteria.
Chlamydia General	BIOM	3773; 3768; 2223; 2218; 2213; 942; 866; 840; 624; 622; 620; 555; 470; 430			Bacteria
Chlamydia General 1	XTRA	430,470,555,622,840,866,942,2213,2218,2223,3768,3773,			Bacteria.
Chlamydia Pneumoniae		*May cause:* **Alzheimer's • Asthma • Atherosclerosis • Chronic fatigue syndrome • Chronic obstructive pulmonary disease • Coronary heart disease • Metabolic syndrome • Multiple sclerosis • Myocardial infarction • Stroke • Tourette syndrome • Pulmonary cancer**			
Chlamydia Pneumoniae	XTRA	676755.5555, 565758.5766	Biofilm. From Newport. Wave=square, Duty=82.4%.	Lung	Biofilm
Chlamydia Pneumoniae 1	CAFL	471,942.9,1885.9,3771.7,7543.4,	As mentioned above	Lung	Bacteria.
Chlamydia Pneumoniae 2	CAFL	470,940.1,1880.1,3760.3,7530.5,	As mentioned above	Lung	Bacteria.
Chlamydia Pneumoniae 3	CAFL	470,471.66,941.8,943.3,3767.3,3773.3,	As mentioned above	Lung	Bacteria.
Chlamydia Pneumoniae 1	XTRA	471,479,620,940.1,942,942.89,1880.09,1885.9,1886,3760.3,3771.69,3772,4710.5,7520.5,7543.7643.39,14702.25=900,	As mentioned above	Lung	Bacteria.
Chlamydia Pneumoniae 2	XTRA	470.89,471.66,479,620,940,941.79,943.29,1880,1886,3760.3,3767.3,3773.3,4710.5,7520.5,7543.39,	As mentioned above	Lung	Bacteria.
Chlamydia Pneumoniae 3	XTRA	471.5,942.89,1885.9,3771.69,7543.39,	As mentioned above	Lung	Bacteria.
Chlamydia Pneumoniae 4	XTRA	470,479,620,940,942.89,1880.09,1885.9,3760.3,3771.69,4710.5,7520.5,7543.39,	As mentioned above	Lung	Bacteria.
Chlamydia Pneumoniae 8	XTRA	470,940.1,1880.09,3760.3,7520.5,	As mentioned above	Lung	Bacteria.
Chlamydia Pneumoniae	BIOM	7543.4; 7520.5; 3777.3; 3767.3; 3760.3; 1886; 1880; 941.8; 943.3; 941.8; 479; 471.66; 470.9		Lung	Bacteria.
Chlamydophila Pneumoniae	RL	875	From Dr. Richard Loyd.	Lung	Bacteria.
Chlamydia Trachomatis	CAFL	430,620,624,840,2213,866,555.7,2222.8,	Usually a sexually-transmitted bacterial infection causing trachoma, inclusion conjunctivitis, lymphogranuloma venereum, urethritis, and proctitis. See Trachoma.		Bacteria.
Chlamydia Trachomatis	HC	379700-383950=3600,	As mentioned above		Bacteria.
Chlamydia Trachomatis	BIOM	430; 620; 624; 840; 866; 1111.4; 555.7; 2213; 2223; 944.40			Bacteria.
Trachoma	CAFL	430,620,624,840,866,2213,	Painful and potentially blinding infectious eye disease caused by Chlamydia Trachomatis - see sets.	Eyes	Bacteria.
Trachoma [Chlamydia trachomatis]	EDTFL	800,1270,7500,65000,125750,229320,415700,563190,709830,978850,	As mentioned above	Eyes	Bacteria.
Chlamydia Infections	XTRA	430,620,624,840,2213,			Bacteria.
Chlamydia Infections Chlamydiaceae Infections	EDTFL	800,1270,7500,65000,125750,229320,415700,563190,709830,978850,			Bacteria.
Cholera	CAFL	330,843,844,556,1035,968,591,691,	Extremely contagious and serious bacterial infection of small intestines.	Intestines	Bacteria
Cholera	BIO	330,843,844,1035	As mentioned above	Intestines	Bacteria
Cholera	VEGA	843,844	As mentioned above	Intestines	Bacteria
Cholera	EDTFL	60,240,5690,7250,25190,73000,87500,196500,475170,853720	As mentioned above	Intestines	Bacteria
Cholera	BIOM	1035; 968; 961; 851; 844; 843; 691; 591; 556; 330; 880		Intestines	Bacteria

Subject / Argument	Author	Frequencies	Notes	Origin	Target
Cholera 2	XTRA	330,450,556,591,660,690,691,727.5,787,802,84 3,844,880,968,1035,1550,	As mentioned above	Intestines	Bacteria
Cholera 3	XTRA	450,727,787,802,832,880,	As mentioned above	Intestines	Bacteria
Cholera Secondary	CAFL	880,802,450,832,787,727,	As mentioned above	Intestines	Bacteria
Cholera Infantum	EDTFL	60,240,5690,7250,25190,73000,210600,475180, 527050,661710,		Intestines	Bacteria
Cholera Spirillum	Rife	851000, 960873	Also called Vibrio Cholerae. See Cholera sets.	Intestines	Bacteria
Cholera Spirillum	XTRA	312,13296.87,15013.63	Also called Vibrio Cholerae. See Cholera sets.	Intestines	Bacteria
Citrobacter general	RL	755	From Dr. Richard Loyd.		Bacteria
Citrobacter freundii	RL	446	From Dr. Richard Loyd. Is responsible for a number of significant opportunistic infections, of the respiratory tract, urinary tract, blood and several other normally sterile sites in patients.		Bacteria
Clostridium Acetobutylicum	HC	382800-391150=3600,	Used in genetic engineering.		Bacteria
Clostridium Acetobutylicum 1	XTRA	948.87,951.84,969.55,11962.5,12000,12223.44,	As mentioned above		Bacteria
Clostridium Acetobutylicum 2	XTRA	951.84, 19118.22	As mentioned above		Bacteria
Clostridium Botulinum	HC	361000-364550=3600,	Produces the lethal neurotoxin botulinum. See Bacillus Botulinus, Botulinum, and Botulism.		Bacteria
Clostridium Botulinum 1	XTRA	894.83,897.3,903.62,11281.25,11312.5,11392.1 9,	As mentioned above		Bacteria
Clostridium Botulinum 2	XTRA	11281.25	As mentioned above		Bacteria
Clostridium Botulinum 3	XTRA	897.3,18022.91	As mentioned above		Bacteria
Clostridium Difficile	CAFL	387,635,673,678	Also called Clostridium Enterocolitis - see set. Can cause diarrhea following treatment with antibiotics.		Bacteria
Clostridium Difficile	BIOM	387			Bacteria
Clostridium Septicum	HC	362050-365600=3600,	Causes gas gangrene.		Bacteria
Clostridium Septicum 1	XTRA	897.42,902.26,906.23,11314.05,11375,11425,	As mentioned above		Bacteria
Clostridium Septicum 2	XTRA	902.26,18122.49,	As mentioned above		Bacteria
Clostridium Tetani	XTRA	120,244,352,363,458,465,554,600,625,628,650, 660,690,727.5,787,880.1142,14625,	Causes tetanus - see Tetanus sets.		Bacteria
Clostridium Paraputrificum	RL	444	From Dr. Richard Loyd.		Bacteria
Clostridium Perfringens Spores	HC	394200-393100=3600,	Can cause food poisoning, gas gangrene, bacteremia, cholecystitis, and tissue necrosis.		Bacteria
Clostridium Perfringens Spores 1	XTRA	974.39,977.12,12284.37,12318.75,12375,	As mentioned above		Bacteria
Clostridium Perfringens Spores 2	XTRA	981.59, 19715.68	As mentioned above		Bacteria
Clostridium Enterocolitis	EDTFL	150,550,850,5580,120000,315500,472500,5270 00,662710,752700,			Bacteria
Clostridium Infections	EDTFL	70,120,750,930,15090,24400,324850,505000,79 1500,995150,			Bacteria
Enterocolitis [Intestine & Colon]	EDTFL	150,550,850,5580,120000,315500,472500,5270 00,662710,752700,			Bacteria
Corynebacterium Diphtheriae	CAFL	151,200,340,432,490,624,776,788,925,	Bacteria that causes Diphtheria - see sets for this.		Bacteria
Corynebacterium Diphtheriae	HC	340000-344000=3600,	As mentioned above		Bacteria
Corynebacterium Diphtheriae 1	XTRA	151,340,432,590,624,776,788,842.77,847.73,85 2.69,925,21250,21375,21500,	As mentioned above		Bacteria
Corynebacterium Diphtheriae 2	XTRA	842.77,847.73,852.69,21250=1800,21375,	As mentioned above		Bacteria
Corynebacterium Diphtheriae 3	XTRA	847.73, 17027.18	As mentioned above		Bacteria
Diphtheria	Rife	800000, 1090154		Diphtheria	Bacteria
Diphtheria	CAFL	151,200,340,432,490,624,776,788,800,925,1000 ,10000,	Bacteria causing sore throat, fever, rapid heartbeat, nausea, chills, and headache. Toxins may damage heart and nerves.	Diphtheria	Bacteria
Diphtheria	EDTFL	50,250,940,970,7500,35620,117520,402060,675 620,823010	As mentioned above	Diphtheria	Bacteria
Diphtheria	BIOM	1000; 925; 800; 788; 776; 624; 590; 432; 340; 151; 5000; 10000		Diphtheria	Bacteria
Diphtheria 1	XTRA	151,340,432,590,624,776,788,800,925,1000,100 00,	As mentioned above	Diphtheria	Bacteria
Diphtheria 2	XTRA	151,340,432,590,624,776,788,842.77,847.73,85 2.69,925,21250,21375,21500,	As mentioned above	Diphtheria	Bacteria
Corynebacterium minutissimum	RL	488	Dal Dr. Richard Loyd.		Bacteria
Corynebacterium Xerosis	HC	315650-316800=3600,	Can cause Endocarditis, skin infections, and other illnesses.		Bacteria

Subject / Argument	Author	Frequencies	Notes	Origin	Target
Corynebacterium Xerosis 1	XTRA	782.41,783.28,785.26,19728.13,19750,19800,	As mentioned above		Bacteria
Corynebacterium Xerosis 2	XTRA	**783.28,15732.7,**	As mentioned above		Bacteria
Cytophaga Rubra	HC	428100-432200=3600,	Bacteria that breaks down cellulose.		Bacteria
Cytophaga Rubra 1	XTRA	1061.15,1065,85,1071.31,13378.12,134.5,13506.25,	Bacteria that breaks down cellulose.		Bacteria
Cytophaga Rubra 2	XTRA	**1065.85, 21408.43**	Bacteria that breaks down cellulose.		Bacteria
Diplococcus Diphtheriae	HC	357950-364000=3600,	Bacteria causing dental abscesses.	Teeth	Bacteria
Diplococcus Diphtheriae 1	XTRA	887.26,894.83,902.26,11185.94,11281.25,11375,	As mentioned above	Teeth	Bacteria
Diplococcus Diphtheriae 2	XTRA	**894.83, 17973.13**	As mentioned above	Teeth	Bacteria
Diplococcus Pneumoniae_1	HC	351650-386450=3600,	As mentioned above	Teeth	Bacteria
Diplococcus Pneumoniae_2	HC	**365000**	As mentioned above	Teeth	Bacteria
Diplococcus Pneumoniae 1	XTRA	892.35,904.74,17923.34,18172.27,	Also called Streptococcus Pneumoniae - see sets.	Teeth	Bacteria
Diplococcus Pneumoniae 2	XTRA	871.64,892.35,904.74,957.9,11250,12076.55,21978.13,	As mentioned above	Teeth	Bacteria
Ehrlichea Chaffeensis	XTRA	**595.64**	·		Bacteria
Ehrlichea Phagocytophila	XTRA	**586.8**			Bacteria
Ehrlichia 3	XTRA	76,308,375,468,521.2,570,788,862,943,1583,1584,2084.8,	Rickettsial tick-borne bacteria, common in Lyme Disease.		Bacteria
Ehrlichia 4	XTRA	129,521.2,523,549,607,632,720,726,943,1062,1357,2084.8,	Rickettsial tick-borne bacteria, common in Lyme Disease.		Bacteria
Ehrlichia 5	XTRA	7989,4880,4870,1590,1455,4996.9,5054.9,884,846,797,758,693,673,579,578,577,422,417,239,128,	As mentioned above		Bacteria
Ehrlichia Chaffeensis	PROV	300,336.39,382.19,394.69,528.39,672.7,749.2,764.39,918,1200,1317.2,1345.4,1364.9,1369.79,1836,14980.5,	As mentioned above		Bacteria
Ehrlichia Equi	PROV	1.19,250,295,349,354.19,406,469.69,590,637.89,698,939.29,1180,1223.4,1416.9,1878.7,2833.9,3248.3,3757.3,7080.5,	As mentioned above		Bacteria
Ehrlichia Lyme	XTRA	**395**	As mentioned above		Bacteria
Ehrlichiosis	BIOM	129; 632; 943; 1062; 549; 720; 726; 521; 2085; 4170			Bacteria
Ehrlichiosis	EDTFL	80,410,9800,82500,203500,345000,607600,725840,852000,923880	Infection of rickettsial tick-borne bacteria, common in Lyme Disease.		Bacteria
Eikanella Corrodens	RL	**834**	From Dr. Richard Loyd. Oral/dental and upper respiratory bacteria common in head and neck cancers, and human bite infections.		Bacteria
Eikanella Corrodens	HC	379500-384300=3600,	As mentioned above		Bacteria
Eikanella Corrodens 1	XTRA	940.69,946.87,952.58,11859.37,11937.5,12009.37,	As mentioned above		Bacteria
Eikanella Corrodens 2	XTRA	**946.87, 19018.65,**	As mentioned above		Bacteria
Enterobacter Aerogenes	HC	374000-374000=3600,	Hospital-acquired highly resistant pathogen causing Bacteremia (see set) and lower respiratory tract infections.		Bacteria
Enterobacter Aerogenes 1	XTRA	**927.04, 11687.5,**	As mentioned above		Bacteria
Enterobacter Aerogenes 2	XTRA	**927.04, 18620.36,**	As mentioned above		Bacteria
Enterobacter Aerogenes	HC	374000-374000=3600,	As mentioned above		Bacteria
Enterobacter cloacae	RL	**378**	From Dr Richard Loyd. Are nosocomial pathogens that can cause a range of infections such as bacteremia, lower respiratory tract infection, skin and soft tissue infections, urinary tract infections, endocarditis, intra-abdominal infections, septic arthritis, osteomyelitis, and ophthalmic infections.		Bacteria
Enterococcus Faecalis	RL	**834**	From Dr Richard Loyd. Intestinal bacteria that can be commensal (innocuous, coexisting organism), but may also be pathogenic, causing diseases such as neonatal meningitis or endocarditis.		Bacteria
Enterococcus Faecalis	BIOM	**686; 409**			Bacteria
Enterococcus Faecium	RL	**343,686**	From Dr Richard Loyd. Intestinal bacteria that can be commensal (innocuous, coexisting organism), but may also be pathogenic, causing diseases such as neonatal meningitis or endocarditis.		Bacteria
Erwinia Amylovora	HC	347200-352100=3600,	Also called fire blight. Contagious disease of apples, pears, and other Rosaceae family members.		Bacteria
Erwinia Amylovora 1	XTRA	**867.55, 17425.47**	As mentioned above		Bacteria
Erwinia Amylovora 2	XTRA	860.62,867.55,872.76,11003.12,21700,	As mentioned above		Bacteria
Erwinia Carotovora 1	XTRA	**924.57, 18570.58**	Bacterial disease affecting trees and vegetables.		Bacteria
Erwinia Carotovora 2	XTRA	900.02,924.57,934.49,11346.87,11656.25,11781.25,	As mentioned above		Bacteria
E Coli	CAFL	7849,7847,1730,1722,1550,1320,1244,1000,957,934,856,840,832,804,802,799,776,642,634,556,548,413,333,330,327,289,282,	Also called Escherichia Coli. Can infect wounds and urinary tract. Recommended in cancers. May need Adenovirus follow-up.		Bacteria
E Coli 1	CAFL	332.5,798,1729,7847,	As mentioned above		Bacteria

Subject / Argument	Author	Frequencies	Notes	Origin	Target
Escherichia Coli	CAFL	282,289,327,333,413,548,642,799,802,804,832, 957,1320,1550,1722,7849,	As mentioned above		Bacteria
Escherichia Coli (E Coli)	HC	356000	As mentioned above		Bacteria
Escherichia Coli	BIO	282,333,413,957,1320,1722,	As mentioned above		Bacteria
Escherichia coli (E. coli)	RL	468,667	From Dr. Richard Loyd.		Bacteria
Escherichia coli (cancer prevention)	BIOM	7847; 1730; 1712; 1244; 1000; 934; 856; 840; 800; 776; 642; 634; 556; 539; 358; 330			Bacteria
Escherichia coli, basic	BIOM	7849; 7847; 1730; 1722; 1712; 1552; 1550; 1320; 1244; 1242; 1000; 957; 934; 856; 840; 832; 804; 802; 800; 799; 776; 642; 634; 632; 556; 548; 539; 413; 358; 330; 282			Bacteria
E Coli 3	XTRA	802,882.44,974.14,17724.2,19566.31,	As mentioned above		Bacteria
E Coli 4	XTRA	282,298,327,333,413,548,642,660,690,727.5,78 7,799,800,802,804,832,880,957,1320,1550,1552 ,1722,2872,7849,	As mentioned above		Bacteria
E Coli Escherichia Coli	XTRA	282,289,327,332,358,413,539,548,642,798,799, 800,802,804,832,834,882.44,957,971.66,974.14, 1320,1550,1722,1729,7847,7849,11125,12250,1 2281.25,17724.2,19566.31,	As mentioned above		Bacteria
Escherichia Coli 1	XTRA	971.66,974.14,12250,12281.25,	As mentioned above		Bacteria
Escherichia Coli 2	XTRA	882.44,11125	As mentioned above		Bacteria
Escherichia Coli 3	XTRA	282,289,327,330,333,413,548,556,634,642,776, 799,800,802,804,832,840,856,934,957,1000,124 4,1320,1550,1552,1722,1730,7847,7849,	As mentioned above		Bacteria
Escherichia Coli 5	XTRA	330,358,539,556,634,642,776,800,840,856,934, 1000,1244,1712,1730,7847,	As mentioned above		Bacteria
Escherichia Coli 6	XTRA	882.44,974.14,17724.2,19566.31,	As mentioned above		Bacteria
Escherichia Coli Comp	XTRA	282,289,327,330,333,358,413,539,548,556,632, 634,642,776,799,800,802,804,832,840,856,934, 957,1000,1242,1244,1320,1550,1552,1703,1712 ,1722,1730,7847,7849,	As mentioned above		Bacteria
E Coli Mutant Strain	CAFL	556,934,1242,1244,1703,632,634,776,	As mentioned above		Bacteria
Escherichia Coli Mutant Strain	XTRA	556,632,634,776,934,1242,1244,1703,	As mentioned above		Bacteria
Escherichia Coli Infections	EDTFL	130,220,630,13030,55370,121300,320510,6940 00,715700,824310	As mentioned above		Bacteria
B Coli Rod Form	Rife	417000	Rife (1936)=8020. Also called E Coli		Bacteria
Bacillus Coli Rod Form	CUST	800	Crane - Dr. Robert P. Stafford, used to modulate a carrier signal of frequency 3.1MHz.		Bacteria
B Coli Rod	XTRA	3332080	Hoyland MOR. Also called E Coli Rod.		Bacteria
Bacillus Coli Rod Form	CAFL	318,417,683,800,8020,	Also called E Coli or Escherischia Coli. Some strains cause food poisoning.	Intestines	Bacteria
Bacterium Coli	CAFL	642,358,539,	As mentioned above	Intestines	Bacteria
B Coli Rod	XTRA	727,787,800,803,21875,800,8020,13031.25,213 43.75,943,19869.63,12453.12,	Balantidium Coli. Parasitic protozoan species causing Balantidiasis.		Bacteria
Coli Rod	XTRA	8020	See also Bacillus Coli Rod Form and B Coli Rod Form.		Bacteria
Bacterium Coli	BIO	642	Also called Bacillus Coli, B Coli, E Coli, Escherischia Coli. Frequent cause of UTIs and wound infection.		Bacteria
Bacterium Coli 1	XTRA	358,539,642	As mentioned above		Bacteria
Bacterium Coli 2	XTRA	282,333,413,957,1320,1722,	As mentioned above		Bacteria
B Coli Filterable Virus	Rife	770000	Rife (1936)=17220		Bacteria
B Coli Virus	CUST	1552	Crane - Dr. Robert P. Stafford, used to modulate a carrier signal of frequency 3.1MHz.		Bacteria
B Coli Virus	XTRA	3076140	Hoyland MOR. Also called E Coli Rod.		Bacteria
Bacillus Coli Virus	CAFL	770		Intestines	Bacteria
B Coli Virus	XTRA	27,1552,11939.05,12031.25,16759.77,17220,21 686.38,	Bacillus Coli virus.		Bacteria
Coli Virus	XTRA	17220	See also Bacillus Coli Virus and B Coli Virus.		Bacteria
Francisella Tularensis	XTRA	323,324,427,694,823,913,	Tick, deer fly, and arthropod borne highly virulent pathogen causing Tularemia - see sets. Found in lagomorphs, rodents, galliformes, and deer. Easily aerosolized, so likely weaponized.		Bacteria
Tularemia	VEGA	324,427,823	Serious tick and arthropod borne infection with lesions and fever, spreading to lungs, lymphatic system, liver, and spleen. Use Francisella Tularensis.		Bacteria
Tularemia	EDTFL	30,220,2930,40000,222700,326520,477500,667 000,721000,988900	As mentioned above		Bacteria
Tularemia	BIOM	324; 427; 823			Bacteria
Fusobacterium General	RL	953	From Dr. Richard Loyd.		Bacteria

Subject / Argument	Author	Frequencies	Notes	Origin	Target
Fusobacterium Nucleatum	RL	377	From Dr. Richard Loyd. It can promote the growth of colorectal cancer.		Bacteria
Fusobacterium-Periodontitis	XTRA	**655557.5776**	Biofilm. From Newport.. Also for Lemierre's Syndrome.		Biofilm
Fusobacterium polymorphum	RL	948	From Dr. Richard Loyd.		Bacteria
Fusobacterium Infections	EDTFL	110,490,970,17300,29530,422500,602500,7153 50,803500,924370	Bacteria causing periodontal disease, Lemierre's Syndrome, and skin ulcers - see appropriate sets. Implicated in colon cancers.		Bacteria
Necrobacillosis	EDTFL	70,410,730,4830,67510,220530,325870,451230, 704940,815080	As mentioned above		Bacteria
Sphaerophorus Infections	EDTFL	60,320,900,85700,150000,222700,225000,4545 00,515100,687620	As mentioned above		Bacteria
Gaffkya Tetragena	HC	344850-352500=3600,	Bacteria found in lobsters that can (rarely) infect man, causing septicemia, meningitis, pneumonia, penile ulcer, and ulcerative stomatitis.		Bacteria
Gaffkya Tetragena 1	XTRA	854.79,867.55,873.75,11015.62,21553.13,21875	As mentioned above		Bacteria
Gaffkya Tetragena 2	XTRA	**867.55,17425.47**	As mentioned above		Bacteria
Gardnerella	CAFL	320,695,782,995,329,485,	Also called Gardnerella Vaginalis- see sets. Bacteria that can infect and inflame the vaginal mucosa.	Vagina	Bacteria
Gardnerella	VEGA	782	As mentioned above	Vagina	Bacteria
Gardnerella	XTRA	320,329,485,695,782,995,	As mentioned above	Vagina	Bacteria
Gardnerella 1	XTRA	320,329,485,695,782,995,16927.59,20812.5=12 00,21250,	As mentioned above	Vagina	Bacteria
Gardnerella 2	XTRA	320,329,485,695,782,825.41,842.77,849.1,995,1 6927.59,20812.5,21250,21409.38,	As mentioned above	Vagina	Bacteria
Gardnerella Vaginalis	HC	333000-342550=3600,	As mentioned above	Vagina	Bacteria
Gardenerella Vaginalis	BIOM	320; 695; 782; 995; 329; 485			
Gardnerella Vaginalis 1	XTRA	**842.77, 16927.59**	As mentioned above	Vagina	Bacteria
Gardnerella Vaginalis 2	XTRA	825.41,842.77,849.1,20812.5,21250,21409.38,	As mentioned above	Vagina	Bacteria
Gardnerella Vaginalis 3	XTRA	**320,782**	As mentioned above	Vagina	Bacteria
Gonococcus	XTRA	600,625,650,660,690,712,727.5,827.52,829.89,8 34.1,927.89,14562.5,16628.88,20865.63,20875, 21031.25,	Also called Neisseria gonorrhoeae. Bacterium that causes Gonorrhea - see sets. Also see Gonorrhea Neisseria.	M. Genitals	Bacteria
Neisseria Gonorrhea	HC	333850-336500=3600,	Bacteria that causes Gonorrhea.	M. Genitals	Bacteria
Gonorrhea Neisseria	XTRA	**927,89,16628.88,**	As mentioned above	M. Genitals	Bacteria
Gonorrhea	Rife	**233000,600000,150649**	Crane=712. Sexually transmitted infection caused by Gonococcus bacterium.	Gonorrhea	Bacteria
Gonorrhea	CUST	712	Crane - Dr. Robert P. Stafford, used to modulate a carrier signal of frequency 3.1MHz.	Gonorrhea	Bacteria
Gonorrhea	XTRA	834	Hoyland MOR.	Gonorrhea	Bacteria
Gonorrhea	CAFL	**660,600,712**	As mentioned above	Gonorrhea	Bacteria
Gonorrhea	EDTFL	80,350,55610,119870,232210,308290,455520,5 85370,697500,825910	As mentioned above	Gonorrhea	Bacteria
Gonorrhea	BIOM	7120; 6000; 2330; 712; 660; 150		Gonorrhea	Bacteria
Gonorrhea 1	XTRA	600,625,650,660,690,712,727.5,927.89,14563.5, 16628.88,20865.63=1200,20875,	As mentioned above	Gonorrhea	Bacteria
Gonorrhea 2	XTRA	150,233,600,660,712,1500,2330,6000,7120,	As mentioned above	Gonorrhea	Bacteria
Gonorrhea 5	XTRA	600,660,727,787,880,5000,	As mentioned above	Gonorrhea	Bacteria
Gonorrhea 6	XTRA	712,1990,14562.5,18750,18831.13,	As mentioned above	Gonorrhea	Bacteria
Gordona Sputi	XTRA	381.19,400.6,429.1,435.39,762.29,801.2,858.2,8 70.7,1524.7,1602.29,1716.4,3049,3204.59,3432. 8,3483,17410.5,	Also called Gordonia Sputi. Bacterium that can cause Bacteremia - see set.		Bacteria
Granulicatella adiacens	RL	364	From Dr. Richard Loyd. Is part of the nutritionally variant streptococci (NVS)		Bacteria
Helicobacter Pylori		*May cause : **Alzheimer's disease • Anxiety disorder • Atherosclerosis • Autoimmune diseases • Stomach ulcers • Metabolic syndrome • Obesity • Psoriasis • Sarcoidosis • Stroke • Stomach cancer • Pancreatic cancer • Anemia Iron-Deficiency.***		
Campylobacter Pyloridis	HC	352000-357200=3600,	Bacteria causing gastric problems. Now named Helicobacter (or Heliobacter) Pylori.		Bacteria
Campylobacter Pyloridis 1	XTRA	**879.96,17674.4**	As mentioned above		Bacteria
Campylobacter Pyloridis 2	XTRA	872.51,879.96,885,4,11093.75,11162.5,22000,	As mentioned above		Bacteria
Heliobacter Pylori 2	CAFL	2950,2819,2779,2167,880,728,705,695,676=60 0,	Also called Heliobacter Pylori. See Ulcer sets. Usually present in Morgellons.	Stomach	Bacteria
Heliobacter Pylori 3	CAFL	**2167,728,880,2950**	As mentioned above	Stomach	Bacteria
Helicobacter Pylori	BIOM	2950.0; 2819.0; 2779.0; 2167.0; 880.0; 728.0; 705.0; 695.0; 676.0; 352.0; 347.0		Stomach	Bacteria
Helicobacter Pylori	EDTFL	70,410,730,750,7500,20000,57500,154000,2255 20,322060	As mentioned above	Stomach	Bacteria
Heliobacter Pylori 1	XTRA	347,352,676=600,695,705,728,880,2167,2779,2 819,2950,	As mentioned above	Stomach	Bacteria

Subject / Argument	Author	Frequencies	Notes	Origin	Target
Heliobacter Pylori 4	XTRA	695,705,2779,2819	As mentioned above	Stomach	Bacteria
Heliobacter Pylori 5	XTRA	0.2,0.4,0.59,0.8	As mentioned above	Stomach	Bacteria
Heliobacterium Pylori Ulcer	CAFL	676	As mentioned above	Stomach	Bacteria
Hemobartonella Felis	BIO	603,957	Gram-negative bacterium that causes severe anemia in cats and can infect humans.		Bacteria
Kingella Kingae	RL	889	From Dr. Richard Loyd. Is a common etiology of pediatric bacteremia and the leading agent of osteomyelitis and septic arthritis in children aged 6 to 36 months.		Bacteria
Klebsiella Pneumoniae	CAFL	412,413,746,765,766,776,779,783,818,840,	Gram-negative bacteria normally present in mouth, skin e intestines that causes serious lung conditions when inhaled - Vedi Pneumonia set.	Lung	Bacteria
Klebsiella Pneumoniae	HC	393450-404660=3600,	As mentioned above	Lung	Bacteria
Klebsiella Pneumoniae 2nd	HC	419000	As mentioned above	Lung	Bacteria
Klebsiella Pneumoniae	RL	446	From Dr. Richard Loyd.	Lung	Bacteria
Klebsiella Pneumoniae	BIOM	993.98; 818; 783; 779.5; 766; 765; 746; 413; 412		Lung	Bacteria
Klebsiella Pneumoniae	XTRA	412,766	As mentioned above	Lung	Bacteria
Klebsiella Pneumoniae 1	XTRA	412,413,660,690,709.2,727.5,746,765,766,779,7 83,818,840,3838.5,12295.3,12531.25,13028.12, 13093.75,19964.61,20860.77,	As mentioned above	Lung	Bacteria
Klebsiella Pneumoniae 2	XTRA	20,450,452,550,578,600,625,650,683,688,776,7 87,802,880,975,1238,1474,1550,1862,2688,122 95.3,12531.25,13028.12,13093.75,19964.61,208 60.77,	As mentioned above	Lung	Bacteria
Klebsiella Pneumoniae 3	XTRA	1033.39,1038.59,1045.78,13028.12,13093.75,13 184.37,	As mentioned above	Lung	Bacteria
Klebsiella Pneumoniae 4	XTRA	975.26,993.98,1003.04,12295.3,12531.25,12645 .62,	As mentioned above	Lung	Bacteria
Klebsiella Pneumoniae 5	XTRA	993.98,1038.59,19964.61,20860.77,	As mentioned above	Lung	Bacteria
Klebsiella Pneumoniae	XTRA	688876.5767	Biofilm. From Newport. Bioweapon. As mentioned above	Lung	Biofilm
Klebsiella oxytoca	RL	567	From Dr. Richard Loyd. It is a leading cause of hospital infection globally.	Lung	Bacteria
Klebsiella Infections	EDTFL	170,180,650,970,7500,11950,40000,152000,524 940,689930	As mentioned above	Lung	Bacteria
Lactobacillus Acidophilus	HC	346050-351650=3600,	As mentioned above		Bacteria
Lactobacillus Acidophilus	EDTFL	110,240,570,281830,301090,392430,431190,67 2530,703540,821690	Naturally occurring GI tract bacteria, with some strains having beneficial probiotic effects.		Bacteria
Lactobacillus Acidophilus 1	XTRA	13517.57	As mentioned above		Bacteria
Lactobacillus Acidophilus 2	XTRA	865,17375.68	As mentioned above		Bacteria
Lactobacillus Acidophilus 3	XTRA	857.76,865.08,871.64,21628.13,21812.5,21978. 13,	As mentioned above		Bacteria
Lactic-acid bacteria	BIOM	512; 526; 798; 951; 5412			Bacteria
Legionella	CAFL	723,724,897,975,8120,8856,690,693,	Gram-negative bacteria causing Legionnaires' Disease. Associated with condensed or treated water that migrate to lung tissue and produce severe respiratory problems, fever, headache, abdominal pain, and may affect kidneys and liver.	Lung	Bacteria
Legionella	VEGA	723	As mentioned above	Lung	Bacteria
Legionella Pneumophila	XTRA	660,690,693,723,724,727.5,897,975,8120,8856,	As mentioned above	Lung	Bacteria
Legionella Pneumophila A		5666555.5554	Biofilm. From Newport. Wave=square, Duty=82.4%. Bioweapon. Run Legionella Pneumophila Toxin immediately after. Use both every 3 days, 5 times in all.	Lung	Biofilm
Legionella Pneumophila Toxin		6877677.6657	Biofilm toxin. From Newport. Bioweapon. Run Legionella Pneumophila A before this. Use both every 3 days, 5 times in all.	Lung	Biofilm
Legionellosis	EDTFL	270,460,750,8880,12710,57800,301200,617500, 747500,891350	Also called Legionnaires' Disease.	Lung	Bacteria
Legionellosis	BIOM	723; 724; 897; 975; 8120; 8856; 693			Bacteria
Legionellosis	XTRA	660,690,693,723,724,727.5,897,975,8120,8856,	As mentioned above	Lung	Bacteria
Leptospira Interrogans Spirochete	HC	397050-401100=3600,	Gram-negative spirochete causing Leptospirosis.		Bacteria
Leptospirosis	CAFL	612,663,	Spirochete disease spread through animal urine that can cause meningitis, jaundice, anemia, miscarriage, and death.	Spleen	Bacteria
Leptospirosis	EDTFL	140,550,950,35710,71250,82700,142500,39350 0,632410,719340	As mentioned above		Bacteria
Leptospirosis	BIOM	612; 663			Bacteria
Leptospirosis 1	XTRA	600,612,663,984.19,989.01,994.23,12407.8,124 68.75,12534.37,19865.04,	As mentioned above		Bacteria
Leptospirosis PC	BIO	612	As mentioned above		Bacteria

Subject / Argument	Author	Frequencies	Notes	Origin	Target
Leptotrichia buccalis	RL	488	From Dr. Richard Loyd.		Bacteria
Listeria Monocytogenes	XTRA	377,471,626,628,634,714,724,744,2162,7867,	Bacteria causing Listeriosis - see sets.		Bacteria
Listeria Monocytogenes	RL	852	From Dr. Richard Loyd.		Bacteria
Listeriose	CAFL	377,471,626,628,634,774,2162,7867,714,724,	Usually caused by eating food contaminated with Listeria Monocytogenes (see set). Causes sepsis and meningitis. Also see Listeriosis, Streptococcus General, and Infections sets.		Bacteria
Listeriose	VEGA	471,774,2162,	As mentioned above		Bacteria
Listeriose	BIOM	377; 471; 626; 628; 634; 774; 7867; 714; 724	Circling disease		Bacteria
Listeria Infections	EDTFL	160,550,850,7500,32500,35670,97500,375540,5 15700,660410			Bacteria
Morgan	BIO	778	Resistant enterobacterium, usually hospital-acquired, causing multiple infections.		Bacteria
Morgan Bacterium	CAFL	726,778,784,787,788,988,	As mentioned above		Bacteria
Mycobacterium Abscessus	RL	588	From Dr. Richard Loyd. It has been known to contaminate medications and products, including medical devices.		Bacteria
Mycobacterium Avium	CAFL	642.2,700.9,769.6,803.4,818.5,1001.2,858.2,786 .7,625.9,674.3,953.6,1180,1148.3,773.3,615.7,6 08.4,770.6,896.9,694.1,680.8,632.2,619.7,680.4, 857.6,860.2,590,825.7,824,825,826,827,828,830 ,937.4,529.3,1058.6,2117.1,617.8,1235.7,2471.3 ,1037.5,2075,	Genus of Actinobacteria causing lymphatic or GI tract lesions, mainly in the immunocompromised.		Bacteria
Mycobacterium avium subspecies paratuberculosis	RL	686	From Dr. Richard Loyd. Also called Mycobacterium paratuberculosis.		Bacteria
Mycobacterium Chimaera	EDTFL	120,550,860,7500,96500,275160,434160,52700 0,637320,700250,			Bacteria
Mycobacterium intracellulare	RL	978	From Dr. Richard Loyd. Mycobacterium avium-intracellulare infection (MAI) is an atypical mycobacterial infection, i.e. one with nontuberculous mycobacteria or NTM, caused by Mycobacterium avium complex (MAC), which is made of two Mycobacterium species.		Bacteria
Mycobacterium Intracellulare	EDTFL	140,7500,30160,67500,96500,275160,434160,5 27000,647570,700250,			Bacteria
Mycobacterium Avium (MAC)	EDTFL	140,7500,30160,67500,96500,275160,434160,5 27000,663710,752700			Bacteria
Nontuberculous mycobacteria (MAC)	EDTFL	140,7500,30160,67500,96500,275160,434160,5 27000,663710,752700			Bacteria
Mycobacterium Leprae	CAFL	117.5,236.6,709,1004,1419.8,5679.16063,	Mycobacterium which causes Handen's Disease (leprosy).		Bacteria
Mycobacterium Phlei	HC	409650-410650=3600,	Mycobacterium which covers itself with mycolic acid, making it extremely difficult to kill.		Bacteria
Mycobacterium Infections	XTRA	60,5440,9600,35440,37040,25714,438800,3030 0,38000,40000,	Genus of Actinobacteria. Members cause TB, leprosy, skin disease, lymph and GI tract lesions.		Bacteria
Mycobacterium Infections	KHZ	60,320,600,2850,8250,39550,129500,341500,70 0570,825000,	As mentioned above		Bacteria
Leprosy	Rife	743000,251926	Crane=600, Rife (1936)=6000.	Leprosy	Bacteria
Leprosy	CAFL	600,10000	Chronic infectious disease caused by the bacterium Mycobacterium leprae	Leprosy	Bacteria
Leprosy Secondary Infection	CAFL	1600,1550,1500,880,832,802,787,776,760,727,7 00,690,666,650,625,600,465,444,20,500,450,44 0,428,660,	As mentioned above	Leprosy	Bacteria
Hansen's Disease [Leprosy]	EDTFL	30,410,15190,87500,122060,312330,532410,65 5200,750300,927100,	As mentioned above	Leprosy	Bacteria
Leprosy	EDTFL	30,410,15190,87500,122060,312330,532410,65 5200,750300,927100		Leprosy	Bacteria
Leprosy (Hansen's Disease)	XTRA	600,	As mentioned above	Leprosy	Bacteria
Hansen's Disease	XTRA	20,428,440,444,450,465,500,600,625,650,660,6 90,700,727.5,760,776,787,802,832,880,1500,15 50,1600,1865,	As mentioned above	Leprosy	Bacteria
Mycoplasma General	CAFL	7344,2950,2900,2842,1147,1113,1067,1062,104 5,969.9,865,829.3,800.4,790,783.6,779.9,690.7, 690,686.6,684.1,679.2,673.9,664,644,610,484,2 54,	Can be useful for lung, sinus, and other problems which do not respond to other sets.		Bacteria
Mycoplasma	HC	322850-323900=3600,	Very small cell wall-deficient bacteria causing respiratory, pelvic inflammatory, and other diseases.		Bacteria
Mycoplasma 2nd	HC	342750-349300=3600,	As mentioned above		Bacteria
Mycoplasma	XTRA	388.6,543.6,777.2,1087.2,1554.5,2174.3,3109,4 348.6,6217.9,	As mentioned above		Bacteria
Mycoplasma basic	BIOM	7344; 2950; 2900; 2842; 1147; 1113; 1067; 1062; 1045; 986; 969.9; 880.2; 878.2; 865; 829.3; 800; 790; 784; 779.9; 706.7; 690.7; 690; 686.6; 684.1; 679.2; 673.9; 664; 644; 610; 484; 254			Bacteria

Subject / Argument	Author	Frequencies	Notes	Origin	Target
Mycoplasma Species Self-Test	XTRA	962.77,748.03,772.9,705.68,790.8,797.8,779.07, 2688.3,798.7,2174.3,770.9,2838.5,832.64305.9	All species 60 secs each. Run in Contact or Plasma Modes. Note running frequency when 'hits' are felt, then use Reverse Lookup.		Bacteria
Mycoplasma Arthritis	XTRA	962.77			Bacteria
Mycoplasma Conjunctivitis	XTRA	748.03			Bacteria
Mycoplasma Faucium	XTRA	772.9	May be found in brain abscesses.		Bacteria
Mycoplasma Fermentans	CAFL	2900,864,790,690,610,484,986,644,254,	Experimental. May be a factor in ALS, Chronic Fatigue, Alzheimer's, Parkinson's, MS, and Lyme.		Bacteria
Mycoplasma Fermentans	BIOM	2900; 878; 880; 864; 790; 706.7; 690; 610; 484; 986; 644; 254			Bacteria
Mycoplasma Fermentans 2	XTRA	705.68			Bacteria
Mycoplasma Fermentans Incognitus	XTRA	779.07, 2688,3	US Patent No. 5,242,820, assignee American Registry of Pathology/US Army.		Bacteria
Mycoplasma Fermentans Incognitus	PROV	254,484,610,644,660,690,706.7,727.5,790,864,8 78.2,880.2,986.2,2900,5044=1020,5355=600,	Very small cell wall-deficient bacteria causing respiratory, pelvic inflammatory, and other diseases. This strain is implicated in AIDS/HIV.		Bacteria
Mycoplasma Genitalium	XTRA	790.8	Causes UTIs and genital tract infections.		Bacteria
Mycoplasma Hominis	RL	876	Dal Dr. Richard Loyd.		Bacteria
Mycoplasma Hominis	XTRA	797.8	STI causing Pelvic Inflammatory Disease, Vaginosis. In the male, it can instead cause infertility, urethritis, prostatitis and pyelonephritis (see sets).		Bacteria
Mycoplasma Hyorhinis	RL	689	From Dr. Richard Loyd. This bacterium is often found as a commensal in the respiratory tract of pigs, and rarely in the skin of humans.		Bacteria
Mycoplasma Lipophilum	XTRA	798.7			Bacteria
Mycoplasma Lyme Disease	XTRA	660,690,728,254,484,610,644,790,864,986,2900 ,	Very small cell wall-deficient bacteria causing respiratory, pelvic inflammatory, and other diseases.		Bacteria
Mycoplasma Penetrans	XTRA	2174.3	STI causing Pelvic Inflammatory Disease - see set.		Bacteria
Mycoplasma Pirum	XTRA	770.9	Found in HIV infections and the immunocompromised.		Bacteria
Mycoplasma Pneumonia	BIO	688,	Also called walking pneumonia. Contagious, bacterial pneumonia of children and young adults. See Pneumonia Walking, and use Streptococcus Pneumoniae.	Lung	Bacteria
Mycoplasma Pneumonia	BIOM	688; 975; 777; 2688; 660; 709.2; 2838.5; 2404.2; 601; 300.5; 150.3; 75.1		Lung	Bacteria
Mycoplasma Pulmonis 1	XTRA	75.09,150.3,300.5,601,2404,	Bacteria carried by pets. Causes pneumonia-like disease.	Lung	Bacteria
Mycoplasma Pulmonis 2	XTRA	38467,38464,38476,38451,	As mentioned above	Lung	Bacteria
Mycoplasma Salivarium	BIOM	253; 279; 420; 453; 761; 832			Bacteria
Mycoplasma Salivarium	XTRA	832.6	Immunomodulator found in disorders of eyes, ears, oral spaces, brain, pleural cavity, and in chronic and septic Arthritis - see sets.		Bacteria
Mycoplasma Salivarium 1	XTRA	32384,35712,53760,57984,48704,53248,	Implicated in eye/ear disorders, oral infections, septic arthritis, and periodontal disease. Run each frequency for 18 min after building up.		Bacteria
Mycoplasma Spermatophilum	XTRA	4305.9	Found in human sperm and cervixes.		Bacteria
L-Form Bacteria (Mycoplasma) Gram (-) Mycoplasma Bacterial Infections, Gram (-)	EDTFL	120,550,860,7500,12500,307250,435370,58750 0,795570,901030			Bacteria
Mycoplasma Infections	KHZ	190,400,950,2500,32500,97500,160030,532500, 817540,923010,	Batteri carenti di parete cellulare, molto piccoli, che causano malattie respiratorie, infiammatorie pelviche e altre malattie.		Bacteria
Neisseria mucosa	RL	678	From Dr. Richard Loyd. Mucosa endocarditis have been reported along with symptoms such as painful finger nodules, fever, headache, and tremors.		Bacteria
Nanobacter	CAFL	634	Nanobacterium sanguineum, found in calcium deposits in arteries, kidneys, gallbladder, muscles, and joints and in autoimmune diseases like lupus, psoriasis, scleroderma, etc. Immunomodulator present in cancer and Morgellons/Lyme.		Bacteria
Nanobacter	XTRA	634,317,1268,1902	As mentioned above		Bacteria
Nanobacter 2	XTRA	6771.59,6772.13,6749,6773.44,6772.29,6725.50 ,5965.19,5198.33,5543.65,5631.24,9916.73,879 8.81,8661.95,4628.34,4128.50,2931.45,2208.53, 2100.67,	As mentioned above		Bacteria
Nanobacter 3	XTRA	13543.18,13543.89,13544.26,13544.49,13546.4 8,13546.88,13544.59,13545.21,13546.95,11930. 39,10396.66,9916.73,8798.81,8661.95,4628.34, 4128.50,2931.45,2208.53,2100.67,	As mentioned above		Bacteria
Nanobacteria	BIOM	6773.44; 9916.73; 8661.95; 4628.34; 4128.5; 2931.4; 2208.53; 1902; 1268; 634; 317			Bacteria
Nanobacterium Sanguineum TR	XTRA	7635.45,6653.86,6346.71,5631.24,5543.65,2962 .14,2642.24,1876.13,1413.46,1344.43,1902,317,	As mentioned above		Bacteria

Subject / Argument	Author	Frequencies	Notes	Origin	Target
Nocardia Asteroides	CAFL	228,231,237,694,719,747,887,2890,	Micro-organism causing nocardosis, an infectious pulmonary disease with abscesses in lungs. Found in Parkin's Disease. See Streptothrix set.	Lung	Bacteria
Nocarcila Asteroldes	VEGA	237	As mentioned above	Lung	Bacteria
Nocardia Asteroides	HC	354950-355350=3600,	As mentioned above	Lung	Bacteria
Nocardiasis	BIOM	228; 231; 237; 694; 719; 747; 880.2; 887; 2890		Lung	Bacteria
Nocardia Infections [Gram +]	EDTFL	120,550,860,7500,12500,275290,307250,43537 0,587500,795520,	As mentioned above	Lung	Bacteria
Ornithosis	CAFL	233,331,332,583,859,1217,	Also called Psittacosis, or Parrot Fever - see sets. Infectious pneumonia transmitted by certain birds.	Lung	Bacteria
Ornithosis [Psittacosis]	EDTFL	60,5070,17400,18000,32500,65560,95000,3058 60,712230,993410,	As mentioned above	Lung	Bacteria
Ornithosis	BIO	331,583,1217	As mentioned above	Lung	Bacteria
Ornithosis	VEGA	583	As mentioned above	Lung	Bacteria
Parrot Fever	CAFL	233,338,332,583,859,1217,	Bacterial disease of parrots and other birds transmissible to man and causing atypical pneumonia. See Ornithosis, and Psittacosis sets.	Lung	Bacteria
Parrot disease	BIOM	233; 331; 332; 583; 859; 1216.9		Lung	Bacteria
Psittacosis	CAFL	233,331,332,583,859,1217,	As mentioned above	Lung	Bacteria
Psittacosis	EDTFL	60,5070,17400,18000,32500,65560,95000,3058 60,712230,993410	As mentioned above	Lung	Bacteria
Psittacosis	BIO	583,1217	As mentioned above	Lung	Bacteria
Porphyromonas gingivalis	RL	867,379	From Dr. Richard Loyd. Common dental bacteria.	Teeth	Bacteria.
Propionibacterium Acnes	HC	383750-389000=3600,	Bacterial cause of Acne (see programs), which can also cause Prostate enlarged, Sciatica, Back pain, chronic Blepharitis and Endophthalmitis		Bacteria.
Propionibacterium Acnes 1	XTRA	11992.19,12156.25,12093.75,951.22,964.23,959 .27,	As mentioned above		Bacteria.
Propionibacterium Acnes 2	XTRA	5996.1=1200,6046.89=360,19267.59,959.27,	As mentioned above		Bacteria.
Propionibacterium Acnes 3	XTRA	5996.1-6078.1=1200,6046.89=360,	As mentioned above		Bacteria.
Propionibacterium Acnes 4	XTRA	19267.59,959.27	As mentioned above		Bacteria.
Cutibacterium acnes	RL	368	From Dr. Richard Loyd. Was Propionibacterium acnes.		Bacteria.
Prevotella Copri	RL	478	From Dr. Richard Loyd. It is a common human intestinal microbe associated with chronic rheumatoid arthritis and psoriatic arthritis.		Bacteria.
Prevotella Denticola	RL	765	From Dr. Richard Loyd. Ils isolated from the human mouth, where it is suspected to cause disease.		Bacteria.
Prevotella Intermedia	RL	836	From Dr. Richard Loyd. Is a gram-negative, obligate anaerobic pathogenic bacterium involved in periodontal infections, including gingivitis and periodontitis, and often found in acute necrotizing ulcerative gingivitis. It is commonly isolated from dental abscesses.		Bacteria.
Prevotella Loescheii	RL	966	From Dr. Richard Loyd. Colonizes the gut and plays an important role in periodontal infections.		Bacteria.
Pseudomonas	BIO	174,482,5311	Drug-resistant bacteria often found in wounds, burns, and infections of urinary tract.		Bacteria
Pseudomonas	VEGA	5311,482	As mentioned above		Bacteria
Pseudomonas aeruginosa	BIOM	405; 482; 633; 739.8; 785; 825.42; 1032; 2959.4; 3865; 5311; 6646; 191; 178; 731			Bacteria
Pseudomonas Fluorescens	CAFL	175.5,248.5,351.4,468.5,2810.9,11243.6,	Usually affects the immunocompromised. Used as a biocontrol agent.		Bacteria
Pseudomonas Infections	EDTFL	190,230,730,880,5360,147250,327250,480500,6 95810,875360	Diseases caused by Pseudomonas spp.		Bacteria
Pseudomonas Pyocyanea	CAFL	437	Also called Pseudomonas Aeruginosa.		Bacteria
Pseudomonas Aeruginosa	HC	331250-334600=3600,	Drug-resistant pathogen commonly acquired in hospitals. Causes Pneumonia, Septic Shock, UTIs, GI tract, skin, and soft tissue infections.		Bacteria
Pseudomonas Aeruginosa	RL	985	From Dr. Richard Loyd.		Bacteria
Pseudomonas Aeruginosa Wound	XTRA	20703.13,20912.5,20812.5,821.09,829.38,825.4 1,	As mentioned above		Bacteria
Folliculitis Hot Tub	CAFL	174,482,5311	Follicular infection by Pseudomonas Aeruginosa, a bacterium common in hot tubs and water slides.	Skin	Bacteria
Hot Tub Folliculitis 1	XTRA	174,178,191,405,482,633,731,739.79,785,1132, 2959,3965,5311,6645,	As mentioned above	Hair	Bacteria
Hot Tub Folliculitis 2	XTRA	437,825.41,16579.09	As mentioned above	Hair	Bacteria
Hot Tub Folliculitis 3	XTRA	174,178,191,405	As mentioned above	Hair	Bacteria
Hot Tub Folliculitis 4	XTRA	501,687,737,743,774,857,875,986,1273,	As mentioned above	Hair	Bacteria
Hot Tub Folliculitis 5	CAFL	174,178,191,405,437,482,501,633,687,731,743, 774,785,857,1132,1273,3965,5311,6646,	As mentioned above	Hair	Bacteria

Subject / Argument	Author	Frequencies	Notes	Origin	Target
Pseudomonas Mallei	CAFL	687,857,875,1273,501,743,774,	Causes Glanders, a blue pus infection of the respiratory system and mouth. Occasionally transmitted to humans by equines. See Glanders, Farcy, Mellei, and Melioidosis sets.		Bacteria
Mallei	BIO	1273	Pseudomonas Mallei. Causes Glanders (AKA Farcy).		Bacteria
Burkholderia Infections	EDTFL	190,1220,4330,17250,63210,119420,341230,40 3030,435000,711170	Bacteria found mostly in equine animals that can cause serious diseases in humans. Likely weaponised.		Bacteria
Glanders	EDTFL	80,350,750,7700,32580,174500,407500,632000, 723540,885550	As mentioned above	Glanders	Bacteria
Melioidosis	EDTFL	30,120,930,7500,30000,147500,262500,315610, 505680,756500	Infectious disease due to Burkholderia pseudomallei (formerly Pseudomonas pseudomallei) causing pain in chest, bones, or joints; cough; skin infections, lung nodules and pneumonia.		Bacteria
Whitmore's Disease [Melioidosis}	EDTFL	30,120,930,7500,30000,147500,262500,315610, 505680,756500,	As mentioned above		Bacteria
Proteus	CAFL	424,434,834	Urinary tract pathogen.		Bacteria
Proteus	BIOM	424; 434; 832.86			Bacteria
Proteus Vulgaris	HC	408750-416450=3600,	Urinary tract pathogen.		Bacteria
Proteus Vulgaris	RL	634	Dal Dr. Richard Loyd.		Bacteria
Proteus Mirabilis	HC	320550-326000=3600,	Bacteria which can produce high levels of urease, hydrolyzing urea to ammonia, thus making urine more alkaline, which can cause Kidney Stones - see sets for this and Kidney Calculi.		Bacteria
Proteus Mirabilis 1	XTRA	20034.38,20375,20250,794.55,808.07,803.12,	As mentioned above		Bacteria
Proteus Mirabilis 2	XTRA	16131.01,803.12	As mentioned above		Bacteria
Pyelitis Proteus	CAFL	434,594,776	Bacteria commonly found in hospital-borne conditions.	Kidney	Bacteria
Pyelitis Proteus 2	XTRA	594	As mentioned above		Bacteria
Rhizobium Meliloti	HC	330000	Nitrogen-fixing bacterium symbiotic with legumes.		Bacteria
Rickettsia	BIO	129,632,943,1062	Pleomorphic bacteria transmitted by many arthropods, including chiggers, ticks, fleas, mites, and lice, as well as leeches and protists, causing Typhus, Rocky Mountain Spotted Fever - Febris Wolhynia.		Bacteria
Rickettsia	VEGA	129,943	As mentioned above		Bacteria
Rickettsia 1	XTRA	129,521,523,549,607,632,720,726,943,1062,135 7,2084.8,	As mentioned above		Bacteria
Rickettsia 2	XTRA	129,521.2,549,632,720,726,943,1062,2084.8,20 85,	As mentioned above		Bacteria
Rickettsia 3	XTRA	129,632,943,1062=300,	As mentioned above		Bacteria
Rickettsia 4	XTRA	129,943	As mentioned above		Bacteria
Rickettsia Rickettsii 1	XTRA	76,308,375,468,521.2,570,788,862,943,1583,15 84,2084.8,	Tick-transmitted causative agent of Rocky Mountain Spotted Fever - see set.		Bacteria
Rickettsia Rickettsii 2	XTRA	129,549,632,720,726,1062,	As mentioned above		Bacteria
Rickettsia Rickettsii 3	XTRA	128,239,417,422,577,578,579,673,693,758,797, 846,1455,1590,4870,4880,4996.89,5054.98,798 9,	As mentioned above		Bacteria
Rickettsia Conorii	RL	866	From Dr. Richard Loyd. Is a Gram-negative, obligate intracellular bacterium that causes human disease called Boutonneuse fever, Mediterranean spotted fever, Israeli tick typhus, Astrakhan spotted fever, Kenya tick typhus, Indian tick typhus, or other names that designate the locality of occurrence while having distinct clinical features.		Bacteria
Rickettsia Infections	EDTFL	150,190,900,55750,322060,477500,527000,662 710,742000,988900			Bacteria
Febris Wolhynia	CAFL	547	Rickettsia illness transmitted by lice fleas, ticks, and mites which is debilitating and conducive to relapse.		Bacteria
Febris Wolyhnia	CAFL	547,356	As mentioned above		Bacteria
Q Fever	CAFL	523,1357,607,129,632,943,1062,549,720,726,	Infectious disease caused by contact with animals with Rickettsia and Coxiella Burnetii. Symptoms may include headache, fever, chills, and sweats. See Rickettsia, and Typhoid Fever sets.		Bacteria
Q Fever	BIO	1357	As mentioned above		Bacteria
Q Fever	EDTFL	50,350,750,930,5250,7500,323590,793500,8756 90,951170	As mentioned above		Bacteria
Rocky Mountain Spotted Fever	CAFL	375,862,943,788,468,308,	Potentially lethal tick-borne rickettsial illness with sudden onset of fever, headache, and muscle pain, followed by rash. Also see Lyme sets.		Bacteria
Rocky Mountain Spotted Fever	EDTFL	70,140,5620,37500,100000,275160,525710,655 200,750000,926700	As mentioned above		Bacteria
Sao Paulo Typhus	EDTFL	60,180,780,7100,8510,55710,96600,657110,749 000,987230,			Bacteria
Typhus, Sao Paulo	EDTFL	60,180,780,7100,8510,55710,346000,628000,83 3700,925680			Bacteria
Rocky Mountain Spotted Fever	VEGA	943	As mentioned above		Bacteria

Subject / Argument	Author	Frequencies	Notes	Origin	Target
Rocky Mountain Spotted Fever	BIO	375,862,943	As mentioned above		Bacteria
Rocky Mountain Spotted Fever and Lyme V	CAFL	128,239,417,422,577,578,579,673,693,758,797, 846,884,1455,1590,4870,4880,7989,39975,4043 9,	As mentioned above		Bacteria
Rhodococcus	CAFL	124,835,432,764,337,682,720,	Bacteria which can infect the immunocompromised. Also see Mycobacterium Infections sets, and try Diphtheria sets.		Bacteria
Rhodococcus	BIO	124,835	As mentioned above		Bacteria
Salmonella	CAFL	713.3,718.2	Bacteria causing food poisoning and paratyphoid fever (similar to typhoid fever).		Bacteria
Common Salmonella	BIOM	8655.5; 7770.5; 6786.5; 1634; 1522; 1244; 972; 773; 762; 754; 752; 719; 718.2; 717; 713.3; 711; 707; 693; 664; 643; 546; 420; 165; 92; 59			Bacteria
Salmonella Comp	CAFL	59,92,165,420,546,643,664,693,707,711,713.3,7 17,718.2,719,752,754,762,773,972,1244,1522,1 634,6787,7771,8656,	All strains.		Bacteria
Salmonella	VEGA	1522	As mentioned above		Bacteria
Salmonella Type B	BIO	546,1634	As mentioned above		Bacteria
Salmonella Enteriditis	HC	329000-329000=3600,	As mentioned above		Bacteria
Salmonella Enteriditis 1	XTRA	815.5, 20562.5	As mentioned above		Bacteria
Salmonella Enteriditis 2	XTRA	760,815.5,16379.95,20562.5,	As mentioned above		Bacteria
Salmonella Enteriditis 3	XTRA	815.5, 16379.95	As mentioned above		Bacteria
Salmonella Enteriditis Gut	EDTFL	40,70,520,680,800,2750,351200,532410,613320 ,709800	As mentioned above		Bacteria
Salmonella Paratyphi	HC	365050-370100=3600,	As mentioned above		Bacteria
Salmonella paratyphi	EDTFL	40,70,520,680,800,2750,325780,519340,691270 ,754190			Bacteria
Salmonella Paratyphi 1	XTRA	776,904.87,912.17,917.38,11407.8,11500,11565 .62,18321.63,	As mentioned above		Bacteria
Salmonella Paratyphi 2	XTRA	904.87,912.17,917.38,11407.8,11500,11656.62,	As mentioned above		Bacteria
Salmonella Paratyphi B	CAFL	59,92,643,707,717,719,752,972,7771,1244,6787 ,165,711,	As mentioned above		Bacteria
Salmonella Paratyphi B	VEGA	717,643,972,707,59,92,7771,	As mentioned above		Bacteria
Salmonella Typhi	CAFL	420,664,8656,773	As mentioned above		Bacteria
Salmonella Typhi 1	XTRA	660,690,712,714,727.5,802,804,824,1550,1770, 1800,1862,1865,3205,11289.05,11875,	As mentioned above		Bacteria
Salmonella Typhi 2	XTRA	420,664,773,8656	As mentioned above		Bacteria
Salmonella Typhi	BIOM	420; 664; 8656; 773	As mentioned above		Bacteria
Salmonella Typhimurium	CAFL	693,754,762	As mentioned above		Bacteria
Salmonella Typhimurium_1	HC	382300-386550=3600,	As mentioned above		Bacteria
Salmonella Typhimurium_2	HC	386000	As mentioned above		Bacteria
Salmonella Typhimurium 1	XTRA	947.62,956.79,958.15,11946.87,12062.5,12079. 69,	As mentioned above		Bacteria
Salmonella Typhimurium 2	XTRA	954.32,956.79,19168.02,19217.81,	As mentioned above		Bacteria
Salmonella Typhimurium	BIOM	693; 754; 762	As mentioned above		Bacteria
Salmonella Typhimurium Nervousness	XTRA	947.62,954.32,958.15,11946.87,12031.25,12079 .69,	As mentioned above		Bacteria
Salmonella Typhi	XTRA	655555.5555	Biofilm. From Newport. Bioweapon. 'Contaminates' some vaccines. Can cause Typhoid Fever (see sets), GI tract/lung problems, liver and spleen enlargement.		Biofilm
Salmonella Infections	EDTFL	40,70,520,680,800,2750,5000,15360,325540,53 3630	Bacteria causing food poisoning or blood infections in sub-Saharan Africa.		Bacteria
Salmonellosis	EDTFL	40,70,520,680,800,2750,297500,425950,675310 ,827000			Bacteria
Salmonellosis (Paratyphoid B)	BIOM	59; 92; 643; 707; 717; 719; 752; 972; 7771; 1244; 6787; 165; 711			Bacteria
Salmonella typhimurium food poisoning	EDTFL	40,70,520,680,800,2750,525750,619340,896010 ,982450,			Bacteria
Salmonellosis complex	BIOM	8656; 7771; 6787; 1634; 1522; 1244; 972; 773; 762; 754; 752; 719; 718.2; 717; 713.3; 711; 707; 693; 664; 643; 546; 420; 165; 92; 59			Bacteria
Typhoid Bacteria MOR	CUST	712	Crane - Dr. Robert P. Stafford, used to modulate a carrier signal of frequency 3.1MHz.		Bacteria
Typhoid Virus	CUST	1862	Crane - Dr. Robert P. Stafford, used to modulate a carrier signal of frequency 3.1MHz.		Bacteria

Subject / Argument	Author	Frequencies	Notes	Origin	Target
Typhoid Virus	XTRA	1865	Use Salmonella Typhimurium, Salmonella Typhi, and Rickettsia sets. See Q Fever set.		Bacteria
Typhoid Virus 1	XTRA	**1862**,1865,11289.05,11299.21,18620,	vedi sopra		Bacteria
Typhoid Virus 2	XTRA	**1862**,11289.05,11875,	As mentioned above		Bacteria
Typhoid	XTRA	2890360	Hoyland MOR.	Typhoid	Bacteria
Typhoid General	XTRA	**690,802,1550,1800**	Use Salmonella Typhimurium, Salmonella Typhi, and Rickettsia sets. See Q Fever set.	Typhoid	Bacteria
Typhoid Fever	EDTFL	70,350,700,45000,78250,114690,323000,63708 0,845870,973700	As mentioned above	Typhoid	Bacteria
Enteric Fever [Typhoid Fever]	EDTFL	70,350,700,45000,78250,114690,323000,63708 0,845870,973700,		Typhoid	Bacteria
Typhus Typhus, Abdominal	EDTFL	60,180,780,7100,8510,55710,96600,657110,749 000,987230	Use Rickettsia, and Lice Infestations sets.	Typhoid	Bacteria
Typhoid Fever	CAFL	3205,824,1550,802,690,1800,**1862**,712,714,186 0,1862,1864,1866,1868,	Typhus infection-related symptoms causing high fever, headache, and rash. Use Salmonella Typhi, and Rickettsia sets. See Q Fever set.	Typhoid	Bacteria
Typhoid Fever General	XTRA	**20,690,770,1570**	As mentioned above	Typhoid	Bacteria
Typhoid Fever 1	XTRA	21.5,**1862**,11289.05,13617.03,18620,18906.25,	As mentioned above	Typhoid	Bacteria
Typhoid Fever 2	XTRA	660,690,**712**,714,727.5,802,804,824,1550,1770, 1800,**1862**,1865,3205,11289.05,11875,	As mentioned above	Typhoid	Bacteria
Typhoid Fever 3	XTRA	690,**712**,714,760,802,824,869,900,1445,1550,18 00,1860,**1862**,1864,1866,1868,3205,6900,9680, 13944,18620,	As mentioned above	Typhoid	Bacteria
Typhoid Fever Filter Passing	Rife	1445000	Rife (1936)=18620.	Typhoid	Bacteria
Typhoid Fever Filter Passing	XTRA	11289.05	As mentioned above	Typhoid	Bacteria
Typhoid Rod	XTRA	3037800	Hoyland MOR. - As mentioned above		Bacteria
Typhoid Rod	XTRA	**6900,11875,12100.78**	As mentioned above		Bacteria
Typhoid Fever Rod Form	Rife	760000	Rife (1936)=6900, 900000, 868984. As mentioned above		Bacteria
Typhoid Fever Rod 1	XTRA	345,712,6900,11875,13577.55,14062.5,	As mentioned above		Bacteria
Typhoid Fever Rod 2	XTRA	11875,	As mentioned above		Bacteria
Typhus Epidemic Louse-Borne	EDTFL	60,180,780,7100,8510,55710,152010,321260,66 9710,823010	As mentioned above		Bacteria
Brill-Zinsser Disease [Typhus]	EDTFL	60,180,780,7100,8510,55710,96600,657110,749 000,987230,	As mentioned above		Bacteria
Serratia liquefaciens	RL	867	From Dr. Richard Loyd.		Bacteria
Serratia Marcescens 1	XTRA	866.2,970.03,872.76,11003.12,21840.63,21937. 5,	Hospital-acquired bacteria causing bacteremia, urinary tract, eye, and wound infections. Weaponised, and common in Morgellons.		Bacteria
Serratia Marcescens	XTRA	20010.1057,24755.6555	Biofilm. From Newport. Bioweapon.		Biofilm
Shigella	CAFL	621,762,769,770,1550,802,832,	Can cause acute Dysentery, and Diarrhea (see sets) as well as chronically infect nerves, brain, and spinal cord.		Bacteria
Shigella Dysenteriae	HC	390089	Causes severe Dysentery - see sets. Specific single frequency.		Bacteria
Shigella dysenteriae intestinal [dysentery]	EDTFL	120,200,900,47500,52500,110250,425140,5700 00,841000,932000,	As mentioned above		Bacteria
Shigella flexneri depression [dysentery]	EDTFL	120,200,900,47500,52500,110250,425140,5700 00,841000,932000,			Bacteria
Depression Shigella Flexneri 1	XTRA	976.62, 12312.5			Bacteria
Depression Shigella Flexneri 2	XTRA	976.62, 19616.09			Bacteria
Shigella sonnei invades tumors	EDTFL	40,410,17500,45680,57500,65190,92500,93500, 222530,315500	Causes shigellosis, with acute fever, acute abdominal cramping, cramping rectal pain, nausea, watery diarrhea, or blood, mucus, or pus in stool. Invades tumors.		Bacteria
Shigellosis	BIOM	621; 762; 769; 770; 832; 335; 335; 966.93; 976.63			Bacteria
Shigella Infections (GEN)	EDTFL	40,410,17500,65190,222530,315500,322520,52 7000,667000,752700	Causes GI tract problems, mainly Diarrhea - see appropriate sets.		Bacteria
Sinus Bacteria	PROV	548	Use for runny nose. See Lung sinus bacteria set. Use Streptococcus pneumoniae and the appropriate Sinusitis and Rhinitis sets.	Respiratory	Bacteria
Sphaerotilus Natans	HC	388400-393450=3600,	Commonly called sewage Fungus, this is actually tightly sheathed filamentous bacteria that can cause metal corrosion.		Bacteria
Spirillum Serpens	HC	378350-382800=3600,	Species of pathogenic Spirillaceae bacteria.		Bacteria
Staphylococcus General 1	CAFL	48,146,160,300.2,424,727,736,738.3,740.7,742. 2,786,943,	Can cause boils, carbuncles, abscesses, tooth infection, heart disease, and infect tumors.		Bacteria
Staphylococci	CUST	728	Crane - Dr. Robert P. Stafford, used to modulate a carrier signal of frequency 3.1MHz.		Bacteria
Staphylococcus	XTRA	3343620	Hoyland MOR.		Bacteria
Staphylococcus	XTRA	**563,611,727**	As mentioned above		Bacteria

Subject / Argument	Author	Frequencies	Notes	Origin	Target
Staphylococcus Aureus	XTRA	786.5	As mentioned above		Bacteria
Staphylococcus Aureus	CAFL	8697,1050,943,824.4,786,745,738,727,647,644, 424,	As mentioned above		Bacteria
Staphylococcus Aureus	HC	376270-380850=3600,	As mentioned above		Bacteria
Staphylococcus Aureus	RL	576	From Dr. Richard Loyd.		Bacteria
Staphylococcus Aureus	VEGA	727,943	As mentioned above		Bacteria
Staphylococcus Aureus	BIOM	8697; 7270; 1050; 999; 943; 824.4; 784; 745; 738; 728; 647; 644; 555; 478; 424			Bacteria
Staphylococcus Aureus 1	XTRA	424,478,555,644,647,727,728,738,745,784,786, 787,824,943,999,1050,7270,8697,	As mentioned above		Bacteria
Staphylococcus Aureus 2	XTRA	936.97,944.39,18819.5,18968.86,	As mentioned above		Bacteria
Staphylococcus Aureus 3	XTRA	96	As mentioned above		Bacteria
Staphylococcus Aureus Basal Cell Special	ODD	727,943,8697,424,786,670,2280,2116,1744,	As mentioned above		Bacteria
Staphylococcus Aureus MRSA	XTRA	20,727,787,802,880,10000	As mentioned above		Bacteria
MRSA	RL	466	From Dr. Richard Loyd. Methicillin-Resistant Staphylococcus Aureus refers to a group of Gram-positive bacteria that are genetically distinct from other strains of Staphylococcus aureus.		Bacteria
Methicillin Resistant Staphylococcus (MRSA)	EDTFL	140,300,950,178720,375170,477500,527000,66 7000,761850,988900,			Bacteria
Staphylococcus Aureus CA/HA Octal	XTRA	9504799.449697,4752399.724849,	Community/hospital-acquired MRSA.		Bacteria
Staphylococcus Aureus CA/HA Scalar	XTRA	9714538.431825,483658.389067,	As mentioned above		Bacteria
Staphylococcus Aureus CA/HA Wavelength	XTRA	4752399.72	As mentioned above		Bacteria
Staphylococcus Aureus Culture	XTRA	932.67,936.97,944.02,11758.44,11812.5,11901. 55,	As mentioned above		Bacteria
Staphylococcus Aureus Slide	XTRA	944.39,11906.25	As mentioned above		Bacteria
Staphylococcus Coagulae Positive	BIO	643	Also called Staphylococcus Aureus.		Bacteria
Staphylococcus Aureus	XTRA	876657.7655	Biofilm. From Newport. Bioweapon. MRSA.		Biofilm
Staphylococcus Pyogenes Aureus	Rife	478000	Rife (1936)=7270, 998740, 555171. Now called Staphylococcus Aureus.		Bacteria
Staphylococcus Pyogenes Aureus 2	XTRA	540,728,7270,14937.5,15605.3,17349.09	Now called Staphylococcus Aureus.		Bacteria
Staphylococcus Pyogenes Aureus 3	XTRA	14937.5	Now called Staphylococcus Aureus.		Bacteria
Staphylococcus Pyogenes Albus	Rife	549070	Now called Staphylococcus Epidermis.		Bacteria
Staphylococcus Pyogenes Albus 1	XTRA	333,424,523,644,647,660,690,727.5,738,744,74 5,768,786,932.67,936.97,943,944.02,944.39,105 0,5906.25,8697,11758.44,11812.5,11901.55,119 06.25,14937.5,18819.5,18968.86	As mentioned above		Bacteria
Staphylococcus Auricularis	RL	866	From Dr. Richard Loyd. This species was originally isolated from the exterior of a human ear and is weakly hemolytic.		Bacteria
Staphylococcus Capitis	RL	366	From Dr. Richard Loyd. It is part of the normal flora of the skin.		Bacteria
Staphylococcus Caprae	RL	788	From Dr. Richard Loyd.		Bacteria
Staphylococcus, complex	BIOM	8697; 8646; 7270; 7160; 2600; 1902; 1089; 1060; 999; 985; 960; 958; 934; 884; 878; 876; 824.4; 786; 1050; 1010; 784; 745; 738; 728; 718; 686; 678; 674; 647; 644; 643; 639; 634; 576; 563; 555; 550; 478; 424			Bacteria
Staph Epidermidis	RL	488,1232	From Dr. Richard Loyd. Is a common cause of infections involving surgical wound infections, and bacteremia in immunocompromised patients.		Bacteria
Staphylococcus Epidermis	XTRA	7755766.6555	Biofilm. From Newport. Causes Bacteremia, Inflammation, pus secretion, fever, headache, fatigue, anorexia, Dyspnea, Septicemia, and Endocarditis - see appropriate sets. Use Bisphenol A after this.		Biofilm
Staphylococcus Haemolyticus	CAFL	388.2,1036.4,31092,4397.1,6218.5,12437,	Skin pathogen found at armpits, groin, and perineum.		Bacteria
Staphylococcus Lugdunensis	RL	657	From Dr. Richard Loyd. It can cause skin and soft tissue infections.		Bacteria
Staphylococcus Saprophyticus	RL	745	From Dr. Richard Loyd. Is a common cause of community-acquired urinary tract infections.		Bacteria
Staphylococcus Warneri	RL	768	From Dr. Richard Loyd. It is part of the normal flora of the skin.		Bacteria

Subject / Argument	Author	Frequencies	Notes	Origin	Target
Staphylococci Infection	CAFL	424,453,550,639,643,674,678,727,786,943,960, 1050,1089,1109,2600,7160,8697,			Bacteria
Staphylococci Infection 1	CAFL	**20,643,727,943,**			Bacteria
Staphylococcal Infections	EDTFL	140,300,950,178720,375170,477500,527000,66 7000,761850,988900			Bacteria
Staph Infections	XTRA	**727**			Bacteria
Staphylococcus/streptococcus infection	BIOM	9647; 7160; 2431; 1902; 1109; 1060; 1050; 1010; 985; 958; 934; 718; 576; 563; 542; 453; 436; 423; 411; 134; 128			Bacteria
Stemonius	HC	**211000**			Bacteria
Streptococcus and Staphylococci V	CAFL	128,134,333,411,423,436,453,542,563,576,643, 686,718,727,786,935,958,1010,1050,1060,1109, 1902,2431,7160,9647,40887,			Bacteria
Staph and Strep	BIOM	2170.0; 1800.0; 1600.0; 1550.0; 802.0; 1500.0; 880.0; 832.0; 802.0; 787.0; 776.0; 727.0; 465.0; 444.0; 522.0; 146.0; 428.0			Bacteria
Staphylococcal and Streptococcal Infection-2	BIOM	9645.5; 7159.5; 2431; 1902; 1109; 1059.9; 1049.9; 1009.9; 985; 958; 934; 786; 727; 718; 686; 643; 576; 563; 542; 453; 436; 423; 411; 333; 134; 128			Bacteria
Streptococcus		*May cause : **Anorexia nervosa** • **ADHD** • **Obsessive – compulsive disorder** • **Tourette syndrome** • **Colorectal cancer.***			
Streptococci	CUST	880	Crane - Dr. Robert P. Stafford, used to modulate a carrier signal of frequency 3.1MHz.		Bacteria
Streptococcus Sweep TR	XTRA	5632.8152-5763,5763-6053.125,	Sweep for strep pneumonia, group G, and pyogenes strains.		Bacteria
Streptococcus	XTRA	**3595750**	Hoyland MOR.		Bacteria
Streptococcus	BIO	**563,611,727**	As mentioned above		Bacteria
Streptococcus	VEGA	**727**	As mentioned above		Bacteria
Basic Streptococcus	BIOM	2000; 1266; 885; 884; 883; 882; 881; 880; 879; 878; 877; 876; 875; 848; 802; 800; 787; 784; 727			Bacteria
Alpha Streptococcus 1	XTRA	916.51,941.92,955.3,11554.69,11875,12043.75,	Streptococcus species causing oxidation of iron in hemoglobin.		Bacteria
Alpha Streptococcus 2	XTRA	916.51,929.52,955.3,11554.69,11718.75,12043. 75,	As mentioned above		Bacteria
Alpha Streptococcus 3	XTRA	929.52,941.92,18670.15,18919.09,	As mentioned above		Bacteria
Alpha Streptococcus_1	HC	369750-385400=3600,	As mentioned above		Bacteria
Alpha Streptococcus_2	HC	**375000**	As mentioned above		Bacteria
Beta Streptococcus 1	XTRA	943.4,954.32,960.26,11893.75,12031.25,12106. 25,	Destroys red blood cells.		Bacteria
Beta Streptococcus 2	XTRA	**954.32,19168.02**	As mentioned above		Bacteria
Beta Streptococcus	HC	380600-387400=3600,	As mentioned above		Bacteria
Streptococcus Pneumoniae	CAFL	231,232,**776**,766,728,846,8865,	Pathogen causing Pneumonia, Bronchitis, Rhinitis, acute Sinusitis, Otitis Media, Conjunctivitis, Meningitis, Bacteremia, Sepsis, Osteomyelitis, septic Arthritis, Endocarditis, Peritonitis, Pericarditis, Cellulitis, and Brain Abscess.		Bacteria
Streptococcus Pneumoniae	HC	366850-370200=3600,	As mentioned above		Bacteria
Streptococcus Pneumoniae	RL	**845**	From Dr. Richard Loyd.		Bacteria
Streptococcus Pneumoniae	EDTFL	130,550,950,5220,25510,42500,162520,492570, 791480,877930			Bacteria
Parasites: Streptococcus pneumoniae	EDTFL	130,550,950,5220,25510,42500,162520,492570, 791480,877930,	As mentioned above		Bacteria
Streptococcus pneumonia (pneumococcus)	BIOM	158; 174; 801; 231; 232; 683; 688; 776; 766; 728; 846; 1552; 8865			Bacteria
Pneumococci	CUST	**776**	Crane - Dr. Robert P. Stafford, used to modulate a carrier signal of frequency 3.1MHz.		Bacteria
Pneumococcus	CAFL	231,232,683,846,8865,	As mentioned above		Bacteria
Pneumococcus	VEGA	**683**	As mentioned above		Bacteria
Pneumococcus	BIOM	158; 174; 645; 801; 231; 232; 683; 688; 776; 766; 728; 846; 1552; 8865			Bacteria
Pneumococcus Mixed Flora	BIO	**158,174,645,801**	As mentioned above		Bacteria
Pneumococcus Mixed Flora	VEGA	**158,645,801**	As mentioned above		Bacteria
Pneumococcal [Streptococcus pneumoniae]	EDTFL	130,550,950,5220,25510,42500,162520,492570, 791480,877930,			Bacteria
Streptococcus Pyogenes (a *Group A* strep)	RL	**838,886**	From Dr. Richard Loyd. Group A is responsible for diseases that include sore throat (acute pharyngitis) and skin and soft tissue infections such as impetigo and cellulite.		Bacteria
Streptococcus Pyogenes	*Rife*	**720000**	Crane=**880**, Rife (1936)=8450.		Bacteria

Subject / Argument	Author	Frequencies	Notes	Origin	Target
Streptococcus Pyogenes	CAFL	625.48,2501.9,616,776,735,845,660,10000,**880**, 787,727,465,20,	Also called Group A beta-haemolytic Strep (GAS). Causes Sore Throat, skin inflammation, Scarlet Fever, Pharyngitis, Impetigo, Erysipelas, Frozen Shoulder, Cellulitis, Septicemia, Toxic Shock Syndrome, and acute Glomerulonephritis - see sets, and Beta Streptococcus. Use General Antiseptic.		Bacteria
Streptococcus Pyogenes	HC	360500-375300=3600,	As mentioned above		Bacteria
Streptococcus Pyogenes	BIOM	10000.0; 5003.5; 8449.5; 2502.0; 2111.0; 1213.9; 880.0; 880.0; 845.0; 787.0; 776.0; 735.0; 727.0; 720.0; 660.0; 625.5; 616.0; 465.0; 20.0			Bacteria
Parasites: Streptococcus pyogenes (tooth)	EDTFL	170,550,950,5250,25000,37500,162500,397500, 536420,702530	As mentioned above		Bacteria
Streptococcus Pyogenes 1	XTRA	142,**880**,8450,11250,12500,16493.86,18968.75,	As mentioned above		Bacteria
Streptococcus Pyogenes 2	XTRA	893.59,924.57,930.27,11265.62,11656.25,11728 .12,	As mentioned above		Bacteria
Streptococcus Pyogenes 3	XTRA	20=1200,465,660,690,727.5,784,787,875=1200, **880**,2000,10000,11250,11265.62=1200,11656.2 5,18570.58,	As mentioned above		Bacteria
Streptococcus Pyogenes 4	XTRA	20,465,616,625.5,660,720,727,735,776,787,845, **880**,1214,2111,2502,5004,8450,10000,	As mentioned above		Bacteria
Streptococcus Pyogenes 5	XTRA	924.57,18570.58,	As mentioned above		Bacteria
Streptococcus Pyogenes 6	XTRA	**11273.33**	As mentioned above		Bacteria
Streptococcus Pyogenes 7	XTRA	**11250**	As mentioned above		Bacteria
Scarlet Fever	CAFL	437,**880**,787,727,690,666,	Causes rash, strawberry tongue, sore throat, swollen glands, headache, and fever. Use Streptococcus Pyogenes.		Bacteria
Scarlet Fever	EDTFL	140,220,760,2580,193110,247560,385210,5216 80,657300,729340	As mentioned above		Bacteria
Streptococcus agalactiae (*Group B* strep)	RL	476,843	From Dr. Richard Loyd. May cause meningitis or septicaemia as well as localized infections such as subcutaneous abscesses, urinary tract infection or arthritis.		Bacteria
Group C					Bacteria
Streptococcus Dysgalactiae	RL	258	From Dr. Richard Loyd. Is most frequently encountered as a commensal of the alimentary tract, genital tract, or less commonly, as a part of the skin flora.		Bacteria
Group D					Bacteria
Streptococcus gallolyticus (was bovis)	RL	889	From Dr. Richard Loyd. Is associated with urinary tract infections, endocarditis, sepsis, and colorectal cancer.		Bacteria
Streptococcus Species *Group G*	HC	368150-368850=3600,	Usually, but not exclusively, beta-hemolytic. Includes Streptococcus Canis. Also see Streptococcus Sweep TR set.		Bacteria
Parasites: Streptococcus sp. group G (tooth)	EDTFL	170,550,950,5250,25000,37500,175440,375430, 375910,598220,	As mentioned above		Bacteria
Viridans					Bacteria
Streptococcus Viridans	CAFL	445,935,1010,1060,8478,457,465,777,778,1214, 1216,	Alpha-haemolytic species causing dental caries and Endocarditis - see appropriate sets, and Alpha Streptococcus.		Bacteria
Streptococcus viridans general	RL	554	From Dr. Richard Loyd.		Bacteria
Streptococcus anginosus	RL	566,587	From Dr. Richard Loyd. Are capable of causing serious pyogenic infections, with a tendency for abscess formation.		Bacteria
Streptococcus Enterococcinum	CAFL	686,409	Can cause infection in the digestive and urinary tracts.		Bacteria
Streptococcus Haemolytic	CAFL	128,134,318,334,368,443,535,542,675,691,710, 712,728,786,**880**,1203,1415,1522,1902,	Blood infection by Streptococcus.		Bacteria
Streptococcus Haemolytic	VEGA	535,1522	As mentioned above		Bacteria
Streptococcus Hemolytic	BIOM	728.0; 880.0; 786.0; 712.0; 128.0; 134.0; 334.0; 443.0; 535.0; 542.0; 675.0; 1415.0; 1522.0; 1902.0; 691.0; 710.0; 1202.9; 368.0; 318.0			Bacteria
Streptococcus Haemolyticus basic	BIOM	2000; 1902; 1522; 1415; 1266; 1203; 881; 878; 877; 876; 875; 848; 802; 800; 786; 784; 728; 712; 710; 691; 675; 542; 535; 368; 318			Bacteria
Streptococcus Haemolyticus alpha	BIOM	941.9; 425; 433; 445; 941.9; 935; 1010; 1060; 457; 465; 777; 778; 1214; 1216; 8478			Bacteria
Streptococcus Haemolyticus beta	BIOM	10000; 5004; 8450; 2502; 2111; 1214; 954.3; 924.6; 845; 735; 720; 660; 625.5; 616; 465			Bacteria
Streptococcus intermedius	RL	975	From Dr. Richard Loyd.		Bacteria
Streptococcus Lactis	HC	382000-387000=3600,	Species used to make dairy products. Has been genetically modified.		Bacteria
Lactococcus lactis	RL	774	From Dr. Richard Loyd. Previously Streptococcus lactis		Bacteria

Subject / Argument	Author	Frequencies	Notes	Origin	Target
Streptococcus Mitis Abscesses Stiff Knees	HC	313800-321100=3600,	Alpha-haemolytic species found in the throat, oropharyngeal spaces, causing Endocarditis - see sets. Can also infect joints. Also see Alpha Streptococcus sets.		Bacteria
Streptococcus Mitis	XTRA	565655.5555	Biofilm. From Newport. Bioweapon, delivered via anesthesia.		Bacteria
Streptococcus Mutans	RL	885	From Dr. Richard Loyd.		Bacteria
Streptococcus Mutans	BIOM	108; 114; 433; 437; 488; 625; 687; 833; 883; 994; 8686; 8777; 9676; 660; 732; 745; 754; 764			Bacteria
Streptococcus Mutant Strain	CAFL	114,437,625,883,994,	Species causing dental caries and Endocarditis - see appropriate sets.		Bacteria
Streptococcus Mutant Strain Secondary	CAFL	108,433,488,660,687,732,745,754,764,833,8686 ,8777,9676,	As mentioned above		Bacteria
Streptococcus oralis	RL	354	From Dr. Richard Loyd.		Bacteria
Streptococcus Pepto	CAFL	201,629	Can cause brain, liver, breast, and lung abscesses, as well as generalized necrotizing soft tissue infections.		Bacteria
Streptococcus Salivarius	RL	836	From Dr. Richard Loyd.		Bacteria
Streptococcus sanguinis	RL	565	From Dr. Richard Loyd. Previously Streptococcus sanguis		Bacteria
Peptostreptococchi	BIOM	201; 629			Bacteria
Streptococco TR Scansione	XTRA	5632.8152-5763,5763-6053.125,	Sweep for strep pneumonia, group G e pyogenes strains.	Sweep	Bacteria
Streptococcus Infection General	CAFL	2000,1266,885,884,883,882,881,**880**,879,878,87 7,876,875,848,802,800,787,784,727,	Streptococcus family. See General antiseptic, and other Streptococcus sets.		Bacteria
Streptococcal Infections	EDTFL	160,550,950,5220,25510,42500,162520,492570, 675510,828530	As mentioned above		Bacteria
Streptococcal Infections	KHZ	150,700,2500,5250,47500,70000,275000,42575 0,842000,932000,	As mentioned above		Bacteria
Streptococcal Infections	XTRA	880	As mentioned above		Bacteria
Erysipelas	CAFL	616,776,735,845,660,10000,880,787,727,465,20 ,	Infection normally with red facial, arm, or leg rash. Usually due to Streptococcus Pyogenes (see sets) or other family members (see Streptococcal Infections).	Skin	Bacteria
Erysipelas	EDTFL	280,650,5150,10570,42500,65330,95700,22533 0,455420,800310	As mentioned above	Skin	Bacteria
Erysipelas	VEGA	845,616	As mentioned above	Skin	Bacteria
Erysipelas	XTRA	616,845	As mentioned above	Skin	Bacteria
Erysipelas 1	XTRA	20,465,616,660,690,727.5,735,776,787,845,880, 2000,10000,	As mentioned above	Skin	Bacteria
Erysipelas 2	XTRA	20,465,660,727,787,880,10000,	As mentioned above	Skin	Bacteria
Erysipelas 3	XTRA	20,465,600,660,727,787,880,2000,10000,	As mentioned above	Skin	Bacteria
Erysipelatous inflammation	BIOM	660; 725; 10000; 880; 787; 727; 465; 20		Skin	Bacteria
Streptomyces Griseus	CAFL	333,887	Soil bacteria which yields the antibiotic Streptomycin.		Bacteria
Streptomyces Griseus	VEGA	887	As mentioned above		Bacteria
Clostridium Tetani	XTRA	120,244,352,363,458,465,554,600,625,628,650, 660,690,727.5,787,880.1142,14625,	Causes tetanus - see Tetanus sets.		Bacteria
Tetanus	Rife	234000	Rife (1936)=1200, 700000, 15779. Infectious disease of the central nervous system caused by Clostridium Tetani - see this set.	Tetanus	Bacteria
Tetanus	CUST	120	Crane - Dr. Robert P. Stafford, used to modulate a carrier signal of frequency 3.1MHz.	Tetanus	Bacteria
Tetanus	CAFL	20,400,880,244,600,554,120,352,1142,363,458, 465,628,	As mentioned above	Tetanus	Bacteria
Tetanus	XTRA	3276000	Hoyland MOR.	Tetanus	Bacteria
Tetanus	BIO	352,554,1142	As mentioned above	Tetanus	Bacteria
Tetanus	EDTFL	40,550,7250,50000,97500,222300,434590,5176 00,687620,717000	As mentioned above	Tetanus	Bacteria
Tetanus Secondary	CAFL	880,787,727	As mentioned above	Tetanus	Bacteria
Tetanus Antitoxin	BIO	363,458	As mentioned above	Tetanus	Bacteria
Tetragenus	CAFL	393,433,2712	Micrococcus Tetragenus causes lung infections and septicemia, usually in the immunocompromised.		Bacteria
Tetragenus	VEGA	393,2712	As mentioned above		Bacteria
Thermi Bacteria	BIO	233,441	Thermithiobacillus is found in hot sulfur baths and springs.		Bacteria
Treponema	CUST	660	Crane - Dr. Robert P. Stafford, used to modulate a carrier signal of frequency 3.1MHz.		Bacteria
Treponema 1	XTRA	6600	Spirochete causing syphilis. Has also been used for Lyme treatment. Use Syphilis, and see Luesinum and Syphilinum sets.		Bacteria
Treponema 2	XTRA	20,600,625,626,650,**660**,10000,			Bacteria
Treponema Denticola	RL	842	From Dr. Richard Loyd. Spirochete causing dental infection. Usually present in Morgellons.		Bacteria
Treponema Pallidum	CAFL	660,902	Spirochete causing syphilis. Has been used in Lyme treatment. Use Syphilis, and see Luesinum and Syphilinum sets.		Bacteria
Treponema Pallidum	HC	346850-347400=3600,			Bacteria

Subject / Argument	Author	Frequencies	Notes	Origin	Target
Parasites: Treponema pallidum causes syphilis	EDTFL	100,250,680,2750,5750,7600,325750,374300,58 6220,748600,	vedi sopra		Bacteria
Treponema Pallidum 1	XTRA	20=1200,120,177,600,625,650,658,660,690,700 ,727.5,902,12338.12,17276.11,21685.01=1200, 21687.5,			Bacteria
Syphilis	CAFL	177,650,625,600,660,658,	Sexually transmitted infection (STI) caused by the bacterium Treponema pallidum.	Syphilis	Bacteria
Syphilis	EDTFL	320,600,32500,67500,97500,325750,374300,58 6220,748600,	As mentioned above	Syphilis	Bacteria
Great Pox [Syphilis]	EDTFL	320,600,6000,32500,67500,97500,325750,3743 00,586220,748600,		Syphilis	Bacteria
Syphilis	XTRA	3154800	Hoyland MOR.	Syphilis	Bacteria
Syphilis (Treponema Pallidum)	Rife	789000	Crane=660, Rife (1936)=6600, 900000.	Syphilis	Bacteria
Syphilis	BIOM	6600; 789; 900; 2776; 177; 650; 625; 600; 660; 658		Syphilis	Bacteria
Syphilis, Congenital	EDTFL	320,600,6000,32500,67500,97500,325750,3743 00,586220,748600,	As mentioned above	Syphilis	Bacteria
Yaws [Treponema Palladium]	EDTFL	100,250,680,2750,5750,7600,325750,374300,58 6220,748600,	Tropical infection of skin, bones, and joints caused by Treponema Pallidum (see set) spirochete.	Syphilis	Bacteria
Frambesia [YAWS]	EDTFL	100,250,680,2750,5750,7600,325750,374300,58 6220,748600,	As mentioned above	Syphilis	Bacteria
Typhus, Scrub	EDTFL	60,180,780,7100,8510,55710,152010,321260,66 9710,823010,	Form of typhus, usually caused by chigger bite.		Bacteria
Tsutsugamushi Disease [Rickettsia]	EDTFL	150,190,900,55750,322060,477500,527000,662 710,742000,988900,	As mentioned above		Bacteria
Mycobacterium Tuberculosis		May cause : **Autoimmune diseases • Stroke**			
Mycobacterium Tuberculosis	HC	430550-434200=3600,	Mycobacterium which causes tuberculosis (TB). Also see Tuberculosis sets, and Tuberculinum.		Bacteria
Mycobacterium Tuberculosis 1	XTRA	1067.23,1070.81,1076.26,13454.69,13500,1356 8.75,	As mentioned above		Bacteria
Mycobacterium Tuberculosis 1	XTRA	13454.69,13568.75,13500,1067.23,1076.26,107 0.82,	As mentioned above		Bacteria
Mycobacterium Tuberculosis 2	XTRA	1070.81,21508	As mentioned above		Bacteria
Mycobacterium Tuberculosis 2	XTRA	21508,1070.81=360,	As mentioned above		Bacteria
Koch's bacillus	BIOM	5; 72			Bacteria
Tuberculinum	CAFL	332,522,664,731,737,748,1085,1099,1700,761,	Homeopathic nosode for Tuberculosis. See Tuberculosis, and Tuberculosis General.		Bacteria
Tuberculinum	VEGA	522,	As mentioned above		Bacteria
Tuberculinum nosod	BIOM	332; 1085; 1099; 1700; 761			Bacteria
Tuberculosis General	CAFL	20,216,369,541,583,666,690,720,727,740,784,8 02,803,1500,1513,1550,1552,1600,1840,	Infectious disease usually due to Mycobacterium Tuberculosis, affecting lungs and other parts of body.	Tuberculosis	Bacteria
Tuberculosis	XTRA	20,	As mentioned above	Tuberculosis	Bacteria
Tuberculosis	EDTFL	140,7500,30160,67500,96500,275160,434160,5 27000,663710,752700	As mentioned above	Tuberculosis	Bacteria
Tuberculosis basic	BIOM	72; 216; 369; 541; 690; 776; 799; 802; 803; 804; 1552; 1550; 1513; 2365; 2127; 2008; 8030		Tuberculosis	Bacteria
Tuberculosis, Spinal	EDTFL	140,7500,30160,67500,96500,52500,425160,57 1000,841000,932000		Tuberculosis	Bacteria
Tuberculosis Secondary Complications	CAFL	776,2127,2008,465	As mentioned above	Tuberculosis	Bacteria
Tuberculosis Aviare	CAFL	303,332,342,438,440,532,3113,6515,697,698,72 0,731,741,748,770,	As mentioned above	Tuberculosis	Bacteria
TB Aviare	VEGA	532	As mentioned above	Tuberculosis	Bacteria
Tuberculosis Aviare	BIOM	303; 332; 342; 438; 440; 532; 3133; 6515; 697; 698; 720; 731; 741; 748; 770; 757		Tuberculosis	Bacteria
Tuberculosis Bovine	BIO	523,3353	As mentioned above	Tuberculosis	Bacteria
Tuberculosis Bovine	CAFL	229,523,625,635,838,877,3353,748,757,	As mentioned above	Tuberculosis	Bacteria
Tuberculosis Bovine	BIOM	229; 523; 625; 635; 877; 3353; 748			Bacteria
TB Bovine	VEGA	523,3353	As mentioned above	Tuberculosis	Bacteria
Tuberculosis cutis	BIOM	93			Bacteria
Tuberculosis Klebsiella	BIO	221,1132,1644,2313,6516,		Tuberculosis	Bacteria
Tuberculosis Klebsiella	CAFL	217,220,221,686,1132,1644,2313,6516,729,748,	As mentioned above	Tuberculosis	Bacteria
Tuberculosis Klebsiella	BIOM	217; 220; 221; 1032; 1644; 2313; 6516; 729; 748			Bacteria

Subject / Argument	Author	Frequencies	Notes	Origin	Target
TB Klebsiella	VEGA	221,1132,1644,2313,6516,	As mentioned above	Tuberculosis	Bacteria
Tuberculosis Rod Form	Rife	369000	Rife (1936)=8300, 583000, 541142.	Tuberculosis	Bacteria
Tuberculosis Rod Form	CUST	803	Crane - Dr. Robert P. Stafford, used to modulate a carrier signal of frequency 3.1MHz.	Tuberculosis	Bacteria
Tuberculosis Rod E Coli Infections	CAFL	799,802,804,1550,1513,	As mentioned above	Tuberculosis	Bacteria
Tuberculosis Rod Form	CAFL	369,541,583,802,803,1513,8030,	As mentioned above	Tuberculosis	Bacteria
Tuberculosis Virus Form	Rife	16000	Crane=1552. - As mentioned above	Tuberculosis	Bacteria
Tuberculosis Virus	CUST	1552	Crane - Dr. Robert P. Stafford, used to modulate a carrier signal of frequency 3.1MHz.	Tuberculosis	Bacteria
Tuberculosis Virus	XTRA	3076000	Hoyland MOR. - As mentioned above	Tuberculosis	Bacteria
Tuberculosis Virus Form	CAFL	2565,1552	As mentioned above	Tuberculosis	Bacteria
Urea Plasma	CAFL	756	Ureaplasma is a non-STI bacterium causing Vaginosis, Pelvic Inflammatory Disease, and (non-gonoccal) Urethritis - see sets.		Bacteria
Urea Plasma 2	XTRA	776.2	vedi sopra		Bacteria
Ureaplasmosis	BIOM	2900; 864; 790; 756; 690; 610; 484; 986; 644; 254			Bacteria
Veillonella Dispar	HC	401750-405200=3600,	Gram-negative bacteria involved in dental caries and joint infections, usually together with Streptococcus spp. See Streptococcus Mutant Strain, and Streptococcus Viridans.		Bacteria
Vibrio parahaemolyticus	RL	474	From Dr. Richard Loyd. Is a bacterium found in brackish, saltwater, which, when ingested, causes gastrointestinal illness in humans.		Bacteria
Parasites: Veillonella dispar	EDTFL	20,230,730,2500,5250,7000,32500,95910,175410,475430	As mentioned above		Bacteria
Whipple Disease Whipple's Disease	EDTFL	40,520,750,2500,5070,47500,175160,525710,759830,932410	It is a rare systemic disease caused by the Tropheryma whipplei bacterium. The main symptoms are arthritis, weight loss, abdominal pain and diarrhea.		Bacteria
Lipodystrophy, Intestinal	EDTFL	500,570,870,12330,42500,152500,287800,424370,567700,985900,			Bacteria
Yersinia Pestis	BIO	333	Also called Pasteurella pestis. Causes Bubonic Plague. Spread primarily by rats and their fleas. May also be involved in arthritis.		Bacteria
Yersinia Pestis 1	XTRA	160,210,216,333,338,492,496,500,504,508,512,1600,5000,5120,	As mentioned above		Bacteria
Yersinia Pestis 2	XTRA	20,210,216,333,500,523,660,690,727.5,768,786,787,880,	As mentioned above		Bacteria
Yersinia Pestis 3	XTRA	337.6	As mentioned above		Bacteria
Yersinia Infections	EDTFL	40,120,950,13390,13930,50000,165800,493200,722700,905370	As mentioned above		Bacteria
Yersinosis [Yersinia Bacteria]	EDTFL	40,120,950,13390,13930,50000,165800,493200,722700,905370,	As mentioned above		Bacteria
Yersinosis	BIOM	5120; 5000; 1600; 512; 508; 504; 500; 496; 492; 338; 333; 210; 216; 160			Bacteria
Plague	CAFL	210,216,333,500	See Bubonic Plague and Yersinia Pestis sets.		Bacteria.
Bubonic Plague Secondary Infections	CAFL	880,787,727,20	As mentioned above		Bacteria
Bubonic Plague Yersinia Pestis	CAFL	210,216,333,500	As mentioned above		Bacteria
Plague	BIO	333	Yersinia pestis. Bubonic plague, spread primarily by rats and their fleas.		Bacteria.
Plague	EDTFL	40,180,300,700,7600,45730,71400,95300,219320,379940			Bacteria
Bubonic Plague	EDTFL	40,180,300,700,42500,71400,95300,232040,390500,429930,	See Bubonic Plague and Yersinia Pestis sets.		Bacteria.
Meningeal Plague	EDTFL	40,260,750,12050,177500,252500,385000,404920,625610,853720	As mentioned above		Bacteria.
Pneumonic Plague	EDTFL	40,180,300,700,7600,45730,71400,95300,219320,379940,	As mentioned above		Bacteria.
Pulmonic Plague	EDTFL	40,180,300,700,42500,71400,95300,232040,390500,429930,	As mentioned above		Bacteria.
Bubonic Plague	Rife	160000,512466,	As mentioned above		Bacteria
Bubonic Plague	XTRA	500	As mentioned above		Bacteria
Bubonic Plague 1	XTRA	20,210,216,333,500,523,660,690,727.5,768,786,787,880,	As mentioned above		Bacteria
Bubonic Plague 2	XTRA	585,16014.55,20000,	As mentioned above		Bacteria
Black Death	XTRA	20,210,216,333,500,523,660,690,727.5,768,786,787,880,	Also see Bubonic Plague, Plague, and Yersinia Pestis.		Bacteria

17d - Virus and Diseases

Note: *diseases caused by pathogens are indicated in blue*

Subject / Argument	Author	Frequencies	Notes	Origin	Target
Virus (General)	EDTFL	30,250,450,950,22500,30280,77500,293050,313350,625230			Virus
Virus General 4	XTRA	344,447,564,633,834,944,3443,6534,7884,10423,12534,17884,21436,			Virus
Common Viruses TR1	BIOM	10000; 7344; 5000; 2950; 2900; 2650; 2600; 1550; 1234; 430; 620; 624; 646; 866; 5147.5; 2213; 1918; 742.4; 303; 23.2; 20; 864; 790; 690; 610; 470			Virus
Common Viruses TR2	BIOM	484; 986; 644; 254; 30; 33; 6000; 599; 611; 613; 2127; 2080; 2050; 2013; 2008; 2003; 2000; 1850; 880; 803; 800; 787; 727; 660; 484; 465; 440; 35; 500; 200; 68			Virus
Virus Comprehensive, Includes H1N1, H5N1, Ebola, Rhinoviruses, Rotaviruses, Influenza A-B	EDTFL	30,250,450,950,6150,22500,30280,51330,77500,313350			Virus
Slow Virus Diseases	EDTFL	50,950,7500,8000,40000,57500,125750,325170,522530,655200	Diseases that, after long latency, follow a slow, progressive course over months or years, often of central nervous system.		Virus
RNA Virus Infections	EDTFL	80,400,850,2740,5000,55160,269710,555300,707000,825500	Viruses with RNA as genetic material which can cause Ebola, SARS, Influenza, Hepatitis C, West Nile Fever, Polio, and Measles - see sets.		Virus
Retroviruses	BIOM	465; 448; 800; 10000			Virus
Human Retrovirus [HIV]	EDTFL	140,320,970,2500,11090,20000,57500,225000,423010,565370,			Virus
HERV	XTRA	419,4	Human Endogenous Retrovirus.		Virus
Retrovirus Variants	CAFL	2489,465,727,787,880,448,800,10000,	Family of viruses replicating in host cells through reverse transcription. Can cause cancers/leukemia, hepatitis, and HIV. See Cancer Cells, Xenotropic Murine Leukemia Virus, Human T Lymphotropic Virus, HIV, and Hepatitis B sets.		Virus
BX- BY Virus			See Chapter 17d - Cancer		Virus

HERPES are divided into three subfamilies: **Alphaherpesvirinae, Betaherpesvirinae, and Gammaherpesvirinae.**

To these three subfamilies belong the eight currently known human herpes viruses (HHV):

1) HHV-1 Herpes Simplex Virus 1 (HSV-1);
2) HHV-2 Herpes Simplex Virus 2 (HSV-2);
3) HHV-3 Varicella-zoster virus (VZV);
4) HHV-4 Epstein-Barr Virus (EBV);
5) HHV-5 Cytomegalovirus (CMV);
6) HHV-6 Human Herpesvirus 6;
7) HHV-7 Human Herpesvirus 7;
8) HHV-8 Human Herpesvirus 8 (or KSHV or Kaposi's Sarcoma Virus).

Subject / Argument	Author	Frequencies	Notes	Origin	Target
Herpes General	XTRA	1552,2489,2950,2347,	As mentioned above	Herpes	Virus
Herpes General 3	CAFL	2950=900,1900,1577,1550,1489,1488=900,629,464,450,383,304,165,141,	Primarily orofacial. Use General Antiseptic set and see Herpex Simplex (type 1/i) sets.	Herpes	Virus
Herpes General 4	XTRA	304,464,1488,1489,1550,1577,1900,2950,18500,	As mentioned above	Herpes	Virus
Herpes General V	CAFL	141,165,383,450,629,	As mentioned above	Herpes	Virus
Herpes General 5	XTRA	360,361,362,363,364,365,366,367,368,369,373,528,532,540,556,665,685,716,717,718,731,732,733,776,808,832,846,848,880,888,1402,1488=900,1489,8778,	As mentioned above	Genitals	Virus
Herpes General 6	CAFL	304,464,1488=900,1489,1550,1577,1900,1950,37000,	As mentioned above	Herpes	Virus
Herpes, general	BIOM	3742; 2950; 2062; 1900; 1871; 1614; 1577; 1550; 1489; 1488; 1043; 944; 936; 895; 822; 785; 748; 664; 629; 589; 476; 468; 464; 450; 384; 322; 304; 165; 141		Herpes	Virus
Herpes General Secondary	CAFL	37000	As mentioned above	Herpes	Virus
Herpes General Secondary	XTRA	18500	As mentioned above	Herpes	Virus
Herpes Type C	BIO	395,424,460,533,554,701,745,2450,		Herpes	Virus
Herpes TR	BIOM	2950; 322; 476; 468; 589; 664; 785; 822; 895; 936; 944; 1042.9; 1614; 1871; 2062; 1489; 3742; 748		Herpes	Virus
Water Blisters Herpes	BIOM	727; 787; 880; 1550		Herpes	Virus

Subject / Argument	Author	Frequencies	Notes	Origin	Target
Herpesviridae Infections	EDTFL	120,550,950,291230,292000,372500,416600,418000,420200,824370	Herpes viral infections. Use General Antiseptic set.	Herpes	Virus
Herpesvirus Infections	EDTFL	120,550,950,291230,292000,372500,416600,571000,865830,937410	Herpes viral infections. Use General Antiseptic set.	Herpes	Virus

Herpes Simplex (HHV-1)		*May cause : **Alzheimer's disease • Bipolar disorder • Coronary heart disease • Dementia • Metabolic syndrome***			
Herpes Simplex i 1	CAFL	339,343,480,591,657,699,700,734,778,782,843,1614,	Primarily orofacial. Use General Antiseptic set and see Herpex Simplex (type 1/i) sets.	H. Simplex	Virus
Herpes Simplex i 2	CAFL	428,465,727,787,880,1500,1550,1800,1850,2489,	As mentioned above	H. Simplex	Virus
Herpes Simplex i 3	CAFL	470,647,648,650,656,658,660,847,5641,8650,	As mentioned above	H. Simplex	Virus
Herpes Simplex i 4	CAFL	**2950**	As mentioned above	H. Simplex	Virus
Herpes Simplex I	CAFL	322,476,589,664,785,822,895,944,1043,1614,2062,1489,2950=1200,	Secondary. Primarily orofacial. First try Herpes General sets. Use General Antiseptic set.	H. Simplex	Virus
Herpes Simplex RTI	CAFL	186,372,427,446,465,484,503,522,541,560,579,598,617,636,655,674,693,712,731,750,769,788,807,826,845,864,883,902,921,940,959,978,997,1016,1035,1054,1073,1488,1550,1568,1644,1865,1909,2489,2976,3176,5000,5310,	Based on RTI's Herpes set; most freqs contract spread. Use for Measles, Chicken pox, Smallpox, Mononucleosis, Shingles, Rubella, cold sores, Epstein Barr, Variola, Stomatitis, and Pyorrhea.	H. Simplex	Virus
Herpes Type 1 Anec Comp	CAFL	339,343,428,467.8,480,591,648,652,656,660,700,727,734,778,782,787,843,847,880,935.5,1500,1614,1800,1850,1871,2489,2950,3742,5641,7484,8650,	Combines most anecdotal frequencies for Herpes Simplex i.	H. Simplex	Virus
Herpes Simplex 1	EDTFL	40,300,620,51250,117250,245560,367500,625220,816720,905000	As mentioned above	H. Simplex	Virus
Herpes Simplex 1	HC	291250-293050=3600,	As mentioned above	H. Simplex	Virus
Herpes Simplex 1 2nd	HC	345350-345760=3600,	As mentioned above	H. Simplex	Virus
HSV-1	RL	**467**	From Dr. Richard Loyd. Herpes simplex virus 1 and 2.	H. Simplex	Virus
Herpes Simplex General Virus	XTRA	322,343,476,822,843,1043,1614,2062,	As mentioned above	H. Simplex	Virus
Herpes simplex type 1 basic	BIOM	8650; 7484; 5641; 3742; 2950; 2489; 1871; 1850; 1800; 1614; 1500; 935.5; 847; 843; 787; 782; 734; 700; 660; 656; 652; 648; 591; 480; 468; 428; 343; 339		H. Simplex	Virus
Herpes simplex type 1 secondary	BIOM	10000; 5000; 2489; 186; 372; 427; 446; 465; 484; 503; 541; 560; 579; 598; 617; 636; 655; 674; 693; 712; 731; 769; 788; 807; 826; 845; 864; 883; 902; 921; 940; 959; 978; 997; 1016; 1035; 1054; 1073; 1488; 1550; 1568; 1644; 1865; 1909; 2976; 5310; 5952		H. Simplex	Virus
Herpes Simplex Encephalitis	EDTFL	110,7550,50800,97150,151340,252500,472500,525330,650000,974500,		H. Simplex	Virus
Encephalitis Herpes Simplex	EDTFL	110,7550,50800,97150,151340,252500,472500,525330,650000,974500		H. Simplex	Virus
Herpetic Acute Necrotizing Encephalitis	EDTFL	110,7550,50800,97150,151340,252500,472500,525330,650000,974500,		H. Simplex	Virus
Meningoencephalitis [Herpes]	EDTFL	110,7550,50800,97150,151340,252500,472500,525330,650000,974500,	Inflammation of the tissue of brain and spinal cord due to Herpes Simplex - see sets.	H. Simplex	Virus
Herpes Eczema	XTRA	**727,787,1550,5000**	Also called Eczema herpeticum. Rare but severe infection at skin damage sites. Also see Herpes Simplex (type 1/i) programs.	H. Simplex	Virus
Herpes Furunculosis Secondary	XTRA	**727,787**	Herpes infection appearing together with furunculosis. See Herpes Simplex (type 1/i), Furunculosis, and Boils.	H. Simplex	Virus
Herpes Furunculosis Skin Disease	XTRA	**200,1000,1550**	As mentioned above	H. Simplex	Virus
Mouth Eruptions Herpes Sores	CAFL	304,464,1488,1489,1550,1577,1900,2720,2950,	Use General Antiseptic set and see Herpex Simplex (type 1/i) sets.	Mouth	Virus
Herpes Simplex, Labial	EDTFL	40,300,620,51250,117250,245560,367500,625220,816720,905000		Mouth	Virus
Herpes stomatitis	BIOM	2489; 1850; 1800; 1550; 1500; 880; 787; 727; 702; 677; 672; 591; 568; 465; 428; 278; 234		Mouth	Virus
Herpes Mouth Sores	XTRA	428,465,660,690,727.5,787,802,880,1500,1550,1800,1850,2489,	As mentioned above	Mouth	Virus

Herpes Simplex Virus 2 (HHV-2)		*May cause : **genital infections, increased body temperature and joint pain.***			
Herpes Type 2A	CAFL	**532,848**	Primarily genital. Also use General Antiseptic set.	Genitals	Virus

Subject / Argument	Author	Frequencies	Notes	Origin	Target
Herpes Type 2A Secondary	CAFL	360,362,364,366,368,370,373,528,540,665,685, 716,717,718,731,732,733,776,846,880,888,1402 ,8778,	As mentioned above	Genitals	Virus
Herpes Type 2 Comp	CAFL	362,366,370,373,528,532,540,556,665,685,717, 732,776,808,880,888,1402,8778,	As mentioned above	Genitals	Virus
Herpes Simplex 2	EDTFL	40,300,620,51250,117250,245560,367500,6252 20,816720,905000	As mentioned above	Genitals	Virus
Herpes Simplex 1	HC	291250-293050=3600,		Genitals	Virus
Herpes Simplex 2_1	HC	353900-362900=3600,	As mentioned above	Genitals	Virus
Herpes Simplex II	BIO	556,832	As mentioned above	Genitals	Virus
Herpes Simplex IU.2	BIO	808	As mentioned above	Genitals	Virus
Herpes Simplex 2	EDTF	120,550,950,291250,293050,292000,353900,36 2900,360000,355000	As mentioned above	Genitals	Virus
HSV-II	RL	556	Dal Dr. Richard Loyd.	Genitals	Virus
Herpes simplex type 2 basic	BIOM	8778; 1900; 1402; 892.4; 888; 880; 848; 846; 832; 808; 776; 717; 685; 665; 556; 540; 532; 528; 373; 370; 366; 362		Genitals	Virus
Herpes simplex type 2 secondary	BIOM	360; 362; 364; 366; 368; 370; 373; 528; 685; 846; 880; 888; 8778; 540; 665; 716; 717; 718; 731; 732; 733; 776; 1402		Genitals	Virus
Herpes type 2 genital	BIOM	141; 878; 898; 5310; 440; 171; 660; 590; 1175		Genitals	Virus
Genital Herpes	BIOM	141.0; 878.0; 898.0; 5309.5; 440.0; 171.0; 660.0; 590.0; 1174.9	As mentioned above	Genitals	Virus
Herpes Genitalis	EDTFL	40,260,680,2250,10890,145220,320250,425910, 657770,825220	As mentioned above	Genitals	Virus
Herpes Progenitalis	CAFL	141,171,440,590,660,878,898,1175,5310,	As mentioned above	Genitals	Virus
Herpes Progenitalis 1	CAFL	141,171,440,556,590,660,832,878,898,1175,531 0,	As mentioned above	Genitals	Virus

Human Herpesvirus 3 (HHV-3)		*May cause : **pain, burning, itching or tightness in the affected skin area which initially presents erythema and fluid-filled blisters.***			
Herpes Zoster Virus	CAFL	134,223,333,345,411,423,425,436,446,453,542, 554,563,572,573,574,576,643,668,686,716,718, 738,786,787,934,958,1544,1577,2323,2431,334 3,7160,40887,	It is caused by the reactivation of the varicella-zoster virus (VZV).	H. Zoster	Virus
Herpes Zoster 1	CAFL	664=600,787,802,880,914,1489,1500,1489,150 0,1550,1600,2170,2489,3343,	Use for Chicken Pox and Shingles - see sets for both, and for Varicella.	H. Zoster	Virus
Herpes Zoster 9	CAFL	580,664=600,787,802,880,914,1160,1500,1600, 2170,2320,3343,	As mentioned above	H. Zoster	Virus
Herpes Zoster	VEGA	1557,574	As mentioned above	H. Zoster	Virus
Herpes Zoster Secondary	CAFL	20,304,464,574,728,800,802,1550,1557,1800,18 65,2128,2720,5000,	As mentioned above	H. Zoster	Virus
Herpes simplex type 3	BIOM	470; 647; 648; 650; 652; 654; 656; 658; 660; 847; 5641; 8650		H. Zoster	Virus
Herpes zoster	BIOM	3343; 2720; 2320; 2170; 1865; 1800; 1600; 1557; 1500; 1160; 914; 664; 580; 574; 20		H. Zoster	Virus
Herpes Zoster	BIOM	2720.0; 2170.0; 1865.0; 1800.0; 1600.0; 1550.0; 1500.0; 880.0; 802.0; 787.0; 727.0; 20.0		H. Zoster	Virus
Herpes zoster, secondary	BIOM	134; 223; 304; 345; 411; 423; 425; 436; 446; 453; 542; 554; 563; 572; 573; 576; 668; 934; 958; 1544; 1577; 2128; 2323; 2431; 3343; 7160		H. Zoster	Virus
Herpes Zoster Oticus	KHZ	120,450,950,5780,137500,372500,495220,7342 50,824370,	Reactivation of Herpes Zoster virus (see sets) in ganglion of facial nerve, causing paralysis, pain, and taste loss. Also see Geniculate Herpes Zoster.	H. Zoster	Virus
Shingles	CAFL	664,787,802,880,914,1500,1600,2170,3343,	Due to Herpes virus that causes Chicken Pox during childhood and Shingles in adulthood.	H. Zoster	Virus
Shingles	BIOM	1557; 574; 1900; 1550; 727; 787; 880		H. Zoster	Virus
Shingles [Herpes Zoster]	EDTFL	120,550,950,291230,292000,293050,367500,62 5220,816720,824370,		H. Zoster	Virus
Herpes Zoster Herpes Zoster "shingles" Herpes Zoster Oticus	EDTFL	120,550,950,291230,292000,293050,367500,62 5220,816720,824370	Reactivation of Herpes Zoster virus (see sets) in ganglion of facial nerve, causing paralysis, pain, and taste loss. Also see Herpes Zoster Oticus.	H. Zoster	Virus
Geniculate Herpes [Zoster]	EDTFL	120,550,950,291230,292000,293050,367500,62 5220,816720,824370,		H. Zoster	Virus
Zona [V. Herpes Zoster]	EDTFL	120,550,950,291230,292000,293050,367500,62 5220,816720,824370,		H. Zoster	Virus
Varicella/Shingles	RL	898	From Dr. Richard Loyd.	H. Zoster	Virus
Ramsay Hunt Paralysis	EDTFL	70,180,1650,7930,102530,165500,320530,6912 70,753070,912330	As mentioned above	H. Zoster	Virus
Chicken Pox	CAFL	664,787,802,880,914,1500,1600,2170,3343,	Very contagious disease, caused by the varicella-zoster virus (VVZ).	H. Zoster	Virus

Subject / Argument	Author	Frequencies	Notes	Origin	Target
Chicken Pox	BIO	**787,3343**	As mentioned above	H. Zoster	Virus
Chicken Pox	BIOM	7160; 3343; 2431; 2323; 1577; 1544; 958; 934; 738; 718; 716; 668; 643; 576; 573; 572; 563; 554; 542; 453; 446; 436; 425; 423; 411; 345; 223; 134; 1		H. Zoster	Virus
Chicken Pox	EDTFL	140,220,700,6210,102500,247500,372500,5056 10,625620,956160	As mentioned above	H. Zoster	Virus
Varicella [Chickenpox]	EDTFL	140,220,700,6210,102500,247500,372500,5056 10,625620,956160,		H. Zoster	Virus
Chicken Pox 1	XTRA	3.89,580,664,787,802,833,880,914,1160,1500,1 600,2170,2320,3343,	As mentioned above	H. Zoster	Virus
Chicken Pox 2	XTRA	3.89,802,833,10000,	As mentioned above	H. Zoster	Virus
Chicken Pox 3	XTRA	20,304,464,574,728,800,802,1550,1557,1800,18 65,2128,2720,5000,	As mentioned above	H. Zoster	Virus
Chicken Pox 6	XTRA	20,727,787,880,3343,5000,	As mentioned above	H. Zoster	Virus
Chicken Pox 8	XTRA	664,787,802,880,914,1500,1600,2170,3343,	As mentioned above	H. Zoster	Virus
Chicken Pox Varicella	XTRA	**802.1550**	As mentioned above	H. Zoster	Virus
Varicella	CAFL	664,787,802,880,914,1500,1600,2170,3343,	Varicella-zoster virus or Human herpesvirus 3 (HHV-3) disease.	H. Zoster	Virus
Varicella	BIO	**345,668,716,738**	The Herpes virus that causes chicken pox during childhood and Shingles (Herpes zoster) in adulthood.	H. Zoster	Virus
Varicella	VEGA	**345,668,716**		H. Zoster	Virus
HHV-4 Epstein Barr Virus		*May cause:* **Mononucleosis** • **Autoimmune diseases** • **Chronic obstructive pulmonary disease** • **Seasonal affective disorder** • **Lupus** • **Multiple sclerosis** • **Ulcerative rectocolitis** • **Rheumatoid arthritis** • **Sjögren syndrome** • **Ankylosing spondylitis** • **Crohn's disease** • **Celiac disease** • **Type 1 diabetes** • **Breast cancer** • **Burkitt's lymphoma** • **Esophageal cancer** • **Hodgkin's lymphoma** • **Nasopharyngeal carcinoma.**			
EBV	CAFL	105,172,253,274,380,660,663,667,669,738,825, 1013,1920,6618,8768,	Also called **Human Herpesvirus 4** or Glandular Fever. Causes Mononucleosis and is associated with certain cancers and HIV.	EBV	Virus
Epstein Barr Virus 1	CAFL	428,465,660,727,776,778,787,880,	As mentioned above	EBV	Virus
Epstein Barr Virus 2	CAFL	105,172,253,274,380,660,663,667,669,738,825, 1013,1920,6618,8768,	As mentioned above	EBV	Virus
Epstein Barr Virus Secondary	CAFL	744,776,778,465,880,787,727,1032,1920,380,	As mentioned above	EBV	Virus
Epstein Barr Virus_1	HC	372500-382350=3600,	As mentioned above	EBV	Virus
Epstein Barr Virus_2	HC	**375000**	As mentioned above	EBV	Virus
Epstein Barr Virus	BIO	105,172,253,660,663,669,744,825,1032,1920,	As mentioned above	EBV	Virus
EBV 1	XTRA	105,172,253,274,380,660,663,667,669,738,825, 1013,1920,6618,8768,	As mentioned above	EBV	Virus
EBV 2	XTRA	929.52,941.92,18670.15,18919.09,	As mentioned above	EBV	Virus
EBV 3	XTRA	**660,663,669**	As mentioned above	EBV	Virus
EBV Secondary	XTRA	465,727,744,776,778,787,880,1032,1920,	As mentioned above	EBV	Virus
Epstein Barr	XTRA	428,465,660,727,776,787,880,	As mentioned above	EBV	Virus
Epstein Barr Virus 1	XTRA	1.1,4.9,6.29,20,27.5,35,72,73,105,120,148,172,2 20,253,274,410,424,428,465,660,663,664,667,6 69,690,727.5,738,744,776,778,787,825,880,101 3,1032,1920,2127.5,6618,8768,11640.62,11718. 75=1200,11875,18670.15,18919.09	As mentioned above	EBV	Virus
Epstein Barr Virus 2	XTRA	95,125,330,444,788,802,1550,1800,1865,2720,1 0000,11640.62=1800,11718.75=1200,11875,18 670.15,18919.09,	As mentioned above	EBV	Virus
Epstein Barr Virus 3	XTRA	105,172,253,660,663,669,744,825,1032,1920,	As mentioned above	EBV	Virus
Epstein Barr Virus 4	XTRA	**12695.3**	As mentioned above	EBV	Virus
Epstein Barr Virus 5	XTRA	105,172,253,274,660,663,667,669,738,825,1013 ,1920,6618,8768,	As mentioned above	EBV	Virus
Epstein Barr Virus 6	XTRA	428,465,660,727,776,778,787,880,	As mentioned above	EBV	Virus
Epstein Barr Virus 8	XTRA	95,125,330,444,788,802,1550,1800,1865,2720,1 0000,	As mentioned above	EBV	Virus
Epstein Barr Virus 9	XTRA	923.34,941.92,947.75,11640.62,11875,11948.44	As mentioned above	EBV	Virus
Epstein Barr Virus A	XTRA	923.34,929.52,947.75,11718.75,11948,	As mentioned above	EBV	Virus
Epstein Barr Virus B	XTRA	929.52,941.92,18670.15,18919.09,	As mentioned above	EBV	Virus
Epstein Barr Virus Lyme	XTRA	**880**	As mentioned above	EBV	Virus
Epstein-Barr Virus-2	BIOM	8767.5; 6617.5; 1920; 1920; 1031.9; 1012.9; 880; 825; 787; 778; 776; 744; 738; 727; 669; 465; 274; 253; 172; 105; 667; 663; 660		EBV	Virus
Mononucleosis	CAFL	105,172,253,274,660,663,667,669,738,825,1013 ,1920,6618,8768,	Causes Asthenia - high fever - swollen lymph nodes - pharyngitis	Mononucleosis	Virus

Subject / Argument	Author	Frequencies	Notes	Origin	Target
Infectious Mononucleosis	BIOM	8767.5; 6617.5; 2950; 1920; 1031.9; 1012.9; 776; 738; 669; 667; 663; 660; 428; 274; 253; 172; 105		Mononucleosis	Virus
Epstein-Barr Virus Infections	EDTFL	120,250,51620,72250,105170,237320,421510,602500,725000,822350,		Mononucleosis	Virus
Infectious Mononucleosis	EDTFL	1420,4370,5500,13930,122500,304250,312600,336000,397100,432000	Symptoms vary with age. Also see Epstein Barr Virus, and EBV.	Mononucleosis	Virus
Glandular Fever	EDTFL	70,320,620,850,5000,22500,60000,352930,422530,563190	As mentioned above	Mononucleosis	Virus
Kissing Disease [EBV Infections]	EDTFL	120,250,51620,72250,105170,237320,421510,602500,725000,822350,	As mentioned above	Mononucleosis	Virus
Epstein Barr Virus Infections	KHZ	70,520,700,930,2500,15830,126010,325350,519340,791280,	As mentioned above	Mononucleosis	Virus
Infectious Mononucleosis 1	XTRA	1.1,4.9,6.29,20,27.5,35,72,73,105,148,172,220,253,274,410,428,465,660,663,667,669,690,727.5,738,744,776,778,787,825,880,1013,1032,1920,2127.5,6618,8768,	As mentioned above	Mononucleosis	Virus
Infectious Mononucleosis 2	XTRA	95,125,330,444,788,802,1550,1800,1865,2720,10000,	As mentioned above	Mononucleosis	Virus
Infectious Mononucleosis 4	XTRA	95,125,330,444,1865,788,802,1550,1800,2720,10000,11640=1680,11718.75,11875,18919.09,18670.15,	As mentioned above	Mononucleosis	Virus
Glandular Fever	CAFL	10000,20,	Also called Infections Mononucleosis - see sets. Also see Mononucleosis, Epstein Barr Virus, EBV, Cytomegalovirus, and CMV.	Mononucleosis	Virus
Glandular Fever 2	XTRA	20,727,787,880,5000,	As mentioned above		Virus
Glandular Fever Parathyroid	XTRA	20,10000	Parathyroid support in Infections Mononucleosis.	Parathyroid	Virus
Glandular Fever Thyroid	CAFL	10000,20,16000	Experimental. Thyroid support in Infections Mononucleosis.	Thyroid	Virus
Glandular Fever Adrenals	XTRA	20,10000,12000	Adrenals support in Infections Mononucleosis.	Adrenals	Virus

HHV-5 Cytomegalovirus		May cause : **Anxiety disorder • Atherosclerosis • Autism • Autoimmune diseases • Dementia • Depression • Diabetes mellitus type 2 • Guillain–Barré syndrome • Lupus • Macular degeneration• Metabolic syndrome • Myocardial infarction • Brain tumor.**			
CMV	CAFL	126,597,629,682,1045,2145,8848,8856,	Cytomegalovirus, also known as **Salivary Gland Virus** or **Human Herpes Type 5.**	CMV	Virus
Cytomegalovirus	CAFL	126,597,629,682,1045,8848,8856,	As mentioned above	CMV	Virus
CMV	BIO	126,597,1045,2145	As mentioned above	CMV	Virus
CMV	VEGA	2145	As mentioned above	CMV	Virus
CMV 1	XTRA	126,597,629,682,1045,2145,8848,8856,	As mentioned above	CMV	Virus
CMV 2	XTRA	1013.8,20362.9	As mentioned above	CMV	Virus
Citomegalovirus-2	BIOM	8855.5; 8847.5; 2146; 2144; 2145; 1045; 682; 629; 597; 126; 2145		CMV	Virus
Cytomegalovirus CMV 1	XTRA	249=360,418=360,647=360,799877.8777,799877.87,799877.88,799877.4-799878.4=1000, 677787.7878,677787.78,677787.79,677787.3-677788.3=1000,77665.5666,77665.56,77665.57,77665-77666=1000,	As mentioned above (Spooky2)	CMV	Virus
Cytomegalovirus CMV 1	XTRA	126,597,629,682,1013,1045,2145,8848,8856,11856,11881,12144,12146.5,12146.75,12191.25,12537,20362.9,20757,	As mentioned above	CMV	Virus
Cytomegalovirus CMV 2	XTRA	68,70,120,126,249,418,597,629,647,682,850,999.79,1045,2144,2145,2146,6380-6418,6689-6754,8848,8856,9500,11856, 11881,12144,12146.5,12146.75,12191.25,12537,12604.69,20757,88000,141200,297500,409000,425950,675310,827000,20330-20451,1012-1019,3190-3209	Herpes Type 5. Duty Cycle=72. Dr H Clark's frequencies included.	CMV	Virus
Cytomegalovirus CMV 3	XTRA	1013.81, 20362.91	As mentioned above	CMV	Virus
Cytomegalovirus (CMV) Antigen	HC	403350-410750=3600,	Causes immune system to produce CMV antibodies. Also called Salivary Gland Virus or (human) Herpes Type 5 - see sets.	CMV	Virus
Cytomegalovirus CMV Antigen	XTRA	999.79,1013.8,1018.14,12604.69,12781.25,12835.94,	As mentioned above	CMV	Virus
Herpes Type 5	CAFL	126,597,629,682,1045,8848,8856,	Also called **Cytomegalovirus** (CMV) - see sets. Causes Infectious Mononucleosis, and retinitis.	CMV	Virus
Herpes Type 5	BIO	126,597, 1045,2145	As mentioned above	CMV	Virus
HHV5 2	XTRA	20362.91,1013.81,12537,41514,47425,47524,48579,48586,48587,48765,	As mentioned above	CMV	Virus
HHV5	XTRA	126,597,629,682,1045,2145,8848,8856,	As mentioned above	CMV	Virus
Cytomegaloviral infection	BIOM	126; 597; 629; 682; 1045; 2146; 2144; 2145; 8848; 8856		CMV	Virus

Subject / Argument	Author	Frequencies	Notes	Origin	Target
Cytomegalovirus [Inclusion D.] Cytomegalic Inclusion Disease	EDTFL	210,230,10530,17500,28210,41900,62500,1500 00,326070,975310,		CMV	Virus
Salivary Gland Virus Disease	EDTFL	80,240,570,6500,10720,36210,142500,321000,4 15700,775680		CMV	Virus
Salivary Gland Virus	BIO	126,597, 1045,2145	Causes Infectious Mononucleosis (see sets), and retinitis.	Mouth	Virus
Human Herpesvirus 6 (HHV-6)		*May cause : ADHD • Chronic fatigue syndrome • Epilepsy • Infertility • Multiple sclerosis*			
HHV6	XTRA	228,1820,3640.1,7281	Also called **Roseolovirus**. Causes Sixth Disease - see Exanthema Subitum set.	HHV6	Virus
Herpes Type 6 1	XTRA	227.3, 454.5, 1818.09, 3636.19	Also called Roseolovirus. Causes Sixth Disease - see Exanthema Subitum set.	HHV6	Virus
Herpes Type 6 2	XTRA	228,1820, 3640,7281	As mentioned above	HHV6	Virus
Herpes Type 6a	XTRA	3740.7	As mentioned above	HHV6	Virus
Exanthema Subitum	EDTFL	140,570,81300,104710,221500,337500,570510, 691510,775480,971550		HHV6	Virus
Roseola Infantum	EDTFL	50,370,900,2500,3000,73300,95750,175000,269 350,355080	Also called Roseola, or Sixth Disease. Febrile condition in very young children with red skin rash and three-day fever.	HHV6	Virus
Herpes simplex type 7	BIOM	232; 237; 1214; 1243; 1244; 1271; 5411		HHV7	Virus
Herpes simplex type 8	BIOM	263.3; 526.6; 2106.4; 4213		HHV8	Virus
Adenovirus	CAFL	333,523,786,768,959,962,666,	Can cause upper respiratory and ear infections, tonsillitis, conjunctivitis, or croup. Other strains may be responsible for other diseases such as gastroenteritis, cystitis and, less frequently, neurological infections.	Adenovirus	Virus
Adenovirus	HC	393000	As mentioned above	Adenovirus	Virus
Adenovirus 2nd	HC	371450-386900=3600,	As mentioned above	Adenovirus	Virus
Adenovirus 3rd	HC	371000	As mentioned above	Adenovirus	Virus
Adenovirus 4th	HC	334000	As mentioned above	Adenovirus	Virus
Adenovirus 5th	HC	568000	As mentioned above	Adenovirus	Virus
Adenovirus	BIO	333,523,786	As mentioned above	Adenovirus	Virus
Adenovirus	VEGA	333,786	As mentioned above	Adenovirus	Virus
Adenovirus	RL	739	By Dr. Richard Loyd. As mentioned above	Adenovirus	Virus
Adenovirus-36	RL	864	By Dr. Richard Loyd. Human adenovirus 36 has long been recognized as the cause of respiratory and ocular infections in humans.	Adenovirus	Virus
Adenovirus 36	BIOM	8875; 6140; 5859; 5797; 5219		Adenovirus	Virus
Adenovirus 41	BIOM	10000; 3176; 9624; 959; 786; 768; 666; 523; 333		Adenovirus	Virus
Adenovirus 66	BIOM	10000; 3176; 8874.5; 6139.5; 5858.5; 5796.5; 5218.5; 1289; 1160.9; 1031.9; 903; 774; 645; 516; 387; 258; 129		Adenovirus	Virus
Adenovirus 1	XTRA	333,523,666,768,786,950.6,958.79,959,959.6,96 0.39,962,967.6,969.3,11593.75,11607.8,11718.7 5,12281.25,14364.52,16628.88,17750,18471,18 670.15,19566.31,20875,	As mentioned above	Adenovirus	Virus
Adenovirus 2nd	XTRA	920.73,929.52,959.02,11607.8,11718.75,12090. 62,	As mentioned above	Adenovirus	Virus
Adenovirus infection, basic	BIOM	10000; 7767; 7762; 7702; 7009; 7001; 6989; 5000; 4868; 2720; 2050; 1395; 1062; 1060; 1034; 1009; 969; 968; 960; 952; 951; 942; 555; 523; 300; 180; 160; 72; 48; 26		Adenovirus	Virus
Adenoviridae Infections Adenovirus Infections	EDTFL	180,520,800,37500,93200,150000,392900,5093 60,755000,866150,	As mentioned above	Adenovirus	Virus
Arbovirus Infections	EDTFL KHZ	70,680,2330,35000,87500,476500,527000,6670 00,753230,987230,	Group of viruses transmitted by arthropods, causing **Dengue Fever, Yellow Fever, Encephalitis, and West Nile Fever.**	Arbovirus	Virus
Encephalitis Arbovirus	KHZ	150,230,600,950,7500,150890,455340,527500,8 96500,917200,	Inflammation of the tissue of brain and spinal cord due to arthropod-transmitted viruses.	Arbovirus	Virus
Dengue Dengue Fever	EDTFL	190,210,680,2470,7500,43000,153000,324450,3 75690,519340,	Tropical infectious disease caused by the **Dengue virus**.	Arbovirus	Virus
Dengue-fever	BIOM	160; 500; 5000; 7344; 4412; 1234; 740; 423; 330; 10000; 5000; 30		Arbovirus	Virus
Dengue Fever 1	XTRA	148,149,206,211,216,423,846,1194,1195,1196,1 692,3383,3389,	Also called Breakbone Fever. Mosquito-borne viral disease with fever, headache, muscle and joint pain.	Arbovirus	Virus
Dengue Fever 2	XTRA	30,160,330,500,727,740,787,880,1234,1550,160 0,2627,4412,5000,5275,7344,10000,10551.5,	As mentioned above	Arbovirus	Virus
Yellow Fever	ETDFL	110,350,870,7270,24000,35680,87500,93500,23 4510,519340	Severe viral infection which can damage the liver, kidneys, heart, and entire GI tract.	Arbovirus	Virus

Subject / Argument	Author	Frequencies	Notes	Origin	Target
Yellow fever	BIOM	20; 142; 178; 232; 432; 734; 1187; 733; 779; 996; 10000		Arbovirus	Virus
Yellow Fever	VEGA	432,734	Caused by a virus known as **Flavivirus**.	Arbovirus	Virus
Yellow Fever	XTRA	0.67,20	As mentioned above	Arbovirus	Virus
Black Vomit	XTRA	0.67,20,60,72,95,142,178,232,432,660,690,727.5,733,734,779,880,1187,10000,	See Yellow Fever.	Arbovirus	Virus
West Nile 1	CAFL	413,826,1239,3303,465,841,8410,	Mosquito-borne Arbovirus infection causing fever, rash, pain, nausea, and, in some, severe neurological diseases including paralysis. Also see Arbovirus Infections, and Encephalitis Arbovirus.	Arbovirus	Virus
West Nile Fever	EDTFL	100,350,17300,37500,210400,327590,476500,665340,789000,987230	As mentioned above	Arbovirus	Virus
Alphavirus Infections	EDTFL	120,780,12710,55000,90000,175050,425000,576000,822000,932000,	Viral group causing infectious arthritis, encephalitis, fever, and rashes.		Virus
Ross River Virus Infections	EDTFL	40,70,150,550,2230,4210,13980,90510,350000,432140			Virus
Astrovirus	RL	586	From Dr. Richard Loyd. Astroviruses are a type of virus that was first discovered in 1975.		Virus
Bird Flu Virus	XTRA	728,800,880,7760,8000,8250,	H5N1. Subtype of Influenza A virus.		Virus
Borna Virus		*May cause:* **depression**, **bipolar disease**, *and other* **mental problems**. *It can make people tired, anxious, manic, and sometimes violent.*			
Borna Disease Virus BDV	XTRA	776,787,802,832,840,880,1550,1570,1998,2008,2052,2127.5,2489,2490,5000,	Zoonotic virus that can infect nerve cells, causing Borna Disease - see set.	Borna	Virus
Borna Disease	EDTFL	130,570,780,930,32500,217500,552710,743010,815910,913520	Infectious neuro syndrome causing abnormal behaviour and possible death, due to BDV - see set.	Borna	Virus
Bunyavirus / Bunyaviridae Infections	EDTFL	70,220,620,2100,5100,40000,475030,527000,667000,742000	Viruses transmitted by ticks and arthropods causing fevers, hemhorrhagic fevers, and encephalitis.		Virus
Caliciviridae Infections	EDTFL	60,250,5000,7000,25750,87500,225000,450000,515150,687620	Family of viruses causing disease in humans (usually gastroenteritis) and animals. Includes Norwalk Virus.		Virus
Chikungunya Virus	RL	663	Dal Dr. Richard Loyd.		Virus
Corona Virus Sars	XTRA	152.19,155,304.39,309.89,456.5,464.89,608.7,619.89,760.89,774.79,1217.5,1239.7,1369.59,1394.7,2435,2479.5,4870,4959,9740,9918,	Upper respiratory and GI tract infections.	Corona	Virus
Corona Virus	XTRA	145.9,165.69,291.69,331.39,437.6,497.1,583.5,662.7,1167,1312.79,1325.5,1491.2,2333.9,2651,4667.8,5301.89,9335.6,	Upper respiratory and GI tract infections.	Corona	Virus
Coronavirus	RL	655	Dal Dr. Richard Loyd.	Corona	Virus
COVID-19 (SARS-CoV-2)	RL	568	Dal Dr. Richard Loyd.	Corona	Virus
Coronaviral infection	BIOM	9918; 6740; 4959; 4870; 2479.5; 2435; 1394.7; 1369.6; 1239.7; 1217.5; 774.8; 760.9; 619.9; 608.7; 464.9; 456.5; 155; 10		Corona	Virus
Coronaviridae Infections [COVID Infections]	EDTFL	50,200,33400,72540,305370,452550,509750,621730,738500,900400,		Corona	Virus
Coronavirus [Human 1] 229E [HCoV-229E, OC43]	EDTFL	40,240,33400,72540,305370,443500,512500,621730,775000,900400,		Corona	Virus
Coronavirus [Human 2] NL63 [HCoV-NL63, HKU1]	EDTFL	50,200,33400,72540,305370,443220,507000,621730,735000,900400,		Corona	Virus
Coronavirus [Middle East RS] [MERS-CoV]	EDTFL	50,200,33400,75500,308500,441500,507000,621730,735000,900400,		Corona	Virus
Coronavirus [Novel] [2019-nCoV]	EDTFL	50,200,33400,72540,305370,452550,509750,621730,738500,900400,		Corona	Virus
Coronavirus [SARS] NL63 [HCoV-NL63, HKU1]	EDTFL	50,200,33400,72540,305370,443220,507000,621730,735000,900400,		Corona	Virus
Coronavirus [COVID19] [2019-nCoV]	EDTFL	50,200,33400,72540,305370,452550,509750,621730,738500,900400,		Corona	Virus
Coronavirus [COVID19] Variants Omnicron, Delta, Alpha	EDTFL	70,230,72540,86030,274330,305370,509750,621730,738500,900400,		Corona	Virus
Coronavirus [COVID19] Post immunization complications	EDTFL	190,200,7250,45750,96500,325000,519340,655200,750000,922530,		Corona	Virus
Coxsackie General	CAFL	612,136,144,232,380,422,424,435,921,923,769,1189,595,676,	Infects heart, pleura, pancreas, and liver, causing pleurodynia, myocarditis, pericarditis, and hepatitis. Found with Bacteroides fragilis. Also see Mumps.	Coxsackie	Virus
Coxsackie	VEGA	136,232,422,424,435,921,923,	As mentioned above	Coxsackie	Virus
Coxsackie	XTRA	136,144,232,380,422,424,435,595,676,769,921,923,1189,	As mentioned above	Coxsackie	Virus
Coxsackie A9	BIOM	1189.9; 923; 921; 857; 769; 705; 676; 612; 595; 534; 424; 422; 380; 232; 144; 136		Coxsackie	Virus

Subject / Argument	Author	Frequencies	Notes	Origin	Target
Coxsackie A16	RL	889	From Dr. Richard Loyd.	Coxsackie	Virus
Coxsackie B1	HC	360500-366100=3600,	As mentioned above	Coxsackie	Virus
Coxsackie B1	CAFL	353,384,834,587,723,	As mentioned above	Coxsackie	Virus
Coxsackie B1	VEGA	834	As mentioned above	Coxsackie	Virus
Coxsackie virus type B1	BIOM	353; 384; 834; 587; 723; 902		Coxsackie	Virus
Coxsackie B2	CAFL	705,534,867	As mentioned above	Coxsackie	Virus
Coxsackie B2	VEGA	705,534	As mentioned above	Coxsackie	Virus
Coxsackie virus type B2	BIOM	705; 534; 867		Coxsackie	Virus
Coxsackie B3	CAFL	612,487,868,653,654,	As mentioned above	Coxsackie	Virus
Coxsackie virus type B3	BIOM	612; 487; 868; 653; 654		Coxsackie	Virus
Coxsackie B4	HC	361450-363700=3600,	As mentioned above	Coxsackie	Virus
Coxsackie B4	CAFL	421,353,540,8632	As mentioned above	Coxsackie	Virus
Coxsackie B4	VEGA	421	As mentioned above	Coxsackie	Virus
Coxsackie virus type B4	BIOM	421; 353; 540; 898.55; 8632		Coxsackie	Virus
Coxsackie B5	CAFL	462,1043,1083,569,647,708,774,		Coxsackie	Virus
Coxsackie B5	VEGA	462,1043,1083,	As mentioned above	Coxsackie	Virus
Coxsackie virus type B5	BIOM	462; 1043; 1083; 569; 647; 708; 774		Coxsackie	Virus
Coxsackie B6	CAFL	488,736,814,343,551,657,668,669,		Coxsackie	Virus
Coxsackie B6	VEGA	736,814	As mentioned above	Coxsackie	Virus
Coxsackie virus type B6	BIOM	488; 736; 814; 343; 551; 657; 668; 669		Coxsackie	Virus
Coxsackie Virus Infections	EDTFL	50,200,15750,45000,93400,376290,512330,689 930,759830,925710,	As mentioned above	Coxsackie	Virus
Breakbone Fever	XTRA	148,149,206,211,216,423,846,1194,1195,1196,1 692,3383,3389,	Common name for Dengue Fever.		Virus
Ebola Virus	XTRA	169,234,239,244,479,957,1195,1914,1828,	Virus causing Ebola, also called Hemorrhagic Shock.	Ebola	Virus
Ebola 1	XTRA	30,1200,15200,35000,22500,25665,4000,36827, 38660,37357,	Also called Hemorrhagic Fever. Use with 3.1MHz carrier (not needed in Remote Mode).	Ebola	Virus
Ebola 2	XTRA	2890,5950,27875,30000,38567,25000,23110,35 200,27747,37998,	As mentioned above	Ebola	Virus
Ebola Fever1	BIOM	1114.7; 2229.6; 633.5; 2.2; 2.2; 752.3; 1504.6; 3009.2; 10; 2.2; 2.2; 702.4; 1404.6; 2809.4; 749.3; 1498.6; 2997.4; 10; 2.2		Ebola	Virus
Ebola Fever2	BIOM	762; 1523.8; 3047.8; 1019.7; 2039.6; 822.9; 1645.8; 3291.6; 1107.1; 2214.2; 779.3; 1558.6; 3117; 10; 2.2; 2.2; 667.5; 1334.8; 2669.8; 681.8; 1363.6; 2727.2; 836.9		Ebola	Virus
Ebola Virus Infections	EDTFL	550,900,5150,55340,151090,387500,452500,62 1810,870560,921020		Ebola	Virus
Hemorrhagic Shock		40,550,910,93500,210500,212960,325430,5157 00,682450,755480		Ebola	Virus
Ebola Hemorrhagic Fever	XTRA	169,234,239,244,479,957,1195,1914,3828,		Ebola	Virus
Echo Virus	CAFL	922,788,765,722,625,620,614,613,612,611,610, 609,608,607,606,605,604,603,514,461,	Virus causing meningitis, particularly in children.	Echo	Virus
Echo Virus Meningitis	XTRA	461,514,603,604,605,606,607,608,609,610,611, 612,613,614,620,625,722,765,788,922,	As mentioned above	Echo	Virus
Echo Virus (Endometritis Tuberculosa)	VEGA	620	Virus causing uterine infections and meningitis. Also see Tuberculosis, Dysmenorrhea, Menstrual Problems, and Enteric Cytopathic Human Orphan Virus.	Echo	Virus
Echovirus infections	BIOM	922; 788; 765; 620; 614; 613; 612; 611; 610; 609; 607; 606; 605; 604; 603; 514; 461		Echo	Virus
Enteric Cytopathic Human Orphan Virus	XTRA	461,514,600,620,625,650,722,765,788,922,	Also called Echo (ECHO) Virus - see sets.		Virus
Ecthyma, Contagious	EDTFL	260,650,5710,11090,42500,65830,92500,23425 0,452590,815870	Also called Orf Disease. Viral skin disease mainly found in sheep and goats, but which can infect man.		Virus
Enterovirus		*May cause : Amyotrophic lateral sclerosis • ADHD • Autoimmune diseases • Carcinoid tumors • Chronic fatigue syndrome • Crohn's disease • Diabetes mellitus type 1 • Diabetes mellitus type 2 • Dilated cardiomyopathy • Guillain–Barré syndrome • Hypertension • Myocardial infarction • Schizophrenia • Carcinoid tumors.*			
Enterovirus	CAFL	20,136,144,232,283,322,380,423,435,461,487,5 15,595,608,610,612,620,625,654,676,721,733,7 42,766,776,788,822,845,868,922,1044,1189,142 2,1488,1500,1850,2632,3636,5000,	Generic term meaning small virus. Includes Echo, Coxsackie, and Polio.	Enterovirus	Virus
Enterovirus D68	RL	678	From Dr. Richard Loyd.	Enterovirus	Virus
Enterovirus infections	BIOM	3636; 2632; 1850; 1488; 1422; 1189; 1044; 922; 868; 845; 822; 788; 776; 742; 733; 721; 676; 654; 620; 612; 610; 608; 595; 515; 487; 461; 435; 423; 380; 322; 283; 232; 144; 136; 20		Enterovirus	Virus

Subject / Argument	Author	Frequencies	Notes	Origin	Target
Enterovirus Infection Non Polio	XTRA	461,514,600,620,625,650,722,765,788,922,	Generic term meaning small virus. Includes Echo and Coxsackie.	Enterovirus	Virus
Foot and Mouth Syndrome	CAFL	232,237,1214,1243,1244,1271,5411,	Viral contagious disease mainly in children, with fever and rash at hands, feet, and mouth. May be a factor in ALS. Use Coxsackie, and Enterovirus sets.		Virus
Foot and Mouth	VEGA	232,237,1214,1244,1271,5411,	As mentioned above		Virus
Foot and Mouth Disease	XTRA	232,237,558.37,585.91,1116.75,1171.83,1214,1243,1244,1271,5411,	As mentioned above		Virus
Foot and Mouth [coxsackievirus]	EDTFL	50,200,15750,45000,93400,376290,512330,689930,759830,925710,	As mentioned above		Virus
Hand Foot and Mouth Syndrome	BIO	232,237,1214,1243,1244,1271,5411,	As mentioned above		Virus
Hantavirus	RL	689	From Dr. Richard Loyd. It causes a rare but serious lung disease called Hantavirus pulmonary syndrome (HPS).		Virus
Hantavirus Infections	EDTFL	60,260,900,9000,10890,45910,125290,526160,652420,750000	Rodent viruses which can infect humans and cause life-threatening illnesses.		Virus
Hemorrhagic Fevers, Viral	EDTFL	40,550,910,93500,210500,212960,321510,471210,567210,647070	Viruses causing this include Ebola, Marburg, Lassa, Rift Valley Fever, and Hantavirus, among others.		Virus
Marburg virus (Hemorrhagic Fever Virus)	EDTFL	40,550,910,93500,210500,212960,321510,471210,567210,647070			Virus
Hendra Virus Disease	EDTFL	210,250,4530,42690,112250,329700,412500,643740,825520,971000			Virus
Nipah Virus Encephalitis	EDTFL	150,830,1700,6970,12590,62300,421000,465000,895000,951300	Bat virus capable of causing illness and death in equines, domestic animals, and humans.		Virus
Paramyxoviridae Infections	EDTFL	80,370,780,900,7520,10310,140000,232500,725470,925370			Virus
Hepatitis General	CAFL	1550,1351,922,880,802,727,477,329,317,224,28,	As mentioned above	Hepatitis	Virus
Hepatitis General 1 Virus	CAFL	166,213,224,317,321,334,477,528,534,558,562,563,781,786,842,876,878,922,934,987,	As mentioned above	Hepatitis	Virus
Hepatitis General Secondary	CAFL	284,458,477,534,768,777,788,922,1041,9670,	As mentioned above	Hepatitis	Virus
Hepatitis	BIO	224,317,1351	Infectious inflammation of liver. Also run Hepatitis General, Blood Purify, and Parasites Schistosoma Mansoni sets if necessary.	Hepatitis	Virus
Hepatitis New Numbers	BIO	477,922	As mentioned above	Hepatitis	Virus
Hepatitis	VEGA	224,317	As mentioned above	Hepatitis	Virus
Hepatitis	XTRA	1.19,28,727,802,880,1550,	As mentioned above	Hepatitis	Virus
Common Hepatitis	BIOM	1550; 1351; 922; 880; 802; 727; 477; 329; 317; 224; 28		Hepatitis	Virus
Secondary Common Hepatitis	BIOM	284; 458; 477; 534; 788; 922; 9669.5; 768; 777; 1040.9		Hepatitis	Virus
Hepatitis, Viral, Human	EDTFL	150,860,5290,27500,45560,95220,182500,233450,418000,420800	Infectious inflammation of liver.	Hepatitis	Virus
Hepatitis, Chronic Hepatitis, Chronic, Cryptogenic Hepatitis A, B, C Hepatitis, Comprehensive Hep A, B, C	EDTFL	200,870,5290,27500,45560,95220,182500,414550,418800,421800		Hepatitis	Virus
Hepatitis General 2	XTRA	224,317,1351	As mentioned above	Hepatitis	Virus
Hepatitis General 3	XTRA	28,224,317,329,470.6,477,483.3,660,690,727.5,802,1550,880,922,941.39,966.6,1351,1882.7,1933.2,329,9889,1351,1882.7,1933.2,329,9889,	As mentioned above	Hepatitis	Virus
Hepatitis General 4	XTRA	28,224,317,329,477,727,802,880,922,1351,1550,	As mentioned above	Hepatitis	Virus
Hepatitis General 5	XTRA	166,213,224,317,321,334,477,528,534,558,562,563,781,786,842,876,878,922,934,987,	As mentioned above	Hepatitis	Virus
Hepatitis General 7	XTRA	1.19,28,224,317,447,727,787,800,880,1550,2189,	As mentioned above	Hepatitis	Virus
Hepatitis General 8	XTRA	477,922	As mentioned above	Hepatitis	Virus
Entero Hepatitis	VEGA	552,932,953	Inflammation of liver and intestine.	Hepatitis	Virus
Hepatitis Type A - HAV virus		May cause : fever, malaise, nausea, abdominal pain and jaundice, accompanied by elevations of transaminases and bilirubin.			
Hepatitis A 2	CAFL	321,346,414,423,487,558,578,693,786,878,3220,717,	Infectious inflammation of liver (from blood or body fluids). Also run Hepatitis General, Blood Purify, and Parasites Schistosoma Mansoni sets if necessary.	Hepatitis A	Virus
Hepatitis Type A	BIO	321,3220	As mentioned above	Hepatitis A	Virus

Subject / Argument	Author	Frequencies	Notes	Origin	Target
Hepatitis A	BIOM	3220; 1550; 1357; 922; 880; 878; 802; 786; 717; 683; 578; 558; 487; 477; 423; 414; 346; 329; 317; 221; 214		Hepatitis A	Virus
Hepatitis A	EDTFL	200,230,5290,18200,57500,95220,182500,41455 0,712500,822000	As mentioned above	Hepatitis A	Virus
Hepatitis A 1	XTRA	321,333,346,414,423,487,523,558,578,693,717, 768,786,878,3220,	As mentioned above	Hepatitis A	Virus
Hepatitis Antigen A	XTRA	587666.5565	From Newport. Follow with Vaccine Toxins set.	Hepatitis A	Virus
Hepatitis Type B - HBV virus		*May cause :* **Vasculitis • Hepatocellular carcinoma • Pancreatic cancer**			
Hepatitis B 2	CAFL	334,433,767,869,876,477,574,752,779,	Infectious inflammation of liver (from blood or body fluids).	Hepatitis B	Virus
Hepatitis B	BIOM	1550; 1351; 987; 934; 922; 880; 878; 876; 869; 842; 802; 786; 781; 779; 767; 752; 727; 574; 563; 562; 558; 534; 528; 477; 423; 334; 329; 321; 317; 224; 213; 166; 28		Hepatitis B	Virus
Hepatitis B	EDTFL	200,230,5290,18200,57500,95220,182500,41455 0,719940,822530	As mentioned above	Hepatitis B	Virus
Hepatitis B 1	XTRA	1023.72,1027.56,1043.05,12906.25,12954.69,13 150,	As mentioned above	Hepatitis B	Virus
Hepatitis B 3	XTRA	1023.72, 20562.06	As mentioned above	Hepatitis B	Virus
Hepatitis Type B	XTRA	433		Hepatitis B	Virus
Hepatitis B Antigen	HC	414550-420800=3600,	As mentioned above	Hepatitis B	Virus
Hepatitis Type C - HCV virus		*May cause :* **Vasculitis • Diabetes mellitus type 2 • Hodgkin's lymphoma • Hepatocellular carcinoma.**			
Hepatitis C 4	CAFL	10000,5000,3220,3176,2489,1865,1600,1550,15 00,880,802,665,650,600,444,250,166,146,125,9 5,72,28,20,	Infectious inflammation of liver.	Hepatitis C	Virus
Hepatitis C 6	CAFL	3176,2489,2189,1865,1600,1550,1371,933,931, 929,802,650,633,625,528,444,329,317,250,224, 166,146,125,95,72,28,20,	As mentioned above	Hepatitis C	Virus
Hepatitis C	BIOM	10000; 5000; 3220; 2489; 2189; 1865; 1600; 1550; 1371; 933; 931; 929; 665; 650; 633; 528; 444; 329; 317; 250; 224; 166; 146; 95; 72; 28; 20		Hepatitis C	Virus
Hepatitis C	EDTFL	130,230,5290,18200,57500,95220,182500,41455 0,719940,822530	As mentioned above	Hepatitis C	Virus
Hepatitis C 1	XTRA	166,244,317,727,728,787,880,2189,	As mentioned above	Hepatitis C	Virus
Hepatitis C 2	XTRA	166,224,317,727,728,787,880,2189,	As mentioned above	Hepatitis C	Virus
Hepatitis C 3	XTRA	166,224,317,329,482.6,528,633,929,930,931,93 2,933,965.1,1371,1930.29,2189,	As mentioned above	Hepatitis C	Virus
Hepatitis Type C	XTRA	166	As mentioned above	Hepatitis C	Virus
Complex Hepatitis C	BIOM	10000; 5000; 3176; 9888.5; 2720; 2489; 2189; 2128; 2082; 1865; 1600; 1550; 1371; 1351; 987; 933; 931; 929; 922; 877; 842; 802; 786; 781; 728; 650; 633; 625; 562; 530; 477; 465; 444; 333; 317; 250; 224; 166; 146; 125; 95; 72; 28		Hepatitis C	Virus
HIV Virus		*May cause : Autoimmune diseases • Dementia • Vasculitis • ADHD • Hodgkin's lymphoma • Kaposi's Sarcoma • Non-Hodgkin lymphoma •*			
HIV	CAFL	683,714,3554,830,450,	Retrovirus causing HIV Infection and AIDS.	HIV	Virus
HIV	HC	365000	As mentioned above	HIV	Virus
HIV	BIO	683,714,3554	As mentioned above	HIV	Virus
HIV Virus	XTRA	1.2	As mentioned above	HIV	Virus
HIV	VEGA	683,3554,714	As mentioned above	HIV	Virus
HIV 1	XTRA	243,646,725,732,844,2432,6353,	As mentioned above	HIV	Virus
HIV 2	XTRA	245,314,725,965,1230,	As mentioned above	HIV	Virus
HIV 3	XTRA	111,392,633,714,776,834,1220,1675,2664,3806, 6230,8225,	As mentioned above	HIV	Virus
HIV 4	XTRA	444,683,714,2323,3554,	As mentioned above	HIV	Virus
HIV 5	XTRA	83,235,645,2323,3432,4093,5532,	As mentioned above	HIV	Virus
HIV 6	XTRA	183,702,747,2245	As mentioned above	HIV	Virus
HIV 8	XTRA	904.74,11406.25	As mentioned above	HIV	Virus
HIV 9	XTRA	904.74,18172.27	As mentioned above	HIV	Virus
AIDS	BIOM	683; 714; 3554; 904; 830; 450; 74		AIDS	Virus
AIDS	BIOM	249; 418; 465; 727; 787; 880; 1113; 1550; 1500; 2128; 2489; 3100; 3175; 3475; 6121		AIDS	Virus
HIV AIDS HTLV-III Infections (HIV) HTLV-III-LAV Infections (HIV)	EDTFL	140,320,970,2500,11090,20000,57500,225000,4 23060,565360	Human T-Lymphotropic Virus	AIDS	Virus

Subject / Argument	Author	Frequencies	Notes	Origin	Target
T-Lymphotropic Virus Type III	EDTFL	20,410,22500,57500,324160,476500,527000,667000,749000,986220		AIDS	Virus
AIDS/HIV	EDTFL	180,240,22000,30000,47500,162820,365000,388900,434000,456110,	Acquired immune deficiency.	AIDS	Virus
HIV Related Infections	EDTFL	140,320,970,2500,11090,20000,57500,225000,423010,565370	As mentioned above	AIDS	Virus
HIV Infections	KHZ	150,180,870,5580,22000,30000,47500,162820,388900,456110,	As mentioned above	AIDS	Virus
Human T Lymphotropic Virus1	CAFL	243,646,725,732,844,2432,6353,	Causes leukemia/lymphoma and nerve demyelination. Use for MS and autoimmune disorders.		Virus
Human T Lymphotropic Virus2	CAFL	245,314,725,965,1230,	Causes leukemia/lymphoma and nerve demyelination. Use for Gulf War Syndrome.		Virus
Human T Lymphotropic Virus3	CAFL	111,392,633,714,776,837,1220,1675,2664,3806,6230,8225,	Causes leukemia/lymphoma and nerve demyelination. Use for AIDS.		Virus
Human T Lymphotropic Virus4	CAFL	**444,2323**	Causes leukemia/lymphoma and nerve demyelination.		Virus
Human T Lymphotropic Virus5	CAFL	83,235,645,2323,3432,4093,5532,	Causes leukemia/lymphoma and nerve demyelination. Use for HIV.		Virus
Human T Lymphotropic Virus6	CAFL	**183,702,747,2245**	As mentioned above		Virus
T Lymph Virus	XTRA	111,243,245,314,392,633,646,714,725,732,776,837,844,965,1220,1230,1675,2432,2664,3806,6230,6353,8225,	Human T-Lymphotropic Virus. Family of viruses causing T Cell Leukemia (see sets), and the demyelinating disease HTLV-I associated myelopathy/tropical spastic paraparesis (HAM/TSP).		Virus
Influenza			See Colds Diseases Section 3h - Flu		Virus
Lassa Fever	EDTFL	200,250,750,2500,3000,5580,175540,324300,425690,571000	Infectious disease caused by a viral agent belonging to the Arenavirus family. Acute viral hemorrhagic fever similar to Ebola and with multiple symptoms.		Virus
Lyssavirus	XTRA	20,120,547,660,690,727.5,787,793,808,880,	Genus of RNA viruses which includes Rabies - see sets.		Virus
Meningococcus Virus	BIO	**720**	Virus infecting the membranes that envelop the brain and spinal cord.		Virus
Mumps	CAFL	152,242,642,674,922,	Acute viral inflammation of the salivary glands, caused by viruses of the genus Rubulavirus. See Coxsackie set.	Mumps	Virus
Mumps Secondary	CAFL	190,235,516,1243,1660,2630,3142,9667,729,741,759,761,1170,	As mentioned above	Mumps	Virus
Mumps Tertiary	CAFL	10000,727,2720,2489,2127,2008,428,880,787,727,20,	As mentioned above	Mumps	Virus
Mumps	BIO	152,190,235,242,516,642,674,922,1243,1660,2630,3142,	As mentioned above	Mumps	Virus
Mumps	VEGA	242,516,642,922,2630,3142,	As mentioned above	Mumps	Virus
Mumps	EDTFL	70,330,700,45000,78240,114620,323000,637080,845380,913500,	As mentioned above	Mumps	Virus
Parotitis, Epidemic	EDTFL	70,330,700,45000,78240,114620,323000,637080,845380,913500	As mentioned above	Mumps	Virus
Epidemic parotitis	BIOM	10000; 727; 2720; 2489; 2127; 428; 880; 787; 727; 20; 242; 152; 674; 642; 922		Mumps	Virus
Epidemic parotitis, secondary	BIOM	516; 1170; 1243; 1660; 2008; 2630; 2489; 3142; 9667		Mumps	Virus
Mumps	XTRA	**14**	As mentioned above	Mumps	Virus
Mumps Antigen	HC	377600-384650=3600,		Mumps	Virus
Mumps Vaccine	BIO	273,551,711,730,1419,		Mumps	Virus
Mumps Vaccine	VEGA	**711,551,1419**		Mumps	Virus
Norovirus	RL	**394**	From Dr. Richard Loyd. Referred to as the winter vomiting virus, it is the most common cause of gastroenteritis.		Virus
Papilloma	EDTFL	80,490,650,7530,12850,17500,72500,226070,475470,527000	Virus causing warts, or lesions leading to cancers of reproductive system, genitals, anus, and oropharynx. See appropriate Cancer, and Human Papilloma Virus HPV sets.	Papilloma	Virus
Papillomavirus	BIO	**907**	As mentioned above	Papilloma	Virus
Human papilloma virus 1	BIOM	725; 2432; 243; 6353; 844; 732; 646; 245; 314; 111; 392; 714; 776; 837; 965; 1230; 1675; 2664; 3806; 633; 1220; 6230; 8225; 444; 2323; 235; 645; 3432; 4093; 5532; 702; 747; 2245; 183	As mentioned above	Papilloma	Virus
Human papilloma virus 2	BIOM	45; 489; 847; 907; 256; 5657; 1011; 9258; 1051; 9609; 466; 110; 767; 404; 265; 9609; 9258; 5657; 1051; 1011; 907; 874	As mentioned above	Papilloma	Virus
Human papilloma virus 3	BIOM	5657; 2170; 953; 915; 907; 874; 466; 110	As mentioned above	Papilloma	Virus
Papillomavirus	PROV	67265,64734,16970,9609,9258,5657,1051,1011,907,874,767,489,466,404,265,110,45,	As mentioned above	Papilloma	Virus
Papilloma HPV 6a	XTRA	**1130.09, 2260.19**	As mentioned above	Papilloma	Virus
Papilloma HPV 6b	XTRA	**1145.5, 2291.09**	As mentioned above	Papilloma	Virus

Subject / Argument	Author	Frequencies	Notes	Origin	Target
Papilloma HPV 11	XTRA	1141.29, 2282.69	As mentioned above	Papilloma	Virus
Papilloma HPV 16	XTRA	1145.2, 2290.5	As mentioned above	Papilloma	Virus
Papilloma HPV 18	XTRA	1152.09, 2304.19	As mentioned above	Papilloma	Virus
Papilloma HPV 33	XTRA	1144.5, 2289	As mentioned above	Papilloma	Virus
HPV skin wart virus	RL	857	From Dr. Richard Loyd.	Papilloma	Virus
Papillomavirus Infections	EDTFL	80,490,650,7530,12850,17500,72500,226070,475470,527000	As mentioned above	Papilloma	Virus
Human Papilloma Virus (HPV)	EDTFL	80,490,650,7530,12850,17500,72500,226070,475470,527000,		Papilloma	Virus
Papilloma, Squamous Cell	EDTFL	80,490,650,7530,27500,52500,225370,434170,517500,687620	As mentioned above	Papilloma	Virus
Human Papilloma Virus HPV	XTRA	45,110,265,404,466,489,767,874,907,1002.15,1011,1051,5667,9258,9609,20218.9,	As mentioned above	Papilloma	Virus
Paramyxovirus	BIOM	8920.5; 8089.4; 4460.2; 4044.7; 2230.1; 2022.3; 1115.1; 1011.2; 557.5; 505.6; 278.8; 252.8; 139.4; 126.4	Causes respiratory disease in children.		Virus
Pneumovirus	CAFL	278,336,712	Causes bronchiolitis and pneumonia in infants. See Respiratory syncitial virus set.		Virus
Polio	CAFL	135,283,742,776,1500,2632,1850,	Caused by infection with a virus belonging to the enterovirus genus, known as **Poliovirus**.	Polio	Virus
Polio Secondary Complications	CAFL	1550,802,428,1500,880,787,727,	Poliomyelitis. Also called Infantile Paralysis - see sets.	Polio	Virus
Polio	BIO	742,1500,2632	As mentioned above	Polio	Virus
Poliomyelitis, complex	BIOM	10000; 5000; 2632; 1850; 1550; 1500; 880; 804; 802; 787; 776; 742; 727; 428; 283; 135; 13; 9.35; 8.25		Polio	Virus
Polio	EDTFL	50,240,970,970,7500,35620,117520,402060,675620,823010	As mentioned above	Polio	Virus
Poliomyelitis Poliomyelitis, Nonpoliovirus Poliomyelitis, Preparalytic	EDTFL	50,240,970,970,7500,35620,157500,525830,757770,975340		Polio	Virus
Post polio syndrome	EDTFL	50,240,970,970,7500,35620,117520,402060,675620,823010,	As mentioned above	Polio	Virus
Infantile Paralysis	CAFL	1500,880,787,727,776,5000,10000,	Also called Polio.	Polio	Virus
Infantile Paralysis 2	XTRA	727,776,787,880,1500,10000,	Also called Polio.	Polio	Virus
Polyomavirus Infections	EDTFL	70,360,700,45000,77260,114690,320000,637090,805810,973200	Family of viruses including Simian Virus 40 (see set), JC virus, BK virus, and Merkel Cell virus.		Virus
Polyomavirus Infections	KHZ XTRA	130,500,6750,71250,105150,347500,572500,690000,775870,826900,	As mentioned above		Virus
Measles	CAFL	727,787,880,342,442,443,467,520,521,552,1489,745,757,763,712,	Also called Rubeola - see sets. Highly contagious condition with fever, cough, rhinitis, red eyes, followed by white oral spots and red skin rash.	Measles	Virus
Measles	VEGA	467,520,1489	Disease caused by a virus, the **Paramyxovirus** of the genus Morbillivirus.	Measles	Virus
Measles	ETDFL	110,890,1700,6970,12890,62300,423000,465000,895000,951300		Measles	Virus
Rubeola	ETDFL	190,600,1220,17250,63210,119420,287210,403030,435000,711170	As mentioned above	Measles	Virus
Measles	KHZ	60,260,750,2250,7500,52500,124940,452590,515680,687620,	As mentioned above	Measles	Virus
Measles	XTRA	333	As mentioned above	Measles	Virus
Measles Rubeola	CAFL	342,467,520,784,787,962,1489,	**9-Day Measles**. Infectious disease with rash, cough, runny nose, eye inflammation, and fever. Also see Measles Rubeola, and Measles.	Measles	Virus
Measles (Day 9)	BIOM	342; 467; 520; 784; 787; 962; 1489; 431; 459; 510; 517; 796; 967; 368; 734; 772; 431; 459; 510; 517; 796; 967; 368; 734; 772	As mentioned above	Measles	Virus
Rubeola	BIO	342,467,520,1489	As mentioned above	Measles	Virus
Measels-Rubella Vaccine	BIOM	429; 459; 832; 926; 505		Measles	Virus
Measles Vaccine	CAFL	214,725,747,783,962,		Measles	Virus
Measles Vaccine	VEGA	962		Measles	Virus
Rubella	CAFL	431,459,510,517,727,787,880,	Also called Rubella, or **3-Day Measles**. Infectious disease with rash, sore throat, itching, fatigue, and swollen lymph nodes. See Measles Rubella, and Rubella sets.	Rubella	Virus
Measles (Day 3)	BIOM	431; 459; 510; 517; 796; 967; 368; 734; 772; 431; 459; 510; 517; 796; 967; 368; 734; 772	As mentioned above	Rubella	Virus
Measles Rubella	CAFL	431,459,510,517,796,967,368,734,772,	Infectious disease, of viral origin due to the **Rubella virus**.	Rubella	Virus
German Measles Rubella	CAFL	368,510,517,734,772,796,967,	As mentioned above	Rubella	Virus
German Measles Secondary	CAFL	727,787,880	As mentioned above	Rubella	Virus
Measles Rubella	BIO	431,510	As mentioned above	Rubella	Virus
German Measles	VEGA	517	As mentioned above	Rubella	Virus

Subject / Argument	Author	Frequencies	Notes	Origin	Target
Rubella	ETDFL	130,520,620,9000,13610,155870,362520,45303 0,775910,925580	As mentioned above	Rubella	Virus
German Measles	ETDFL	110,890,1700,6970,12890,72500,96500,269710, 375370,377980,		German M.	Virus
German Measles Rubella 1	XTRA	368,431,459,510,517,734,772,796,967,	As mentioned above	German M.	Virus
German Measles 1	XTRA	20=1380,342,344,368,420=1380,431,459,510,5 17,520,660,690,727.5,735,772,784,796,880,943, 967,1489,	As mentioned above	German M.	Virus
German Measles 2	XTRA	727,787,880	As mentioned above	German M.	Virus
Rubella Vaccine	VEGA	459		German M.	Virus
German Measles Rubella Vaccine	XTRA	429,459,505,832,926,	Vaccine detox	German M.	Virus
Reoviridae [Respiratory Virus]	ETDF	550,610,780,970,5870,57050,152030,524370,60 1270,781090,	Double-stranded RNA family of viruses that can affect the gastrointestinal system (such as Rotavirus) and the respiratory tract.		Virus
Reovirus	RL	967	From Dr. Richard Loyd.		Virus
Rhinovirus	RL	865	From Dr. Richard Loyd.They are the causative agents of the most common colds.		Virus
Rotavirus	RL	666	From Dr. Richard Loyd. Rotaviruses are the most common cause of diarrhoeal disease among infants and young children.	Rotavirus	Virus
RotaVirus	BIOM	8449.5; 5003.5; 2502; 2111; 1213.9; 885; 875; 880; 845; 787; 776; 735; 727; 720; 660; 625.5; 616; 465; 9100.5; 7344; 1234; 906; 880; 832; 802; 787; 776; 765; 727; 697; 688; 683; 526; 284; 46; 20		Rotavirus	Virus
Rotavirus	ETDF	180,320,950,7500,25750,52500,425140,570000, 841000,932000		Rotavirus	Virus
Sars 1	CAFL	162,563,1556,1559,2286,3735,5235,5513,5613, 5763,6157,8015,9563,33566,255616,	Also use Streptococcus Pneumoniae set.	Sars	Virus
Sars 2	CAFL	499.25,524.47,563,597.68,648,654.4,689.14,701 .6,720.36,769.62,779.5,937.76,998.5,1001.86,10 48.94,1143,	As mentioned above	Sars	Virus
Acute Respiratory Viral Infections 1	BIOM	2.2; 10.0; 12.5; 19.5; 26.0; 49.0; 55.0; 92.5		Sars	Virus
Acute Respiratory Viral Infections 2	BIOM	0.9; 1.75; 2; 2.5; 2.93; 3.6; 4; 4.9; 5.5; 5.9; 6.5; 7.7; 8; 9.4; 9.44; 12; 12.5; 13.5; 13.75; 18; 21; 21.5; 25.5; 26		Sars	Virus
Acute Respiratory Viral Infections 3	BIOM	26.5; 32.5; 46.; 52.75; 53; 53.5; 62; 62.5; 66; 69; 74; 75.5; 76.5; 79; 81; 85; 86; 87.5; 90; 91.5; 92; 94; 94.5; 95.5; 98.8; 100		Sars	Virus
Acute Respiratory Viral Infections 4	BIOM	0.7; 0.9; 2.5; 2.65; 3.3; 9.8; 56.0; 69.0		Sars	Virus
Acute Respiratory Viral Infections 5	BIOM	2.5; 3.6; 3.9; 5.0; 6.3; 8.1; 34.0; 92.0		Sars	Virus
Respiratory Syncytial Virus	CAFL	336,712,278	Common virus causing respiratory tract infections. Also see Lung, Bronchial, Pneumovirus, and other appropriate sets.	RSV	Virus
Respiratory Syncytial Virus	BIOM	336; 712; 278; 942		RSV	
Respiratory Syncytial Virus	HC	378950-383150=3600,	As mentioned above	RSV	Virus
Respiratory Syncytial Virus Infections	EDTFL	550,610,780,970,5870,57050,152030,524370,60 1270,781090	As mentioned above	RSV	Virus
RSV	RL	995	From Dr. Richard Loyd. As mentioned above	RSV	Virus
Simian Virus 40	XTRA	79333.9,83173.3,95443,93806.5,132112,134443 ,138591.3,140781,141346,148107,335175,3554 36,385643,	From Dr. Jeff Sutherland. SV40 plays a role in an aggressive lung cancer called Mesothelioma (see set). Also found in Astrocytomas, Ependymomas, Glioblastomas, Medulloblastomas, and Papillomas of the choroid plexus (see appropriate sets).Probable cause of celiac disease.		Virus
Tobacco Mosaic Virus	HC	427150-429550=3600,	RNA virus that infects many plant types. Also used in micro-batteries.		Virus
Parasites: Tobacco mosaic virus	ETDF	680,900,2500,5500,13930,93500,385150,38595 0,386400,388000	As mentioned above		Virus
Smallpox	CAFL	3222,2544,2132,1644,1550,876,832,802,569,54 2,511,476,142,	Also called Variola. Extremely contagious viral disease marked by fever, prostration, and a rash of small blisters. Also see Herpes Simplex RTI set.	Small Pox	Virus
Smallpox	BIOM	3222; 2544; 2132; 1644; 1550; 876; 832; 802; 569; 542; 511; 476; 142; 33		Small Pox	Virus
Smallpox Secondary	CAFL	334,360,471,647,506,711,880,787,727,20,	Smallpox virus (Variola virus) disease	Small Pox	Virus
Smallpox, secondary	BIOM	334; 360; 471; 647; 506; 711; 880; 787; 727; 20		Small Pox	Virus
Variola	CAFL	142,476,511,542,569,802,832,876,1550,1644,21 32,2544,3222,	As mentioned above	Small Pox	Virus
Smallpox	ETDF	70,370,12710,47500,97500,225750,377910,519 380,691270,753070	As mentioned above	Small Pox	Virus

Subject / Argument	Author	Frequencies	Notes	Origin	Target
Variola Major	ETDF	70,370,12710,47500,97500,225750,377910,519 380,691270,753070,	As mentioned above	Small Pox	Virus
Smallpox Variola	BIO	142,476,511,876,1644,2132,2544,	Also known as Smallpox - see sets. Also see Variolinum, and Herpes Simplex RTI.	Small Pox	Virus
Variola	VEGA	511,2132,2544,876,	As mentioned above	Small Pox	Virus
Variola Minor	ETDF	70,370,12710,47500,97500,225750,377910,519 380,691270,753070,	Attenuated form of smallpox.	Small Pox	Virus
Alastrim	ETDF	80,410,5500,35180,62500,93500,215000,49603 0,682450,753070	As mentioned above	Small Pox	Virus
Xenotropic Murine Leukemia Virus (XMRV)	*May cause:* **Autism, Fibromyalgia, Multiple Sclerosis, Amyotrophic Lateral Sclerosis, Parkinson's, Chronic Fatigue Syndrome (CFS), Prostate cancer.**				
Xenotropic Murine Leukemia Virus	XTRA	448	XMRV - found in Lyme Disease and Chronic Fatigue Syndrome. Also see Retrovirus Variants set.	XMRV	Virus
Xenotropic Murine Leukemia Virus	XTRA	4673.6	As mentioned above	XMRV	Virus
ZIKA Virus	ETDFL	1230,2340,11250,22260,43200,123740,336200, 628390,721330,802330	Virus transmitted by mosquitoes.	XMRV	Virus

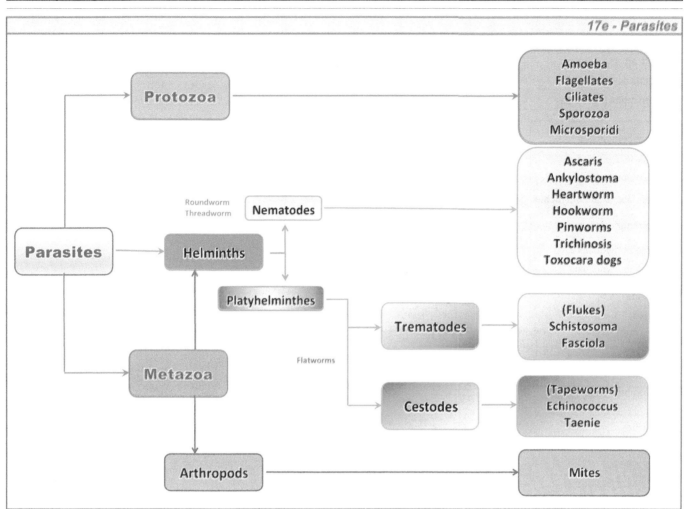

Subject / Argument	Author	Frequencies	Notes		Target
Parasite Detoxification			See Section **2c - Detox**		Parasites
Dr. Hulda Clark Parasite General	EDTFL	160,300,680,900,2500,5500,13930,93500,35672 0,451170			Parasites
Parasites: (Dr. Hulda Clark Parasite General, Comprehensive)	EDTFL	60,240,780,830,2500,10890,22500,124370,3750 00,515700			Parasites
Parasites General	CAFL	20,64,72,96,112,120,152,651,732,1360,2720,10 000,	Pancreatic, liver, and intestinal flukes.		Parasites
Parasites General 1	CAFL	4412,2112,1862,1550,800,732,728,712,688,676, 644,422,128,120,			Parasites
Parasites General 2	CAFL	10000,3176,1998,1865,1840,880,800,780,770,7 40,728,727,690,665,660,465,444,440,125,120,9 5,80,72,47,			Parasites
Parasites General Comprehensive	CAFL	20,64,72,96,112,120,125,128,152,240,334,422,4 42,465,524,644,651,688,712,728,732,800,854,8 80,1550,1864,2112,2400,2720,4412,5000,			Parasites
Parasites General Alternative V	CAFL	102,172,344,411,422,524,591,604,605,633,732, 741,749,827,829,854,942,967,1522,4122,			Parasites
Parasites: general	EDTFL	680,900,2500,5500,13930,93500,386400,45190 0,455000,457100			Parasites
Parasites: general comprehensive	EDTFL	680,900,2500,5500,13930,93500,386400,42140 0,424000,426300			Parasites
Parasites	XTRA	444,125,95,72,20,1865,			Parasites
Parasites General 4	XTRA	187,294,387,453,562,697,752,772,844,947,1113 ,3437,			Parasites
Blood Parasites		847; 867; 329; 419; 635; 7390.5; 5515.5; 9888.5			Parasites
Digestive tract parasites		142; 275; 435; 524; 651; 676; 763; 830; 854; 945; 1850; 2000; 2003; 2013; 2082; 2128; 2150; 6578; 6641; 6672; 6766			Parasites

Subject / Argument	Author	Frequencies	Notes	Origin	Target
Intestinal Parasites		524; 651; 676; 844; 848; 854; 2128; 2084; 2150; 6765.5			Parasites
Worms	Rife	2400			Parasites
Helminth eggs	BIOM	164; 793; 969; 5243			
Helminthiasis	EDTFL	70,460,510,730,7500,22000,57500,150000,2155 30,322060	Infection of worms like tapeworm, flukes, or roundworm. See appropriate set if parasite has been identified.		Parasites
Nematomorpha [Horsehair worm]	EDTFL	180,190,730,9000,11090,22500,106000,115700, 377910,470120,			Parasites
Macracanthorhynchus	HC	438850-442800=3600,	Acanthocephalan parasite living in the intestines of pigs and other suids, and occasionally in humans or dogs, causing enteritis, gastritis, or peritonitis.		Parasites
Parasites: Macracanthorhynchus	EDTFL	680,900,2500,5500,13930,93500,386400,39800 0,400000,402650	As mentioned above		Parasites
Parasites Macracanthorhynchus	KHZ	120,230,600,2500,10890,2750,30000,122530,21 0500,455820,	As mentioned above		Parasites
Macracanthorhynchus	XTRA	1087.79,1090.65,1097.58,13714.05,13750,1383 7.5,	As mentioned above		Parasites
Macracanthorhynchus 2	XTRA	1828,1830,1832,1834,1838,1840,1842,1844,184 6,1848,1850,1852,1854,1856,1858,1860,	As mentioned above		Parasites
Macracanthorhynchosis	BIOM	1090.7			Parasites
Rope Worm	EDTFL	70,500,1000,7200,17500,127500,335290,52515 0,705250,813670	Intestinal parasites, or worms, which often lead to very severe disorders.	Intestines	Ropeworm
Ropeworm	RL	1359	From Dr. Richard Loyd. Large GI parasite in Morgellons/Lyme.	Intestines	Ropeworm

17f - Protozoa and Diseases

Subject / Argument	Author	Frequencies	Notes	Origin	Target
Protozoa	CAFL	432,753,5776	Group of unicellular eukaryotic organisms.		Protozoa
Protozoan Infections	EDTFL	130,570,830,2250,5710,32500,97500,332410,37 2000,520000	Disorders caused by unicellular eukaryotic organisms, including Malaria, Amoebiasis, Giardiasis, Toxoplasmosis, Cryptosporidiosis, Trichomoniasis, Chagas Disease, Leishmaniasis, and others. See sets.		Protozoa
Histomoniasis	EDTFL	80,410,1000,5780,7250,15870,92500,215700,32 3580,519340	As mentioned above		Protozoa
Amoeba	BIO	310,333,532,732,827,1522,	A single-celled, sometimes infectious microorganism (also spelled Ameba).		Amoeba
Amoeba General	CAFL	310,333,532,732,769,827,1522,	As mentioned above		Amoeba
Parasites and Amoebas 4	XTRA	1865,444,125,95,72,20,			Amoeba
Amoeba Hepar Abscess	CAFL	344,605	Liver abcess caused by amebic infection. Also spelled Ameba.	Liver	Amoeba
Amoebiasis	BIOM	148; 166; 308; 309.9; 344; 393; 631; 732; 769; 778; 827; 954.3; 981.6; 1522			Amoeba
Amoebiasis	EDTFL	520,2500,40000,95000,376290,476500,527000, 665340,752700,987250,	Also spelled Amebiasis.		Amoeba
Amebiasis, oral	BIOM	1084.7			Amoeba
Amebiasis, secondary	BIOM	1552; 1550; 943; 880; 832; 802; 787; 727; 690; 660; 465; 786; 768; 523; 333			Amoeba
Iodamoebiasis [entamoeba infection]	EDTFL	2500,13930,204510,337300,388950,389000,390 700,408150,409000,411150,	As mentioned above		Amoeba
Ameboma	EDTFL	520,2500,40000,95000,376290,476500,527000, 665340,752700,987230,	Intestinal disease		Ameba
Babesia	PROV	76,570,1583,1584,432,753,5776,	Protozoan causing malaria-like symptoms. Mostly tick-borne, but has been found in blood products.		Protozoa
Babesia	BIOM	5775.5; 2050; 2016; 1584; 1520; 920; 864; 790; 753; 690; 630; 625; 620; 615; 610; 570; 505; 500; 495; 490; 485; 432; 76			Protozoa
Babesia Divergens	XTRA	470.46	As mentioned above		Protozoa
Babesia Lyme	XTRA	76,570,753,1583,1584,5776,650,	As mentioned above		Protozoa
Babesia Microti	RL	646	From Dr. Richard Loyd. Is a parasitic blood-borne piroplasm transmitted by deer ticks.		Protozoa
Babesia Microti - WA	XTRA	465.7, 467.7	As mentioned above		Protozoa
Babesia	BIOM	5775.5; 2050; 2016; 1584; 1520; 920; 864; 790; 753; 690; 630; 625; 620; 615; 610; 570; 505; 500; 495; 490; 485; 432; 8			Protozoa
Babesiasis	EDTFL	40,180,700,900,7500,45750,71500,95000,21934 0,379930,	Malaria-like illness caused by Babesia.		Protozoa
Piroplasmosis	EDTFL	60,260,650,5150,7400,42500,92500,475950,526 000,661710	As mentioned above		Protozoa
Babesiosis	XTRA	76,432,570,753,1583,1584,5776,	As mentioned above		Protozoa
Besnoitia (Lung Sect.) Protozoan	HC	352800-361400=3600,	Protozoan causing pedunculated lesions in skin, nasal cavity, and larynx.		Protozoa

Subject / Argument	Author	Frequencies	Notes	Origin	Target
Parasites: Besnoitia (lung section) protozoan	EDTFL	680,900,2500,5500,13930,122500,322600,397600,401000,403250	As mentioned above		Protozoa
Besnoitia 1	XTRA	874.5,887.38,895.82,11025,11187.5,11293.75,	As mentioned above		Protozoa
Besnoitia 2	XTRA	887.38,17823.77	As mentioned above		Protozoa
Blastocystis Hominis	CAFL	365,595,844,848,1201,1243,5777,11425,11841,11967,13145,13469,21776,	Protozoan causing GI tract problems. Often misdiagnosed as Irritable Bowel Syndrome (IBS).	Intestines	Protozoa
Blastocystis Hominis	BIO	365,595,844,848,1201,1243,	As mentioned above	Intestines	Protozoa
Blastocystis Hominis	VEGA	848,365,844,595	As mentioned above	Intestines	Protozoa
Blastocystis Hominis	XTRA	210,365,595,844,848,1201,1243,5777,11425,11841,11967,13145,13469,21776,	As mentioned above	Intestines	Protozoa
Blastocystis Hominis	BIOM	365; 595; 844; 1201; 1243; 5777		Intestines	Protozoa
Blastocystis hominis infections	EDTFL	180,230,970,7500,32500,175000,453720,515110,684810,712420,	As mentioned above	Intestines	Protozoa
Blepharisma	CAFL	31320	Ciliate water-dwelling protist		Protozoa
Blepharisma	HC	405650-407450=3600,	Ciliate water-dwelling protist.		Protozoa
Blepharisma	XTRA	1007.61,3120,20233.43	Ciliate water-dwelling protist.		Protozoa
Chilomastix Cysts (Rat)	HC	388950-390700=3600,	Protozoan which lives in the GI tract.		Protozoa
Chilomastix Cysts (Rat) 2nd	HC	425200-427300=3600,	Protozoan which lives in the GI tract.		Protozoa
Parasites: Chilomastix cysts (rat)	EDTFL	680,900,2500,13930,198510,323300,376900,404900,408000,409150	GI tract protozoan not considered parasitic by medicine, but occurring with other parasite infections.		Protozoa
Chilomastix Cysts (Rat)	XTRA	1053.97,1055,95,1059.17,13287.5,13312.5,13353.12,	Protozoan which lives in the GI tract.		Protozoa
Chilomastix Amoeba Cysts	XTRA	964.23,1055.95,19367.16,21209.29,	Protozoan which lives in the GI tract.		Protozoa
Chilomonas Whole Mount	HC	393750-400000=3600,	GI tract protozoan not considered parasitic by medicine, but occurring with other parasite infections.		Protozoa
Parasites: Chilomonas, whole mount	EDTFL	680,900,2500,13930,204510,331000,337300,403850,408000,409700	As mentioned above		Protozoa
Chilomonas Whole Mount	XTRA	976,986.53,991.5,12304.69,12437.5,12500,	As mentioned above		Protozoa
Chilomonas 2	XTRA	986.53,19815.25	As mentioned above		Protozoa
Coccidiosis	XTRA	336,337,20000=2400,	Parasitic disease of GI tract caused by coccidian protozoa.		Protozoa
Cryptosporidium Parvum	XTRA	432,482,660,690,727.5,753,4122,5776,	Parasitic protozoa causing diarrhea. See Cryptosporidiosis.		Protozoa
Cryptosporidium	CAFL	220,482,575,4122,698,711,893,895,1276,5690	As mentioned above	Intestines	Protozoa
Cryptosporidium	VEGA	482,4122,	As mentioned above		Protozoa
Cryptosporidiosis	BIOM	220; 482; 575; 4122; 698; 711; 893; 895; 1276; 5690			Protozoa
Cryptosporidiosis	EDTFL	40,230,820,9800,67500,212500,215500,435290,695750,875950,	GI tract infection caused by the protozoan parasite Cryptosporidium - see sets.		Protozoa
Cyclospora	CAFL	543,316,992,751,268,2144,	Parasitic protist that infects the GI tract.	Intestines	Protozoa
Cyclospora	XTRA	268,316,543,751,992,2144,	As mentioned above	Intestines	Protozoa
Cyclosporiasis	BIOM	543; 316; 992; 751; 268; 2144			Protozoa
Cyclosporiasis	EDTFL	180,250,930,7500,10530,95950,322530,419340,564280,642060,	GI tract infection due to parasitic protist Cyclospora.	Intestines	Protozoa
Cystoisospora belli	RL	886	From Dr. Richard Loyd. Is a parasite that causes an intestinal disease known as cystoisosporiasis.	Intestines	Protozoa
Dientamoeba Fragilis	HC	401350-406050=3600,	GI tract parasitic amoeba causing pain, diarrhea, weight loss, and fever. See Dientamoebiasis.		Protozoa
Dientamoeba fragilis	RL	676	From Dr. Richard Loyd.		Protozoa
Dientamoeba Fragilis 1	XTRA	1001.41, 20113.97,	As mentioned above		Protozoa
Dientamoeba Fragilis 2	XTRA	994.85,1001.41,1006.5,12542.19,12625,12689.05,	As mentioned above		Protozoa
Parasites: Dientamoeba fragilis	EDTFL	680,900,2500,13930,204510,331000,337300,424250,428000,430650	As mentioned above		Protozoa
Dientamebiasis	BIOM	1001.4			Protozoa
Dientamoebiasis	EDTFL	520,2500,40000,95000,376290,476500,527000,665340,752700,987230,	GI tract parasitic amoeba infection causing pain, diarrhea, weight loss, and fever.		Protozoa
Endolimax Nana Trophozoites and Cysts	HC	394250-397100=3600,	As mentioned above		Amoeba
Endolimax Nana Trophozoites and Cysts 2nd	HC	430500-433350=3600,	Genus of amoeba causing diarrhea, whose presence indicates ingestion of fecal matter.		Amoeba
Parasites: Endolimax nana trophozoites and cysts	EDTFL	680,900,2500,5500,13930,122500,322600,401350,404000,406050	As mentioned above		Amoeba
Endolimax Nana Trophozoites Cysts 1	XTRA	981.59,1070.81,19715.68,21508,	As mentioned above		Amoeba

Subject / Argument	Author	Frequencies	Notes	Origin	Target
Endolimax Nana Trophozoites Cysts 2	XTRA	1067.09,1070.81,1074.17,13453.12,13500,13542.19,	As mentioned above		Amoeba
Endolimax Nana Trophozoites Cysts 3	XTRA	977.25,981.59,984.3,12320.3,12375,12409.37,	As mentioned above		Amoeba
Entamoeba Coli Trophozoites	HC	397000-400350=3600,	Life cycle stage of GI tract parasitic amoeba.		Amoeba
Parasites: Entamoeba coli trophozoites	EDTFL	2500,13930,204510,337300,388950,389000,390700,408150,409000,411150	As mentioned above		Amoeba
Entamoeba Coli Trophozoites 1	XTRA	981.59,984.05,992.37,12375,12406.25,12510.94,	As mentioned above		Amoeba
Entamoeba Coli Trophozoites 2	XTRA	**981.59,19715.68**	As mentioned above		Amoeba
Entamoeba gingivalis	RL	**477**	From Dr. Richard Loyd.		Amoeba
Entamoeba Gingivalis Trophozoite	HC	433800-441000=3600,	Life cycle stage of dental parasitic amoeba.		Amoeba
Parasites: Entamoeba gingivalis trophozoite	EDTFL	680,900,2500,5500,13930,122500,322600,409950,414000,416000	As mentioned above		Amoeba
Entamoeba Gingivalis Trophozoites	XTRA	1075.27,1085.69,1093.13,13556.25,13687.5,13781.25,	As mentioned above		Amoeba
Parasites Entamoeba Gingivalis Trophozoite	XTRA	810,1420,4320,5500,13930,122500,322600,433800,441000,438000,	Life cycle stage of protozoan found in dental spaces.		Amoeba
Entamoeba Histolytica	CAFL	148,166,308,393,631,778,	GI tract parasitic amoeba causing tissue destruction, particularly liver damage - use Liver Support sets.	Liver	Amoeba
Entamoeba Histolytica	VEGA	**148,166,308**	As mentioned above	Liver	Amoeba
Entamoeba Histolytica	BIOM	148; 166; 308; 393; 631; 778		Liver	Amoeba
Entamoeba Histolytica 2	BIOM	1552; 880; 802; 1550; 832; 787; 727; 690; 660; 465; 786; 768; 523; 333		Liver	Amoeba
Entamoeba Histolytica 2	XTRA	333,465,523,660,690,727.5,768,786,787,802,832,880,1550,1552,	As mentioned above	Liver	Amoeba
Entamoeba Histolytica 3	XTRA	148,166,303,333,393,465,523,631,660,690,727.5,768,778,786,787,802,832,880,954.32,1550,1552,19168.02,	As mentioned above	Liver	Amoeba
Entamoeba Histolytica 4	XTRA	148,166,308,393,631,778,	As mentioned above	Liver	Amoeba
Entamoeba Histolytica Secondary	XTRA	333,465,523,660,690,727,768,786,787,802,832,880,1550,1552,	As mentioned above	Liver	Amoeba
Entamoeba Histolytica Trophozoite	HC	381100-367800=3600,	As mentioned above	Liver	Amoeba
Parasites: Entamoeba histolytica trophozoite	EDTFL	2500,13930,204510,337300,388950,389000,390700,418550,421000,423900	As mentioned above	Liver	Amoeba
Entamoeba Histolytica Trophozoite	XTRA	911.69,944.64,954.32,11493.75,11909.37,12031.25,	As mentioned above	Liver	Amoeba
Euglena	CAFL	432,3215,3225,3325,6448,	Water-dwelling unicellular flagellate protist.		Protozoa
Giardia	CAFL	334,407,812,829,2018,4334,5429,	Also called Giardia Intestinalis, or Lamblia - see sets. Parasitic protozoan that colonizes the GI tract.	Intestines	Protozoa
Parasites Giardia	CAFL	334,4334,5429,829,812,2018,407,	As mentioned above	Intestines	Protozoa
Parasites: giardia	EDTFL	170,320,850,2750,17500,47300,75500,97500,151070,451040	As mentioned above	Intestines	Protozoa
Parasites: giardia lamblia type 2	EDTFL	150,380,930,2520,31200,47300,75500,97500,151070,451040,	As mentioned above	Intestines	Protozoa
Parasites: giardia lamblia (trophozoites)	EDTFL	170,320,850,2750,17500,47300,75500,97500,151070,451040,	As mentioned above	Intestines	Protozoa
Giardia Lamblia Trophozoites	HC	421400-426300=3600,	Life cycle stage of parasitic protozoan that colonizes the GI tract.	Intestines	Protozoa
Giardia Parasites	XTRA	334,407,721,812,829,1442,2018,2163,4334,5429,5768,	As mentioned above	Intestines	Protozoa
Giardia Lamblia	XTRA	1044.54,1050.99,1056.69,13168.75,13250,13321.87,	As mentioned above	Intestines	Protozoa
Giardia Intestinalis	XTRA	200=900,334,407,829,1000,2018,4334,5429,13168.75=1200,13250,13454.09,13763.75,14459.37,21109.72,	As mentioned above	Intestines	Protozoa
Giardia Parasites Lamblia	XTRA	**1050.99, 21109.72,**	As mentioned above	Intestines	Protozoa
Lamblia 1	XTRA	334,407,812,829,2018,4334,5429,	As mentioned above	Intestines	Protozoa
Lamblia 2	XTRA	**1050.99,21109.72,**	As mentioned above	Intestines	Protozoa
Lamblia 3	XTRA	334,407,721,812,829,1442,2018,2163,4334,5429,5768,	As mentioned above	Intestines	Protozoa
Giardia	XTRA	**6888887.7777, 6888887.7877**	Biofilm. From Newport. Wave=square, Duty=82.4%, Repeat Set=13. Parasitic protozoan that colonizes GI tract, and causes B12 deficiency.	Intestines	Biofilm

Subject / Argument	Author	Frequencies	Notes	Origin	Target
Lambliasis	BIOM	5768; 5429; 4334; 2163; 2018; 1442; 829; 812; 721; 407; 334		Intestines	Protozoa
Giardiasis [giardia parasite]	EDTFL	170,320,850,2750,17500,47300,75500,97500,151070,451040,	Infection by Giardia Lamblia.	Intestines	Protozoa
Lambliasis	EDTFL	190,300,620,2500,7500,8000,55230,150000,325540,325700		Intestines	Protozoa
Beaver Fever [Giardiasis]	EDTFL	170,320,850,2750,17500,47300,75500,97500,151070,451040,		Intestines	Protozoa
Histomonas Meleagridis	HC	376550-373700=3600,	Parasitic protozoan affecting birds and farmyard poultry which can infect the liver.		Protozoa
Histomonas Meleagridis 1	XTRA	926.3,933.37,934.49,11678.12,11767.19,11781.25,	As mentioned above		Protozoa
Histomonas Meleagridis 2	XTRA	934.49,18769.72	As mentioned above		Protozoa
Parasites: Iodamoeba butschlii	EDTFL	680,900,2500,5500,13930,93500,386400,424450,427000,429550	Parasitic intestinal amoeba.		Protozoa
Iodamoeba Butschlii	XTRA	1103.03,11077.62,	As mentioned above		Protozoa
Iodamoeba Butschlii Trophozoites and Cysts	XTRA	1085.31,1103.03,1111.72,13682.8,13906.25,14015.62,	Life cycle stages of parasitic intestinal amoeba.		Protozoa
Leishmania Amastigote	XTRA	565555.5544	Apply=Frequencies Directly. Use Malt (best) or Malt extract to digest this. Dowsed by Newport. Reported in Morgellons.		Protozoa
Parasites Leishmania Braziliensis	CAFL	787	Protozoan spread by sandflies causing skin, mouth, and nasal conditions.		Protozoa
Leishmania Braziliensis	HC	400050-405100=3600,	As mentioned above		Protozoa
Parasites: Leishmania braziliensis	EDTFL	680,900,2500,5500,13930,93500,386400,386800,393200,395500	As mentioned above		Protozoa
Leishmania Braziliensis	XTRA	991.62,998.94,1004.13,12501.55,12593.75,12659.37,	As mentioned above		Protozoa
Parasites Leishmania Donovani	CAFL	525,781	Protozoan spread by sandflies causing spleen and liver enlargement, and infection of bone marrow.		Protozoa
Leishmania Donovani	HC	398000-402650=3600,	As mentioned above		Protozoa
Parasites: Leishmania donovani	EDTFL	130,220,930,5500,17500,32500,52500,70000,92500,122530	As mentioned above		Protozoa
Leishmania Donovani	XTRA	986.53,991.5,998.07,12437.5,12500,12582.8,	As mentioned above		Protozoa
Leishman-Donovan Bodies	BIO	525	As mentioned above		Protozoa
Leishmania Mexicana	HC	400200-403800=3600,	Protozoan spread by sandflies causing milder form of Leishmaniasis. This can be more serious in those with defective T-cell immunity. See Leishmania Mexicana, and Leishmaniasis programs.		Protozoa
Parasites: Leishmania mexicana	EDTFL	40,320,650,900,5750,7500,37500,150000,375410,496010	As mentioned above		Protozoa
Leishmania Mexicana	XTRA	992,996.46,1000.91,12506.25,12562.5,12618.75	As mentioned above		Protozoa
Parasites Leishmania Tropica	CAFL	791	Protozoan spread by sandflies causing skin problems. See Leishmania Tropica, and Leishmaniasis sets.		Protozoa
Leishmania Tropica	HC	402100-407400=3600,	As mentioned above		Protozoa
Parasites: Leishmania tropica	EDTFL	160,300,570,950,2500,5500,20000,150000,319340,478500	vedi sopra		Protozoa
Leishmania Tropica	XTRA	996.71,1003.88,1009.84,12565.62,12656.25,12731.25,	As mentioned above		Protozoa
Leishmania Virus New	XTRA	428.3,856.6,1713.09	RNA virus found to be present in some species of Leishmania.		Protozoa
Leishmania Virus Old	XTRA	431.8,863.6,1727.2,	As mentioned above		Protozoa
Leishmaniasis	BIOM	787; 525; 781; 791			Protozoa
Leishmaniasis [Leishmania Tropica]	ETDFL	160,300,570,950,2500,5500,20000,150000,319340,478500,	Leishmania infection. Also see species-specific Leishmania sets.		Protozoa
Leucocytozoon	HC	397460-402550=3600,	Parasitic protozoan in birds and poultry.		Protozoa
Parasites: Leucocytozoon	ETDFL	680,900,2500,5500,398150,402000,404750,437850,445000,448500	As mentioned above		Protozoa
Leucocytozoon 1	XTRA	985.2,991.5,997.82,12420.62,125000,12579.69,	As mentioned above		Protozoa
Leucocytozoon 2	XTRA	991.5,19914.83,	As mentioned above		Protozoa
Plasmodium Cynomolgi	HC	417300-424500=3600,	Malaria protozoan.		Protozoa
Parasites: Plasmodium cynomolgi	ETDFL	680,900,2500,5500,13930,93500,356900,362000,364350,386400	As mentioned above		Protozoa
Plasmodium Falciparum Smear	HC	372300-373800=3600,	As mentioned above		Protozoa
Parasites: Plasmodium falciparum smear	ETDFL	680,900,2500,5500,13930,93500,386400,436300,440000,442100	As mentioned above		Protozoa
Plasmodium Vivax Smear	HC	438150-445100=3600,	As mentioned above		Protozoa

Subject / Argument	Author	Frequencies	Notes	Origin	Target
Parasites: Plasmodium vivax smear	ETDFL	680,900,2500,5500,13930,93500,437800,44700 0,452000,454200	As mentioned above		Protozoa
Malaria	CAFL	4,20,28,222,550,713,880,930,1032,1433,1444,1 445,455,743,	Mosquito-borne infectious disease with fever, anemia, and spleen enlargement, caused by parasitic Plasmodium protozoans.	Malaria	Protozoa
Malaria 1	CAFL	**20,555**	As mentioned above	Malaria	Protozoa
Malaria 2	CAFL	**20,28,787,880**	As mentioned above	Malaria	Protozoa
Malaria Falciparum 1	CAFL	1518,1348,1473,1002,1019,	As mentioned above	Malaria	Protozoa
Malaria	BIOM	4; 20; 28; 222; 550; 555; 713; 880; 930; 1032; 1433; 1444; 1445; 455; 743		Malaria	Protozoa
Malaria Falciparum	BIOM	1518; 1348; 1473; 1002; 1019		Malaria	Protozoa
Malaria	ETDFL	180,370,710,920,36510,182580,392110,507380, 672130,721220	Complication of malaria that can lead to kidney failur.	Malaria	Protozoa
Blackwater Fever	ETDFL	190,350,13020,90000,326800,355080,475160,6 67000,789000,986220	As mentioned above	Malaria	Protozoa
Marsh Fever	ETDFL	50,460,950,7500,32500,50000,67600,125910,31 9340,855820	As mentioned above	Malaria	Protozoa
Plasmodium Infections	ETDFL	680,900,2500,5500,13930,93500,356900,36200 0,364350,386400,	As mentioned above	Malaria	Protozoa
Malaria	BIO	222,550,713,930,1032,1433,	As mentioned above	Malaria	Protozoa
Malaria	XTRA	**555**	As mentioned above	Malaria	Protozoa
Malaria 1	XTRA	4,20,28,222,455,550,713,743,880,930,1032,143 3,1444,1445,	As mentioned above	Malaria	Protozoa
Malaria 2	XTRA	20,728,787,800,880,	As mentioned above	Malaria	Protozoa
Malaria 3	XTRA	**20,555**	As mentioned above	Malaria	Protozoa
Malaria 4	XTRA	20,222,455,550,555,713,743,930,1002,1019,103 2,1348,1433,1473,1518,	As mentioned above	Malaria	Protozoa
Malaria Chicken Pox	XTRA	**20**		Malaria	Protozoa
Myxosoma	HC	409600-416950=3600,	Myxosporean parasite of salmonids (salmon, trout, etc.)		Protozoa
Parasites: Myxosoma	ETDFL	680,900,2500,5500,13930,93500,386400,40210 0,405000,407400	As mentioned above		Protozoa
Naegleria Fowleri	HC	356900-364350=3600,	Freshwater parasitic protist amoeba, commonly called 'brain-eating amoeba.'		Amoeba
Parasites: Naegleria fowleri	ETDFL	680,900,2500,5500,13930,93500,386400,39745 0,400000,402550	As mentioned above		Amoeba
Paramecium Caudatum	CAFL	**4500,1150,2298**	Eukaryotic unicellular organism.		Protozoa
Protomyxzoa Rheumatica	XTRA	1583,515,515-521=1260,	Experimental. Protozoan parasite found in Lyme and Morgellons.		Protozoa
Protomyxzoa Rheumatica Spectrum Sweep	XTRA	517.544 - 518.456	As mentioned above		Protozoi
Sarcocystis	HC	450550-454950=3600,	Parasitic protozoan from undercooked meat with Nausea, Abdominal Pain, and Diarrhea (sometimes severe), and, rarely, Vasculitis and Myositis. See sets for these.		Protozoa
Parasites: Sarcocystis	ETDFL	680,900,2500,5500,13930,93500,372300,37300 0,373800,386400	As mentioned above		Protozoa
Sarcocystis neurona (EPM in horses)	RL	**432**	From Dr. Richard Loyd.		Protozoa
Sarcocystis 1	XTRA	14079.69,14217.19,14125,1116.79,1127.71,112 0.4,	As mentioned above		Protozoa
Sarcocystis 2	XTRA	**11251.87,1120.4**	As mentioned above		Protozoa
Toxoplasma gondii		*May cause:* **Alzheimer's disease • Depression • Parkinson's disease • Tourette syndrome**			
Toxoplasma (Human Strain)	HC	**395000**	Parasitic protozoan causing Toxoplasmosis.		Protozoa
Parasites: Toxoplasma [human strain]	ETDFL	130,570,830,2250,5710,32500,97500,332410,37 2000,520000,			Protozoa
Toxoplasma Special	ODD	12343.74,19665.88,979.11,434,853,	As mentioned above		Protozoa
Toxoplasmosis	BIOM	**434; 852; 979.1**			Protozoa
Toxoplasmosis	ETDFL	140,300,5500,24500,40000,93500,517500,6530 00,772290,956030	Infectious disease, caused by the protozoan Toxoplasma gondii, obligate intracellular parasite spread among mammals and birds.		Protozoa
Toxoplasma gondii Infection	ETDFL	140,300,5500,24500,40000,93500,332410,4751 10,667000,752700			Protozoa
Toxoplasmosis	VEGA	**434,852**	As mentioned above		Protozoa
Trichomonas	CAFL	**610,692,980**	Parasitic protozoan, usually sexually transmitted, causing vaginal irritation with discharge and itching.	Vagina	Protozoa
Trichomonas	BIOM	414; 542; 610; 642; 652; 692; 800; 832; 845; 866; 942; 980; 728; 784; 880; 464		Vagina	Protozoa
Trichomonas Vaginalis	HC	378000-383600=3600,	As mentioned above	Vagina	Protozoa
Parasites: Trichomonas vaginalis	ETDFL	680,900,2500,5500,13930,93500,386800,39840 0,400000,402000	Sexually transmitted infection of protozoan causing vaginitis in women and urethritis in men.	Vagina	Protozoa

Subject / Argument	Author	Frequencies	Notes	Origin	Target
Trichomoniasis	BIOM	610; 692; 980; 800; 728; 784; 880; 944.4		Vagina	Protozoa
Trichomonas [Vaginalis protozoa infection]	ETDFL	680,900,2500,5500,13930,93500,386800,398400,400000,402000,	As mentioned above	Vagina	Protozoa
Troglodytella Abrassari	HC	377750-385200=3600,	Parasitic GI protozoan found in primates. Also see Protozoan Infections, and Protozoa sets.		Protozoa
Troglodytella Abrassari 2nd	HC	416900-422200=3600,	As mentioned above		Protozoa
Parasites: Troglodytella abrassari	ETDFL	680,900,2500,5500,13930,93500,386400,388000,395000,422000	As mentioned above		Protozoa
Trypanosoma Brucei	HC	423200-431400=3600,	Protozoan causing Sleeping Sickness - see set.		Protozoa
Parasites: Trypanosoma brucei	ETDFL	680,900,2500,5500,13930,93500,346850,347000,347400,386400	As mentioned above		Protozoa
Trypanosoma Cruzi (Brain Tissue)	HC	460200-465650=3600,	Protozoan causing Chagas Disease (see set). cardiac, GI tract, and peripheral nervous system disorders.		Protozoa
Parasites: Trypanosoma cruzi (brain tissue)	ETDFL	680,900,2500,5500,13930,93500,386400,403850,404500,405570	As mentioned above		Protozoa
Trypanosoma Cruzi (Brain Tissue)	XTRA	14381.25,14451.55,14468.75,1140.72,1154.23,1147.66,	As mentioned above		Protozoa
Parasites Trypanosoma Cruzi Brain Tissue	XTRA	11525.7, 1147.66	As mentioned above		Protozoa
Trypanosoma Equiperdum_1	HC	434600-451250=3600,	Protozoan causing equine diseases.		Protozoa
Trypanosoma Equiperdum_2	HC	442000	As mentioned above		Protozoa
Trypanosoma Equiperdum_3	HC	434600-451250=3600,	As mentioned above		Protozoa
Parasites: Trypanosoma Equiperdum	ETDFL	80,400,730,900,2500,5170,12710,97500,250000,422530	As mentioned above		Protozoa
Parasites: trypanosoma equiperdum	ETDFL	680,900,2500,5500,13930,93500,378000,381000,383600,386400	As mentioned above		Protozoa
Trypanosoma Gambiense	BIO	255,316	Variety of Trypanosoma Brucei causing slow onset of Trypanosomiasis.		Protozoa
Trypanosoma Gambiense	CAFL	255,316,403,700,724,	As mentioned above		Protozoa
Trypanosoma Gambiense	HC	393750-398700=3600,	As mentioned above		Protozoa
Parasites: Trypanosoma gambiense	ETDFL	130,570,850,5170,37100,102790,352500,591020,652930,952590,	As mentioned above		Protozoa
Trypanosoma Lewisi	HC	424500-426000=3600,	Protozoan found in rats and carried by their fleas which can cause disease in humans.		Protozoa
Parasites: trypanosoma lewisi	ETDFL	680,900,2500,5500,13930,93500,386400,423200,429000,431400	As mentioned above		Protozoa
Parasites: Trypanosoma lewisi (blood smear)	ETDFL	240,700,970,2500,27500,45830,67500,97500,325360,451170	As mentioned above		Protozoa
Parasites: trypanosoma lewisi (blood smear)	ETDFL	680,900,2500,5500,93500,383000,385200,416900,419000,422200	As mentioned above		Protozoa
Trypanosoma Rhodesiense	HC	423500-428550=3600,	Variety of Trypanosoma Brucei.		Protozoa
Parasites: Trypanosoma Rhodesiense	ETDFL	130,230,750,850,5250,7250,45000,87500,95360,150000	As mentioned above		Protozoa
Parasites: trypanosoma rhodesiense	ETDFL	60,570,850,5250,7000,20000,52500,90000,356720,425430	As mentioned above		Protozoa
Parasites: trypanosoma rhodesiense	ETDFL	680,900,2500,5500,13930,93500,386400,460200,463000,465650	As mentioned above		Protozoa
Chagas Disease [Trypanosomiasis]	EDTFL	1620,1920,2590,27500,41500,61200,261290,402150,607200,620100,	Also called American Trypanosomiasis. Tropical parasitic disease caused by Trypanosoma Cruzi - see sets for this and Trypanosomiasis.		Protozoa
Chagas Disease A	XTRA	53763.8956,11000.1187,17777.7856,6576.3757	Biofilm-related. Bioweapon. From Newport.		Biofilm
Chagas Disease Biofilm	XTRA	657755.5578	Biofilm. From Newport. Use after Chagas Disease A. If no flare-up present, may be used alone.		Biofilm
African Sleeping Sickness	EDTFL	60,830,970,5160,20000,65000,175110,475110,476500,527000,	Conditions caused by Trypanosoma protozoans, including Sleeping Sickness, and Chagas Disease. Also see Protozoan Infections.		Protozoa
Trypanosomiasis	BIOM	255; 316; 403; 656; 700; 724; 780; 981.6988			Protozoa
Trypanosomiasis {Trypanosoma Protazoa]					
Trypanosomiasis, African Parasite	EDTFL	680,900,2500,5500,13930,93500,378000,381000,383600,386400,	As mentioned above		Protozoa
Trypanosomiasis, South American Parasite					
African Trypanosomiasis	CAFL	656,988,780,	Also called Sleeping Sickness. Protozoan disease caused by Trypanosoma Brucei.		Protozoa

Subject / Argument	Author	Frequencies	Notes	Origin	Target
Nagana [Trypanosoma Infection]	EDTFL	680,900,2500,5500,13930,93500,346850,34700 0,347400,386400,	As mentioned above		Protozoa

Nematodes - Roundworm - Threadworm

Subject / Argument	Author	Frequencies	Notes	Origin	Target
Nematodes	BIO	771	Roundworms.		Roundworm
Nematoda, general	BIOM	104; 535; 543; 688; 728; 771; 799; 1077; 2322; 5050; 5868; 6187.5; 6436; 6468.8; 6436			Roundworm
Parasites Nematode	KHZ	70,120,680,950,2500,7500,27500,92500,269710 ,497610,	Also see Parasites Roundworm.		Roundworm
Anisakiasis	EDTFL KHZ	40,230,780,5620,15050,35330,67500,125000,22 5000,733000,	Due to eating raw/undercooked fish infected with parasitic nematode.		Roundworm
Roundworm	CAFL	20,104,112,120,128,240,332,422,543,650,688,7 21,732,772,827,942,3212,452,4412,5897,7159,	Also called Nematodes. Also see Parasites Nematode, and Parasites Roundworm(s) sets.		Roundworm
Parasites Roundworm General	CAFL	20,104,112,120,128,152,240,332,422,543,650,6 88,721,732,772,827,835,942,2720,3212,4152,44 12,5897,7159,	As mentioned above		Roundworm
Round Worms	BIO	240,650,688	As mentioned above		Roundworm
Round Worms	VEGA	650	As mentioned above		Roundworm
Parasites: roundworms	EDTFL	680,900,2500,9200,13930,25300,93500,417300, 422000,424500	As mentioned above		Roundworm
Parasites Threadworm	CAFL	332,422,721,732,749,942,3212,4412,	Roundworm which can infect human skin, lungs, and GI tract. Common in Morgellons. See Strongyloides, Parasites Strongyloides, Parasites Threadworm, and Strongyloidiasis.		Roundworm
Threadworm	BIO	422,423,732,4412	Common GI parasitic worm, with itching of anus. See Enterobius Vermicularis, Pinworm, and Anal Itching sets.	Anus	Roundworm
Threadworm	VEGA	423,732,4412	As mentioned above	Anus	Roundworm
Parasites: threadworms	EDTFL	680,900,2500,5500,13930,93500,386400,39890 0,400000,402000	As mentioned above	Anus	Roundworm
Hookworm	CAFL	6.8,440,2008,5868,6436,	Blood-feeding roundworm. See Parasites Hookworm, Creeping Eruption, and Larva Migrans.		Roundworm
Hookworm disease	BIOM	6.8; 440; 2008; 5868; 6436			Roundworm
Parasites Hookworm	CAFL	6.8,440,2008,6436,5868,	As mentioned above		Roundworm
Parasites: hookworm	EDTFL	170,460,10880,55160,96500,350000,567000,69 2330,810200,982110,	As mentioned above		Roundworm
Hookworm Infections	EDTFL	170,460,10880,55160,96500,350000,567000,69 2330,810200,982110	Infection by blood-feeding roundworms. See Hookworm, Creeping Eruption, and Larva Migrans.		Roundworm
Bunostomiasis	EDTFL	100,580,780,5250,21800,49480,158000,342060, 475160,533000	As mentioned above		Roundworm
Ancylostoma Braziliense	HC	397600-403250=3600,	Hookworm in dogs and cats. Can cause Cutaneous Larval Migration in humans. See Hookworm, Creeping Eruption, and Larva Migrans.		Roundworm
Ancylostoma Braziliense	XTRA	985.54,993.98,999.55,12425,12531.25,12601.55 ,	As mentioned above		Roundworm
Parasites Ancylostoma Braziliense Adult	XTRA	680,900,2500,5500,13930,122500,322600,3976 00,403250,401000,	As mentioned above		Roundworm
Parasites: Ancylostoma braziliense (adult)	EDTFL	80,380,760,900,7520,10320,140000,232500,725 470,925370	As mentioned above		Roundworm
Larva Migrans [Hookworm Infection]	EDTFL	170,460,10880,55160,96500,350000,567000,69 2330,810200,982110,	It is caused by Ancylostoma infection		Roundworm
Ancylostoma Caninum_1	HC	383100-402900=3600,	Hookworm in dogs. Can cause Cutaneous Larval Migration in humans. See Hookworm, Creeping Eruption, and Larva Migrans.	Dog	Roundworm
Ancylostoma Caninum_2	HC	393000	As mentioned above	Dog	Roundworm
Ancylostoma Caninum_3	HC	383100-402900=3600,	As mentioned above	Dog	Roundworm
Parasites: Ancylostoma caninum	EDTFL	80,390,780,950,7520,10320,140000,232500,725 470,925370	As mentioned above	Dog	Roundworm
Ancylostoma Caninum 1	XTRA	949.61,991.5,998.69,11971.87,12500,12590.62,	As mentioned above	Dog	Roundworm
Ancylostoma Caninum 2	XTRA	949.61,974.14,998.69,11971.87,12281.25,12590 .62,	As mentioned above	Dog	Roundworm
Ancylostoma Caninum 3	XTRA	949.61,956.79,998.69,11971.87,12062.5,12590. 62,	As mentioned above	Dog	Roundworm
Angiostrongylus Cantonensis Angiostrongyliasis	EDTFL	680,900,2500,9200,13930,25300,93500,417300, 422000,424500	It is a parasitic nematode that causes angiostrongyliasis, the most common cause of eosinophilic meningitis		Roundworm
Rat Lungworm Disease	EDTFL	680,900,2500,9200,13930,25300,93500,417300, 422000,424500	The nematode commonly resides in the pulmonary arteries of rats, hence the name.		Roundworm

Subject / Argument	Author	Frequencies	Notes	Origin	Target
Parasites Ascaris	CAFL	442,8146,751,1146,797,152,	Roundworm (nematode) usually found in small intestine.	Intestines	Roundworm
Ascaris Megalocephala (Male)	HC	403850-409700=3600,	As mentioned above	Intestines	Roundworm
Parasites: Ascaris megalocephala (male)	EDTFL	680,900,2500,5500,13930,93500,386400,387000,388000,422000	As mentioned above	Intestines	Roundworm
Ascaris Megalocephala All Stages	XTRA	128159.7732=300,111.1211,8810.5764=360,22450.8855=300,34688.1655=300,	First freq wakes hibernating parasites, last two kill Candida tropicalis (needed by this). Multiple treatments over many days may be needed.	Intestines	Roundworm
Ascaris Larvae	HC	404900-409150=3600,	Parasitic roundworm Ascaris lumbricoides.	Intestines	Roundworm
Ascaris Larvae	XTRA	1003.64,1011.33,1014.17,12653.12,12750,12785.94,	As mentioned above	Intestines	Roundworm
Ascaris Lumbricoides All Stages	XTRA	471910.2143=1200,55455.4555=120,7456.5499=240,4777.5565=360,	SRH4. Use cloves to calm parasites between treatments.	Intestines	Roundworm
Ascariasis	BIOM	152; 442; 751; 797; 1011.3; 1146; 8146		Intestines	Roundworm
Ascariasis	EDTFL KHZ	60,1330,5270,10890,90000,379930,425000,571000,829000,932000,	Caused by the parasitic roundworm Ascaris Lumbricoides.	Intestines	Roundworm
Baylisascaris	RL	763	From Dr. Richard Loyd. Infection with the raccoon roundworm, Baylisascaris procyonis.	Intestines	Roundworm
Parasites: Capillaria hepatica (liver section)	EDTFL	680,900,2500,13930,123530,383100,386000,393000,400000,402900	Nematode inhabiting the liver.	Liver	Roundworm
Parasites Capillaria Hepatica	XTRA	1060.91, 21308.86	As mentioned above	Liver	Roundworm
Capillariasis	BIOM	940; 947; 982; 987; 4000; 706; 4000; 706; 4000			Roundworm
Dracunculiasis	EDTFL	80,410,800,2500,7500,30000,65310,125000,355720,422530	Subcutaneous parasitosis, caused by guinea worm (Dracunculus medinensis). Causes slowly moving burning pain, fever, nausea, and vomiting.		Roundworm
Guinea Worm Infection	EDTFL	40,250,690,48140,142790,219270,322200,592200,765290,822340	As mentioned above		Roundworm
Parasites Enterobiasis	CAFL	20,120,773,826,827,835,4152,	Intestinal worms which cause itching of anal and perineal areas. See Anal Itching, and Pruritis sets. Pinworms.	Anus	Roundworm
Enterobius Vermicularis	HC	420950-425300=3600,	As mentioned above	Anus	Roundworm
Parasites: Enterobius vermicularis	EDTFL	680,900,2500,5500,13930,122500,322600,425500,427000,428750	As mentioned above	Anus	Roundworm
Enterobius Vermicularis 2	XTRA	1043.43,1048.5,1054.21,13154.69,13218.75,13290.62,	As mentioned above	Anus	Roundworm
Enterobius Vermicularis 1	XTRA	422,423,732,733,827,835,4412,13154.69=1800,13218.75,21059.93,	As mentioned above	Anus	Roundworm
Enterobiasis	CAFL	20,222,773,826,827,835,4152,	As mentioned above	Anus	Roundworm
Enterobiasis	BIOM	112; 120; 773; 826; 827; 835; 4152		Anus	Roundworm
Enterobiasis	VEGA	773,827,835	As mentioned above	Anus	Roundworm
Filariose	BIO	112,120	Also called Filariasis - see set. Parasitic infection of roundworm spread by blood-feeding flies. Also see Round Worms, Roundworm, and Parasites Roundworm sets		Roundworm
Parasites Filariose	CAFL	112,120,332,753	Worms in blood and organs of mammals - larvae passed by biting insects.	Blood Organs	Roundworm
Parasites: filariose	EDTFL	680,900,2500,5500,13930,93500,386400,427700,434000,435100,	As mentioned above		Roundworm
Brugia malayi	RL	334	From Dr. Richard Loyd. Parasite that causes lymphatic filariasis, otherwise known as "elephantiasis".		Roundworm
Microfilaria bolivarensis	RL	466	From Dr. Richard Loyd. A New Species of Filaria from Man in Venezuela .		Roundworm
Filariasis	BIOM	112; 120; 332; 753; 1090.7			Roundworm
Filariasis	EDTFL	110,550,960,5500,17500,37500,162500,383500,421000,645250	Parasitic infection of roundworm spread by blood-feeding flies. Also see Round Worms, Roundworm, and Parasites Roundworm sets		Roundworm
Filarioidea Infections	EDTFL	90,250,970,9000,73860,123200,257500,302580,592490,875430	As mentioned above		Roundworm
Elaeophoriasis	EDTFL	150,180,930,2750,125320,246200,405000,731500,826500,921340	As mentioned above		Roundworm
Haemonchus Contortus	HC	386800-395000=3600,	Parasitic GI tract nematode in cattle, sheep, and goats.		Roundworm
Parasites: Haemonchus contortus	EDTFL	40,320,650,900,5870,7500,37500,421400,424000,426300	As mentioned above		Roundworm
Parasites: Haemonchus contortus	EDTFL	160,300,680,930,2500,5500,13930,93500,356720,451170	As mentioned above		Roundworm
Haemonchus Contortus	XTRA	958.77,974.14,979.11,12087.5,12281.25,12343.75,	As mentioned above		Roundworm
Haemonchus Contortus	BIOM	974.2			Roundworm

Subject / Argument	Author	Frequencies	Notes	Origin	Target
Heartworms	CAFL	200,535,799,1077,2322,	Also called Dog Heartworm. Parasitic mosquito-borne filaria that can infect other animals, and humans. See Dirofilaria Immitis and Parasites Heartworms.		Roundworm
Parasites Heartworms	CAFL	543,2322,200,535,1077,799,	As mentioned above		Roundworm
Dirofilaria Immitis	CAFL	200,535,543,799,1077,2322,	As mentioned above		Roundworm
Dirofilaria Immitis Dog Heartworm	HC	408150-411150=3600,	As mentioned above		Roundworm
Heartworms	BIO	543,2322	As mentioned above		Roundworm
Parasites: heartworms	ETDFL	160,300,570,850,2750,12330,20000,150000,326070,479500	As mentioned above		Roundworm
Parasites: Dirofilaria immitis/dog heartworm	ETDFL	2500,13930,204510,337300,388950,389000,390700,425200,426000,427300	As mentioned above		Roundworm
Dirofilaria Immitis 1	XTRA	1011.7,1013.8,1019.13,12754.69,12781.25,12848.44,	As mentioned above		Roundworm
Dirofilaria Immitis 2	XTRA	200,535,543,728,799,1077,2322,	As mentioned above		Roundworm
Dirofilaria Immitis 3	XTRA	200,535,543,799,1077,2322,	As mentioned above		Roundworm
Dirofilariasis	BIOM	728; 1013.8; 543; 2322; 200; 535; 1077; 799; 728; 1013.8			Roundworm
Loa Loa	HC	360551	Parasitic roundworm commonly called 'eye worm,' transmitted by deer fly and mango fly. Also see Loiasis, Filariasis, Filariose, and other Roundworm sets.		Roundworm
Parasites: Loa loa	ETDFL	680,900,2500,5500,13930,93500,386400,400050,403000,405100	As mentioned above		Roundworm
Loa Loa	XTRA	893.72	As mentioned above		Roundworm
Loaiasis	BIOM	894.8			Roundworm
Loaiasis	ETDFL	680,900,2500,5500,13930,93500,386400,400050,403000,405100,	Skin and eye disease due to loa loa nematode worm transmitted by deer fly and mango fly.	Skin and eye	Roundworm
Loiasis [Loa Loa Parasite]	ETDFL	680,900,2500,5500,13930,93500,386400,400050,403000,405100,	As mentioned above	Skin and eye	Roundworm
Onchocerca Volvulus (Tumor)	HC	435300-442100=3600,	Nematode that causes Onchocerciasis - see sets. Larvae form tumor-like nodules in subcutaneous tissue.		Roundworm
Parasites: Onchocerca volvulus (tumor)	ETDFL	680,900,2500,5500,13930,93500,360550,361000,386400,388000	As mentioned above		Roundworm
Onchocerciasis [Roundworm]	ETDFL	680,900,2500,9200,13930,25300,93500,417300,422000,424500,	Infection by Onchocerca Volvulus - see set.		Roundworm
Onchocerciasis 2	XTRA	2250=720,13600,15000,40000,31477,39660,10300,36469,35444,	As mentioned above		Roundworm
Parasites: Pinworm	ETDFL	680,900,2500,5500,13930,93500,386400,409600,414000,416950	Common GI parasitic worm, with Anal Itching (see set). Also see Enterobius Vermicularis, Enterobiasis, Parasites Enterobiasis, and Threadworm sets.	Anus	Roundworm
Pin Worms [Pinworm]	ETDFL	680,900,2500,5500,13930,93500,386400,409600,414000,416950,		Anus	Roundworm
Passalurus Ambiguus_1	HC	428800-444150=3600,	Pinworms found in rabbits and hares.		Roundworm
Passalurus Ambiguus_2	HC	437000	As mentioned above		Roundworm
Parasites: Passalurus ambiguus	ETDFL	680,900,2500,5500,13930,93500,386400,437350,440000,442100	As mentioned above		Roundworm
Stephanurus Dentalus (Ova)	HC	467350-463100=3600,	Eggs of large kidney worm parasitizing swine.		Roundworm
Parasites: Stephanurus denta_us (ova)	ETDFL	680,900,2500,5500,13930,93500,386400,387000,388000,473000	As mentioned above		Roundworm
Parasites Strongyloides	CAFL	332,422,721,732,749,942,3212,4412,	Roundworm which can infect human skin, lungs, and GI tract. Common in Morgellons. See Parasites Threadworm.		Roundworm
Parasites Strongyloides Secondary	CAFL	380,698,722,738,746,752,776,1113,	As mentioned above		Roundworm
Strongyloides	BIO	332,422,721,942,3212,	As mentioned above		Roundworm
Strongyloides (Filariform Larva)	HC	398400-402000=3600,	As mentioned above		Roundworm
Parasites: Strongyloides (filariform larva)	ETDFL	120,680,2500,60000,122530,300000,496010,655200,750000,912330,	As mentioned above		Roundworm
Strongyloidiasis	ETDFL	120,680,2500,60000,122530,300000,496010,655200,750000,912330	As mentioned above		Roundworm
Toxocariasis	ETDFL	250,870,5120,85000,100000,355720,425160,571000,837000,937410	Infection in humans of dog, cat, or fox roundworm. Major cause of blindness, and may provoke rheumatic, neurologic, or asthmatic symptoms.		Roundworm
Trichinella Spiralis Muscle	HC	403850-405570=3600,	Nematode commonly found in undercooked pork causing Trichinosis.		Roundworm
Trichinella	BIOM	101.0; 541.0; 822.0; 1053.9; 1372.0			Roundworm
Parasites: Trichinella spiralis (muscle)	ETDFL	100,250,680,2750,5750,7600,96500,215700,475000,527000	As mentioned above		Roundworm

Subject / Argument	Author	Frequencies	Notes	Origin	Target
Trichinella Spiralis Muscle	XTRA	12620.3,12674.05,12640.62,1001.03,1005.3,1002.65,	As mentioned above		Roundworm
Parasites Trichinella Spiralis	XTRA	1002.65, 20138.86	As mentioned above		Roundworm
Parasites Trichinosis	CAFL	101,541,822,1054,1372,	As mentioned above		Roundworm
Trichinosis	BIOM	101; 541; 822; 1002.66; 1054; 1372		Intestines	Roundworm
Trichinosis	BIO	101,541,822,1054,1372,	Caused by ingestion of Trichinella Spiralis, usually in undercooked pork.	Intestines	Roundworm
Trichinosis	VEGA	541,1372	As mentioned above	Intestines	Roundworm
Trichinosis [Trichinella Roundworm infection]	EDTFL	100,250,680,2500,5870,7500,96500,215700,475000,527000,	As mentioned above	Intestines	Roundworm
Trichinelliasis	EDTFL	100,250,680,2500,5870,7500,96500,215700,475000,527000,		Intestines	Roundworm
Trichinosis 1	XTRA	101,230,541,822,1054,1372,12620.3=1800,12640.62,20138.86,	As mentioned above	Intestines	Roundworm
Trichinosis 3	XTRA	5411372	As mentioned above	Intestines	Roundworm
Trichuris Species Male	HC	388300-408900=3600,	Type of Roundworm called Whipworm - see sets.		Roundworm
Parasites: Trichuris spiralis (male)	EDTFL	680,900,2500,5500,13930,93500,386400,420550,427150,428000	As mentioned above		Roundworm
Parasites Trichuris	KHZ	50,120,750,800,5170,17500,67500,222530,225910,454370,	As mentioned above		Roundworm
Trichuris Species Male	XTRA	12134.37,12778.12,12687.5,962.5,1013.55,1006.37,	As mentioned above		Roundworm
Turbatrix	CAFL	104	Also called vinegar eels. Non-parasitic nematodes feeding on mother of vinegar, filtered by suppliers. See Turbatrix.		Roundworm
Parasites: Turbatrix	EDTFL	130,570,850,5750,7500,20000,52500,90000,358570,475440	As mentioned above		Roundworm
Parasites: turbatrix	EDTFL	120,150,620,830,2750,10530,15910,96500,225410,524370	As mentioned above		Roundworm
Parasites Whipworm	XTRA	13134.37,12687.5,20213.54,	Type of Roundworm - see sets. Also see Parasites Trichuris and Trichuris Species Male sets.		Roundworm
Whipworm Infections	EDTFL	60,320,900,32500,67500,97000,325750,519340,691270,754190	As mentioned above		Roundworm

					Trematodes
Trematodes	BIOM	6765.5; 6671.5; 6640.5; 6577.5; 2150; 2128; 2082; 2013; 2008; 2003; 2000; 1850; 945; 854; 846; 763; 676; 664; 651; 524; 435; 435; 275; 143; 142			Trematodes
Blood trematodes	BIOM	157; 329; 419; 469; 635; 847; 867; 5516; 6889; 7391			Trematodes
Small intestine trematodes	BIOM	524; 651; 676; 2084; 2128; 2150; 6766			Trematodes
Clonorchis Sinensis	HC	425700-428750=3600,	Blood fluke. Also see Parasites Clonorchis Sinensis.	Blood	Trematodes
Clonorchis Sinensis	XTRA	1055.2,1058.43,1062.75,13303.12,13343.75,13398.44,	Blood fluke.	Blood	Trematodes
Parasites: Clonorchis sinensis	EDTFL	680,900,2500,13930,204510,331000,337300,458800,460000,462900	Liver fluke.	Liver	Trematodes
Parasites Clonorchis Sinensis 1	XTRA	1058.43, 21259.08	Liver fluke.	Liver	Trematodes
Clonorchiasis	BIOM	1058.4			Trematodes
Cryptocotyle Lingua (Adult)	HC	409950-416000=3600,	Parasitic trematode in fish that can infect humans.		Trematodes
Parasites: Cryptocotyle lingua (adult)	EDTFL	680,900,2500,13930,204510,331000,337300,352800,358000,361400	As mentioned above		Trematodes
Cryptocotyle Lingua (Adult)	XTRA	1016.15,1026.2,1031.16,12810.94,12937.5,13000,	As mentioned above		Trematodes
Echinoparyphium Recurvatum	HC	418550-423900=3600,	Type of fluke normally found in domesticated birds.		Trematodes
Parasites: Echinoporyphium recurvatum	EDTFL	2500,13930,204510,337300,388950,389000,390700,393750,398000,400000	As mentioned above		Trematodes
Echinoparyphium Recurvatum	XTRA	1037.48,1043.54,1050.74,13079.69,13156.25,13246.87,	As mentioned above		Trematodes
Parasites Echinoparyphium Recurvatum	XTRA	2500,13930,204510,337300,388950,390700,389000,418550,423900,421000,	Fluke usually found in European freshwater snails.		Trematodes
Echinostoma Revolutum	HC	425500-429650=3600,	Type of fluke ingested from undercooked snails, shellfish, and frogs.		Trematodes
Parasites: Echinostoma revolutum	EDTFL	680,900,2500,5500,13930,122500,322400,425700,427000,428750	As mentioned above		Trematodes
Echinostoma Revolutum	XTRA	1054.71,1060.91,1065,13296.87,13375,13426.55,	As mentioned above		Trematodes
Flukes	XTRA	143,275,435,524,651,676,763,854,945,	All species. Also see appropriate fluke sets for species/organ.		Trematodes

Subject / Argument	Author	Frequencies	Notes	Origin	Target
Parasites General Flukes	CAFL	142,275,435,524,651,676,763,830,846,854,945, 1850,2000,2003,2008,2013,2082,2150,6578,664 1,6672,6766,	Pancreatic, liver, and intestinal flukes.		Trematodes
Parasites: flukes general	EDTFL	680,900,2500,5500,13930,93500,386400,42730 0,432000,433000			Trematodes
Parasites Blood Flukes	CAFL	329,419,635,847,5516,7391,9889,		Blood	Trematodes
Parasites: flukes blood	EDTFL	680,900,2500,5500,13930,93500,386400,42735 0,434000,435200		Blood	Trematodes
Parasites Brain and Spinal Flukes	CAFL	421,434		Nerve	Trematodes
Parasites Lymph Flukes	CAFL	157,10050	Vedi anche Liver flukes.	Lymph	Trematodes
Parasites: flukes lymph	EDTFL	30,240,700,1290,12330,27500,35410,142000,35 7770,475910		Lymph	Trematodes
Parasites Liver Flukes	CAFL	143,238,275,676,763,6641,6672,	Liver fluke life cycle stage.	Liver	Trematodes
Parasites: flukes liver	EDTFL	190,520,780,1220,5200,13390,17500,72500,234 250,425430	As mentioned above	Liver	Trematodes
Fasciola Hepatica	BIO	143,275	As mentioned above	Liver	Trematodes
Parasites: Fasciola Hepatica	ETDFL	1420,4320,5500,13930,122500,322600,394250, 396000,397100,432000	As mentioned above	Liver	Trematodes
Fasciola Hepatica 1	XTRA	13167.19,13353.12,13281.25,1044.42,1059.17,1 053.47,	As mentioned above	Liver	Trematodes
Fasciola Hepatica 2	XTRA	1044.42,1053.47,1059.17,13167.19,13281.25,13 353.12,	As mentioned above	Liver	Trematodes
Parasites: Fasciola hepatica cercariae	ETDFL	1420,4320,5500,13930,122500,322600,394250, 396000,397100,432000	Intermediate stage of sheep liver fluke.	Liver	Trematodes
Fasciola Hepatica Cercariae	XTRA	1050.5,1058.43,1067.34,13243.75,13343.75,134 56.25,	As mentioned above	Liver	Trematodes
Parasites Fasciola Hepatica Cercariae	XTRA	1058.43, 21259.08	As mentioned above	Liver	Trematodes
Fasciola Hepatica Miracidia	HC	421750-424700=3600,	Free-living sheep liver fluke larvae.	Liver	Trematodes
Parasites: Fasciola hepatica miracidia	ETDFL	680,900,2500,5500,13930,93500,386400,42095 0,423000,426300	As mentioned above	Liver	Trematodes
Fasciola Hepatica Miracidia	XTRA	1045.41,1048.5,1052.73,13179.69,13218.75,132 71.87,	As mentioned above	Liver	Trematodes
Parasites Fasciola Hepatica Miracidia 1	XTRA	1048.5, 21059.93,	As mentioned above	Liver	Trematodes
Fasciola Hepatica Rediae	HC	420600-427500=3600,	Free-living sheep liver fluke larvae with sucker.	Liver	Trematodes
Parasites: Fasciola Hepatica Rediae	ETDFL	680,900,2500,5500,13930,93500,386400,42035 0,421000,422300	As mentioned above	Liver	Trematodes
Fasciola Hepatica Rediae	XTRA	1042.55,1053.47,1059.67,13153.75,13281.25,13 359.37,	As mentioned above	Liver	Trematodes
Fasciola Hepatica Eggs	HC	422000-427600=3600,	Egg stage of liver fluke.	Liver	Trematodes
Parasites: Fasciola hepatica eggs	ETDFL	1420,4320,5500,13930,122500,322600,381100, 385000,387000,394250	As mentioned above	Liver	Trematodes
Fasciola Hepatica Eggs	XTRA	1046.02,1053.47,1059.91,13187.5,13281.25,133 62.5,	As mentioned above	Liver	Trematodes
Parasites Fasciola Hepatica Eggs	XTRA	1053.47, 21159.5,	As mentioned above	Liver	Trematodes
Fascioliasis	BIOM	1048.5; 1053.5; 1058.4		Liver	Trematodes
Fascioliasis	ETDFL	150,570,81300,103710,221500,337500,570510, 691510,775480,971550	Liver fluke infection.	Liver	Trematodes
Parasites Sheep Liver Flukes	CAFL	826,830,834,	As mentioned above	Animal	Trematodes
Parasites: flukes sheep liver	ETDFL	110,320,900,2530,17500,47430,78100,90000,15 7000,425410	As mentioned above	Animal	Trematodes
Eurytrema Pancreaticum	HC	420350-422300=3600,	Pancreatic fluke in sheep, goats, pigs, cattle, donkeys, and camels that can infect man.	Pancreas	Trematodes
Parasites: Eurytrema pancreaticum	ETDFL	810,1420,4320,5500,13930,122500,322600,433 800,438000,441000	As mentioned above	Pancreas	Trematodes
Eurytrema Pancreaticum	XTRA	1850,2000,2003,2008,2013,2050,2080,6578,131 35.94=1200,13156.25,20960.36,	As mentioned above	Pancreas	Trematodes
Eurytrematosis	BIOM	1043.6; 1046.8; 1041.9		Pancreas	Trematodes
Parasites Pancreatic Flukes	CAFL	1850,2000,2003,2008,2013,2050,2080,6578,	Experimental	Pancreas	Trematodes
Parasites: flukes pancreatic	ETDFL	140,320,870,2580,17500,44430,72500,92500,15 1000,453720	As mentioned above	Pancreas	Trematodes
Parasites Intestinal Flukes	CAFL	524,651,676,844,848,2008,2084,2128,2150,676 6,	Experimental.	Intestines	Trematodes
Parasites: flukes intestinal	ETDFL	230,500,2800,5230,11910,91110,401430,43400 0,443210,454250		Intestines	Trematodes

Subject / Argument	Author	Frequencies	Notes	Origin	Target
Fluke Intestinal	XTRA	15,55,524,651,676,844,848,854,2000,2084,2128,2150,6766,	Also see Fasciolopsis Buski, Parasites Intestinal Flukes, and Parasites General Flukes.	Intestines	Trematodes
Flukeworm	BIO	524,854	Parasitic Flatworms, including tapeworms, that invade many body areas. Also see appropriate fluke sets for species/organ.		Trematodes
Fasciolopsis Fluke	XTRA	15,55,1070.81,1075.77,2000,21508,21607.59,	Large common human intestinal fluke, also found in pigs. See Fluke Intestinal, Parasites Flukes Intestinal, and Parasites Intestinal Flukes.	Intestines	Trematodes
Fasciolopsis Buski Adult	CAFL	846,847.7,2000	As mentioned above	Intestines	Trematodes
Fasciolopsis Buski Adult	HC	427700-435100=3600,	As mentioned above	Intestines	Trematodes
Parasites: Fasciolopsis buski adult	EDTFL	680,900,2500,5500,13930,93500,386400,423800,427000,430600	As mentioned above	Intestines	Trematodes
Fasciolopsis Buski Adult 2	XTRA	1060.16,1075.77,1078.5,13365.62,13652.5,13596.87,	As mentioned above	Intestines	Trematodes
Fasciolopsis Cercariae	HC	429500-435250=3600,	Intermediate stage of intestinal fluke.	Intestines	Trematodes
Parasites: Fasciolopsis cercariae	EDTFL	680,900,2500,5500,13930,93500,386400,422000,425000,427600	As mentioned above	Intestines	Trematodes
Fasciolopsis Cercariae	XTRA	1064.61,1075.77,1078.88,13421.87,13562.5,13601.55,	As mentioned above	Intestines	Trematodes
Fasciolopsis Miracidia	HC	427350-435200=3600,	Life cycle stage of large common human intestinal fluke, also found in pigs.	Intestines	Trematodes
Parasites: Fasciolopsis miracidia	EDTFL	680,900,2500,5500,13930,93500,386400,421750,423000,424700	As mentioned above	Intestines	Trematodes
Fasciolopsis Miracidia	XTRA	1059.28,1075.77,1978.75,13354.69,13562.5,13600,	As mentioned above	Intestines	Trematodes
Fasciolopsis Rediae	HC	427300-433000=3600,	Free-living liver fluke larvae with sucker.	Intestines	Trematodes
Parasites: Fasciolopsis rediae	EDTFL	680,900,2500,5500,13930,93500,386400,420600,425000,427500	As mentioned above	Intestines	Trematodes
Fasciolopsis Rediae	XTRA	1059.17,1070.81,1073.29,13353.12,13500,13531.25,	As mentioned above	Intestines	Trematodes
Fasciolopsis Buski Eggs	CAFL	15,846,847.7	Egg stage of fluke.	Intestines	Trematodes
Fasciolopsis Buski Eggs	HC	427350-435450=3600,	As mentioned above	Intestines	Trematodes
Parasites: Fasciolopsis buski eggs	EDTFL	680,900,2500,5500,13930,93500,386400,421350,425000,427300	As mentioned above	Intestines	Trematodes
Fasciolopsis Buski Eggs 2	XTRA	1059.28,1075.77,1079.36,13354.69,13562.5,13607.8,	As mentioned above	Intestines	Trematodes
Fischoederius Elongatus	HC	441750-443200=3600,	Bovine fluke found in GI tract.	Animal	Trematodes
Parasites: fischoedrius elongatus	EDTFL	680,900,2500,5500,13930,93500,386400,427350,434000,435450	As mentioned above		Trematodes
Fischoederius Elongatus	XTRA	1094.99,1095.6,1098.57,13804.69,13812.5,13850,	As mentioned above	Animal	Trematodes
Parasites: Flatworms	EDTFL	680,900,2500,5500,13930,93500,386400,429500,434000,436250	Flukes		Trematodes
Gastrothylax Elongatus	HC	451900-457100=3600,	Type of intestinal fluke. Fluke that infects ruminants and can infect man.		Trematodes
Parasites: Gastrothylax elongatus	EDTFL	180,400,800,5500,27500,45370,72500,92500,132000,478500	As mentioned above		Trematodes
Gastrothylax Elongatus	XTRA	1120.15,1127.82,1133.03,14218.75,14284.37,	As mentioned above		Trematodes
Gyrodactylus	HC	378750-381800=3600,	Ectoparasitic fluke found in sea fish.		Trematodes
Parasites: Gyrodactylus	EDTFL	520,680,970,2500,27500,35910,95430,375370,533630,653690	As mentioned above		Trematodes
Parasites: gyrodactylus	EDTFL	50,120,900,5500,15410,27500,45000,421400,424000,426300	As mentioned above		Trematodes
Gyrodactylus	XTRA	938.83,941.92,946.38,11835.94,11875,11931.25,	As mentioned above		Trematodes
Parasites: Hasstile sig. tricolor (adult)	EDTFL	680,900,2500,5500,13930,93500,378750,380000,381800,386400	Rabbit fluke		Trematodes
Parasites: Hypodereum conoideum	EDTFL	410,600,850,5170,22500,57500,322060,475430,575440,627000	Is a species of digenetic trematodes in the family Echinostomatidae.		Trematodes
Metagonimus Yokogawai	HC	437350-442100=3600,	Tiny intestinal fluke associated with raw or undercooked fish.		Trematodes
Parasites: Metagonimus Yokogawai	EDTFL	680,900,2500,5500,13930,93500,386400,400200,402000,403800	Fluke found in fish which can infect man.		Trematodes
Paragonimus Westermani Adult_1	HC	437800-454200=3600,	Also called Japanese Lung Fluke. Food-borne parasitic flatworm. See Parasites Paragonimus Westermani.		Trematodes
Paragonimus Westermani Adult_2	HC	447000	As mentioned above		Trematodes

Subject / Argument	Author	Frequencies	Notes	Origin	Target
Parasites: Paragonimus Westermanii adult	EDTFL	680,900,2500,5500,13930,93500,386400,43885 0,440000,442800	As mentioned above		Trematodes
Paragonimiasis	BIOM	1108; 1120.4			Trematodes
Prostnogonimus Macrorchis Egg	HC	396850-404750=3600,	Is an avian parasite found in regions of the United States and Canada near the Great Lakes.		Trematodes
Parasites: Prosthogonimus macrorchis(eggs)	EDTFL	70,520,750,970,2500,12330,22500,65430,32206 0,475430	As mentioned above		Trematodes
Parasites Schistosoma Haematobium	CAFL	847,867,635,	Blood flukes. Associated with bladder problems. Also see Schistosoma Haematobium, and Blood Fluke sets.	Blood	Trematodes
Schistosoma Haematobium	HC	473000	Blood fluke. Associated with bladder problems. Also see Parasites Schistosoma Haematobium, and Blood Fluke sets.	Blood	Trematodes
Parasites: Schistosoma haematobium	ETDFL	680,900,2500,5500,13930,93500,386400,40575 0,407000,409150	As mentioned above	Blood	Trematodes
Parasites: schistosoma haematobium	ETDFL	680,900,2500,5500,13930,93500,386400,45055 0,452000,454950	As mentioned above	Blood	Trematodes
Parasites: schistosoma haematobium (blood flukes)	ETDFL	60,520,620,930,2500,15440,42500,100000,3762 90,450000	As mentioned above	Blood	Trematodes
Schistosoma Mansoni	BIOM	329; 9888.5		Blood	Trematodes
Schistosoma Mansoni	HC	353000	Blood fluke which can cause symptoms identical to Hepatitis C. Also see Parasites Schistosoma Mansoni, and Blood Flukes sets.	Blood	Trematodes
Parasites Schistosoma Mansoni	CAFL	329,9889	As mentioned above	Blood	Trematodes
Parasites: Schistosoma mansoni	ETDFL	680,900,2500,5500,13930,93500,386400,39685 0,401000,404750	As mentioned above	Blood	Trematodes
Parasites: schistosoma mansoni	ETDFL	70,120,800,5500,15000,27500,510200,667500,8 90520,907500	As mentioned above	Blood	Trematodes
Schistosoma Mansoni 1	XTRA	329,9889,1035.49,1087.17,1089.25,1238.74,125 7.39,1261.5,1272.83,1350.21,1431.24,1564.68,1 734.89,1799.56,1910.33,11031.25,	As mentioned above	Blood	Trematodes
Bilharziasis	ETDFL	140,260,5620,42500,65110,90000,517400,6882 90,712230,997870	Blood fluke infection. Also see Blood Flukes, Bilharzia.	Blood	Trematodes
Schistosomiasis [Katayama Flatworm]	ETDFL	680,900,2500,5500,13930,93500,386400,42950 0,434000,436250,	As mentioned above	Blood	Trematodes
Schistosomiasis, intestinal	BIOM	329; 464; 6889		Blood	Trematodes
Schistosomiasis, urinary	BIOM	174; 635; 847; 867; 1172.5		Blood	Trematodes
Urocleidus	HC	442350-450000=3600,	Fluke found in fish.		Trematodes
Parasites: Urocleidus	ETDFL	680,900,2500,5500,13930,93500,386400,40175 0,403000,405200	As mentioned above		Trematodes
Parasites: urocleidus	ETDFL	70,220,680,970,2250,5750,25430,125000,22632 0,456500	As mentioned above		Trematodes
Parasites: urocleidus	ETDFL	130,570,850,7500,13610,15910,52500,90000,35 7770,534250	As mentioned above		Trematodes

					Cestodes
Cestodes, main	BIOM	142; 187; 523; 624; 662; 803; 843; 848; 854; 1223; 3032			Cestodes
Cestode Infections	ETDFL	130,300,5500,21500,40000,91500,332410,4751 10,667000,752700	Tapeworm infections		Cestodes
Bertielliasis [Tapeworm]	ETDFL	680,900,2500,5500,13930,93500,360500,37300 0,375300,386400,	As mentioned above		Cestodes
Cenuriasis	ETDFL	30,500,47500,150000,214350,325190,451170,5 17500,687620,992000	As mentioned above		Cestodes
Dipylidiasis	ETDFL	120,250,20000,125190,377910,414180,515170, 683000,712000,993410	As mentioned above		Cestodes
Raillietiniasis	ETDFL	120,580,800,5070,15000,90000,375050,410250, 564280,824960	As mentioned above		Cestodes
Cysticercus Fasciolaris	XTRA	1081.73,1090.76,13637.5,13751.55,	Encysted larval cat tapeworm, usually in muscle.		Cestodes
Cysticercosis	EDTFL	30,200,700,7500,12330,325500,440000,672500, 797500,925950,	Infection of brain by Taenia solium, a pork tapeworm.		Cestodes
Cysticercosis, Brain	EDTFL	30,200,700,7500,12330,18300,155030,517500,6 96500,893000,	As mentioned above	Brain	Cestodes
Cysticercosis, Nerves	EDTFL	30,500,850,5250,77250,112780,321100,511880, 725370,825000,	As mentioned above		Cestodes
Central Nervous System Cysticercosis	EDTFL	30,500,850,5250,77250,112780,321100,511880, 725370,825000	As mentioned above		Cestodes
Neurocysticercosis	EDTFL	30,200,700,7500,12330,18300,155030,517500,6 96500,893000,	As mentioned above	Brain	Cestodes

Subject / Argument	Author	Frequencies	Notes	Origin	Target
Diphyllobothrium Erinacei	XTRA	1158.2,1208.51,14601.55,15235.94,	Tapeworm. Also called Spirometra Erinaceieuropaei.		Cestodes
Diphyllobothrium Latum	XTRA	1122.63,1170.71,14153.12,14759.37,	Tapeworm that causes Diphyllobothriasis.		Cestodes
Diphyllobothriasis	EDTFL	40,370,830,2500,30000,67520,192200,475310,6 75690,819340	Infection caused by Diphyllobothrium tapeworm, commonly Diphyllobothrium Latum.		Cestodes
Dipylidium Caninum 1	XTRA	1089.53,1101.3,13735.94,13884.37,	Dog tapeworm that occasionally infects cats and children.		Cestodes
Dipylidium Caninum 2	XTRA	1120.26,1170.33,14123.44,14754.69,	As mentioned above		Cestodes
Echinococcus Granulosus 1	XTRA	1093.5,1106.75,13785.94,13953.12,	Tapeworm in dogs, wolves, cats, and rodents that can infect man.		Cestodes
Echinococcus Granulosus 2	XTRA	142,164,187,333,453,522,523,542,562,624,662, 663,768,786,803,843,854,1223,1360,3032,5122, 5522,	As mentioned above		Cestodes
Echinococcus Granulosus 3	XTRA	1119.4,1143.94,14112.5,14421.87,	As mentioned above		Cestodes
Echinococcus Multilocularis	XTRA	1129.94,1136.14,14245.3,14323.44,	As mentioned above		Cestodes
Echinococcus Granulosus Larval	XTRA	410	Larval stage of tapeworm in dogs, wolves, cats, and rodents that can infect man.		Cestodes
Cyst Hydatid	CAFL	164,187,453,523,542,623,803,843,854,1223,303 2,5522,	Tapeworm. See Echinococcus, Tapeworm, Taenia, and Hymenolepis sets.	Intestines	Cestodes
Cyst Hydatid	EDTFL	60,200,730,830,12330,20000,85000,95310,1225 30,150000,	As mentioned above		Cestodes
Cyst Hydatid 1	XTRA	164,187,453,523,542,623,803,843,854,1223,136 0,3032,5522=600,	As mentioned above		Cestodes
Cyst Hydatid 2	XTRA	164,453,542,623,5522=900,	As mentioned above		Cestodes
Cyst Hydatid Secondary	XTRA	142,187,624,662,	As mentioned above		Cestodes
Echinococcosis	BIOM	164; 453; 542; 623; 5523			Cestodes
Hydatidosis [Echinococcosis]	EDTFL	680,900,2500,5500,13930,93500,360500,37300 0,375300,386400,	Infestation of Echinococcus tapeworms. Also called Hydatid disease.		Cestodes
Echinococcosis [Tapeworm]	EDTFL	680,900,2500,5500,13930,93500,360500,37300 0,375300,386400,	As mentioned above		Cestodes
Hymenolepis Cysticercoides	XTRA	1184.83,1194.14,14937.5,15054.69,	Larval stage of dwarf tapeworm. Can exist free-form or encysted.		Cestodes
Hymenolepis Diminuta	XTRA	1103.03,1192.65,13906.25,15035.94,	Rat tapeworm which can be passed to man by accidental ingestion of insects.		Cestodes
Hymenolepiasis	BIOM	981.6; 1070.8			Cestodes
Parasites Tapeworms	CAFL	164,453,523,542,623,843,854,1223,803,3032,	Tapeworms found in dogs, wolves, cats, and rodents that can infect humans. Dr. Hulda Clark recommended a zapper for tapeworm.	Intestines	Cestodes
Parasites Tapeworms Secondary	CAFL	142,187,624,662	As mentioned above	Intestines	Cestodes
Parasites Tapeworms Echinococcinum	CAFL	164,453,542,623	As mentioned above	Intestines	Cestodes
Tapeworm	VEGA	522,562,843,1223,3032,5522,	As mentioned above		Cestodes
Parasites: tapeworms	EDTFL	680,900,2500,5500,13930,93500,360500,37300 0,375300,386400	As mentioned above		Cestodes
Parasites: tapeworms echinococcinum (dog and cats)	EDTFL	680,900,2500,5500,13930,93500,368000,36815 0,368850,386400	As mentioned above	Animals	Cestodes
Tapeworm Infection	EDTFL	680,900,2500,5500,13930,93500,360500,37300 0,375300,386400,	As mentioned above		Cestodes
Taenia	CAFL	164,187,453,542,623,803,843,854,1223,3032,55 22,		Intestines	Cestodes
Taenia	VEGA	187		Intestines	Cestodes
Parasites Taenia	CAFL	164,187,453,523,542,623,803,843,854,1223,303 2,5522,	Dr. Hulda Clark recommended a zapper for tapeworm.	Intestines	Cestodes
Parasites: Taenia	EDTFL	680,900,2500,5500,13930,93500,366850,36800 0,370200,386400	use Parasites, tapeworms		Cestodes
Taeniasis	EDTFL	40,260,730,2250,7400,30000,270280,333920,65 4320,779500	Caused by infection of tapeworm - pork, beef, or Taenia Asiatica. See Parasites Taenia, Taenia, Parasites Tapeworm, Tapeworm, Cysticercosis, and Neurocysticercosis sets.		Cestodes
Taenia Infections	EDTFL	110,490,730,2250,7400,30000,270280,333920,7 91030,905070	As mentioned above		Cestodes

					Arthropods

Subject / Argument	Author	Frequencies	Notes	Origin	Target
Arthropod Diseases	EDTFL KHZ	60,850,7800,25000,52500,275090,426900,5710 00,829000,937410,	Diseases transmitted by arthropods.		Mite
Arthropod-Borne Encephalitis	EDTFL	150,230,900,950,7500,150890,455340,527500,8 96500,917200			Mite
Mite Infestations	EDTFL	30,120,930,7500,132330,247520,362540,59655 0,695610,819340			Mite
Meal Mite	HC	718000	Also called Flour or Grain Mites. Cause Grocer's, Baker's, and Grain Itch.		Mite

Subject / Argument	Author	Frequencies	Notes	Origin	Target
Meal Mite	XTRA	1779.74,11218.75	As mentioned above		Mite
Dermatophagoides Dust Mite	HC	707000	Mite living in human homes which lives on dead skin flakes and whose droppings are allergenic.		Mite
Mite Dust	XTRA	11046.87,1752.48	As mentioned above		Mite
Ornithonyssus Bird Mite_2	HC	878000	Avian parasitic mite which will readily feed on human blood.		Mite
Ornithonyssus Bird Mite_1	HC	877000	As mentioned above		Mite
Mite Bird	XTRA	13703.12,13718.75	As mentioned above		Mite
Ornithonyssus Bird Mite 1	XTRA	13703.12,2173.86	As mentioned above		Mite
Ornithonyssus Bird Mite 2	XTRA	13718.75,2176.34	As mentioned above		Mite
Demodex Folliculorum Follicle Mite	HC	682000	Human parasitic mite found in hair follicles, also called Face Mite, and Eyelash Mite.		Mite
Demodex Folliculorum Follicle Mite	XTRA	1090.5,21312.5	As mentioned above		Mite
Demodex Folliculorum	RL	476	From Dr. Richard Loyd.		Mite
Mite Follicle	XTRA	21312.5,1690.5	Demodex. Also see Follicular Mange, and Mange sets.		Mite
Scabies	CAFL	90,110,253	Itc - contagious infection of the skin caused from Sarcoptes scabiei.	Skin	Mite
Scabies	EDTFL	350,930,7200,17500,52500,70000,215700,326500,434000,523010	Contagious skin infection caused by the mite Sarcoptes scabiei.	Skin	Mite
Parasites Scabies	CAFL	90,94,98,102,106,110,253,693=600,920,1436,2871,5742,90-110=1800,	Sarcoptic mange is a contagious dermatitis found in many animals caused by scabies mites. Also see Scabies, and Sarcoptes Scabiei Itch sets.	Skin	Mite
Parasites: Scabies	EDTFL	350,930,7200,17500,52500,70000,215700,326500,434000,523010,	As mentioned above	Skin	Mite
Parasites Follicular Mange	CAFL	253,693,701,774,	Due to Demodex mites. See Follicular Mange.	Hair Skin	Mite
Parasites: follicular mange	EDTFL	70,320,970,2380,15330,46370,73200,87520,153000,415700	As mentioned above	Hair Skin	Mite
Ectoparasitic Infestations [Parasite General]	EDTFL	60,240,780,830,2500,10890,22500,124370,375000,515700,	Infestation of skin parasites or mites.	Skin	Mite

17h - Diseases caused by insects and animals

Subject / Argument	Author	Frequencies	Notes	Origin	Target
Lice Infestations [Head & Body Lice]	EDTFL	70,120,600,870,2250,125520,387500,525000,707500,816500,			Insect
Pediculosis	EDTFL	190,230,3650,62500,162500,219110,322400,472530,888030,937390			Insect
Head Lice	EDTFL	70,120,600,870,2250,125520,387500,525000,707500,816500			Insect
Fleas	CAFL	2374,2750			Insect
Collembola	XTRA	70,700,907500,907.500,90-110	Apply=Frequencies Directly. If no effect, try .02% Feathering. Removes collembola infestations, reported in Morgellons.		Insect
Collembola Comp	XTRA	70,700,907500,907.500,90-111,69-71,699-701,907480-907520	Removes collembola infestations, reported in Morgellons.		Insect
Collembola Sweep	XTRA	907450-907500	Removes collembola infestations, reported in Morgellons.		Insect
Yellow Fly	CAFL	996	Also called Deer Fly. Blood-feeding pest causing diseases in humans and animals.		Insect
Household Insect Mix	BIO	723			Insect
Household Insect Mix	CAFL	723,100			Insect
Household Insect Mix	VEGA	723			Insect
Roaches	CAFL	100	Unknow, but may target a symbiote.		Insect
Myiasis	XTRA	1950,7840,9600,13920,24750,31500,37993,35044,40000,30070	Infestation of fly larvae (maggots). Also called Fly Strike. Often seen in Morgellons.		Parasites
Myiasis	EDTFL	60,350,620,970,12500,27500,325870,325950,623010,815580	As mentioned above		Parasites
Maggot Infestations	EDTFL	40,250,970,48140,142790,219270,322200,592200,765290,822340			Parasites
Zoonoses	EDTFL	160,560,780,930,2750,7500,22500,40000,120,225710	Infectious animal diseases that can be contracted by humans. These include Rabies, West Nile Fever, Lyme Disease, Bubonic Plague, and Rocky Mountain Spotted Fever (see sets).		Insect
Araneae Thrush	XTRA	727,787,880	Thrush due to spider species bite.		Insect
Bites Insects	XTRA	727,787,880,5000			Insect
Biting of Insects	CAFL	727,880			Insect
Insect Bites General 2	XTRA	660,690,727.5,880			Insect
Insect bites	BIOM	30; 727; 740; 787; 880; 1234; 1550; 4412; 5000; 7344; 10000			Insect
Ant bites	BIOM	376; 724; 727; 728; 787; 880; 5000			Insect
Gnat bites	BIOM	80			Insect
Blackfly bite	BIOM	2167			Insect
Pappataci Fever	EDTFL	40,320,580,850,30250,173210,301800,402850,410700,475470	Viral febrile arboviral infection caused by sandfly bites.		Insect

Subject / Argument	Author	Frequencies	Notes	Origin	Target
Sandfly Fever	EDTFL	120,570,2940,8150,9180,233400,582300,69730 0,771000,922590	As mentioned above		Insect
Phlebotomus Fever	EDTFL	70,410,730,5850,72500,135000,367500,550300, 725340,921020	As mentioned above		Insect
Black Widow Spider	CAFL	376,728	Bite		Insect
Black Widow Spider	XTRA	376,660,690,727.5	Bite.		Insect
Brown Recluse Spider 1	XTRA	724,884,1830,3260,11996.34,13888.55,14500= 1800,15004,	Bite		Insect
Brown Recluse Spider 2	XTRA	724,884,1830,3260,15004=300,	For bite.		Insect
Brown Recluse Spider	CAFL	724	For bite.		Insect
Deer Tick	CAFL	271,289,671,737,738,773,7989,	Tick bites.		Insect
Deer Tick 2	XTRA	271,289,671,737,738,773,	Tick bites.		Insect
Blacklegged tick		271; 289; 671; 737; 738; 773; 7989			Insect
Tick-Borne Diseases	EDTFL	140,250,600,2250,20140,32500,46900,62870,67 110,135520,			Insect
Tick Paralysis	EDTFL	140,250,600,2250,30500,112330,319340,52571 0,753070,900000,			Insect
Ruko Tick	CAFL	6634,285,308	Obscure biting tick, indicating possible Ruko genetic involvement in Morgellons.		Insect
Monkeypox	EDTFL	120,350,930,22500,97500,225750,377910,5193 80,691270,753070,	Zoonotic viral disease transmitted via animal bite or blood contact. Symptoms similar to Smallpox, to which it is related.	Viral	Animal
Rabies	BIO	547,793	Also known as hydrophobia. See Lyssavirus, and Lyssinum sets.	Viral	Animal
Rabies	CAFL	20,120,547,793	As mentioned above	Viral	Animal
Rabies	BIOM	793			Animal
Rabies	EDTFL	130,580,730,2580,5780,145910,372520,428020, 511190,605590	As mentioned above	Viral	Animal
Hydrophobia	EDTFL	120,550,5850,81500,127550,241520,471200,62 5300,853000,915090	As mentioned above	Viral	Animal
Rat-Bite Fever	EDTFL	240,700,940,72500,97500,336420,475190,5270 00,662730,752700	Rare serious condition caused by contact with rodent bites, urine, or secretions. Also try Streptothrix sets.	Viral	Animal
Sodoku [Gram Neg Spirillum]	EDTFL	120,550,860,7500,12500,307250,435370,58750 0,795570,901030,		Viral	Animal

18 - Animals

Subject / Argument	Author	Frequencies	Notes	Origin	Target
Animal Diseases	EDTFL KHZ	50,570,870,2500,5810,92500,424370,561930,70 9830,985900,			Animal
Cattle Diseases [MCD Bovine]	EDTFL	130,250,620,5750,17250,37300,129560,345430, 415700,682020,			Animal
Bovine spongiform encephalopathy	EDTFL	130,250,620,5750,17250,37300,129560,345430, 415700,682020,			Animal
Angiostrongyliasis	EDTFL	680,900,2500,9200,13930,25300,93500,417300, 422000,424500	Angiostrongylus vasorum is a nematode that as an adult, nestles in the cardio-circulatory system of the animal.		Animal
Strongylidosis, basic	BIOM	332; 698; 721; 732; 749; 752; 942; 991.5; 1026.2; 3212; 4412			Animal
Strongylidosis, secondary	BIOM	380; 422; 722; 738; 746; 752; 1113			Animal
Distemper	BIO	242,254,312,442,551,573,624,671,712,940,1269 ,1950,	Viral disease that affects a wide variety of animals.	Virus	Animal
Distemper	VEGA	242,254,312,551,573,671,712,1269,	Viral disease that affects a wide variety of animals.	Virus	Animal
Distemper	XTRA	242,253,254,255,312,442,551,573,624,660,671, 690,712,727.5,760,940,950,1269,1950,8567,	Viral disease that affects a wide variety of animals.	Virus	Animal
Glanders	Rife	986000, 736591	Also called Farcy - see sets. Weaponized zoonotic equine disease with respiratory system and oral lesions caused by Pseudomonas Mallei - see sets.	Glanders	Animal
Glanders	CAFL	501,687,743,774,857,875,1273,		Glanders	Animal
Glanders 2	XTRA	501,687,737,743,774,857,875,986,1273,		Glanders	Animal
Glanders 3	XTRA	20,501,660,687,690,727.5,743,774,787,857,875, 880,1273,		Glanders	Animal
Glanders 4	XTRA	407,11509.22,15406.25,		Glanders	Animal
Glanders, complex	BIOM	6646; 5311; 3865; 2959.4; 1273; 1032; 986; 875; 857; 785; 774; 743; 739.8; 737; 731; 687; 633; 482; 437; 405; 191; 178; 174; 501		Glanders	Animal
Glanders Pseudomonas Mallei	XTRA	20,727,787,880		Glanders	Animal
Farcy	XTRA	20,501,660,687,690,727.5,743,774,787,857,875, 880,1273,	Also called Glanders - see sets. Weaponized zoonotic equine disease with respiratory system and oral lesions caused by Pseudomonas Mallei - see sets.	Glanders	Animal
Parasites: common roundworm of cats and dogs	EDTFL	680,900,2500,9200,13930,25300,93500,417300, 422000,424500,		Parasites	Animal

Subject / Argument	Author	Frequencies	Notes	Origin	Target
Heart Animals	XTRA	3.89,20,73,80,95,125,160,465,727,787,880,3000		Heart	Animal
Heart Tonic Animals	XTRA	1.19,3.89,20,73,80,95,125,160,162,465,727,787, 880,3000,		Heart	Animal
Rift Valley Fever	EDTFL	20,520,760,830,112500,217500,329250,497500, 775280,825000	Viral disease that can cause mild to life-threatening symptoms, usually contracted from infected animals, or by infected mosquito bites.		Animal
Rhinopneumonitis	CAFL	185,367,820,487	Equine respiratory infection usually due to Equine herpesvirus type 1 (EHV-1) or Equine herpesvirus type 4 (EHV-4). Also try Streptococcus Pneumoniae sets.	Nose	Animal
Rhinopneumonitis	BIO	185,367,820	As mentioned above	Nose	Animal
Serum Schweinepest	CAFL	503,246,604,465	Classical swine fever, or hog cholera, a highly contagious disease of swine.		Animal
Serum Schweinepest	VEGA	503	As mentioned above		Animal
Reptile Diseases	EDTFL	110,380,650,970,3500,13450,20000,140000,523 240,608110	Common diseases of reptiles and amphibians.		Animal
Amphibian Diseases	EDTFL KHZ	70,5810,10830,57500,125050,376290,419340,5 60000,642910,930120,			Animal
Bird Diseases [inc H5N1]	EDTFL	30,500,830,5710,79300,192500,467500,652200, 802510,912560,			Animal
Fibroma, Shope	EDTFL	230,1180,2260,13580,308490,425080,511750,6 08020,715830,822410	Oncoviruses that can cause cancer. See appropriate Cancer sets.	Shope	Animal
Papilloma, Shope	EDTFL	80,490,650,7530,12850,17500,72500,226070,47 5470,527000			Animal
Bird Flu Virus	XTRA	728,800,880,7760,8000,8250,	H5N1 is a subtype of Influenza A virus.	Shope	Animal
Bird Tuberculosis	XTRA	529.29,590	Avian TB.		Animal
Dog and Cat Hostility 1	CAFL	3.6			Animal
Cat Diseases	EDTFL	30,650,12330,29000,183230,225170,534500,66 7000,742000,986220	Infections or diseases of cats.	Cats	Animal
Feline flea		430; 834; 2232; 3233		Cats	Animal
Cat liver fluke Opisthorchis felineus	RL	256	From Dr. Richard Loyd.	Cats	Animal
Cat Virus	CAFL	364,379,645,654,786,840,841,842,843,844,845, 847,848,849,857,946,967,6878,		Cats	Animal
Feline Cat Immunodeficiency Virus FIV	XTRA	262,323,372,404,567,712,742,760,773,916,1103 ,1132,3701,	Feline Immunodeficiency Virus - similar to HIV in humans.	Cats	Animal
FIV	BIO	262,323,372,404,567,712,742,760,773,916,1103 ,1132,3701,	As mentioned above	Cats	Animal
FIV	CAFL	262,323,372,404,567,712,742,760,773,916,1103 ,1132,3201,	As mentioned above	Cats	Animal
FIV	VEGA	262,323,372,567,916,	As mentioned above	Cats	Animal
Felis	CAFL	430,834,2232,3233		Cats	Animal
Feli	CAFL	435,742		Cats	Animal
Cancer Feline Cat	XTRA	424,830,901,918	Usually due to Feline Leukemia Virus (FLV). See Feline Cat Immunodeficiency Virus FIV, and Feline Cat Leukemia.	Cats	Animal
Feline Cat Leukemia 1	XTRA	258,332,414,424,544,741,743,830,901,918,997,		Cats	Animal
Feline Cat Leukemia 2	XTRA	424,830,901,918		Cats	Animal
Cancer Leukemia Feline	CAFL	258,332,414,424,544,830,901,918,997,741,743,	Begins in bone marrow, causing white blood cell abnormalities. Use Blood Cleanser.	Cats	Animal
Canine Babesial disease		76; 432; 570; 753; 1583; 1584; 5776; 5775.5			Animal
Canine itch		90; 94; 98; 102; 106; 110; 253; 693; 701; 774; 920; 1436; 2871; 5742			Animal
Canine parvovirus 1,2, type B, mutated		323; 433; 428; 514; 535; 613; 755; 761; 764; 766; 768; 185; 188; 562; 622; 637; 1000; 4027			Animal
Canine Parvovirus	CAFL	185,188,323,428,433,562,613,622,1000,4027,	Parvovirus.	Dog	Animal
Parvovirus Canine	BIO	185,323,562,613,622,1000,4027,		Dog	Animal
Parvovirus Canine	CAFL	637,185,323,562,613,622,1000,4027,		Dogs	Animal
Canine Parvo	VEGA	323,562,622,4027		Dog	Animal
Canine Parvo B	VEGA	323,535,755		Dog	Animal
Canine Parvovirus Type B	CAFL	323,535,613,755,761,764,766,768,		Dog	Animal
Canine Parvo Mutant	VEGA	323	Mutated form of virus mainly affecting dogs.	Dog	Animal
Canine Parvovirus Mutant Strain	CAFL	323,514		Dog	Animal
Toxocara Canis	RL	567	From Dr. Richard Loyd. Also known as dog roundworm, is worldwide-distributed helminth parasite of dogs and other canids.	Dog	Animal

19 - Light frequencies

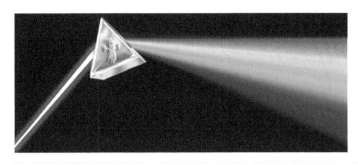

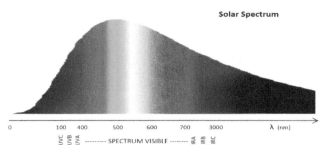

Solar Spectrum

The light is the small part of the spectrum of the electromagnetic waves, that we can perceive with the eyes. The nature of light is twofold: wave and particle; as wave is characterized by wavelength or frequency. The different wavelengths are interpreted by the brain as colors ranging from red with the longest wavelength (lower frequency) to violet of shorter wavelength (higher frequency). The photons, massless, are the elementary particles of light.
The therapies that use light and the colors are varied, these are the most known:

Heliotherapy: it is a very ancient natural circulation, which is based on exposure to sunlight for the treatment of various kinds of disorders including: dermatologic diseases, osteo-articular (activation of Vitamin D), respiratory, hematologic, the system circulatory and mood disorders.

Light Therapy: sunlight stimulates the serotonin and, especially in the Nordic countries where the insolation is very limited, this therapy is frequently used. In the field of chronobiology it is to administer light that plays the best conditions of the entire solar spectrum, through specific lamps, at a specific time, with a few sessions of ten minutes a day. The light through the optic nerve, balance melatonin - serotonin and regulates circadian rhythms sleep - waking, improving mood, appetite and sleep quality. This therapy thus exploits the close connection between the retina and the suprachiasmatic nucleus (nucleus of the hypothalamus, where is located the biological clock of man) to reset the circadian rhythms that are out of phase in certain diseases, such as seasonal depression and the bipolar. This therapy has therefore been found useful for the treatment of depression, bulimia, sleep disorders and circadian rhythm, ADHD, dementia and altered sleep patterns, obsessive - compulsive disorder, headache not migraine and cluster headaches, premenstrual syndrome, Chronic Fatigue syndrome, abnormal sleep patterns to work with night-day shifts, jet lag.

PhotodynamicTherapy (PDT) : or Photochemotherapy, is an innovative technique successfully used especially in the treatment of cutaneous affections for the treatment of various pathological or aesthetic conditions, such as: removal acne, photodamage or injury due to skin aging, actinic or solar keratosis, the pre-cancerous lesions and lesions cancer (basal cell carcinoma, squamous cell carcinoma).
The therapy is based on the irradiation of light at certain frequencies and the application of a photosensitizing substance in the form of cream or administered intravenously, which triggers an oxidative reaction only in causing pathological cells favoring the elimination and replacement with new cells.

Phototherapy: is the use of light to cure a series of especially skin disorders (jaundice, psoriasis, etc.) And as a cosmetic treatment. The patient is exposed to specific light waves for a period of time.

Chromotherapy: is an ancient therapeutic technique natural origin, which studies the meaning of the colors and exploit its therapeutic properties to balance the chakras, relieve psychosomatic disorders and bring the body (which is a set of body, mind and spirit) to a condition of well-being. Our body can absorb the colors in many ways (sun, lighting fixtures, clothes, food, etc.).
The chromotherapy light irradiation is the most effective technique: the electromagnetic waves transmit an energy capable of getting deep into cells causing a series biological reactions, as better described hereinafter.

Chromopuncture: fruit of the brilliant idea of German researcher Peter Mandel (the early 70s), is a form of acupuncture that uses instead of needles, colored lights, which are directed on traditional acupuncture points to treat various diseases. The therapy is also applied on some points located on the ear (chromopuncture headset) demonstrating that in some cases is more effective than the classical auricular puncture, given that the depth reached in the stimulation through the colors, is greater. These stimulations normally arouse a feeling of pain, although bearable, in the ear points that correspond to the energy area of the body affected by the disease.

Biophoton: This is a sensational discovery of the German biophysicist **Fritz Albert Popp**, who was able to show that the cells of any living being, emit very weak light radiation; this light radiation is called biophotons. The emission of electromagnetic energy propagates at the speed of light by means of DNA, which acts as a transceiver station allowing a constant electromagnetic communication, both inter-cellular which with the outside world (also long-distance).
Popp also discovered that healthy bodies emit very coherent bio-photon. While in poor health, bodies emit less coherent photons. The disease would be an interruption in the biophoton communication lines within the body due to parasites, viruses, fungi, pollutants etc. Furthermore, while investigating a particular light radiation with a wavelength equal to 380 nanometers, he discovered that it is associated with the repair of photo-phenomenon. If in fact a cell is damaged (and even almost totally destroyed) by the ultra violet light, it can repair itself alone in a matter of a day if it is exposed to a radiation of the same frequency but of much lower intensity.

Two sets of frequencies, based on the studies of Dr. Fritz Albert Popp, can be found in the chapter of the "cancer" (Cancer Cell Repair Octal and Scalar).

Subject / Argument	Frequencies	Notes
Infrared	300 GHz – 428 THz / 1 mm – 700 nm	Infrared rays are invisible to the human eye but we can perceive them as "heat": it is therefore radiant heat energy. Therapeutic context, the thermal effect of infrared radiation causes vasodilation and benefits the circulatory system, acceleration of metabolic exchange and other effects on the peripheral nervous system and muscles. It is useful to specify that the beneficial effects of irradiation to infrared rays, are much higher than those of simple heat treatments.
Infrared Type C (IRC)	300 GHz - 100 THx / 10000 - 3000 nm	The Far Infrared Ray (**FIR**) are the only ones to transfer energy exclusively in the form of heat, perceived by skin thermoreceptors. Increase the potential difference of the cell membranes and mitochondrial membranes by facilitating exchanges between the cell and the external environment. Favor the restoration of blood flow. *Depth of penetration into the skin up to 5-10 mm.*
Infrared Type B (IRB)	100 - 214 - THz / 3000 - 1400 nm	*Depth of penetration into the skin up to 0.5 mm*
Infrared Type A (IRA)	214 - 428 -THz / 1400 - 700 nm	Are the most used in medical practice and physiotherapy and are indicated for the treatment of trauma, cervical or lumbar osteoarthritis, for disorders that affect the muscular system (stiff neck, back pain and other similar ailments). In addition they are used in case of injury (ie. to treat bed sores), since the radiated heat stimulates the natural regenerative processes of the body. *Depth of penetration into the skin up to 0.1 mm.*
Visible light	428 THz – 749 THz / 700 nm – 400 nm	Is that small part of the spectrum of electromagnetic waves, which we can see. The length (λ) of these electromagnetic waves is by extremely small and, knowing the frequency, can be calculated as follows: $$\lambda = c\,/\,f$$ where **c** is the propagation speed of light equal to 300,000 km / s, and **f** is the wave frequency.
Red Associated element: Earth	400 - 484 THz / 750 - 620 nm It has the length of the lower wave and the more penetrating power. Increases heart rate, breathing, blood pressure, stimulates neuronal activity, endocrine and liver. *This energy level is related to the first chakra Muladhara, or coccyx chakra; It is the color of the fire element and is the most Yang color.*	It stimulates the growth of the cells and has an anti-inflammatory effect; for example wounds heal much faster and is useful for relieving contractures, strains and inflammation of the muscle fibers. It also helps to relieve the pain. *Indications:* lowered immunity, anemia, fatigue, depression, bradycardia, impotence, hypoglycemia, hypotension, hypothyroidism, paresis.
Orange Associated element: water	484-508 THz / 620 - 590 nm It is the color of serenity. It stimulates the thyroid gland and the secretion of breast milk; it has a great power of energy balance and manages to demobilize the crystallization of energy, very important factor for many skin problems, kidney, gall, nerve and intellectuals. *It corresponds to the second sacral chakra, Swadhisthana and is a Yang color.*	It is extremely positive for the psyche plagued by depression, fears, neuroses and mania, but also for anorexic people, because it stimulates in them a natural appetite and helps to regain the love of life. *Indications:* anemia, arteriosclerosis, bradycardia, immune system, impotence, gastric hyposecretion, hypotension, paralysis, drowsiness, constipation, vomiting.
Yellow Associated element: fire	508-526 THz / 590 - 570 nm It has a stimulating effect on the physiological level, but its effect is not as strong and steady as the red; it is an indication of the sense of joy and positivity. It helps mental focus and troubleshooting. *It is the color associated with the third of the solar plexus chakra, Manipura and being linked to the nervous and digestive system, for the Chinese corresponds to the fire element and is a Yang color.*	It helps relieve all digestive disorders, abdominal bloating colitis, cleanses the blood; also acts on motor nerves, it produces energy for the muscles and, thanks to its stimulating activity, also of the nervous system, increases the capacity of the memory, concentration and at the same time of socialization. *Indications:* canker sores, activates the left hemisphere, bronchitis, colitis, diabetes, diarrhea, nervous exhaustion, intoxication, exanthematous diseases, increases attention and night vision, whooping cough, rheumatism, sinusitis, constipation.

Subject / Argument	Author	Frequencies	Notes	Origin	Target
Green Associated element: air		526-606 THz / 570 - 495 nm The green light infuses harmony. It is considered curative broad spectrum and has antiseptic, detoxifying, rebalancing of energies; its calming effect the nervous system, is evident in the need innate in people to immerse themselves in the green nature to have feelings of peace and balance. *The color green is in affinity with the fourth heart charka, Anahata, and for the Chinese is related to the wood element and is a Yin color.*	As beneficial to the overexcited psyche, gives serenity and calm in case of anxiety and stress, calms the cramps and the gastrointestinal disorders (especially gastritis and ulcers); It has a natural antibacterial and disinfectant action. *Indications:* hair loss, headaches, sleep disorders, headaches, palpitations, general rebalancing, sciatica, stress.		
Cyan		606-631 THz / 495 - 475 nm			
Blue Associated element: life, ether, sound		631-668 THz / 475 - 450 nm Is considered the color of relaxation, meditation, serenity, peace (very useful in cases in which the body needs to regenerate after a fatigue or illness) and is connected to the pituitary gland, which governs the entire endocrine system. It has a sedative effect of the nervous system, blood pressure and heart rate as it determines slowing and vasodilation. Has analgesic action, antiseptic and anti-inflammatory acting very well in the immune system and lymphatic system; it is a great tool at osteoarticular level, especially when combined with red. *Is the color linked to the fifth throat chakra, Vishuddha; for Chinese it corresponds to lodge wood and is a Yin color.*	The blue light is able to kill large numbers of bacteria (such as *Streptococcus aureus, Propionibacterium acnes, Pseudomonas aeruginosa, as Porphyromonas gingivalis and Helicobacter pylori*) and treat lesions of the skin such as acne. It has properties to reduce jaundice in newborns (changes the molecular structure of bilirubin making it soluble in water and then eliminating it through bile and urine). Injected directly into the root canal of an infected tooth, it can destroy both Gram positive bacteria and Gram-negative. *Indications:* agitation, anxiety, anxiety, bronchial asthma, hot flashes, anger, conjunctivitis, muscle cramps, dysmenorrhea, headache, pharyngitis, fever, infections, insomnia, hypertension, back pain, rash, palpitations, frozen shoulder, insect bites, tachycardia, ulcers , burns.		
Indigo Associated element: thinking		It 'a great purifier of the blood and acts primarily on the mind, favoring intuition. Is the color linked to meditative vision, it presides over the higher functions of thought and corresponds to the third eye. It has the ability to balance our sense organs to make them more sensitive; also it has a calming effect and anesthetic especially in the airways, nose, or eyes. *It has affinity with the sixth chakra front, Ajna and is a Yin color for Chinese.*	It is useful for all disorders affecting the head, including the eyes, nose and ears. *Indications:* eczema, hyper-emotion, hyperthyroidism, hives, psoriasis.		
Violet Associated element: the light		668-749 THz / 450 - 400 nm It is the color with the highest visible frequency and greater penetration and therefore has always been considered the color of the spirit, stimulating the subtle energies, the unconscious, the creativity, inspiration and intuition. An excess can cause melancholy and loss of the sense of reality and concreteness. Violet is the color of the upper nervous system and the right brain seat of intuition, synthesis and perception. *It is the color of the seventh crown chakra, Sahasrara, which belongs to the pineal gland, and for the Chinese is a Yin color.*	Very useful in cases of inflammation such as neurosis, irritation of the nerves and for disorders of the lymphatic circulation, to stimulate the production of white blood cells and the activity of the spleen, kidneys and bladder, for scalp problems and sciatica. It is helpful for the lack of sleep and calms the states nervous and irritable. *Indications:* anesthetic action, scarring, inflammation of the skin, bacterial and viral diseases, neuralgia, sedative of the nervous system.		

Subject / Argument	Author	Frequencies	Notes	Origin	Target
Ultraviolet		749 THz – 30 PHz / 400 nm – 10 nm	The ultraviolet radiation is a type of light that can not be perceived by the human eye and constitutes about 8% of the solar radiation. Prolonged exposure to these rays can lead to the destruction of the collagen bridges increasing the aging of the skin and at high doses can cause skin cancer (basal cell carcinomas, squamous cell carcinoma and melanoma).		Light
UVA		400 – 315 nm	The UV-A radiation promotes the degradation and excretion of uric acid; its use is therefore recommended in case of gout. Also it causes an increase in antibodies in the blood, thereby increasing the ability of the immune system to respond to infection. They penetrate deeply into the skin, so it is the main responsible for skin aging (wrinkles).		Light
UVB		315 – 280 nm	Exposure is commonly used to treat a number of skin conditions such as vitiligo, acne and psoriasis (the rays penetrating the skin, slows its growth). In addition, the UVB light: - mobilizes calcium phosphate and increases the metabolism of calcium in the bones (in the irradiation applications are therefore indicated for the treatment of fractures); - stimulates the production of "D" vitamin and is therefore essential for the prevention of very serious diseases; - lowers the blood sugar level if is too high; - stimulates the tan.		Light
UVB-NB		311-313 nm	They are UVB but in a very narrow band, so that the therapies which use these frequencies, can obtain the maximum effective dose of radiation, and the minimum dose of harmful radiation. They are used for the treatment of numerous dermatological diseases including psoriasis, vitiligo, atopic dermatitis, cutaneous lymphomas, mycosis fungoides, mastocytosis, nodular prurigo, pityriasis lichenoid etc.		Light
UVC			The UV-C irradiation is extremely dangerous (especially to the eyes) and a carcinogen, but that natural of sunlight, is "completely" screen from the Ozone wing.		Light
UVGI			The Ultraviolet germicidal irradiation, is a particular frequency of the UV-C, able to modify the DNA or RNA of micro-organisms (molds, bacteria and viruses), preventing them from reproducing or be harmful. The germicidal lamps are used to sterilize the workplace and tools used in biology and medicine laboratories, for the disinfection of food, water and air.		Light
VUV			VUV (or ultra-UVC) radiation, unlike conventional UV germicide, neither can penetrate through the outer and dead layer of the skin and therefore does not damage the underlying epithelial cells, nor can penetrate the outer layer of the eye. However, it penetrates and kills bacteria and viruses that live on the skin.		Light

19a - LED and LASER Therapies

The technology of laser light applied to the medical field saw its birth in the late '70s. In the years following the technique has evolved more and more. The use of this technology has expanded, including also LED light sources.

The main difference between the two light sources consists mainly in the fact that while the laser emits a coherent light, ie with all the rays in phase, the LED diodes do not have this characteristic. Both, however, emit monochromatic or single colored light, that is, at a precise wavelength, from infrared to ultraviolet (in the visible range each frequency corresponds to a specific color and vice versa).

In terms of frequencies, the visible spectrum varies between 400 and 1200 teraHertz which corresponds to a wave length ranging from 400 to 800 nm (nanometers) or a comparable size to that of human cells.

In phototherapy and in many other therapeutic applications of monochromatic light, it appears that the differences between the laser and the LED are not appreciable since coherent light is converted into incoherent light when passed through the body. In practice the therapeutic effect depends on the wavelength, the dose and the intensity and therefore little or not at all on the coherence. The absorption depends on the type of tissue that is irradiated and on the wavelength of the light. Light blue, green and yellow are almost completely absorbed by the skin surface. The red light is better transmitted than these and the infrared even better, being able to achieve a penetration depth of up to 10 mm.

For therapeutic medical devices (mainly laser), the shades used are light blue, green, yellow, red and infrared, but especially the red/infrared light, between 630 and 900 nm, which are employed in most medical treatments. In this range of frequencies, the photons activate mainly the final vector of the mitochondrial respiratory chain (cytochrome-c-oxidase).

Mitochondria are organelles present in all animal cells whose main function is that of cell respiration and production of ATP, a coenzyme that can provide power to all cellular reactions and the processes of the body including, for example, the transmission of nerve impulses and muscle contraction. Mitochondria occupy about 10-15 percent of the volume of a living cell.

Therefore, the red monochromatic light with a wavelength from 630 to 660 nm acts by interfering with the mitochondrial respiratory chain of cells and more specifically on the enzymatic structures "cytochrome oxidase". This process results in an increased production of endogenous energy in the form of ATP (increase of 150%) that the cell will use to improve its functions. From the therapeutic point of view, this will manifest itself as an improvement of the functional activity of that tissue "photo-stimulated" and then in a rapid restoration of its integrity. From this knowledge derive many unexpected therapeutic applications.

The flow of light penetrating the tissues causes the biochemical reactions that induce several effects among which are:

- Vasodilation resulting in the increase in local heat, increase in cellular metabolic demands, neuro vegetative stimulation and modification of intra-capillary hydrostatic pressure (lowers blood pressure);

- Increased lymphatic drainage and activation of microcirculation;

- Anti-inflammatory, anti-edema and improvement of the nutritional state of tissues because of the increase in blood flow due to capillary and arteriolar vasodilation;

- Significant acceleration of regenerative processes, acceleration of the healing of wounds, increase in the potential of the nerve cells and a greater production of collagen and elastin;

- Increased production of endorphins and, consequently, treatment of acute and chronic pain;

- Care of trauma , injury to the ligaments, tendons, bones, nerves, skin, dental problems and infections (including herpes).

So the applications are used in neurology, dentistry, dermatology (including cosmetic applications), physical therapy and rehabilitation (including the sports field).

The light can be applied to any part of the body: blood vessels, skin, soft tissues, muscles, bones, brain and with LED devices, also to the eyes. The correct position of the laser probes or those realized with a matrix of laser diodes or LEDs, it is important to avoid energy losses. Normally, the best position is perpendicular to the skin at the point of application and at a distance varying from 1-2 mm to a maximum of 1-5 cm. As already said, the light energy absorption primarily depends on the color of the light (or the wavelength of the beam) and on the constitution of the tissues that are invested by the radius (skin, blood, muscles, bones, etc.). The duration of the application depends on the energy (Joules / cm^2) radiated by the probe as a function of the depth of the tissue to be treated and the type of the beam emission (continuous, pulsating, modulated).

The light can be emitted continuously (e.g. to relieve pain), pulsating (e.g. to stimulate healing) or modulated frequency (e.g. for the application of Rife frequencies). Many authors consider the modulated laser light more effective in terms of therapeutic effects; some combine the continuous emission with frequency modulation by using the patient's reactions.

Finally, there is a wide range of studies (reflex therapy) that examines the effects of frequencies, with the stimulation of the points of acupuncture meridians, chakras, or trigger point (Dr.Nogier, Dr.Bahr, Dr.Reininger, etc.). The laser acupuncture combines the advantages of traditional Chinese acupuncture with modern laser technology. The correct frequency modulation of the laser beam on a point of meridians or acupuncture, stimulates the oscillation of the frequency of the meridian. This therapy is less invasive, less painful and safer than traditional acupuncture.

Later we will analyze the results of these studies using the above laser equipment.

Subject / Argument	Author	Frequencies		Notes		Origin	Target

19b - Nogier Frequencies

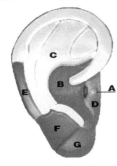

Dr. Paul Nogier (Lyon, 1908 - 1996) may be recognised as the father of Auriculotherapy and frequency therapy. He studied Medicine in Lyon including homeopathy and acupuncture, brain stimulation.

After many years of study and research, he developed experimentally, some frequencies that enter into resonance with some biological receptors and specific exert effects on the body. His research revealed that the outer ear, is energetically connected to the entire body. Although there are no direct nerve connections between the ear and the rest of the body, the nerves from the ear do connect to reflex centers in the brain, which send neurological reflex messages to the spinal cord, and then to nerves connecting to the corresponding part of the body.

Today the results of his work are recognized by the World Health Organization (WHO).

The low frequencies are used for treatment. The high frequencies are used for laser devices (at a higher harmonic - n°128), with an identical action. With respect to the reference frequency, it can be used variations ranging from -30% to + 30%.

The frequencies are used as a carrier of information. If a perfect resonance is reached, there will be a high therapeutic effect.

The left figure shows the frequency zones as discovered by Nogier; the therapeutic effect is obtained by applying a device to modulated laser light on the corresponding ear area.

treatment / laser devices

Nogier Frequency A	XTRA	2.28 / 293.625	Cellular Vitality - Regenerating	Nogier

The frequency corresponds to the Color Orange

Stimulate cell work, without stimulating the cell division. Resonates with the Ectoderm (outermost tissue) that forms skin, glands, nerves, eyes, ears, teeth, brain and spinal cord. Used for traumata, crushing, oedema, hematoma, anoxia, hypoxia, infarct, burns, inflammation, orifices, skin/tissue, epithelial tumors, acute diseases, nerve repair and reduces scar tissue. May be helpful with degenerative disorders. Frequency A is a universal frequency (as is G) to try for any condition. Try D if a chronic condition related to A is not improving.

Nogier Frequency B	XTRA	4.56 / 587.25	Nutritional Metabolism - Regenerating	Nogier

The frequency corresponds to the Color Red

Stimulate functions linked to pluricellularity. Resonates with Endoderm (innermost tissue) that forms the lining of the the auditory tube, the lungs, the bladder, the urethra and the intestinal tract. It also forms the thyroid, thymus, liver, gall bladder and pancreas. Improves nutritional assimilation, allergy problems and balances the parasympathetic nervous system. Used for venous, lymphatic insufficiency, arteritis, auto immune diseases, digestive system (celiac disease, malabsorptions, obesity, metabolic syndrome) osteoarthritic, abdomen, sedation, metabolic problems, chronic diseases circulatory problems, edema and lymph problems. Is used in conjunction with C and G for tendon, ligament, joint and other injuries where reaching secondary levels of tissue is needed.

Nogier Frequency C	XTRA	9.125 / 1174.5	Movement - Muscle Relaxing	Nogier

The frequency corresponds to the Color Yellow

Stimulate the motor and excretion functions. Resonates with Mesoderm (middle tissue) that forms connective tissue such as ligaments, tendons, cartilage, muscle and bone. It also forms the heart, blood and lymph vessels, kidneys, ovaries, testes, spleen and the cortex of the adrenal gland. Used for muscle, bones, joints, circulation, movement disorders, skeletal, myofascial pain atonia, hypertonia (trismus, intestine, arterial spasms, vesical or vesicular atony, constipation, motor diarrhea, blood low pressure). When it used with B and G can be especially good for tendon and ligament injuries. It also helps to relax the major muscle groups. Try D if chronic condition related to C is not improving.

Nogier Frequency D	XTRA	18.25 / 2349	Coordination - Muscle Relaxing	Nogier

The frequency corresponds to the Color Red Tango

Stimulate functions linked to symmetry phenomena, to displacement and locomotion. Helps to balance the two sides of the brain. May also help reduce and handle stress. Used for laterality problems commissural, posture, ocular movements, locomotion (walking disorders), brain, stress balance, relaxation, inter-hemisphere blocks. It is also recommended for chronic conditions not responsive to setting A or C. This setting to be a good supplement to A when healing processes appear static.

Nogier Frequency E	XTRA	36.5 / 4698	Nerves - Analgesic	Nogier

The frequency corresponds to the Color Petrol Blue

Stimulate functions linked with medullar functions. Resonates with the spinal cord and peripheral nervous system, reducing the excitability of nervous tissue. Used for spinal and skin disorders, pain control, nerves, neuralgia, Herpes zoster, spine/brain, reflex arc, medullary disorders and aid in diminishing excess calcification associated with chips, spurs and arthritic conditions.

Nogier Frequency F	XTRA	73.406 / 9344	Emotional Reactions - Regenerating	Nogier

The frequency corresponds to the Color Dark blue

Stimulate functions of the sub cortical cortex. Resonates with the subcorticalor lower regions of the brain, including the thalamus and hypothalamus (centers for body functions). May also help with muscle spasms, facial pain, headaches. Has been used for non-healing bone fractures and to help balance hormones and with activating humoral and endocrine functions. Used for healing, tissue regeneration, bone reconstruction, face, mouth, brain central commands, dys-metabolism, dysesthesia, dyskinesi, bulimia, anorexia, menstruation disorders (amenorrhea, dysmenorrhoea, spaniomenorrhoea), cicatrisation disorders (pseudarthrosis, varicous ulcer), thermoregulation disorders, emotional disorders (depression, psychosomatic, brain frequency).

Nogier Frequency G	XTRA	146.812 / 18688	Intellectual Organization - Analgesic - Muscle Relaxing	Nogier

The frequency corresponds to the Color Magenta

Stimulate the cortical cortex. Resonates with the cerebral cortex of the brain, involved with thinking, imagining and creating. Used for pain of central origin, frontal cortex, tinnitus, muscle strain, intellectual disorders, anxiety, hysteria, psychiatric problems, memory, psychological disorders, nervousness and worry, psychosomatic diseases, cognitive disorders.
Frequency G is a universal frequency (as is A) to try for any condition.

Nogier Frequency L	XTRA	276 /	Equilibrium of the laterality	Nogier

Has an action on disorders linked with bad laterality. Resonates with the sagittal median line of the scalp. Used for the equilibrium of the laterality, dyslexia, dyscalculia, dysorthographia, learning difficulties in school, concentration and memory disorders, disturbed laterality (re-educated left handed persons), nervous depression (linked with a laterality disorder), tobacco-stop, weaning from antidepressant drugs.

Nogier Frequency U	XTRA	1.14 /	Universal/base frequency	Nogier

It is a Universal frequency or also called "U" that would be useful for detoxification and affects all cellular and biological processes where external or unbalancing agents intervene.

The resulting 7 fundamental frequencies, are multiples of 2 (octave division)

Subject / Argument	Author	Frequencies	Notes	Origin	Target
Analgesic		C + D + G or E + G			Nogier
Cicatrisation		A + B + F			Nogier
Muscle relax		E + F or C + D + G			Nogier
Regenerating		A + B + F			Nogier
Relaxation		C + D + G			Nogier

19c - BAHR frequencies

The physician **Dr. Frank Bahr**, Germany, discovered various frequencies which are used since many years. He was a student of Nogier and is today the President of the largest German acupuncture society. He detected more than 14 major bio-frequencies (BAHR 1, BAHR 2) and Chakra frequencies.
The BAHR-Frequencies correspond to ear points and body acupuncture, three skin tissues layers and the nervous system.

Subject / Argument	Author	Frequencies	Disease, part of the body	Origin	Target
Bahr Frequency 1.1	CUST	599.5	Disruption in conversation of acquired energy, disruption in conversation of own energy resources, source of illness, affinity to sympatetic nerve system. Lower tissue layer		Bahr
Bahr Frequency 1.2	CUST	1199	Transfer of energy, neuronal energy and distribution function, hormonal and nerve systems, affinity to parasympathetic nerve system. Central tissue layer		Bahr
Bahr Frequency 1.3	CUST	2398	Boundary and tangential area between man and the environment, biotic points, OmegaRen channel points Surface tissue structures. Omega-Ren-channel		Bahr
Bahr Frequency 1.4	CUST	4796	Omega-Du channel points		Bahr
Bahr Frequency 1.5	CUST	9592	Oscillation frequency, Super Omega		Bahr
Bahr Frequency 1.6	CUST	19184	Left axis, right points		Bahr
Bahr Frequency 1.7	CUST	38360	Right axis, left points		Bahr
Bahr Frequency 2.1	CUST	963,5	Pain		Bahr
Bahr Frequency 2.2	CUST	1131	Hysteria		Bahr
Bahr Frequency 2.3	CUST	7708	Homeopathy		Bahr
Bahr Frequency 2.4	CUST	1927	Anti allergy		Bahr
Bahr Frequency 2.5	CUST	699	Defence		Bahr
Bahr Frequency 2.6	CUST	637	Yang-Energy		Bahr
Bahr Frequency 2.7	CUST	1102	Yin-Energy		Bahr
Chakra			*Apply the chakra frequency directly on the chakra in the correct movement.*		
Bahr Chakra 1	CUST	4023	Root		Bahr
Bahr Chakra 2	CUST	3123	Sacral		Bahr
Bahr Chakra 3	CUST	2398	Solar plexus		Bahr
Bahr Chakra 4	CUST	1589	Heart		Bahr
Bahr Chakra 5	CUST	990	Throat		Bahr
Bahr Chakra 6	CUST	573	**Third eye**		Bahr
Bahr Chakra 7	CUST	232	Crown		Bahr
Bahr Chakra 8	CUST	7695	Qi Master point		Bahr
Bahr Chakra 9	CUST	24	Shaman-Chakra 8		Bahr
Bahr Chakra 10	CUST	7696,5	Shaman-Chakra 9		Bahr
Bahr Chakra 11	CUST	7697	Protection-Chakra general		Bahr
Bahr Chakra 12	CUST	7698	Pocks charge		Bahr
Bahr Chakra 13	CUST	7699	Pest charge		Bahr
Bahr Chakra 14	CUST	7700	Disturbance field / Thymus		Bahr
Bahr Chakra 15	CUST	7707	Upper-Omega		Bahr
Bahr Chakra 16	CUST	7708	Master of constitution (Homeopathy)		Bahr
Bahr Chakra 17	CUST	7710	Inner mental core		Bahr
Bahr Chakra 18	CUST	7713	Life/Karma		Bahr

19d - REININGER frequencies

Dr. Manfred Reininger, Austria, Vice President of the largest Austrian acupuncture society (OGKA), was the first who detected and published the frequencies of the acupuncture meridians. In the course of his studies he found a large number of different frequencies related to the human body, diseases (allergy, tinnitus etc.) and the environment.

Meridian	Author	Frequencies	*Apply the meridian frequencies to acupuncture points on the relevant meridian.*	Origin	Target
Lu , lung	CUST	824			Reininger
LI, large intestine	CUST	553			Reininger
St, stomach	CUST	471			Reininger
SP, spleen pancreas	CUST	702			Reininger

Subject / Argument	Author	Frequencies	Notes	Origin	Target
He, heart	CUST	497			Reininger
SI, small intestine	CUST	791			Reininger
BI, bladder	CUST	667			Reininger
Ki, kidney	CUST	611			Reininger
Ci, circulation (pericard)	CUST	530			Reininger
3H, triple heater	CUST	732			Reininger
Gb, gall bladder	CUST	583			Reininger
Li, liver	CUST	442			Reininger
Anti frequencies			Use the pure frequency e.g. **Allergy** for RAC [1] diagnosis and the Anti frequency e.g. **Anti allergy** for the treatment. Apply as long as the RAC is active or according to the general guideline for local therapy.		
General	CUST	384			Reininger
Psyche	CUST	129			Reininger
Anti Psyche	CUST	4221			Reininger
Vegetative	CUST	112			Reininger
Anti vegetative	CUST	3665			Reininger
Addiction	CUST	112			Reininger
Anti addiction	CUST	3305			Reininger
Carcinoma	CUST	108			Reininger
Anti Carcinoma	CUST	3534			Reininger
Pain	CUST	101			Reininger
Anti pain	CUST	3894			Reininger
Inflammation	CUST	128			Reininger
Anti inflammation	CUST	4189			Reininger
Allergy	CUST	3648			Reininger
Anti Allergy	CUST	933			Reininger
Tinnitus	CUST	125			Reininger
Anti Tinnitus	CUST	4090			Reininger
Viral/Bacterial			Use the pure frequency for RAC [1] diagnosis and the Anti frequency for therapy.		
Viral	CUST	1408			Reininger
Anti viral	CUST	360			Reininger
Bacterial	CUST	1664			Reininger
Anti bacterial	CUST	425			Reininger
Various	CUST				
Regeneration	CUST	640			Reininger
Regeneration blocked by disturbance field	CUST	2503			Reininger
Kidney-Yin	CUST	158			Reininger
Kidney-Yang	CUST	5160			Reininger
Geopathogenic charge	CUST	182			Reininger
Toxic charge	CUST	7680			Reininger

(1) A method to find the exact frequency for the treatment of a disease, it is called "the Nogier Pulse" or **RAC** (Reflex Auriculo Cardial) or VAS (Vascular Autonomic Signal). According to this technique, the physician with one hand radiates the painful area or the corresponding ear area, while with the other hand the patient's pulse. If changing the frequency of the laser is observed a variation of the pulse, it means that that is the right frequency to use. This method is similar to muscle testing used in kinesiology.

Subject / Argument	Author	Frequencies	Notes	Origin	Target

Subject / Argument	Author	Frequencies	Notes	Origin	Target
Colors	CAFL	470,624,640,677,745,800,815,858,920,960,2055 ,2155,	Color decode from Jade machine.		Jade M.
Jade Machine Color Code Blue	CAFL	624,	Healing color system similar to SpectroChrome. Wavelength transposed to frequency.		Jade M.
Jade Machine Color Code Green	CAFL	2055,	As mentioned above		Jade M.
Jade Machine Color Code Indigo	CAFL	640,	As mentioned above		Jade M.
Jade Machine Color Code Lavender	CAFL	677,	As mentioned above		Jade M.
Jade Machine Color Code Light Blue	CAFL	8280,	As mentioned above		Jade M.
Jade Machine Color Code Light Green	CAFL	960,	As mentioned above		Jade M.
Jade Machine Color Code Magenta	CAFL	800,	As mentioned above		Jade M.
Jade Machine Color Code Orange	CAFL	920,	As mentioned above		Jade M.
Jade Machine Color Code Purple	CAFL	745,	As mentioned above		Jade M.
Jade Machine Color Code Red	CAFL	815,	As mentioned above		Jade M.
Jade Machine Color Code Sienna	CAFL	858,	As mentioned above		Jade M.
Jade Machine Color Code Yellow	CAFL	470,	As mentioned above		Jade M.
Green Dye	CAFL	563,2333,			

20 - Chemical Elements and Minerals

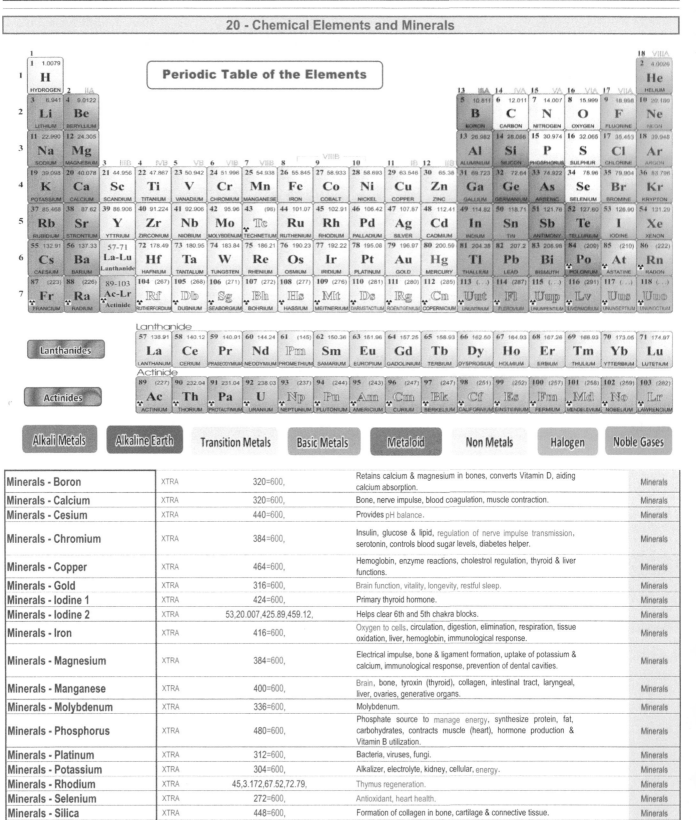

Periodic Table of the Elements

Minerals - Boron	XTRA	320=600,	Retains calcium & magnesium in bones, converts Vitamin D, aiding calcium absorption.	Minerals
Minerals - Calcium	XTRA	320=600,	Bone, nerve impulse, blood coagulation, muscle contraction.	Minerals
Minerals - Cesium	XTRA	440=600,	Provides pH balance.	Minerals
Minerals - Chromium	XTRA	384=600,	Insulin, glucose & lipid, regulation of nerve impulse transmission, serotonin, controls blood sugar levels, diabetes helper.	Minerals
Minerals - Copper	XTRA	464=600,	Hemoglobin, enzyme reactions, cholestrol regulation, thyroid & liver functions.	Minerals
Minerals - Gold	XTRA	316=600,	Brain function, vitality, longevity, restful sleep.	Minerals
Minerals - Iodine 1	XTRA	424=600,	Primary thyroid hormone.	Minerals
Minerals - Iodine 2	XTRA	53,20.007,425.89,459.12,	Helps clear 6th and 5th chakra blocks.	Minerals
Minerals - Iron	XTRA	416=600,	Oxygen to cells, circulation, digestion, elimination, respiration, tissue oxidation, liver, hemoglobin, immunological response.	Minerals
Minerals - Magnesium	XTRA	384=600,	Electrical impulse, bone & ligament formation, uptake of potassium & calcium, immunological response, prevention of dental cavities.	Minerals
Minerals - Manganese	XTRA	400=600,	Brain, bone, tyroxin (thyroid), collagen, intestinal tract, laryngeal, liver, ovaries, generative organs.	Minerals
Minerals - Molybdenum	XTRA	336=600,	Molybdenum.	Minerals
Minerals - Phosphorus	XTRA	480=600,	Phosphate source to manage energy, synthesize protein, fat, carbohydrates, contracts muscle (heart), hormone production & Vitamin B utilization.	Minerals
Minerals - Platinum	XTRA	312=600,	Bacteria, viruses, fungi.	Minerals
Minerals - Potassium	XTRA	304=600,	Alkalizer, electrolyte, kidney, cellular, energy.	Minerals
Minerals - Rhodium	XTRA	45,3.172,67.52,72.79,	Thymus regeneration.	Minerals
Minerals - Selenium	XTRA	272=600,	Antioxidant, heart health.	Minerals
Minerals - Silica	XTRA	448=600,	Formation of collagen in bone, cartilage & connective tissue.	Minerals
Minerals - Silver	XTRA	376=600,	Antibiotic.	Minerals
Minerals - Sodium	XTRA	352=600,	Sodium.	Minerals
Minerals - Sulfur	XTRA	256=600,	Liver, bile, skin, wounds. Also spelled sulphur.	Minerals
Minerals - Vanadium	XTRA	368=600,	Healthy glucose, lipid metabolism, prevention of tooth decay, diabetes helper.	Minerals
Minerals - Zinc 1	XTRA	480=600,	Antiseptic, antibiotic, antioxidant, metabolism of nucleic acid, protein synthesis, mucosal linings, hormone production, prostate gland, regulates hunger, Vitamin A utilization.	Minerals

Subject / Argument	Author	Frequencies	Notes	Origin	Target
Minerals - Zinc 2	XTRA	30,6.254,133.13,143.52,	Helps harmonize body, mind, spirit.		Minerals
Aluminum 1	XTRA	15950,	Toxic metal. Present in chemtrail sprays. See Detox sets.		Minerals
Aluminum 2	XTRA	554.67,597.95,			Minerals
Antimony 121sb	XTRA	509.39,549.13,11684.56,	Heavy metal, binding metal.		Minerals
Antimony 123sb	XTRA	275.86,297.37,12655.27,	Heavy metal, binding metal.		Minerals
Arsenic as	XTRA	364.56,393,16724.61,	Heavy metal.		Minerals
Barium 135ba 1	XTRA	211.46,227.96,19402.34,	Heavy metal. Present in chemtrail sprays. See Detox sets.		Minerals
Barium 137ba 2	XTRA	236.56,255.02,21705.08,			Minerals
Beryllium be	XTRA	299.14,322.49,13723.62,	Toxic heavy metal.		Minerals
Beryllium	XTRA	16350,	Heavy metal. Detox.		Minerals
Bismuth bi	XTRA	342.06,368.75,15692.37,			Minerals
Boron 10b	XTRA	228.75,246.59,20988.27,	Heavy metal.		Minerals
Boron 11b	XTRA	682.97,736.25,15666.02,	Heavy metal.		Minerals
Bromine 79br	XTRA	533.29,574.9,12232.9,	Can cause thyroid problems by replacing iodine.		Minerals
Bromine 81br	XTRA	574.87,619.73,13186.52,	Can cause thyroid problems by replacing iodine.		Minerals
Cadmium 111cd	XTRA	451.38,486.61,20708,			Minerals
Cadmium 113cd	XTRA	472.18,509.02,21662.11,			Minerals
Cadmium	XTRA	14325,	Heavy metal.		Minerals
Calcium 2	XTRA	143.21,154.38,13140.62,			Minerals
Carbon c	XTRA	535.24,577,12277.34,			Minerals
Cesium cs	XTRA	279.22,301,12809.56,	Heavy metal.		Minerals
Chlorine 35cl	XTRA	208.56,224.84,19136.72,	Element, halogen group.		Minerals
Chlorine 37cl	XTRA	173.62,187.15,15929.69,			Minerals
Chromium cr	XTRA	120.31,129.69,11039.05,			Minerals
Chromium vi	XTRA	19600,			Minerals
Chromium	XTRA	383,			Minerals
Cobalt co	XTRA	502.67,541.88,11530.27,			Minerals
Cobalt	XTRA	14075,			Minerals
Copper 63cu	XTRA	564.21,608.23,12941.88,	Metal, essential trace element.		Minerals
Copper 65cu	XTRA	604.41,651.58,13864.26,			Minerals
Fluorine f	XTRA	2.62,158.87,11484.01,	Highly toxic reactive halogen. Compounds used in pharmaceuticals, dental 'care,' PET scanning, and uranium enrichment.		Minerals
Gallium	XTRA	11350,			Minerals
Germanium	XTRA	74.25,80.04,136.25,			Minerals
Gold au	XTRA	36.43,39.28,13375,			Minerals
Gold	XTRA	14750,			Minerals
Hydrogen 1h	XTRA	128.69,294.79,12207.03,	Hydrogen and pH balance.		Minerals
Hydrogen 2h	XTRA	326.77,352.26,14991.2,			Minerals
Hydrogen 3h	XTRA	270.54,477.68,13020.38,			Minerals
Indium	XTRA	12075,	Heavy metal.		Minerals
Iodine 1	XTRA	425.88,459.12,19538.09,			Minerals
Iodine 2	XTRA	424,			Minerals
Iodine	XTRA	2030.464,	Experimental. Derived from molar weight.		Minerals
Iridium	XTRA	14250,	Heavy metal.		Minerals
Iron fe	XTRA	68.78,74.14,12621.09,	Metal. Necessary for blood health.		Minerals
Lead pb	XTRA	445.35,480.08,20430.65,			Minerals
Lead	XTRA	190000,			Minerals
Lithium 6li	XTRA	313.25,337.69,14371.09,	Element.		Minerals
Lithium 7li	XTRA	186.61,955.98,16951.04,	Element.		Minerals
Lithium	XTRA	11975,	Element.		Minerals
Magnesium mg	XTRA	130.27,140.43,11952.14,	Mineral essential for life.		Minerals
Magnesium	XTRA	480,	Mineral essential for life.		Minerals
Magnesium	XTRA	11325,	Mineral essential for life.		Minerals
Manganese 1	XTRA	11425,	Element essential for life.		Minerals
Manganese mn	XTRA	525.01,565.99,12042.96,	Element essential for life.		Minerals
Mercury	XTRA	21850,	Toxic metal element.		Minerals
Mercury 199hg	XTRA	379.48,409.08,17409.18,			Minerals
Mercury 201hg	XTRA	140.46,151.43,12888.67,			Minerals
Molybdenum 95mo	XTRA	138.65,149.47,12722.65,	Metal element essential for life.		Minerals
Molybdenum 97mo	XTRA	141.59,152.65,12992.19,	Metal element essential for life.		Minerals
Molybdenum	XTRA	464,336,	Metal element essential for life.		Minerals
Nickel ni	XTRA	190.21,205.06,17453.13,	Toxic metal element.		Minerals

Subject / Argument	Author	Frequencies	Notes	Origin	Target
Nickel	XTRA	13800,	Toxic metal element.		Minerals
Osmium	XTRA	14800,	Toxic metal element.		Minerals
Oxygen	XTRA	5.772,			Minerals
Ozone Generate	XTRA	78,16,15.99	Experimental. May be contraindicated in Morgellons cases.		Minerals
Palladium	XTRA	18850,	Metal element used in dentistry. Low toxicity, but may be carcinogenic.		Minerals
Phosphorus	XTRA	861.72,928.95,19766.11,	Essential element.		Minerals
Lead pb	XTRA	445.35,480.08,20430.65,			Minerals
Lead	XTRA	190000,			Minerals
Platinum pt	XTRA	457.64,493.36,20955.11,	Metal element. Exposure to salts can cause short-term and long-term problems. Used in chemotherapy and body implants.		Minerals
Platinum	XTRA	14825,			Minerals
Potassium k	XTRA	99.34,107.09,18230.47,	Essential element.		Minerals
Rhodium 85rb	XTRA	205.53,221.56,18857.41,	Metal element.		Minerals
Rhodium 87rb	XTRA	696.52,750.87,15977.04,	Metal element.		Minerals
Rhodium rh	XTRA	67.51,72.79,12390.62,	Metal element.		Minerals
Rubidium	XTRA	12300,	Metal element.		Minerals
Scandium 21	XTRA	517.05,557.4,11860.35,	Metal element.		Minerals
Selenium 34	XTRA	406.41,438.12,18644.52,	Trace mineral element essential for cardiac health.		Minerals
Selenium	XTRA	272,	Trace mineral element essential for cardiac health.		Minerals
Silicon si	XTRA	422.87,455.86,19399.4,	Metal element. Not to be confused with silicone, which is a man-made polymer.		Minerals
Silver	CAFL	15903,	Metal element. Experimental.		Minerals
Silver 2	XTRA	21650,	Metal element.		Minerals
Silver 107ag	XTRA	86.12,92.84,15804.69,	Metal element.		Minerals
Silver 109ag	XTRA	99.03,106.75,18171.88,	Metal element.		Minerals
Sodium Chloride	XTRA	29.22,	Table salt.		Minerals
Sodium na	XTRA	563.05,606.99,12915.53,	Metal element.		Minerals
Strontium sr	XTRA	92.23,99.43,16925.77,			Minerals
Sulfur si	XTRA	163.27,176,14980.46,	Element. Also spelled sulphur.		Minerals
Thallium	XTRA	18300,	Highly toxic metal element.		Minerals
Tantalum	XTRA	12225,	Metal element, toxic at high levels.		Minerals
Tin 115sn	XTRA	696.05,750.37,15966.3,	Metal element.		Minerals
Tin 117sn	XTRA	758.35,817.51,17395.02,	Metal element.		Minerals
Tin 119sn	XTRA	793.4,855.3,18199.22,	Metal element.		Minerals
Tin	XTRA	14925,	Metal element.		Minerals
Titanium 47ti	XTRA	119.98,129.36,11009.77,	Metal element. Commonly used in medical implants.		Minerals
Titanium 49ti	XTRA	120.01,129.37,11011.71,	Metal element. Commonly used in medical implants.		Minerals
Titanium	XTRA	17650,	Metal element. Commonly used in medical implants.		Minerals
Tungsten w	XTRA	88.57,95.48,16253.9,	Metal element.		Minerals
Tungsten	XTRA	11875,	Metal element.		Minerals
Uranium u	XTRA	38.1,41.07,13984.37,	Radioactive metal element.		Minerals
Vanadium 50v	XTRA	212.22,228.78,19472.65,	Metal, trace element.		Minerals
Vanadium 51v	XTRA	559.61,603.27,12836.43,	Metal, trace element.		Minerals
Vanadium	XTRA	16400,	Metal, trace element.		Minerals
Zinc	XTRA	14050,	Metal element, essential mineral.		Minerals
Zinc 2	XTRA	480,	Metal element, essential mineral.		Minerals
Zinc zn	XTRA	133.12,143.52,12214.84,	Metal element, essential mineral.		Minerals
Zirconium zr	XTRA	198.61,214.09,18222.65,	Metal element with no known biological role, although present in all biological systems.		Minerals
Colloidal Silver Generate	XTRA	1000=1800,10000=1800,	Wave=square, Duty Cycle=95%, Amplitude=8, select Inverse+Sync.		
Colloidal Silver Octal	XTRA	4653391.397248,2326695.698624,	Octal sub-harmonics of sub-10nm spheroid colloidal nanoparticles.		
Colloidal Gold Octal	XTRA	7205251.195738,3602625.597869,	Octal sub-harmonics of sub-10nm spheroid colloidal nanoparticles.		
Colloidal Gold Scalar	XTRA	7364246.875738,366644.262680,	Scalar sub-harmonics of sub-10nm spheroid colloidal nanoparticles.		
Colloidal Silver and Gold Octal	XTRA	9088.655073,7036.378121,1173.892841,908.820264,	Octal sub-harmonics of sub-10nm spheroid colloidal nanoparticles.		
Colloidal Silver and Gold Sub-1MHz	XTRA	900656.399467,581673.924656,473582.172629,366644.262680,	Scalar and octal HF sub-harmonics of sub-10nm spheroid colloidal nanoparticles.		
Colloidal Silver and Gold Sub-10KHz	XTRA	72709.240582,56291.024967,23578.268006,18254.142973,	As mentioned above		
Colloidal Silver and Gold Sub-100KHz	XTRA	72709.240582,56291.024967,23578.268006,18254.142973,	As mentioned above		

Subject / Argument	Author	Frequencies	Notes	Origin	Target
		21 - Homeopathy			
Anthracinum	BIO	633,	Homeopathic anthrax nosode.		Homeopathy
Arsenic Alb	CAFL	562,	Homeopathic cell salt.		Homeopathy
Bacillinum	CAFL	132,423,432,785,853,854,921,1027,1042,1932,	Homeopathic nosode.		Homeopathy
Bacillinum	VEGA	132,854,921,1042,1932,	Homeopathic nosode.		Homeopathy
Bacteria Lactis Nosode	CAFL	512,526,798,951,5412,	Homeopathic nosode.		Homeopathy
Bacteria Lactis Nosode	VEGA	512,526,5412,	Homeopathic nosode.		Homeopathy
Baker's Yeast Allergy	CAFL	775,843,	Homeopathy preparation.		Homeopathy
Barley Smut	CAFL	377,224,1447,	Homeopathic preparation for an allergen.		Homeopathy
Barley Smut	BIO	377,	Homeopathic preparation for an allergen.		Homeopathy
Bermuda Smut	CAFL	422,767,847,971,644,780,	Homeopathic preparation for an allergen.		Homeopathy
Bermuda Smut	BIO	971,	Homeopathic preparation for an allergen.		Homeopathy
Botrytis Cinereas	CAFL	1132,212,	Homeopathic preparation from a fungal allergen.		Homeopathy
Botrytis Cinereas	BIO	1132,	Homeopathic preparation from a fungal allergen.		Homeopathy
Botrytis Cinereas	XTRA	212,1132,1545,	Homeopathic preparation from a fungal allergen.		Homeopathy
Botrytis	CAFL	1545,	Homeopathic preparation from a fungal allergen.		Homeopathy
Carbo Animalis	CAFL	444,	Homeopathic remedy from animal bone charcoal.		Homeopathy
Causticum	BIO	540,1013,	A homeopathic remedy.		Homeopathy
Chelidonium	CAFL	162,	Homeopathic remedy.		Homeopathy
Convoforce	CAFL	774,	Homeopathic.		Homeopathy
Coraforce	CAFL	774,	Homeopathic.		Homeopathy
Corallinus	CAFL	533,	Homeopathic.		Homeopathy
Corn Smut	CAFL	546,1642,289,	Homeopathic preparation for an allergen.		Homeopathy
Corn Smut	BIO	546,1642,	Homeopathic preparation for an allergen.		Homeopathy
Corn Smut	VEGA	546,	Homeopathic preparation for an allergen.		Homeopathy
Diptherinum	VEGA	624,	Homeopathic.		Homeopathy
Enterococcinum	CAFL	686,409,	Homeopathic nosode for Streptococcus family organisms found in GI and urinary tracts.		Homeopathy
Enterococcinum	BIO	686,	As mentioned above		Homeopathy
Echinococcinum	BIO	164,453,542,623,	Homeopathic remedy for Echinococcus tapeworms in dogs, wolves, cats, and rodents that can infect man.		Homeopathy
Echinococcinum 2	XTRA	164,453,542,623,5522=900,	As mentioned above		Homeopathy
Epidermophyton Floccinum	BIO	644,766,	Homeopathic remedy for Fungus that attacks skin and nails. Includes athlete's foot.		Homeopathy
Epidermophyton Floccinum 2	XTRA	20,345,465,634,644,660,690,727.5,766,784,802,880,1550,	As mentioned above		Homeopathy
Fel Tauri	BIO	672,	Homeopathic preparation of ox bile.		Homeopathy
Fischpyrogen	BIO	832,	Homeopathic nosode.		Homeopathy
Fluor Alb	CAFL	110,342,420,423,688,757,	Homeopathic cell salt.		Homeopathy
Fluor Alb	VEGA	420,423,424,2222,502,	Homeopathic cell salt.		Homeopathy
Influenza Triple Nosode	BIO	421,632,1242,1422,1922,3122,	Homeopathic.		Homeopathy
Influenza Toxicum	VEGA	854,	Homeopathic nosode for influenza/flu.		Homeopathy
Influenza Bach Poly	CAFL	122,350,487,572,634,768,823,1043,1272,764,771,	Homeopathic nosode for influenza/flu.		Homeopathy
Influenza Bach Poly	VEGA	122,823,	Homeopathic nosode for influenza/flu.		Homeopathy
Influenzum Bach Poly Flu	BIO	122,350,487,634,823,	Homeopathic.		Homeopathy
Influenza Berlin	VEGA	55,430,720,733,	Homeopathic nosode for influenza/flu.		Homeopathy
Influenza Berlin 55	CAFL	430,720,733,787,	Homeopathic nosode for influenza/flu.		Homeopathy
Influenza Vesic	VEGA	203,292,975,	Homeopathic nosode for influenza/flu.		Homeopathy
Influenza Vesic NW	CAFL	332,364,519,588,590,238,239,715,	Homeopathic nosode for influenza/flu.		Homeopathy
Influenza Vesic NW	VEGA	364,	Homeopathic nosode for influenza/flu.		Homeopathy
Influenza Vesic SW	CAFL	433,645,658,824,	Homeopathic nosode for influenza/flu.		Homeopathy
Influenza Vesica General	CAFL	203,292,588,612,975,407,682,	Homeopathic nosode for influenza/flu.		Homeopathy
Vapch Grippe	VEGA	153,343,	Homeopathic nosode for influenza/flu.		Homeopathy
Lac Deflorat	CAFL	230,371,232,2121,	Homeopathic.		Homeopathy
Lac Deflorat	VEGA	230,371,	Homeopathic.		Homeopathy
Luesinum and Syphilinum	CAFL	177,600,625,650,658,660,	Homeopathic. See Syphilis.		Homeopathy
Luesinum and Syphilinum 2	XTRA	177,600,625,650,658,660,789,900,2776,6600,	Homeopathic. See Syphilis.		Homeopathy
Luesinum and Syphilinum 3	XTRA	177,	Homeopathic. See Syphilis.		Homeopathy
Lyssinum	BIO	547,793,	Homeopathic nosode for rabies. Also see Lyssavirus and Rabies sets.		Homeopathy
Medorrhinum	BIO	230,442,554,843,854,1700,1880,2222,	Homeopathic nosode for urethral discharge.		Homeopathy
Medorrhinum	VEGA	442,843,2222,	Homeopathic nosode for urethral discharge.		Homeopathy

Subject / Argument	Author	Frequencies	Notes	Origin	Target
Meningococcinum	BIO	130,517,676,677,	Homeopathic nosode for Meningitis.		Homeopathy
Meningococcinum	VEGA	676,677,517,	Homeopathic nosode for Meningitis.		Homeopathy
Monotospora Languinosa	BIO	788,	Homeopathic remedy for fungal allergen.		Homeopathy
Morbillinum	CAFL	467,520,1489,	Homeopathic noside for Measles.		Homeopathy
Mycogone Species (spp)	CAFL	371,446,748,1123,	Homeopathic allergenic preparation based on Fungus.		Homeopathy
Mycogone Species (spp)	BIO	371,446,1123,	Homeopathic allergenic preparation based on Fungus.		Homeopathy
Myocarditis Necrose	CAFL	706,789,	Homeopathic remedy from heart cells that died as a result of inadequate blood flow to them. See Circulatory Stasis.		Homeopathy
Neurospora Sitophila	CAFL	705,878,	Homeopathic allergenic preparation.		Homeopathy
Neurospora Sitophila	BIO	705,	Homeopathic allergenic preparation.		Homeopathy
Nigrospora Species (spp)	CAFL	302,350,764,	Homeopathic allergenic preparation.		Homeopathy
Nigrospora Species (spp)	BIO	302,	Homeopathic allergenic preparation.		Homeopathy
Ox Bile	BIO	672,	The homeopathic remedy derived from it.		Homeopathy
Pasteurella Combination	BIO	913,	Homeopathic nosode for bacterial diseases spread by animal bites.		Homeopathy
Phoma Destructiva	CAFL	163,815,621,	Homeopathic.		Homeopathy
Phoma Destructlva	VEGA	163,	Homeopathic.		Homeopathy
Prostate Adenominum	PROV	442,688,1875,748,766,920,	Homeopathic remedy for prostate tumor.		Homeopathy
Psorinum	CAFL	786,767,	Homeopathic nosode for psoriasis. Useful for persistent skin itch, especially post-scabies.		Homeopathy
Psorinum	BIO	786,	As mentioned above		Homeopathy
Pullularia Pullulans	CAFL	432,873,1364,684,739,750,	Homeopathic allergy remedy.		Homeopathy
Pullularia Pullulans	BIO	1364,	Homeopathic allergy remedy.		Homeopathy
Pyocyaneus	BIO	437,	Homeopathic nosode for Pseudomonas pyocyanea.		Homeopathy
Pyrogenium 62	CAFL	151,429,594,622,872,497,498,	General homeopathic remedy for pus.		Homeopathy
Pyrogenium 62	VEGA	429,	Homeopathic.		Homeopathy
Pyrogenium Ex Ovo	CAFL	231,1244,1210,1216,	Homeopathic.		Homeopathy
Pyrogenium Fish	CAFL	287,304,	Homeopathic.		Homeopathy
Pyrogenium Mayo	BIO	1625,	Homeopathic.		Homeopathy
Pyrogenium Suits	CAFL	341,356,673,	Homeopathic.		Homeopathy
Sanguis Menstrualis	BIO	591,	Homeopathic nosode.		Homeopathy
Sorghum Smut	BIO	294,	Homeopathic preparation for an allergen.		Homeopathy
Tobacco Mosaic	BIO	233,274,543,782,1052,	Homeopathic preparation for an allergen.		Homeopathy
Tonsillar NOS	BIO	1656,			Homeopathy
Tuberculinum	CAFL	332,522,664,731,737,748,1085,1099,1700,761,	Homeopathic nosode for Tuberculosis.		Homeopathy
Tuberculinum	VEGA	522,			Homeopathy
Vaccininum	BIO	476,	A homeopathic nosode.		Homeopathy
Variolinum	BIO	542,569,832,3222,	Homeopathic smallpox nosode.		Homeopathy
Variolinum	VEGA	542,832,3222,	As mentioned above		Homeopathy

22 - Bach Flower

Frequency-Hz / Pulse AM-Hz

Subject / Argument	Author	Frequencies	Notes	Origin	Target
Agrimony	CUST	310.31 / 1.21	For those who hide their torments behind a cheerful and courteous facade. Addiction, unhappy, anxiety, insomnia.		Bach F.
Aspen	CUST	391.54 / 1.53	For those who are afraid of vague, indistinct things and for no apparent reason. Fear, worries, unknown fears.		Bach F.
Beech	CUST	490.87 / 1.92	For those who want to see more beauty and are sometimes intolerant of others and criticize them. Intolerance, critical, lack of compassion.		Bach F.
Centaury	CUST	384.68 / 1.50	For those who have a lack of will, those who are easily influenced or overly altruistic. Weak-willed, tired, timid, passive, quiet.		Bach F.
Cerato	CUST	291.80 / 1.14	For those who do not have self-confidence and continually ask others for advice. Confirmation, seeking advice, do not trust own wisdom or judgment.		Bach F.
Cherry Plum	CUST	262.01 / 1.02	For those who are afraid of losing reason and self-control. Fear of losing control, temper tantrum, breakdown, abusive, rage, explode.		Bach F.
Chestnut Bud	CUST	425.77 / 1.66	For those who always repeat the same mistakes. Learning, repeating mistakes.		Bach F.
Chicory	CUST	489.22 / 1.91	For those who love possessively, trying to do everything possible to be reciprocated. Possessive, over protective, self-centered, self pity.		Bach F.
Clematis	CUST	415.26 / 1.62	For those who daydream, living more in the future than in reality. Daydreaming, dreaminess, withdrawing, lack of concentration.		Bach F.
Crab Apple	CUST	359.21 / 1.40	For those who need cleansing in the body or mind. Cleansing, poor self image, sense of not being clean, obsessive.		Bach F.
Elm	CUST	463.13 / 1.81	For those who feel overwhelmed with responsibility. Depression overwhelmed by responsibilities, despondent, exhausted.		Bach F.
Gentian	CUST	265.67 / 1.04	For those who abandon themselves to pessimism, they become easily discouraged and depressed. Discouraged, depressed.		Bach F.
Gorse	CUST	424.21 / 1.66	For those who feel great desperation and feel like they are stuck. Hopelessness, despair, pessimism.		Bach F.
Heather	CUST	301.78 / 1.18	For those who don't like being alone and often find an opportunity to talk to others and those who are self-centered. Talkative, demand attention, dislike being alone, lonely.		Bach F.
Holly	CUST	479.48 / 1.87	For those who experience anger, envy and hatred, strong negative feelings towards others. Envy, jealousy, hate, insecurity, suspicious.		Bach F.
Honeysuckle	CUST	275.98 / 1.08	For those who have nostalgia for the past or who is homesick. Homesickness, nostalgia, bereavement.		Bach F.
Hornbeam	CUST	257.45 / 1.01	For those who cannot start the day with the right energy. Weariness, bores, tired, needs strength, overworked, procrastination, doubting own abilities.		Bach F.
Impatiens	CUST	463.06 / 1.81	For those who are impatient and cannot stand interference with their rhythms. Impatience, irritated, nervy, frustration, fidgety, accident-prone, hasty.		Bach F.
Larch	CUST	336.52 / 1.31	For those who have low self-esteem, and are afraid of failing. Lack of confidence, depressed, discouraged, feeling of inferiority.		Bach F.
Mimulus	CUST	492.23 / 1.92	For those with fear or anxiety of known origin. Fear, blushing, stammering, shyness, timid, sensitive, lack of courage.		Bach F.
Mustard	CUST	254.78 / 1.00	For those who feel momentarily unhappy and cannot say why. Depression, deep gloom for no reason.		Bach F.
Oak	CUST	318.03 / 1.24	For those who can't stop working and never give up. Exhaustion, overwork, workaholic, fatigued, over-achiever.		Bach F.
Olive	CUST	431.65 / 1.69	For those who are exhausted from physical or mental fatigue. Lack of energy, fatigue, convalescence.		Bach F.
Pine	CUST	280.93 / 1.10	For those with a strong sense of guilt. Guilt, self-reproach, humble, apologetic, shame, unworthy, undeserving.		Bach F.
Red Chestnut	CUST	292.06 / 1.14	For those who are apprehensive about loved ones. Worried, over-concern, fear.		Bach F.
Rock Rose	CUST	277.99 / 1.09	For those who are seized with great fear and panic. Frozen fear, terror.		Bach F.
Rock Water	CUST	451.74 / 1.76	For those who are very rigid in their way of being and want to be an example. Mental and character flexibility.		Bach F.
Scleranthus	CUST	307.07 / 1.20	For those who are undecided between two choices. Indecision, imbalance, uncertainty, dizziness.		Bach F.
Star of Bethlehem	CUST	276.57 / 1.08	For those who have suffered an emotional shock. Trauma, after effect of shock, post traumatic stress.		Bach F.
Sweet Chestnut	CUST	421.51 / 1.65	For those who experience extreme anxiety, where nothing but destruction is seen. Extreme mental anguish, hopeless despair, intense sorrow.		Bach F.

Subject / Argument	Author	Frequencies	Notes	Origin	Target
Vervain	CUST	409.14 / 1.60	For those who let themselves be carried away too much by enthusiasm and have a strong sense of justice. Over-enthusiasm, hyper-active, fanatical, highly strung.		Bach F.
Vine	CUST	383.91 / 1.50	For those who want to dominate others. Domineering, inflexible, very capable, gifted, bullying, aggressive.		Bach F.
Walnut	CUST	261.26 / 1.02	For those who face big changes and need protection from external influences. Influenzable, hypersensitive, unstable and confused, busy.		Bach F.
Water Violet	CUST	370.22 / 1.45	For those who love to be alone and are sometimes proud. Reserved, asocial, independent, arrogant.		Bach F.
White Chestnut	CUST	247.09 / 0.97	For those who have constant and unwanted thoughts, and want mental peace. Repeated unwanted thoughts, mental arguments, concentration, sleeplessness.		Bach F.
Wild Oat	CUST	430.20 / 1.68	For those who are unsure of the role to play in life. Cross-road in life, decision making, lack of clarity, drifting in life.		Bach F.
Wild Rose	CUST	349.54 / 1.37	For those who abandon themselves to resignation and apathy. Apathy, resignation, lost motivation, lack of ambition.		Bach F.
Willow	CUST	264.74 / 1.03	For those who experience bitterness and resentment. Victim of destiny, suffering for adversity and bad luck.		Bach F.
Rescue Remedy	CUST	277.99,415.26,463.06,262.01,276.57,	Universal first aid, to deal with all emergency situations. Consisting of: Rock Rose, Clematis, Impatiens, Cherry Plum e Star of Bethlehem.		F. Bach

23 - Plants

Subject / Argument	Author	Frequencies	Notes	Origin	Target
Aconite	CAFL	3347,5611,2791,	Used to stimulate lymphocyte production.		Plants
Arnica	BIO	1042,	A healing herb.		Plants
Cannabidiol CBD	XTRA	5031.472	Experimental. Derived from molar weight.		Plants
Catahua	XTRA	422.578	Experimental. Powerful medicinal herb from the Amazon rain-forest, courtesy of a shaman friend of Spooky2.		Plants
Cimicifuga	CAFL	334,594,	Plant family including Black Snakeroot and Black Cohosh.		Plants
Cimicifuga	VEGA	594,	Plant family including Black Snakeroot and Black Cohosh.		Plants
Blue Cohosh	BIO	364,	A healing herb.		Plants
Crocus Sotilus	CAFL	710,	Is a genus of flowering plants in the iris family comprising 90 species of perennials growing from corms.		Plants
Gingerol + Shogaol		14377777.192,13497912.882,	Experimental. Active constituents of ginger. May be useful for Rheumatoid Arthritis, and cancers of blood, lung, bowel, breast, ovaries, and pancreas. Also see appropriate sets. Do NOT use together with NAC.		Plants
Marijuana	XTRA	30,			Plants
Marsh Elder	BIO	474,	Allergen, member of Ragweed family.		Plants
Nasturtium	BIO	143,	A healing herb.		Plants
Penny Royal	VEGA	772,	Healing herb.		Plants
Ragweed	CAFL	473,	Flowering plant whose pollen causes allergic reactions.		Plants
Mannan	BIO	961,	Unknown. May refer to plant polysaccharide related to mannose, or to constituent of yeast cell walls (common in Otitis Media - see sets).		
Mannan	XTRA	661,961,			
Sorghum Syrup	HC	277000,	Sweet syrum made from Sweet Sorghum grass.		

24 - Essential Oils

Bruce Tanio, of Tainio Technology and head of the Department of Agriculture at Eastern Washington University, has developed a Calibrated Frequency Monitor (CFM) that has been used to measure the frequencies of essential oils and their effect on human frequencies when applied to the body.

Subject / Argument	Author	Frequencies	Notes	Origin	Target
Essential Oil - Abundance	XTRA	19500000,	Blend: orange, frankincense, patchouli, clove, ginger, myrrh, cinnamon, spruce. Enhances human magnetic field.	78 MHz.	Essential Oil
Essential Oil - Acceptance	XTRA	12750000,	Blend: rosewood, almond, geranium, frankincense, blue tansy, sandalwood, neroli. Promotes acceptance of self and others, helps with procrastination and denial.	102 MHz	Essential Oil
Essential Oil - Angelica	XTRA	21250000,	Exhaustion, skin, psoriasis, gout, detox, fluid retention.	85 MHz	Essential Oil
Essential Oil - Aroma Life	XTRA	21000000,	Blend: cypress, marjoram, helichrysum, ylang ylang, sesame seed. Energizes life force. Combine with Chakra 2 Heart set.	84 MHz	Essential Oil
Essential Oil - Aroma Siez	XTRA	16000000,	Blend: basil, marjoram, lavender, peppermint, cypress. Soothes soreness after exercise.	64 MHz	Essential Oil
Essential Oil - Awaken	XTRA	22250000,	Blend: almond, Joy, Present Time, Forgiveness, Dream Catcher, Harmony. Promotes awareness and awakening.	89 MHz	Essential Oil
Essential Oil - Basil	XTRA	13000000,	Single: invigorates and refreshes the mind. Infections, healing, fatigue, alertness, concentration.	52 MHz	Essential Oil
Essential Oil - Blue Tansy	XTRA	13125000,	Single: similar qualities to German Chamomile.	105 MHz	Essential Oil
Essential Oil - Brain Power	XTRA	19500000,	Blend: sandalwood, cedarwood, melissa, frankincense, blue cypress, lavender, helichrysum. Clarifies thought and develops focus.	78 MHz	Essential Oil
Essential Oil - Chamomile, German	XTRA	13125000,	Single: skin problems, inflammation, promotes new cell growth, insomnia, stress.	105 MHz	Essential Oil

Subject / Argument	Author	Frequencies	Notes	Origin	Target
Essential Oil - Christmas Spirit	XTRA	13000000,	Blend: orange, cinnamon bark, spruce. Promotes happiness, joy, and security.	104 MHz	Essential Oil
Essential Oil - Citrus Fresh	XTRA	22500000,	Blend: orange, tangerine, mandarin, grapefruit, lemon, spearmint. Immune system. Promotes security, creativity, and joy.	90 MHz	Essential Oil
Essential Oil - Clarity	XTRA	12625000,	Blend: basil, cardamom, rosemary, peppermint, rosewood, geranium, lemon, palmarosa, ylang ylang, bergamot, Roman chamomile, jasmine. Promotes mental sharpness.	101 MHz	Essential Oil
Essential Oil - Di-Gise	XTRA	12750000,	Blend: tarragon, ginger, peppermint, juniper, fennel, lemongrass, anise, patchouli. Supports digestive system.	102 MHz	Essential Oil
Essential Oil - Dragon Time	XTRA	18000000	Blend: clary sage, fennel, lavender, marjoram, yarrow, jasmine. Supports emotions during female monthly cycle.	72 MHz	Essential Oil
Essential Oil - Dream Catcher	XTRA	24500000,	Blend: sandalwood, tangerine, ylang ylang, black pepper, bergamot, juniper, anise, blue tansy. Enhances dreaming and visualisation.	98 MHz	Essential Oil
Essential Oil - En-R-Gee	XTRA	13250000,	Blend: rosemary, juniper, lemongrass, nutmeg, Idaho balsam fir, clove, black pepper. Boosts energy, restores mental alertness.	106 MHz	Essential Oil
Essential Oil - EndoFlex	XTRA	17250000	Blend: sesame seed, spearmint, sage, geranium, myrtle, nutmeg, German chamomile. Glandular, circulatory, respiratory, nervous, reproductive, and other systems. Helps weight control.	138 MHz	Essential Oil
Essential Oil - Envision	XTRA	22500000	Blend: spruce, geranium, orange, lavender, safe, rose. Creativity, resourcefulness, fortitude.	90 MHz	Essential Oil
Essential Oil - Exodus II	XTRA	22500000,	Blend: olive, cassia, myrrh, cinnamon, calamus, hyssop, galbanum, frankincense, spikenard.	180 MHz	Essential Oil
Essential Oil - Forgiveness	XTRA	24000000,	Blend: melissa, geranium, frankincense, rosewood, sandalwood, angelica, lavender, lemon, jasmine, Roman Chamomile, bergamot, ylang ylang, palmarosa, helichrysum, rose, sesame seed. Release hurt and move on.	192 MHz	Essential Oil
Essential Oil - Frankincense	XTRA	18375000	Dry and aging skin, rejuvenation, stress, despair, focus, Alzheimer's, brain function, cancer, asthma, herpes, skin, auto-immune problems, panic attacks.	147 MHz	Essential Oil
Essential Oil - Galbanum	XTRA	14000000,	Supports immune, digestive, respiratory, circulatory and other systems. Skin problems, and aging skin.	56 MHz	Essential Oil
Essential Oil - Gathering	XTRA	24750000,	Blend: lavender, galbanum, frankincense, geranium, ylang ylang, spruce, cinnamon, rose, sandalwood. Unifies spiritually and emotionally.	99 MHz	Essential Oil
Essential Oil - Gentle Baby	XTRA	19000000,	Blend: rosewood, geranium, palmarosa, lavender, Roman chamomile, ylang ylang, lemon, jasmine, bergamot, rose. Helps emotions in pregnancy, calms fretful children, soothes skin.	152 MHz	Essential Oil
Essential Oil - Grounding	XTRA	17500000,	Use damped wave, or for simple waves set X to 5. Blend: white fir, spruce, ylang ylang, pine, cedarwood, angelica, juniper. Helps stability, coping, and positivity.	140 MHz	Essential Oil
Essential Oil - Harmony	XTRA	12625000,	Blend: lavender, sandalwood, ylang ylang, frankincense, orange, angelica, geranium, hyssop, spruce, Spanish sage, rosewood, lemon, jasmine, Roman chamomile, bergamot, palmarosa, rose. Harmonic balance.	101 MHz	Essential Oil
Essential Oil - Helichrysum	XTRA	22625000,	Single: skin problems, sunscreen, cholesterol.	181 MHz	Essential Oil
Essential Oil - Hope	XTRA	24500000,	Blend: almond, melissa, juniper, spruce. Uplifts and balances emotions, overcomes despair and depression.	98 MHz	Essential Oil
Essential Oil - Humility	XTRA	22000000,	Blend: sesame seed, rosewood, ylang ylang, geranium, melissa, frankincense, spikenard, myrrh, rose, neroli. Balances heart and mind, enabling healing, reconnects to spirit.	88 MHz	Essential Oil
Essential Oil - Immupower	XTRA	22250000,	Blend: hyssop, mountain savory, XTRAus, ravensara, frankincense, oregano, clove, cumin, Idaho tansy. Supports immune system, boosts positive energy.	89 MHz	Essential Oil
Essential Oil - Inner Child	XTRA	24500000,	Blend: orange, tangerine, jasmine, ylang ylang, spruce, sandalwood, lemongrass, neroli. Helps reconnect with the true self.	98 MHz	Essential Oil
Essential Oil - Inspiration	XTRA	17625000,	Blend: cedarwood, spruce, rosewood, myrtle, sandalwood, frankincense, mugwort. Enhances spirituality, prayer, meditation, and inner awareness.	141 MHz	Essential Oil
Essential Oil - Into the Future	XTRA	22000000,	Blend: almond, clary sage, ylang ylang, white fir, Idaho tansy, juniper, jasmine, frankincense, orange, cedarwood. Fosters determination to move forward.	88 MHz	Essential Oil
Essential Oil - Joy	XTRA	23500000,	Blend: bergamot, ylang ylang, geranium, rosewood, lemon, mandarin, jasmine, Roman chamomile, palmarosa, rose. Mental and emotional uplift.	188 MHz	Essential Oil
Essential Oil - Juniper	XTRA	24500000,	Single: acne, eczema, skin, diuretic. Supports nerve function.	98 MHz	Essential Oil
Essential Oil - Juva Flex	XTRA	20500000,	Blend: sesame seed, fennel, geranium, rosemary, Roman chamomile, blue tansy, helichrysum. Supports liver, digestive, lymphatic systems. May help cell function.	82 MHz	Essential Oil
Essential Oil - Lavender	XTRA	14750000,	Single: burns, joint pains, insect bites, antibacterial, whooping cough, chicken pox, insomnia, stress, anxiety.	118 MHz	Essential Oil
Essential Oil - Lemon	XTRA	19000000,	Single: antioxidant, antiparasitic.	76 MHz	Essential Oil
Essential Oil - Live With Passion	XTRA	22250000,	Blend: clary sage, ginger, sandalwood, jasmine, angelica, cedarwood, helichrysum, patchouli, neroli, melissa. Revives optimism and zest, improves energy.	89 MHz	Essential Oil

Subject / Argument	Author	Frequencies	Notes	Origin	Target
Essential Oil - M-Grain	XTRA	18000000,	Blend: basil, marjoram, lavender, peppermint, Roman chamomile, helichrysum. Calms and promotes sense of well-being.	72 MHz	Essential Oil
Essential Oil - Magnify Your Purpose	XTRA	24750000,	Blend: sandalwood, rosewood, sage, nutmeg, patchouli, cinnamon bark, ginger. Promotes positivity, creativity, focus, and motivation.	99 MHz	Essential Oil
Essential Oil - Melissa	XTRA	12750000,	Single: Immune system support, skin benefits, calming, cold sores, viral infections. Also called Lemon Balm.	102 MHz	Essential Oil
Essential Oil - Melrose	XTRA	24000000,	Blend: melaleuca, naouli, rosemary, clove. Cuts, scrapes, burns, rashes, skin infections.	48 MHz	Essential Oil
Essential Oil - Mister	XTRA	18375000,	Blend: sage, fennel, lavender, myrtle, peppermint, blue yarrow, sesame seed. Promotes inner body balance in men, and may help stress.	147 MHz	Essential Oil
Essential Oil - Motivation	XTRA	12875000,	Blend: Roman chamomile, spruce, ylang ylang, lavender. Fosters action and accomplishment, enables positivity and progress.	103 MHz	Essential Oil
Essential Oil - Myrrh	XTRA	13125000,	Single: Purifies, restores, revitalizes, uplifts. Helps skin and oral hygiene.	105 MHz	Essential Oil
Essential Oil - PanAway	XTRA	14000000,	Blend: wintergreen, helichrysum, clove, peppermint. Supports circulation, joints, and muscles. Aids cell function.	112 MHz	Essential Oil
Essential Oil - Peace & Calming	XTRA	13125000,	Blend: tangerine, organge, ylang ylang, patchouli, blue tansy. Calms and uplifts. Especially useful with children.	105 MHz	Essential Oil
Essential Oil - Peppermint	XTRA	19500000,	Single: digestion, nausea, migraine, sinusitis, blood oxygenation, liver, respiratory, exhaustion, itching, cooling, allergies, weight control.	78 MHz	Essential Oil
Essential Oil - Present Time	XTRA	24500000,	Blend: ylang ylang, spruce, neroli, almond. Anger, anxiety, depression, fear, grief, guilt, jet lag, lupus, panic, shock, trauma.	98 MHz	Essential Oil
Essential Oil - Purification	XTRA	23000000,	Blend: citronella, lemongrass, rosemary, melaleuca, lavandin, myrtle. Insect bites, skin, cuts, and scrapes.	46 MHz	Essential Oil
Essential Oil - Raven	XTRA	17500000,	Blend: ravensara, lemon, wintergreen, peppermint, eucalyptus radiata. Chest and throat conditions.	70 MHz	Essential Oil
Essential Oil - Ravensara	XTRA	16750000,	Single: sinus, lung, and throat infections, hepatitis, shingles, herpes, and viral infections. Immune system support.	134 MHz	Essential Oil
Essential Oil - RC	XTRA	18750000,	Blend: eucalyptus globulus leaf, myrtus communis, pine leaf, marjoram leaf, eucalyptus radiata leaf, eucalyptus citriodora leaf, lavender, cupressus sempervirens, tsuga canadensis leaf, peppermint. Respiratory and immune system support.	75 MHz	Essential Oil
Essential Oil - Release	XTRA	12750000,	Blend: ylang ylang, lavandin, geranium, sandalwood, blue ansy, olive. Facilitates release of suppressed negative emotions.	102 MHz	Essential Oil
Essential Oil - Relieve It	XTRA	14000000,	Blend: spruce, black pepper fruit, hyssop, peppermint. Relaxes, warms, and soothes aching joints and muscles.	56 MHz	Essential Oil
Essential Oil - Rose	XTRA	20000000,	Single: poison ivy, scarring, hormone balance, PMS, menopause, aphrodisiac, grief, balance, harmony, skin.	320 MHz	Essential Oil
Essential Oil - Sacred Mountain	XTRA	22000000,	Blend: spruce, ylang ylang, fir, cedarwood. Strength, power, and grounding.	176 MHz	Essential Oil
Essential Oil - Sandalwood	XTRA	24000000,	Single: Skin care, uplifting, relaxing. Frequency of aloe essential oil also.	96 MHz	Essential Oil
Essential Oil - SARA	XTRA	12750000,	Blend: ylang ylang, geranium, lavender, orange, blue tansy, cedarwood, rose, white lotus, almond. Helps soothe deep emotional wounds.	102 MHz	Essential Oil
Essential Oil - Sensation	XTRA	22000000,	Blend: ylang ylang, jasmine, geranium, bergamot, coriander. Romantic, uplifting, refreshing.	88 MHz	Essential Oil
Essential Oil - Surrender	XTRA	24500000,	Blend: lavender, Roman chamomile, German chamomile, angelica, mountain savory, lemon, spruce. Relaxes urge to control and helps release negative emotions.	98 MHz	Essential Oil
Essential Oil - Thieves	XTRA	18750000	Blend: clove, lemon, cinnamon, eucalyptus radiata, rosemary. Highly effective immune system and general health support.	150 MHz	Essential Oil
Essential Oil - Three Wise Men	XTRA	18000000,	Blend: sandalwood, juniper, frankincense, spruce, myrrh, almond.	72 MHz	Essential Oil
Essential Oil - Trauma Life	XTRA	23000000,	Blend: frankincense, sandalwood, valerian, lavender, davana, spruce, geranium, helichrysum, citrus hystrix, rose. Helps release buried emotional trauma.	92 MHz	Essential Oil
Essential Oil - Valor	XTRA	23500000,	Blend: spruce, rosewood, blue tansy, frankincense, coconut oil.Corrects body balance and alignment. Fosters strength, courage, and self-esteem in adversity.	47 MHz	Essential Oil
Essential Oil - White Angelica	XTRA	22250000,	Blend: bergamot, geranium, myrrh, sandalwood, rosewood, ylang ylang, spruce, hyssop, melissa, rose, almond. Protects against negative energy and enhances the energy bodies.	89 MHz	Essential Oil
Rose	XTRA	320,	Rosa damascene (essential oil).		Essential Oil

Subject / Argument	Author	Frequencies	Notes	Origin	Target

25 - Planets

Subject / Argument	Author	Frequencies	Notes	Origin	Target
Earth Resonance	XTRA	7.83,	Also called the Schumann Resonance. Use for grounding/calming.		Planets
Schumann Resonance	CAFL	7.83,	Fundamental frequency of the Earth. Relaxing.		Planets
Schumann	XTRA	7.83,14.3,20.8,27.3,33.8,	Earth's fundamental frequency and harmonics. Accelerate/enhance healing, increase stress tolerance, stimulate study, improve mental function, advance learning, boost creative thought and concentration.		Planets
Power of Earth	BIOM	65.65; 61.5; 61.55; 55; 44.96			
Grounding	XTRA	194.71,			
Table of sound frequencies corresponding to the human body.					
Sun - Coccyx	ALT	2.06,			Planets
Sun - Kidneys, Strength	ALT	4.11,	Frequency one octave higher than the previous one.		Planets
Sun - Mouth, Speech, Creativity	ALT	8.22,	Frequency one octave higher than the previous one.		Planets
Sun - Top of Head, Spirit, Liberation, Transcendence	ALT	16.4,	Frequency one octave higher than the previous one.		Planets
Moon - Bladder	ALT	2.57,			Planets
Moon - Stomach, Emotional Acceptance	ALT	5.14,	Frequency one octave higher than the previous one.		Planets
Moon - Nasal Passage, Breathing, Taste	ALT	10.3,	Frequency one octave higher than the previous one.		Planets
Mercury - Genitals	ALT	2.3,			Planets
Mercury - Spleen, Blood, Emotional Impulse	ALT	4.6,	Frequency one octave higher than the previous one.		Planets
Mercury - Upper Lip, Emotions, Conflict Resolution	ALT	9.19,	Frequency one octave higher than the previous one.		Planets
Venus - Liver, Pancreas, Emotional, Appetite/Digestion	ALT	3.84,			Planets
Venus - Shoulders, Strength of Arms, Expansion, Teaching	ALT	7.69,	Frequency one octave higher than the previous one.		Planets
Venus - Cortex, Intelligence	ALT	15.4,	Frequency one octave higher than the previous one.		Planets
Mars - Bara, Pelvic Balance, Emotion Balance and Stability	ALT	3.07,			Planets
Mars - Heart, Love, Warmth	ALT	6.15,	Frequency one octave higher than the previous one.		Planets
Mars - Eyes, Visualization	ALT	12.3,	Frequency one octave higher than the previous one.		Planets
Jupiter - Intestines, Emotional Assimilation, Expansion	ALT	2.67,			Planets
Jupiter - Lungs, Oxygen, Heat	ALT	5.35,	Frequency one octave higher than the previous one.		Planets
Jupiter - Hearing, Formal Concepts	ALT	10.7,	Frequency one octave higher than the previous one.		Planets
Saturn - Ovaries, Vitality, Life at Every Level	ALT	3.44,			Planets
Saturn - Collarbones, Vitality, Overall Balance, Stability	ALT	6.88,	Frequency one octave higher than the previous one.		Planets
Saturn - Frontal Lobes, Seventh Sense, Final Decision	ALT	13.8,	Frequency one octave higher than the previous one.		Planets
Planet - SUN	ALT	126.22,	SUN.		Planets
Planet - Moon	ALT	210.42,	Moon.		Planets
Planet - Mercury	ALT	141.27,	Mercury.		Planets
Planet - Venus	ALT	221.23,	Venus.		Planets
Planet - Mars	ALT	144.72,	Mars.		Planets
Planet - Jupiter	ALT	183.58,	Jupiter.		Planets
Planet - Saturn	ALT	147.85,	Saturn.		Planets
Planet - Uranus	ALT	207.36,	Uranus.		Planets
Planet - Neptune	ALT	211.44,	Neptune.		Planets
Planet - Pluto	ALT	140.25,	Pluto.		Planets

Subject / Argument	Author	Frequencies	Notes	Origin	Target
Planetary Orbits	CAFL	141.27,144.72,183.58,221.23,272.2,280.5,295.7, 414.7,422.8,	Brainwave frequencies, from Mercury to Pluto.		Planets
Astral Projection	XTRA	6.30,63,			Planets
Astral Travel	XTRA	40,22,			Planets
Kings Chamber 438	XTRA	438	Resonant frequency of Giza Pyramid's King's Chamber. This is the correct measured frequency, not 441.		
Kings Chamber	XTRA	441,	Resonant frequency of Giza Pyramid's King's Chamber. Further research shows that this was originally 438, not 441: http://www.bibliotecapleyades.net/piramides/esp_piramide_19.htm		

26 - Meridians

Subject / Argument	Author	Frequencies	Notes	Origin	Target
Meridians - Bladder	XTRA	343.8			Meridians
Meridians - Conception Vessel	XTRA	60			Meridians
Meridians - Gallbladder	XTRA	506.8			Meridians
Meridians - Governing Vessel	XTRA	100.9			Meridians
Meridians - Heart	XTRA	289			Meridians
Meridians - Kidney	XTRA	383.7			Meridians
Meridians - Large Intestine	XTRA	4230			Meridians
Meridians - Liver	XTRA	1032			Meridians
Meridians - Lungs	XTRA	2287			Meridians
Meridians - Pericardium	XTRA	447			Meridians
Meridians - Small Intestine	XTRA	316			Meridians
Meridians - Spleen	XTRA	264.9			Meridians
Meridians - Stomach	XTRA	126.9			Meridians
Meridians - Triple Warmer	XTRA	496			Meridians
Kidney Meridian Balance/Correct	XTRA	9.2,	As mentioned above		Meridians
Acupuncture Disturbance Field	CAFL	5.9,18,	Meridian disruption due to scarring.		Meridians

27 - Chakras

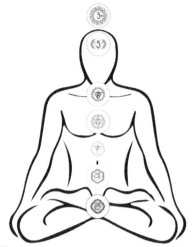

7th Chakra	6th Chakra	5th Chakra	4th Chakra	3rd Chakra	2nd Chakra	1st Chakra
Kundalini Expand	XTRA	55,		(in yoga) latent female energy believed to lie coiled at the base of the spine.		Chakra
Chakra Crown	ALT	172.06,		Frequency of the Platonic Year.		7° Chakra
Chakra 3rd Eye	ALT	221.23,		Venus		6° Chakra
Chakra Throat	ALT	141.27,		Mercury.		5° Chakra
Chakra Heart	ALT	136.10,		Frequency of the Earth Year (OM).		4° Chakra
Chakra Solar Plexus	ALT	126.22,		Sun.		3° Chakra
Chakra Sacral	ALT	210.42,		Frequency of the Synodic Moon.		2° Chakra
Chakra Base	ALT	194.18,		Frequency of the Earth Day.		1° Chakra
Chakra 2 Crown	ALT	**432,**		**432Hz** basis.		7° Chakra
Chakra 2 3rd Eye	ALT	288,		432Hz basis.		6° Chakra
Chakra 2 Throat	ALT	384,		432Hz basis.		5° Chakra
Chakra 2 Heart	ALT	256,		432Hz basis.		4° Chakra
Chakra 2 Solar Plexus	ALT	364,		432Hz basis.		3° Chakra
Chakra 2 Sacral	ALT	606,		432Hz basis.		2° Chakra
Chakra 2 Base	ALT	456,		432Hz basis.		1° Chakra
Third Eye Opening	XTRA	83,		Detox Fluoride, Calcifications, and Pineal sets should be used first.		Chakra
Chakra Base Root	CAFL	20,		Pulse (Gate) at 4Hz.		Chakra
Chakra Chain 2	XTRA	456,606,364,256,384,288,432=360,288,384,256,364,606		432Hz-based. From Dr Pankaj K Mishra.		Chakra
Chakra Balance (Fabian Maman Set)	EDTFL	100,570,15190,52510,119340,356300,427370,561030,641210,930180,				Chakra

Chakra Balance (Fabian Maman Set) Root-F / Sacral-C / Solar-G / Heart-D / Throat-A / 3rd eye-E / Crown-B / Pineal-Bb / Pituitary-BM / Crown Lotus-Bbm.
Letters next to the Chakras are the Music Note representation of the Chakra.
Chakra 7 - 10 express the chakras of the crown, which are represented by the note B. Chakra 8, 9, 10 = Diatonic
Balance the Chakras and You Balance Your Life. Experience the self-healing, self-balancing power of prana.

Chakra / Musical notes / Solfeggio		*See next Sections*			

28 - Musical Scales and Frequencies

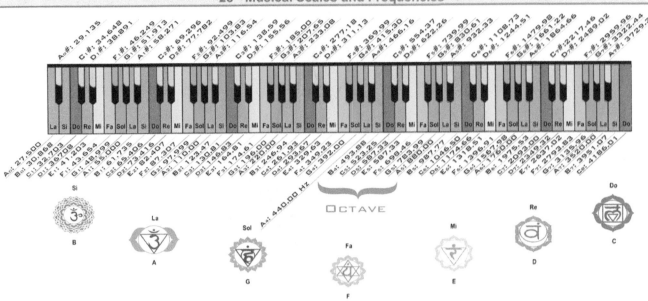

Equations for the Frequency Table

designed by M.

In music, an octave is the interval between one musical pitch and another with double its frequency. According to this rule, if a note has a frequency of 440 Hz (A4), the note one octave above is at 880 Hz and the note one octave below is at 220 Hz.

That is, if F (A_4) = 440 Hz, the frequency of the upper octave will be:

$$F (A_5) = F (A_4) * 2 = 440 * 2 = 880 \text{ Hz}$$

Each octave has 12 notes: C, C#, D, D#, E, F, F#, G, G#, A, A#, B. So there is a coefficient "x" which, multiplied by the frequency of a note, results in the frequency of the note that is in the next semitone.

Since an octave is made up of 12 semitones,

$$F (A_5)= F (A_4) * 2 = F (A_4) * x*x*x*x*x*x*x*x*x*x*x*x$$

Therefore:

$x^{12} = 2$

$x = (2)^{1/12}$ = the twelfth root of 2 = the number which when multiplied by itself 12 times equals 2 = 1.059463094359...

For example:

$$F (A_4) = 440\text{Hz}$$
$$F (A_4\#) = 440\text{Hz} * x = 466.164$$
$$F (B_4) = 440\text{Hz} * x * x = 493.883$$
$$F (C_4) = 440\text{Hz} * x * x * x = 523.251$$

.....

The wavelength of the sound for the notes is found from: $W_n = c/F_n$

where W is the wavelength and c is the speed of sound. The speed of sound depends on temperature, and is approximately 345 m/s at "room temperature.

	La / A	La# / A#	Si / B	Do / C	Do# / C#	Re / D	Re# / D#	Mi / E	Fa / F	Fa# / F#	Sol / G	Sol# / G#	La / A
					Frequencies for equal-tempered scale, A4 = 440 Hz								
A_{-1}	13,750	14,568	15,434	16,352	17,324	18,354	19,445	20,602	21,827	23,125	24,500	25,957	27,500
A_0	27,500	29,135	30,868	32,703	34,648	36,708	38,891	41,203	43,654	46,249	48,999	51,913	55,000
A_1	55,000	58,270	61,735	65,406	69,296	73,416	77,782	82,407	87,307	92,499	97,999	103,826	110,000
A_2	110,000	116,541	123,471	130,813	138,591	146,832	155,563	164,814	174,614	184,997	195,998	207,652	220,000
A_3	220,000	233,082	246,942	261,626	277,183	293,665	311,127	329,628	349,228	369,994	391,995	415,305	440,000
A_4	**440,000**	466,164	493,883	523,251	554,365	587,330	622,254	659,255	698,456	739,989	783,991	830,609	880,000
A_5	880,000	932,328	987,767	1046,502	1108,731	1174,659	1244,508	1318,510	1396,913	1479,978	1567,982	1661,219	1760,000
A_6	1760,000	1864,655	1975,533	2093,005	2217,461	2349,318	2489,016	2637,020	2793,826	2959,955	3135,963	3322,438	3520,000
A_7	3520,000	3729,310	3951,066	4186,009	4434,922	4698,636	4978,032	5274,041	5587,652	5919,911	6271,927	6644,875	7040,000
					Bold frequencies are used in "The Spine Frequencies"								

	La A	La# A#	SI B	Do C	Do# C#	Re D	Re# D#	MI E	Fa F	Fa# F#	Sol G	Sol# G#	La A
						Frequencies for equal-tempered scale, A4 = 432 Hz							
A_{-2}	6,750	7,151	7,577	8,027	8,504	9,010	9,546	10,114	10,715	11,352	12,027	12,742	13,500
A_{-1}	13,500	14,303	15,153	16,054	17,009	18,020	19,092	20,227	21,430	22,704	24,054	25,485	27,000
A_0	27,000	28,606	30,306	32,109	34,018	36,041	38,184	40,454	42,860	45,408	48,109	50,969	54,000
A_1	54,000	57,211	60,613	64,217	68,036	72,081	76,368	80,909	85,720	90,817	96,217	101,938	108,000
A_2	108,000	114,422	121,226	128,434	136,071	144,163	152,735	161,817	171,439	181,634	192,434	203,877	216,000
A_3	216,000	228,844	242,452	256,869	272,143	288,325	305,470	323,634	342,879	363,267	384,868	407,754	432,000
A_4	432,000	457,688	484,904	513,737	544,286	576,651	610,940	647,269	685,757	726,535	769,736	815,507	864,000
A_5	864,000	915,376	969,807	1027,475	1088,572	1153,302	1221,881	1294,537	1371,515	1453,069	1539,473	1631,015	1728,000
A_6	1728,000	1830,752	1939,614	2054,950	2177,144	2306,603	2443,761	2589,075	2743,029	2906,138	3078,946	3262,030	3456,000
A_7	3456,000	3661,504	3879,229	4109,900	4354,287	4613,207	4887,522	5178,149	5486,058	5812,276	6157,892	6524,059	6912,000

Bold frequencies are used in "The Spine Frequencies"

The above frequencies, in addition to "The Spine Frequencies" set (on the last page), can be found in many other programs in this manual.

It should also be noted that by setting these frequencies on a signal generator and connecting a speaker to the latter, you can perform extremely precise tuning or calibration of any musical instrument.

29 - Solfeggio Frequencies

Subject / Argument	Author	Frequencies	Notes	Origin	Target
Remove pain physically and energetically	CUST	174			Sofeggio
Energy fields	CUST	285			Sofeggio
Liberating Guilt and Fear	XTRA	396	Eliminates the feeling of fear and guilt that leads to lower defense mechanisms.	Chakra Base	Sofeggio
Facilitating Change	XTRA	417	Eliminates negative energy from our body and promotes energy rehabilitation of cells and body.	Chakra Sacrale	Sofeggio
Transformation and Miracles	XTRA	528	It helps repair human DNA and keep it in the best condition. It can also lead to transformations and miracles for our life.	Chakra Plesso Solare	Sofeggio
Connecting / Relationships	XTRA	639	Helps solve problems in relationships with family or friends. Helps tune the body and soul.	Chakra Cuore	Sofeggio
Intuition Awakening	XTRA	741	It is used for cleaning and removing toxins from our cells and organs. It can remove electromagnetic radiation from our cells.	Chakra Gola	Sofeggio
Love Unconditional	XTRA	852	It is used to raise awareness and restore mental order. This frequency allows cells to transform into higher energy systems.	Chakra 3° occhio	Sofeggio
Returning to unity	CUST	963		Chakra Corona	Sofeggio
Solfeggio Frequencies	XTRA	396,417,528,639,741,852,	Controversial. Liberate guilt, fear, release emotional patterns, undo situations, facilitate change, transformation, miracles, DNA repair, connecting, relationships, whole-brain interconnection, awaken intuition, non-linear knowing, return to spiritual order, unconditional love.		Sofeggio

Solfeggio tones

Blood Circulation	CUST	337		Sofeggio
Endocrine Function	CUST	537		Sofeggio
Kidney Function	CUST	625		Sofeggio
Pituitary Function	CUST	635		Sofeggio
HGH Production	CUST	645		Sofeggio
Pancreas Function	CUST	654		Sofeggio
Pineal Gland	CUST	662		Sofeggio
Heart Function	CUST	696		Sofeggio
Liver Function	CUST	751		Sofeggio
Thyroid Function	CUST	763		Sofeggio
Nervous System Function	CUST	764		Sofeggio
Immune System Function	CUST	835		Sofeggio
Adrenal Function	CUST	1335		Sofeggio
Spiritual Well Being	CUST	1565		Sofeggio

Subject / Argument	Author	Frequencies	Notes	Origin	Target
		30 - Frequencies of various types			
Final Program	XTRA	465,	A good set to end every Spooky session with.		
Frequency Fatigue	CAFL	10.55,7.83,	Tiredness, not detox, from using frequencies too long.It is very similar to herxing		
Frequency Fatigue 1	XTRA	7.83,10.55,			
Frequency Fatigue 2	XTRA	1.55,			
Interferential 1	XTRA	0.01,	Analgesic therapy of bipolar interferential		
Interferential 2	XTRA	5,			
Interferential 3	XTRA	10,			
Interferential 4	XTRA	50,			
Interferential 5	XTRA	90,			
Interferential Carrier 1	XTRA	4000,			
Interferential Carrier 2	XTRA	4500,			
General Program Emem	CAFL	720,1550,20,4200,	Medley of useful frequencies taken from Emem Rife machine.		
Curva Spic	CAFL	435,	.		
Centering Frequency	XTRA	12,	Balance.		
Miraculous Windfall of Money	XTRA	520,			

Notes

The Spine Frequencies

	Frequency	Parts of body	Symptoms
C1	130.81 128.43	Blood supply to the head, pituitary gland scalp, bones of the face, brain, inner and middle ear, sympathetic nervous system	Headaches, nervousness, insomnia, head colds, high blood pressure, migraine headaches, nervous breakdowns, amnesia, chronic tiredness, dizziness
C2	146.83 144.16	Eyes, optic nerves, auditory nerves, sinuses, mastoid bones, tongue, forehead	Sinus trouble, allergies, pain around the eyes, earaches, fainting spells, certain case of blindness, crossed eyes, deafness
C3	164.81 161.82	Cheeks, outer ear, face bones, teeth, trigeminal nerve.	Neuralgia, neuritis, acne or pimples, eczema
C4	174.61 171.44	Nose, lips, mouth, eustachian tube	Hay fever, runny nose, hearing loss, adenoids
C5	196.00 192.43	Vocal cords, neck glands, pharinxs	Laryngitis, hoarsness, throat conditions such as sore throat or quinsy
C6	220.20 216.1964	Neck muscles, shoulders, tonsils	Stiff neck, pain in upper arm, tonsillitis, croup, chronic cough
C7	246.94 242.45	Thyroid gland, bursae in the shoulders, elbows	Bursitis, colds, thyroid conditions
T1	130.81 128.43	Arms from the elbows down, including hands, wrists and fliger, esophagus and trachea	Asthma, cough, difficult breathing, shortness of breath, pain in lower arms and hands
T2	146.83 144.16	Heart, including its valves and covering, coronary arteries	Functional heart conditions and certain chest conditions
T3	164.81 161.82	Lungs, bronchial tubes, pleura, chest, breast	Bronchitis, pleurisy, pneumonia, congestion, influenza
T4	174.61 171.44	Gallbladder, common duct	Gallbladder conditions, jaundice, shingles
T5	196.00 192.43	Liver, solar plexus, circulation (general)	Liver conditions, fevers, blood pressure problem, poor circulation, arthritis
T6	220.20 216.1964	Stomach	Stomach trobles including: nervous stomach, indigestion, heartburm, dyspepsia
T7	246.94 242.45	Pancreas, duodenum	Ulcers, gastritis
T8	138.57 136.07	Spleen	Lowered resistance
T9	155.56 152.74	Adrenal and suprarenal glands	Allergies, hives
T10	185.00 181.63	Kidneys	Kidney troubles, hardening off the arteries, chronic tiredness, nephritis, pyelitis
T11	207.65 203.88	Kidneys, uterus	Skin conditions such as acne, pimples, eczema, boils
T12	233.08 228.34	Small intestines, lymph circulation	Rheumatism, gas pains, certain types of sterility
L1	138.57 136.07	Large intestines, inguinal rings	Constipation, colitis, dysentery, diarrhea, some ruptures of hernias
L2	155.56 152.74	Appendix, abdomen, upper leg	Cramps, difficult breathing, minor varicose venis
L3	185.00 181.63	Sex organs, uterus, bladder, knees	Bladder troubles, menstrual troubles such as painful or irregular periods, miscarriages, bed wetting, impotency, change of life symptoms, knee pains
L4	207.65 203.88	Prostate gland, muscle of lower back, sciatic nerve	Sciatica, lumbago, difficult painful or too frequent urination, backaches
L5	233.08 228.34	Lower legs, ankles, feet	Poor circulation in the legs, swollen ankles, weak ankles and arches, cold feet, weakness in the legs, leg cramps
Sacrum		Hip bones, buttocks	Sacroiliac conditions, spinal curvatures
Coccyx		Rectum, anus	Hemorrhoids (piles), pruritus (itching), pain at the end of the spine on sitting

designed by M. Allegretti   *in green 440 Hz scale   in red 432 Hz scale*

The Spine Frequencies

In *June Leslie Wieder*'s book "Songs of the Spine", each vertebra has a frequency to which it responds. By transmitting these frequencies in sequence, the aim is to get the spine back into good working conditions - in essence, to realign the vertebrae correctly.

There are two versions of these frequencies, one of which is calibrated to the A=440Hz scale (Wieder's original), and the other to the A=432Hz scale (experimental but based on sound science). Try both and use whichever one produces the best results.

The frequencies may also be used individually or on a parallel Channel together with other frequencies if desired.

ABOUT THE AUTHOR

Marcello Allegretti, professor of Quantum Medicine at Unicamillus International Medical University in Rome, biomedical engineer and naturopath, is an independent scientific researcher, owner of a bioengineering and energy balance laboratory.
Stimulated by a strong personal motivation, he devoted many years to the study of traditional, alternative and complementary medicine, but above all to technologies for the use of electromagnetic waves in the field of energy medicine, that is intended as a means for rebalancing for psycho-physical well-being.
For many years he has been conducting studies and research on Microcurrents, Frequency Imprinting & Scalar Waves.
In the course of his studies, he has designed and built innovative scientific devices, that are highly effective especially in the field of research.

Science director of Power-Waves (www.power-waves.com).

*Author of the book "**The Frequencies of Rifing**" published in the US in March 2016, and successfully sold all over the world, now in its fifth edition.*

*Author of the book "**The Therapeutic Properties of Electromagnetic Waves**" published in the US in September 2018.*

*Author of the book "**Therapeutic Waves**" published in the US in September 2020.*

He is a consultant and referent for Italy of an international team of engineers, designers and technicians for the study, research and development of bioengineering technologies for the use of electromagnetic frequencies

Made in the USA
Las Vegas, NV
16 September 2024